# Evidence-Based Practices in Behavioral Health

**Series editor**

Nirbhay N. Singh, Medical College of Georgia, Augusta University, Augusta, USA

Georgia. His particular interests include psychopharmacology, treatment of persons with chronic severe mental illness, management of co-occurring psychiatric and intellectual disabilities, and improvement of mental health delivery systems.

# About the Contributors

**Anthony O. Ahmed, Ph.D.** is Assistant Professor in the Department of Psychiatry at Weill Cornell Medical College. He held a previous appointment as Assistant Professor at the Medical College of Georgia, Augusta University where he had completed a psychotic disorders postdoctoral fellowship. His research interests include studying recovery and psychosocial functioning in people with schizophrenia and other severe mental illnesses. He has published extensively in this area and provides consultation to clinical teams about the implementation of recovery-based practices.

**Brian Anderson, CPS** is Certified Peer Specialist and Certified Recovery Educator in the Department of Psychiatry and Health Behavior at Augusta University for Project GREAT as well as for SHE PREVAILS (Supporting Health Engagement through Prevention, Recovery, and Empowerment Via ACCESS, Intervention, and Linkage Services). He previously worked with the Charlie Norwood VA Medical Center in Augusta, GA where he assisted in the creation of a Peer Specialist position in 2006. In 2008, Mr. Anderson was named Certified Peer Specialist of the Year. He served as a member of the Planning and Advisory Council for the Georgia Mental Health Consumer Network from 2008 to 2011. He is the author of the book, *Beautiful Scars: My Journey to Wholeness and Healing* (2012). He has appeared several times on Trinity Broadcast Network and Atlanta Live TV and has traveled the country presenting at conferences as a motivational speaker on the topic of recovery. He is currently a member of the Board of Directors for the Georgia Mental Health Consumer Network and is the CEO of Beautiful Scars, LLC.

**Cheryl Anderson, SSW, CPRP** born and raised in ON, Canada, Ms. Anderson began volunteering in the field of Human Services at the age of 14 and eventually became the CEO for the Community Living in Halliburton, Canada. Then she immigrated to the United States and is presently the Director of Recovery and Resiliency Support Services at Marc Community Resources. Ms. Anderson is the past Vice Chair for the Peer and Family Coalition for Arizona, a member of Mercy Maricopa Integrated Care Governance Board for the Behavioral Health system in Maricopa County and is also a member of the City of Mesa's Human Resources Advisory Board. Ms. Anderson has a family member who receives behavioral health services in AZ.

**Andrea Avila, MA** is a graduate student in the Clinical Psychology Training Program and the Law-Psychology Program at University of Nebraska–Lincoln, working toward joint completion of the Ph.D. and J.D. She is a member of the Serious Mental Illness Research Group at UNL. Her research interests focus on therapeutic jurisprudence, law and social policy related to serious mental illness, training corrections personnel in mental health issues, and people with serious mental illness who become involved with the criminal justice system. She is a past Executive Editor of the *Nebraska Law Review*.

**Doug Barshter, MS, CPRP** has been working in the adult behavioral health system for over 30 years in direct and administrative services. He has worked locally and nationally as manager, trainer, consultant, and accreditation surveyor to promote psychiatric rehabilitation principles and quality practices in a variety of organizations. Currently, Mr. Barshter is designing curricula to prepare peer employees in recovery/resilience practices. He is also collaborating with in-house and national experts to enhance the skills of peer employees in integrated healthcare skill sets and improve the supervisory skills of managers overseeing peer-driven services.

**Kathy Bashor, MC** currently serves as the Bureau Chief of the Office of Individual and Family Affairs (OIFA) for the Arizona Department of Health Services, in Phoenix, Arizona. In her role with OIFA she ensures the voice of the individual and family member at every level of the system. Kathy has spent most of her life receiving services in the behavioral health system, including years of hospitalization in state and local hospitals. Kathy is known as fierce advocate working to ensure Arizona adheres to a Recovery-based mental health system.

**Chyrell Bellamy, MSW, Ph.D.** is Assistant Professor of Yale University's Department of Psychiatry and the Director of Peer Services/Research for Yale's Program for Recovery and Community Health. She has experience as a frontline service provider, community educator and organizer, instructor in psychology and social work, community and academic researcher, and as a person in recovery. Her expertise includes developing and conducting community-based research initiatives in partnership with people with lived experience. Her research examines sociocultural pathways of recovery from mental illness, with a particular focus on health disparities; as well as research and practice experience in the area of peer support services; group-work interventions; spirituality; health promotion; and culture and recovery.

**Anneliese C. Boettcher, MS** is a doctoral student in the Combined-Integrated Clinical and Counseling Psychology program at the University of South Alabama in Mobile, AL. She will soon begin her clinical internship at the University of Florida Health Sciences Center. Her research interests include cognitive assessment, knowledge of mTBI sequelae in healthcare professionals, and the intersection of chronic pain, emotional variables, and cognitive functioning.

**Erika Carr, Ph.D.** is Assistant Professor at Yale School of Medicine and is also the Director of the Inpatient Psychology Service at Connecticut Mental Health Center in New Haven, Connecticut. She earned her doctoral degree from the University of Tennessee–Knoxville, and completed her internship at Emory School of Medicine/Grady Hospital. Dr. Carr also completed her postdoctoral fellowship at Yale School of Medicine, specializing in clinical work with those who experience serious mental illness and substance use, as well as homelessness. Her primary research and clinical interests are the sexual objectification of women, serious mental illness, recovery-oriented care, trauma, positive behavioral supports, and psychology training.

**Larry Davidson, Ph.D.** is Professor of Psychology in the Department of Psychiatry of the Yale School of Medicine, where he directs the Program for Recovery and Community Health. He also serves as Senior Policy Advisor for the Connecticut Department of Mental Health and Addiction Services. His research has focused on processes of recovery in serious mental illnesses and addictions and the development, evaluation, and dissemination of social policies and innovative community-based programs to promote recovery and community inclusion among persons with these conditions.

**Maryanne Davidson, DNSc, APRN, CPNP** is Associate Professor and Director of the Undergraduate Program in Nursing at Sacred Heart University. She received both her Masters of Science in Nursing and Doctor of Nursing Science from Yale University School of Nursing and has worked in the fields of psychiatric nursing and pediatrics for over 30 years. Her research interests include individual and family management of chronic illness and perception and management of pediatric eating disorders.

**Jenny L. Devine, JD, MA** is Assistant Federal Defender for the Middle District of Florida, Tampa Division, representing defendants facing trial for federal criminal allegations. She has previously practiced law in Gainesville, FL, and Seattle, Washington, representing indigent criminal defendants as well as individuals with chronic mental illness facing lengthy involuntary civil commitment in hospitals and treatment centers. Ms. Devine received her undergraduate degree *summa cum laude* from the University of Florida and holds both a Master of Arts in History and a Juris Doctor from the University of Florida. She is a member of the Florida Bar, the Washington State Bar, the Middle District of Florida Federal Bar, and is admitted to practice before the Eleventh Circuit Court of Appeals.

**Gina N. Duncan, MD, FAPA** was Clinical Assistant Professor of Psychiatry and Health Behavior at the Medical College of Georgia, Augusta University, Augusta, GA and previously served as the Associate Dean for Admissions for the Medical College of Georgia. She earned her BS from Hampton University and MD from the University of North Carolina School of Medicine in Chapel Hill, NC. She completed her internship and residency at the Massachusetts General Hospital (MGH)/McLean Hospital Adult Psychiatry Residency Program in Boston, MA. Dr. Duncan has served as the psychiatrist on the Medical College of Georgia Department of Psychiatry and Health Behavior's Project GREAT (Georgia Recovery-Based Educational

**Evelyn E. Harris, MSW, LCSW, SCPM** is the Director of Hospital System Quality Management for the Department of Behavioral Health and Developmental Disabilities (DBHDD) for the State of Georgia. Prior to this position, she served as the Project Manager for DBHDD's CRIPA Settlement Agreement with the Department of Justice (DOJ). She is a Licensed Clinical Social Worker (LCSW) and earned her MSW from the University of Georgia. In addition, she earned her certification (SCPM) in Advanced Project Management from Stanford University. She has 25 years of experience in clinical social work, primarily in the field of mental health both in private and public sectors.

**Benjamin D. Hill, Ph.D.** is a clinical neuropsychologist and Assistant Professor in the Psychology Department and core faculty in the Combined-Integrated Clinical and Counseling Psychology doctoral program at the University of South Alabama in Mobile, Alabama. He earned a Masters degree in Experimental Psychology at Wake Forest University and doctoral degree in Clinical Psychology at Louisiana State University and completed his clinical internship at the University of Mississippi Medical Center and postdoctoral fellowship in clinical neuropsychology at the Alpert Medical School of Brown University. His research interests include cognitive assessment and intervention, psychometrics, the interaction of personality and cognitive functioning, and intra-individual variability as a marker of neuropathology. He is Associate Editor for the *Journal of Child and Family Studies,* on the editorial board of *Journal of Attention Disorders,* and is the statistical editor for *Mindfulness.*

**Kristin M. Hunter, MS** is a doctoral candidate in the Counseling Psychology doctoral program at the University of Georgia. She completed her pre-doctoral psychology internship at the APA-accredited Medical College of Georgia-Charlie Norwood Veterans Affairs Medical Center Psychology Internship. Her primary research interests include teaching the mental health recovery model to members of interdisciplinary teams and the utilization of exercise in the maintenance of mental health.

**Monica M. Jackman OTD, MHS, OTR/L** is an occupational therapist and consultant. She has provided therapy to children and adults and has served as a compliance monitor under the Civil Rights for Institutionalized Persons Act in residential facilities throughout the United States. Her research interests include use of the Mindful Engagement Support model for individuals with intellectual and developmental disabilities, and mindfulness-based programs for children and mothers with post-partum mood disorders. She has written curricula and workshops on the Mindful Engagement Support model, and enjoys creating and developing new therapy devices, programs, and interventions. She believes that her most profound clinical insight and understanding have come from the lived experience of recovery from serious mental illness.

**Susan Junck** serves as the Family Community Liaison at the Arizona Department of Health Services, Division of Behavioral Health, Office of Individual and Family Affairs. Susan has been involved with the behavioral health community for over a decade serving as an advocate, manager of family support, human rights liaison, family psycho-education facilitator, and mother of a young man with a serious mental illness. She is also an active volunteer with NAMI (National Alliance on Mental illness) where she has helped hundreds of families who have been affected by mental illness by teaching NAMI Family-to-Family courses and facilitating family support groups. Currently Susan is developing statewide polices for family support programs and family support provider training, certification and supervision requirements.

**Martha Kent, Ph.D.** serves as Research Scientist and Neuropsychologist at the Phoenix VA Health Care System, Arizona. She is a principal investigator working on current studies on brain training for resilience skills in obesity, chronic pain, and PTSD. She has authored papers and chapters in these areas and has edited The Resilience Handbook: Approaches to Stress and Trauma/ (2014). She has developed training, lectures, and seminars for interns, staff, and professional communities. Central to her work is the concept of resilience as the capacity to balance goal-directed action versus stimulus-based responding in evocative contexts of threat, pain, overeating, and addiction.

**Giulio E. Lancioni, Ph.D.** is Professor in the Department of Neuroscience and Sense Organs, University of Bari, Italy. Prior to this position, he spent many years at the Department of Psychology, University of Leiden, The Netherlands. His research interests include development and assessment of assistive technologies, training of social and occupational skills, and evaluation of strategies for examining preference and choice with individuals with severe/profound intellectual and multiple disabilities (including post-coma persons in a minimally conscious state and persons with Alzheimer's disease). He has published widely in these areas and serves on the editorial board of several international journals concerned with these topics.

**P. Alex Mabe, Ph.D.** received his doctoral degree in Clinical Psychology from Florida State University in Tallahassee, FL. Currently, he is Professor, Chief of Psychology, and Director of Psychology Internship Training in the Department of Psychiatry and Health Behavior at the Medical College of Georgia/Augusta University. His publications include over 60 articles/chapters/abstracts in the areas of clinical and pediatric psychology as well as the recovery-oriented mental health care. He has made numerous presentations at national and international professional meetings on topics related to behavioral medicine, recovery-oriented mental health care, child–pediatric psychology, and parent training. He is the principal investigator on a psychology workforce development project funded by the Department of Health and Human Services, Health Resources and Services Administration, Graduate Psychology Education Program. He serves as the Director of Project GREAT (Georgia Recovery-based Educational Approach to Treatment) helping to design and implement workshops and recovery-based practice tools. In 2012, Project GREAT and the Department of Psychiatry and Health Behavior were the recipients of the American College of Psychiatrists' annual award for *Creativity in Psychiatric Education.*

**Colleen McGregor, MADM/MPH** currently serves as an Implementation Manager for the System of Care Unit within the Division of Behavioral Health Services at the Arizona Department of Health Services in Phoenix, AZ. She has dedicated herself both personally and professionally to improving access to comprehensive, high-quality integrated care and is deeply passionate about healthcare system transformation. With more than 20 years of progressive experience in public health and human services in both New York and Arizona, she has been involved, professionally in local, state and national initiatives focused on Primary Care and Behavioral Health service expansion and integration, Health Information Exchange, Transparency and Transformation Initiatives, Medicaid-driven Health Literacy and Patient Engagement projects and most recently, Early Childhood Comprehensive System Change. As an adult with Attention Deficient/Hyperactivity Disorder and a single mother to two amazing children whom both have comprehensive special health care, developmental disabilities and learning needs, she knows, first-hand the impact stigma has on her and her children's lives.

**Elaina Montague, M.A.** is a doctoral student in the Clinical Psychology Training Program at the University of Nebraska–Lincoln. She received her B.A. from the Bernard M. Baruch College, City University of New York, and conducted research on factors that moderate learning success in a neurocognitive remediation program at New York State Psychiatric Institute. She now works in the Serious Mental Illness Research Group at UNL, studying neurocognitive and social cognitive change prior to onset of serious mental illness and among populations with subclinical schizotypy. Her research interests broadly include application of developmental, biological, behavioral, and social perspectives into assessment and treatment of complex mental illness.

**Rachel E. Myers, Ph.D., RN** is Associate Professor of Nursing in the WellStar School of Nursing, College of Health and Human Services at Kennesaw State University, Kennesaw, Georgia, USA. She is also a Certified Diabetes Educator and has worked as a nursing consultant for over 14 years in facilities that serve individuals with mental illness and intellectual and developmental disabilities. Her research interests include mindfulness, health and wellness promotion, disease prevention, and diabetes. She has several publications in these areas, and has presented her research at national and international conferences. She is Associate Editor of *Journal of Child and Family Studies.*

**Jeff Phillips, Ph.D.** is the Director of Psychology at Western State Hospital where he has practiced psychology for over 25 years. He is Visiting Assistant Professor in the Department of Psychiatry and Neurobehavioral Sciences at the University of Virginia. He earned a doctoral degree in Clinical Psychology from Southern Illinois University at Carbondale.

**John W. Reich, Ph.D.** is Emeritus Professor of Psychology at Arizona State University (ASU). His work has focused on the application of social psychological concepts in understanding societal issues and the development of interventions for improving individuals' well-being. He is the former Director of the Social Psychology Graduate Training Program of Arizona State University and is the author or co-editor of six books and over 100 research articles. Dr. Reich is a member of the ASU Resilience Solutions Group (http://www.asu.edu/resilience).

**Michael Rollock, Ph.D.** is Assistant Professor in the Department of Psychiatry and Health Behavior at the Medical College of Georgia, Augusta University, and a licensed clinical psychologist at East Central Regional Hospital, an inpatient psychiatric facility, serving individuals with severe mental illness. He earned his doctoral degree from the University of Massachusetts Boston, and specializes in the application of recovery-oriented interventions at the individual and systemic level. In addition to conducting clinical supervision and courses with psychology and psychiatry residents, he facilitates workshops for healthcare providers. This work focuses on enhancing care by drawing upon principles and practices at the intersection of recovery-oriented cognitive therapy and positive psychology. He served as President of the Augusta Area Psychological Association in 2014–2015.

**Michael S. Shafer, Ph.D.** is Professor in the School of Social Work at Arizona State University's College of Public Service and Community Solutions where he also holds affiliate appointments in the Center for Health Information Research and the School of Criminology and Criminal Justice. Dr. Shafer is the founding director of the Center for Applied Behavioral Health Policy which has, for the past 25 years, conducted cutting-edge research on the adoption and implementation of innovative practices in behavioral health care. Dr. Shafer has authored more than 40 peer-reviewed research articles and generated more than $45 million in grants and contracts that target capacity building and innovation in behavioral health services. Dr. Shafer began his career in mental health as an undergraduate student at Camarillo State Hospital, CA, where he lived and worked for two years as an embedded student.

**Channing Sofko, MA** is a doctoral student in the Combined-Integrated Clinical and Counseling Psychology program at the University of South Alabama in Mobile, Alabama. Her research interests include intra-individual variability in older adults, contributors to healthy cognitive aging, and resiliency factors in individuals with post-traumatic stress disorder. Her clinical interests include neuropsychological assessment as well as work with trauma survivors and with caregivers of individuals diagnosed with dementia.

**Will D. Spaulding, Ph.D.** is Professor of the Clinical Psychology Training Program, Department of Psychology, University of Nebraska–Lincoln. He received his Ph.D. from the University of Arizona in 1976, and was a postdoctoral fellow in Mental Health Teaching and Research in the Department of Psychiatry, University of Rochester School of Medicine and Dentistry. His research has spanned the experimental psychopathology of schizophrenia-spectrum disorders, treatment and rehabilitation outcomes, the nature of recovery, and social policy for severe and disabling mental illness. He is a former chair of the American Psychological Association Task Force on SMI and SED. He is a co-author, with Mary Sullivan and Jeffrey Poland, of *Treatment and Rehabilitation of Severe Mental Illness* (Guilford Press, 2003), and is currently co-editor of the *American Journal of Orthopsychiatry*.

**Lisa St. George, MSW, CRP** is the Director of Recovery Practices at RI International and RI Consulting. With over 30 years of social work experience, Lisa is an expert in developing recovery-focused systems and strong peer support workforces that provide mental health, substance use, and integrated care. She has provided leadership and start-up of many recovery programs in Arizona, California, and New Zealand and has supervised and developed effective and sustainable peer workforces for more than 20 programs and over 600 peer support workers. Her work has transformed multiple systems of care to have a strong recovery focus and vision while working within existing processes and procedures. Wherever she goes, she brings unending belief in the inherent courage, wisdom, and strength of people in recovery. Over the years, Ms. St. George has authored multiple books, articles, and trainings with a recovery focus.

**Vicki Staples, MED, CRP** is the Associate Director for Clinical Initiatives at the Arizona State University's Center for Applied Behavioral Health (CABHP). In this capacity, Ms. Staples has served as project director for a number of system and workforce capacity initiatives, including serving as Co-director of the SAMHSA-funded Pacific Southwest Addiction technology transfer center, and NIMH-funded Educational Outreach initiative, and the Arizona Peer Career Advancement Academy. Prior to joining ASU, Ms. Staples served as the Director of Recovery, Resiliency & Wellness for Arizona Department of Health, Division of Behavioral Health Services where she oversaw system change initiatives. With over 25 years of implementing evidence-supported clinical and recovery services, she continues to focus on increasing collaboration with stakeholders and across service systems, to stimulate practice improvements and promote recovery.

**Thomas Styron, Ph.D.** is Associate Professor of Psychiatry at the Yale School of Medicine. Dr. Styron is also the Executive Director of Community Services Network of Greater New Haven, a consortium of New Haven based not-for-profit community-based providers or recovery-oriented care for people with serious mental illnesses (SMI) and the Director of Psychology Training within the Outpatient Services Division of the Connecticut Mental Health Center. He earned a doctoral degree in Clinical Psychology from the University of Massachusetts–Amherst and completed pre-doctoral and postdoctoral training at Yale. His primary research interests are in the development and promotion of recovery-oriented care for individuals with SMI.

**Mary E. Sullivan, MSW** is Research Specialist in the Department of Psychology, University of Nebraska–Lincoln, and a freelance consultant on mental health services and program development. She received her M.S.W. in

1978, from the School of Social Work, with a Certificate in Health Studies from the Maxwell School of Citizenship and Public Affairs, of Syracuse University. She is a member of the Serious Mental Illness Research Group at UNL. From 1998 until 2009 she was Director of the Community Transition Program, a recovery-oriented psychiatric rehabilitation program in a Nebraska state hospital. Her interests include treatment outcomes and program administration and development in rehabilitation and recovery for serious mental illness. She is a co-author, with Will Spaulding and Jeffrey Poland, of *Treatment and Rehabilitation of Severe Mental Illness* (Guilford Press, 2003).

**Janis Tondora, PsyD** is Assistant Professor in the Department of Psychiatry at the Yale University School of Medicine. Based at the Program for Recovery and Community Health, Dr. Tondora's professional interests focus on the design, implementation, and evaluation of services that promote self-determination, recovery, and community inclusion among individuals living with serious behavioral health disorders. She has provided training and consultation to nearly 20 states seeking to develop person-centered planning models and programs, and has shared her work with the field in numerous publications including a 2009 book co-authored with several colleagues entitled, *A Practical Guide to Recovery-Oriented Practice: Tools for Transforming Mental Health Care*. In 2014, Dr. Tondora released a comprehensive text, *Partnering for Recovery in Mental Health: A Practical Guide to Person-Centered Planning*, which promises to contribute significantly to the implementation of recovery-oriented practice across the behavioral health field.

**Alan S.W. Winton, Ph.D.** was Senior Lecturer in the School of Psychology at Massey University in Palmerston North, New Zealand until his retirement from academia. He continues his research interests in mindfulness procedures and their application in human service delivery systems.

**Alex J. Zautra, Ph.D.** is Arizona State University (ASU) Foundation Professor of Clinical Psychology. He directs ASU's Resilience Solutions Group, and is the Vice-President of the Social Intelligence Institute, a non-profit organization dedicated to the development and testing of social-emotional resilience interventions. He has dedicated his career to the study of biopsychosocial aspects of resilience, and the building of interventions that further adaptation for individuals, organizations, and communities. His work addresses fundamental questions in behavioral health such as the restorative role of positive social engagement and the sources of vulnerability within the person and social relations that increase risk of health and mental health problems. His most recent book, with co-authors Reich and Hall, is entitled *Handbook of Adult Resilience* by Guilford Press. He is also the author of *Emotions, Stress, and Health*, published by Oxford University Press.

# Contributors

**Anthony O. Ahmed** Department of Psychiatry, Weill Cornell Medical College, White Plains, NY, USA

**Brian Anderson** Department of Psychiatry and Health Behavior, Medical College of Georgia, Augusta University, Augusta, GA, USA

**Cheryl Anderson** Marc Community Resources, Mesa, AZ, USA

**Andrea Avila** Department of Psychology, University of Nebraska–Lincoln, Lincoln, NE, USA

**Jack W. Barber** Department of Behavioral Health and Developmental Services, Richmond, VA, USA

**Doug Barshter** Marc Community Resources, Mesa, AZ, USA

**Kathy Bashor** Office of Individual and Family Affairs, AZ Health Care Cost Containment System (AHCCCS), Phoenix, AZ, USA

**Chyrell Bellamy** Department of Psychiatry, Yale University School of Medicine, New Haven, CT, USA

**Anneliese C. Boettcher** Department of Psychology, UCOMM 1500, University of South Alabama, Mobile, AL, USA

**Erika Carr** Department of Psychiatry, Yale University School of Medicine, New Haven, CT, USA

**Larry Davidson** Department of Psychiatry, Yale University School of Medicine, New Haven, CT, USA

**Maryanne Davidson** College of Nursing, Sacred Heart University, Fairfield, CT, USA

**Jenny L. Devine** Office of the Federal Defender, Tampa, FL, USA

**Gina N. Duncan** Department of Psychiatry and Health Behavior, Medical College of Georgia, Augusta University, Augusta, GA, USA

**Christina Dye** Partners in Recovery, Mesa, AZ, USA

**Donna Lee Elm** Office of the Federal Defender, Tampa, FL, USA

**Shady Elsamra** Department of Psychiatry, Yale University School of Medicine, New Haven, CT, USA

**Gareth Fenley** College of Social Work, University of South Carolina, Columbia, SC, USA

**Ellie Fossey** Department of Occupational Therapy, Monash University, Melbourne, Australia

**Michael Franczak** Marc Community Resources, Mesa, AZ, USA

**Evelyn Harris** Division of Behavioral Health and Developmental Disabilities, Atlanta, GA, USA

**Benjamin D. Hill** Department of Psychology, UCOMM 1500, University of South Alabama, Mobile, AL, USA

**Kristin M. Hunter** Department of Counseling and Human Development Services, University of Georgia, Athens, USA

**Monica M. Jackman** Little Lotus Therapy and Consulting, Port St. Lucie, FL, USA

**Susan Junck** Office of Individual and Family Affairs, AZ Health Care Cost Containment System (AHCCCS), Phoenix, AZ, USA

**Martha Kent** Phoenix Veterans Affairs Health, Phoenix, AZ, USA

**Giulio E. Lancioni** Department of Neuroscience and Sense Organs, University of Bari, Bari, Italy

**P. Alex Mabe** Department of Psychiatry and Health Behavior, Medical College of Georgia, Augusta University, Augusta, GA, USA

**Colleen McGregor** Regional Behavioral Health Authority, Mercy Maricopa Integrated Care, Phoenix, AZ, USA

**Elaina Montague** Department of Psychology, University of Nebraska–Lincoln, Lincoln, NE, USA

**Rachel E. Myers** WellStar School of Nursing, Kennesaw State University, Kennesaw, GA, USA

**Jeff Phillips** Department of Psychology, Western State Hospital, Staunton, VA, USA

**John W. Reich** Department of Psychology, Arizona State University, Tempe, AZ, USA

**Michael Rollock** Department of Psychiatry and Health Behavior, Medical College of Georgia, Augusta University, Augusta, GA, USA

**Scott Van Sant** Department of Psychiatry and Health Behavior, Medical College of Georgia, Augusta University, Augusta, GA, USA

**Michael S. Shafer** Center for Applied Behavioral Health Policy, Arizona State University, Phoenix, AZ, USA

**Nirbhay N. Singh** Department of Psychiatry and Health Behavior, Medical College of Georgia, Augusta University, Augusta, GA, USA

**Channing Sofko** Department of Psychology, UCOMM 1500, University of South Alabama, Mobile, AL, USA

**Will D. Spaulding** Department of Psychology, University of Nebraska–Lincoln, Lincoln, NE, USA

**Lisa St. George** RI, International, Phoenix, AZ, USA

**Vicki Staples** Center for Applied Behavioral Health Policy, Arizona State University, Phoenix, AZ, USA

**Thomas Styron** Department of Psychiatry, Yale University School of Medicine, New Haven, CT, USA

**Mary E. Sullivan** Department of Psychology, University of Nebraska–Lincoln, Lincoln, NE, USA

**Janis Tondora** Department of Psychiatry, Yale University School of Medicine, New Haven, CT, USA

**Alan S.W. Winton** Massey University, Palmerston North, New Zealand

**Alex J. Zautra** Department of Psychology, Arizona State University, Tempe, AZ, USA

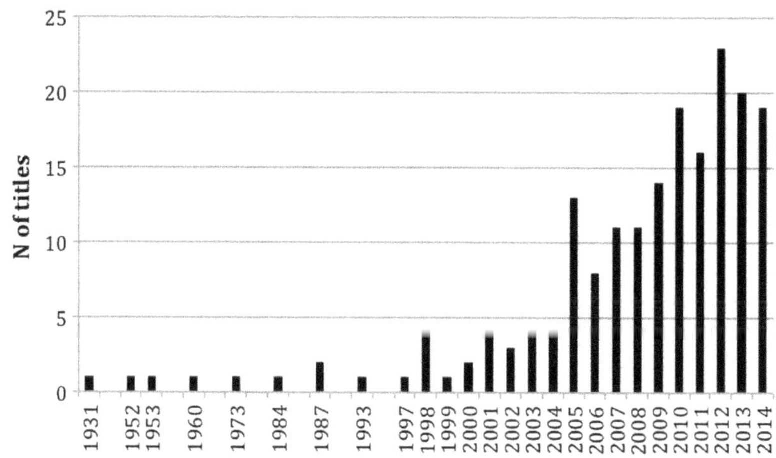


**Fig. 1.1** PsychInfo titles including "recovery" and "mental illness"

that recovery from mental illness is now a real possibility" (President's Commission 2003). The possibility of recovery from severe mental illness is a proposition that is evident in the previous scholarly literature, much of which will be discussed in this chapter, but with the Commission's report, recovery became an acknowledged tenet of national healthcare policy. The year 2005 is the first to reflect the mental health scientific and policy community's response to that development, and, for the purposes of the present discussion, conveniently serves to mark the beginning of the contemporary era of recovery-oriented mental health policy, research, and services.

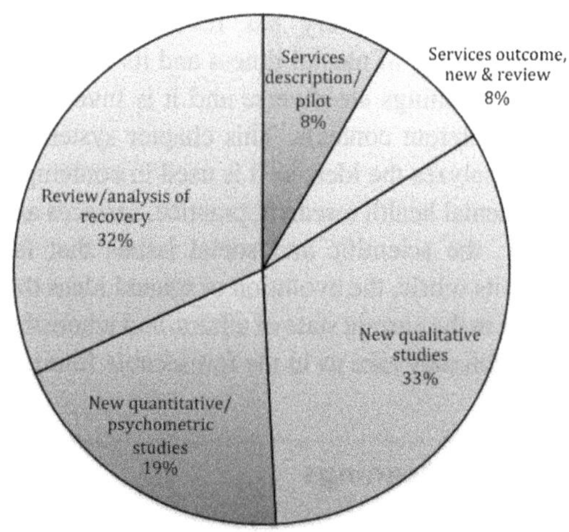


**Fig. 1.2** Methodological distribution of the PsycInfo sample, 2005–2015, $N = 167$ titles

Figure 1.2 shows the methodological make-up of the PsycInfo sample from 2005 until present, including the fourteen 2015 citations omitted from Fig. 1.1. For many veterans of mental health research, the most striking feature is the robust representation of original studies using qualitative or mixed qualitative/quantitative methods. This arguably reflects a more general increase in use of qualitative methods in behavioral and social science, but in addition, many researchers see the partly subjective nature of recovery, as it took shape leading up to the contemporary era, as especially well suited to qualitative analysis. About the same proportion of the sample is theoretical work—review of research and conceptual analysis concerning the idea of recovery itself, and implications for policy, research and practice. Next largest is new empirical studies, using psychometrics and other quantitative paradigms, of the nomothetic dimensions and longitudinal processes of recovery. The two smallest methodological categories are descriptions and/or pilot studies of innovative services or programs, and new controlled analyses or research reviews of service outcomes.

Figure 1.3 shows the topical distribution of the PsycInfo sample. The plurality of the publications is about services—treatment, support, and rehabilitation. Within that category, the largest subcategory is conceptual or theoretical discussions of the relevance to recovery of

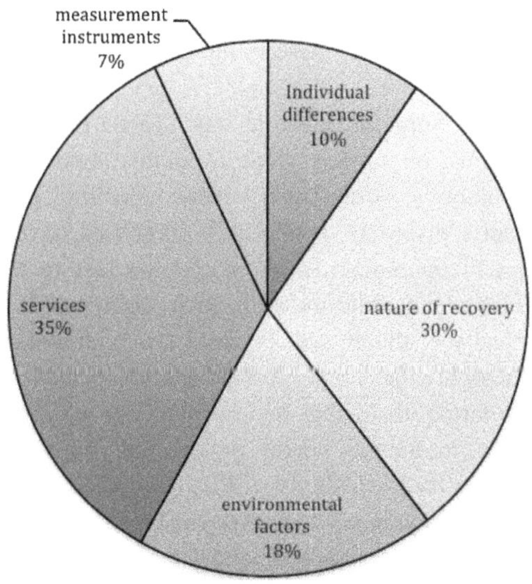


**Fig. 1.3** Topical distribution of the PsycInfo sample, 2005–2015, $N = 167$ titles

traditional or conventional mental health services, including the need for modification of content and clinical practice to make them compatible with recovery principles. This category also includes descriptions of innovative modalities or service packages not yet ready for controlled outcome trials, experimental and quasi-experimental outcome trials, program evaluations, analyses concerning the economics and dissemination of recovery-oriented services, and the training and education of practitioners.

There is not a single entirely new service modality undergoing controlled outcome evaluation in the entire sample. There are several descriptions and pilot studies of previously validated services being modified for specific subpopulations, e.g., elderly people, and accounts of one previously validated illness/wellness management skill training approach, reconfigured for group leaders who are self-identified people with mental illness and not mental health professionals, progressing through pilot studies and controlled trials.

Consistent with the methodological distribution, the next most represented topic is about the nature of recovery itself. This category includes research reviews and original empirical studies using both qualitative and quantitative methods. Subcategories include studies of types of roles and activities associated with recovery (occupational roles and activities, leisure activities, family roles) as well as broader attempts to identify a range of narrative themes and intrapersonal or phenomenological features that characterize recovery. A much smaller category, with both qualitative and quantitative original studies but no research reviews, is about features that may constitute important individual differences in the experience of recovery, including developmental characteristics, course of the illness, and experience with the service system, gender and cultural background. A few of these are quantitative modeling studies that attempt to identify trajectories and pathways leading to recovery outcomes.

Environmental factors that represent either barriers to or facilitators of recovery are the third largest category. These also include research reviews and original studies using qualitative and quantitative methods. Some focus on particular factors, including public attitudes toward mental illness, social support networks, and family characteristics. Others attempt to broadly identify facilitating factors and barriers.

The smallest topical categories are reports concerning development of specific instruments to measure the longitudinal course of recovery, either as a continuous process or a succession of stages, and studies of individual differences possibly relevant to recovery.

In summary, this simple analysis of the scholarly and scientific literature suggests that the past decade has seen new interest in recovery from mental illness, associated with canonization of that idea in national healthcare policy. The scholarly work divides itself into analysis of the recovery process itself, identification of environmental factors that facilitate or inhibit recovery, adapting existing treatment and other services to the new recovery-oriented context, and to a lesser extent, quantitatively measuring recovery and identifying individual differences in how people experience it. There is no evidence in the PsycInfo sample that scholarly interest in recovery has stimulated development of new types of treatment or rehabilitation, but there is considerable interest in how existing services and approaches should accommodate recovery principles. This includes modification of previously validated therapy and skill training modalities, adapting existing approaches to specific subpopulations, specialized education of professionals and other providers, inclusion of people with mental illness in development and testing of services, and provision of services by people with mental illness who are not mental health professionals. Outside the traditional domain of mental health services, there is considerable interest in policy and social interventions to make environments maximally conducive to recovery.

## Healthcare Policy and Government

The milestone New Freedom Commission (2003) was preceded by a 1999 U.S. Surgeon General report that indicted the American mental health system for anachronism, inefficiency, and insensitivity to both scientific advances and consumer needs (U.S. Surgeon General 1999). The report also goes into great detail about the idea of recovery and its development, and discusses new treatment and other approaches needed to overcome the problems. Other federal actions that set the stage for canonization of recovery at the national level included the 1986 Protection and Advocacy for Individuals with Mental Illness Act, which extended federal funding to state agencies originally established to provide legal services and advocacy for people with developmental disabilities and their families. The 1990 Americans with Disabilities Act (ADA) reflected broad public concerns about citizens with all kinds of disabilities. The 1992 ADAMHA Reorganization Act, which broadly reorganized the federal mental health bureaucracy, also brought the states into the policy and planning process, with a new system of block grants that made federal funding contingent on state-level planning councils whose membership includes consumers and family members. Attention to the needs of people with severe and disabling forms of mental illness, including the idea of recovery, began to appear in state-level policy documents describing best practices for that population.

The Surgeon General and New Freedom Commission reports were explicitly about two populations: adults with severe, disabling psychiatric disorders, historically diagnosed mostly as schizophrenia (dementia praecox before the 1930s), and children with such disorders, historically diagnosed mostly as childhood schizophrenia. These populations are named by two terms of art that had been in use since the 1980s in mental health policy and discourse, *serious mental illness* (SMI) for adults, and *severe emotional disturbance* (SED) for children.

In 2003 diagnostic practices for adults distinguished schizophrenia, schizo-affective disorder, bipolar disorder, and severe, chronic depressive disorder, but all have in common an onset in adolescence or later, an episodic course (periods of better and poorer functioning), a psychotic presentation during episodes of exacerbation, and chronic, pervasive impairment at all or most levels of personal and social functioning. In the context of their historical analyses, both reports identified this SMI population as primarily those who were confined in psychiatric hospitals before the deinstitutionalization movement.

For children, the diagnosis of childhood schizophrenia has been abandoned, replaced by several others that still fall under the SED rubric. Generally, policy and practice in child mental health have changed as much as for adults. The child mental health industry is fairly distinct from the industry that serves adults with SMI, and the consumer and advocacy communities are fairly distinct. It is therefore difficult to draw parallels or distinctions between adult and child recovery, and a complete account is beyond the scope of this chapter. Hereafter, for the purposes of this discussion, recovery will mean recovery as experienced by those with adolescent- or adult-onset conditions, i.e., recovery from SMI.

In 2004, the federal Substance Abuse and Mental Health Services Administration (SAMHSA, which had replaced ADAMHA in 1992) sponsored the National Consensus

Conference on Mental Health Recovery and Mental Health Systems Transformation, in collaboration with six other federal agencies. The primary purpose was to create a consensus definition of recovery. Participants included over 110 expert panelists, representing a wide range of stakeholders including consumers, family members, providers, advocates, researchers, academicians, accreditation organization representatives, representatives of the healthcare underwriting industry, state and local public officials, and others. Recovery from mental illness was defined as "a journey of healing and transformation enabling a person with a mental health problem to live a meaningful life in a community of his or her choice while striving to achieve his or her full potential." Ten "fundamental components" of recovery were enumerated, and the list has since become ubiquitous in agency mission statements in the mental health services industry. The fundamental components include: self-direction, person-centered individualization, empowerment, holistic perspective, expectation of nonlinear progress, a strengths-based focus, peer support, respect, personal responsibility of the consumer, and hope for a better future.

## The Public Forum

Public discussion of recovery is another important source of its contemporary meaning. The 1999 Surgeon General Report (pp. 92–98) identified several public organizations that have participated in the mental health policy discourse, beginning with Clifford Beers and the mental hygiene movement in 1908. The organizations include collaborations of citizens and professionals (e.g., Mental Health America, formerly National Mental Health Association), parents and families (e.g., National Alliance on Mental Illness, formerly National Alliance for the Mentally Ill), and self-identified people with mental illness. The last are further categorized as protest-oriented groups, whose members self-identify as "survivors" of psychiatry and/or an oppressive mental health system (e.g., Alliance for the Liberation of Mental Patients, the Insane Liberation Front), and self-help groups (e.g. Schizophrenics Anonymous, National Resource Center on Homelessness and Mental Illness).

The public discourse has not always been consistent with contemporary meanings of recovery. For example, NAMI's founders were a generation who had suffered from the psychoanalytic theory of the "schizophrenogenic mother," essentially attributing SMI to emotionally aloof parenting. Parents' interest in destigmatizing themselves was unfortunately served by the biological reductionism of the so-called neo-Kraepelinian movement in psychiatry (Kutchins and Kirk 1997), which reduced schizophrenia to an incurable neurological disease. Attempts to destigmatize schizophrenia as an imagined character disorder backfired, because incurable diseases are even more stigmatizing (Deacon and Baird 2009; Deacon and Lickel 2009), and obviously inconsistent with recovery. The neo-Kraepelinian preoccupation with drug treatment was equally inconsistent with recovery. As the neo-Kraepelinian era gave way to modern neuroscience, and as self-identified people with mental illness gained membership on the NAMI Board of Directors, NAMI policies and positions became more consistent with recovery.

More recently the public discourse has been facilitated by development of the internet, especially the advent of web logs or *blogs*, essays and discussions posted on web sites, in which multiple discussants can participate over time. Blogs also create a convenient way to study the meanings of recovery associated with the public discourse. For the purposes of this discussion, the authors created a sample of internet websites consisting of the first 35 unduplicated results of a Google search, in July 2015, using the search string "mental health recovery blog," excluding sites that do not actually include a blog page (mostly websites of mental health providers advertising their services). The resulting sample includes four government websites (11 % of the sample), sponsored by the National Institute of Mental Health (NIMH), the Substance Abuse and Mental Health Services Administration (SAMSHA), the Centers for Disease Control

understandings of SA, less infused with spiritual or religious ideas and less committed to the principle of absolute abstinence as the only viable outcome (Burnam and Watkins 2006). Therapist credentials and related components of the SA infrastructure had evolved outside the traditional healthcare disciplines and guilds, sometimes creating an "anti-professional" climate. The authors of the 2006 analysis (Burnam and Watkins 2006) argued that this had not been particularly problematic for treatment of addictions, but there was a growing realization that addictions often occur in conjunction with other psychiatric disorders. Organizational boundaries, service funding channels, and the tensions between SA and mental health communities were significant barriers to joint treatment of SA co-occurring with other disorders. People with co-occurring disorders often "fell through the cracks" between the service systems. Similarly, there was a gross discrepancy between public funding of SA and mental health services, including a prohibition against eligibility for Social Security disability benefits (Supplemental Security Income, SSI) based on SA alone. The obvious solution is integration of services, but this is easier said than done. Most efforts to redress the segregation and disproportionate funding of SA have been carried out at the state level, e.g., through creative manipulation of Medicaid eligibility and funding streams, including new funding streams exclusively for co-occurring disorders.

There has been much progress in developing effective approaches for co-occurring disorders, but the results are unclear, and even troubling, with regard to recovery from SMI. On the one hand, there are many similarities and parallels between the idea of recovery as invoked by the New Freedom Commission and historical ideas about recovery from addiction. These were celebrated in a 2009 SAMHSA publication (Sheedy aand Whitter 2009) identifying all the key elements of recovery from SMI as equally applicable to addictions and co-occurring disorders. Subsequent SAMHSA publications (e.g., SAMSHA 2014) describe recovery without distinguishing between SA, SMI, or other disorders. The term "behavioral health" increasingly replaced "mental health" in agency names and policy language, to include SA and other psychiatric disorders under a common rubric in the healthcare regulatory infrastructure. Differences between recovery from SMI and recovery from co-occurring disorders were further obscured by changes in use of the term SMI itself, devolving from denotation of schizophrenia spectrum disorders and the historical psychiatric institutional population to include virtually any psychiatric diagnosis (Insel 2013). This was an economic boon to the SA services industry, because a co-occurring diagnosis makes more people with SA eligible for public funding of treatment.

However, an (arguably) inadvertent result was diversion of resources away from the SMI population. Since the beginning of the deinstitutionalization and community mental health movements it has proved difficult to incentivize community services for the SMI population sufficiently to recruit providers (Lamb and Bachrach 2001). Stretching the SMI category to include virtually any psychiatric disorder has exacerbated that problem. At the national level, this has generated pointed criticism of SAMHSA policy (Torrey 2015; U.S.G.A.O. 2014), even accusations of abandoning the SMI population. A recent case analysis of state-level consequences of national policy (Laib 2015) portrays a massive transfer of fiscal resources liberated by downsizing of state hospitals, to nongovernmental community providers who serve primarily the "co- occurring disorder" population while actively excluding individuals with SMI.

For people with SMI and SA, disability is generally most directly caused by the SMI, with SA in an exacerbating role. For people with co-occurring SA and non-SMI disorders, the disability generally is caused primarily by the SA. Integrated services for co-occurring disorders are generally joint provision of the separate treatments for SA and for the co-occurring disorder. Effective SA treatment for people with SMI is different in content and approach from treatment for SA or SA co-occurring with other disorders (Drake et al. 2004). Although the abstract principles of recovery may be comparably applicable, recovery from SMI is different from recovery from SA.

The term "rehabilitation," closely associated with "recovery," often appears in both the SA and the SMI literature and policy. However, in SA "rehab" refers to programs derived from Twelve Step or related models, and focused on detoxification and sustained abstinence, whereas in SMI it refers to *psychiatric rehabilitation*, a comprehensive approach combining psychosocial and biomedical components and derived from rehabilitation of physical disabilities (further discussed in a later section of this chapter).

A more complete analysis of the similarities and differences between recovery from SMI and from SA, co-occurring disorders or other mental health conditions is beyond the scope of this chapter. Hereafter, the present discussion of recovery will refer specifically to recovery from SMI, whether co-occurring with SA or not, but it is important to note that obfuscation of the differences, linked to attrition of resources for people with SMI, is an important issue in policy, research, and practice.

## Evolution of Key Concepts

The understanding of recovery portrayed in the New Freedom Commission report, and elaborated in the subsequent decade, was a convergence of several key developments in mental health research, policy, and practice. Historical accounts trace these developments as far back as the moral therapy movement in seventeenth century Western Europe. For present purposes, the late twentieth century provides a sufficient perspective on how current meanings emerged.

### Social Factors in SMI

In the 1950s and 1960s, sociological analyses such as those of Goffman (1961) stimulated public awareness that SMI is more than the intrapersonal processes postulated by both psychoanalytic and biomedical paradigms, dominant at the time. This complemented broader post-modern social criticism (e.g. Foucault 1961/2006) that identified mental illness as a kind of social role imposed by an exploitative culture on vulnerable and disenfranchised individuals. At a more individual level, experimental psychology also reinforced the idea that mental illness is at least partly the result of interpersonal processes. Analysis of the behavior of institutionalized patients using Skinner's operant learning paradigm showed that it is shaped by rewards and punishments unsystematically meted out by direct care staff (Gelfand et al. 1967). The new methods of experimental social psychology revealed that patients' understanding of their situation influences in turn the perceptions and judgments of their caregivers (Braginsky et al. 1969). These were highly counterintuitive findings at a time when the mainstream understanding of SMI emphasized irrationality and detachment from reality.

In the 1960s, the experimental findings were translated into a treatment approach, *token economy*, which effectively re-established adaptive social behavior in institutionalized patients (Ayllon and Azrin 1968). A decade later, in what was at the time the largest controlled treatment trial in the history of psychiatry (Paul and Lentz 1977), a treatment program based on token economy and related principles of social learning theory proved overwhelmingly superior to standard institutional treatment, not only in re-establishing personal and social functioning, but in leaving the institution for a stable community tenure.

Tragically, the successes of the early learning-based programs in psychiatric institutions were largely ignored. This is partially attributable to the deinstitutionalization movement of the 1970s, when most expected that institutional facilities would soon be nonexistent. In addition, analysis of the economics of the mental health industry (Magaro et al. 1978) reinforced the sociological ideas of the previous decade: mental illness, and by implication recovery from mental illness, is in large part an interpersonal process, recovery is not necessarily profitable for service providers, and effective recovery approaches are sometimes incompatible with the traditional power hierarchies of the mental health professions. This is echoed in the New Freedom Commission's first principle for transforming the mental health system, which without such context may seem a platitude: "First, services and treatment must be consumer and family centered, geared to give consumers real and meaningful choices about treatment options and providers—not oriented to the requirements of bureaucracy." Sadly, failure to realize this principle has been a major barrier to disseminating recovery-oriented practices and developing recovery-oriented services.

Today the legacy of earlier research on social factors is evident in the recovery movement, in its rejection of the limiting social role of "mental patient," whether imposed by the service system, the patient's family, practitioners, the culture at large, or the people with mental illness themselves. People in the "mental patient" role do not participate in community life. Participation in community life, a central value of recovery, includes participation in the community's economy—not just the monetary economy, but the social and emotional economy as well, the myriad social contracts that give meaning to our lives. Social learning theory gives us a scientific perspective on those economies, how they are disrupted by mental illness, and how we can use them in pursuit of recovery goals. Mental illness does not obliterate a person's ability to participate in economies, and with appropriate assistance and acquisition of key skills, such participation is within reach.

Just as important, *absence* of the economic benefits of community participation *does* compromise normal motivation to perform normal social roles. Recovery is most facilitated when the social environment provides incentives to reject dependent social roles, but the incentives must be engineered to be accessible to people at every stage of their recovery, in accordance with their abilities. A concrete example is the relationship between disability pensions and vocational functioning—when the former becomes a disincentive for pursuing one's own work- and independence-related recovery goals, the system is not optimally recovery-oriented. Less concretely, this also means that interests within the mental health industry that benefit from the dependence and disability of its clients must be confronted and changed, at individual, organizational, and political levels.

## Deinstitutionalization

Deinstitutionalization was itself a convergence of the sociological insights of the 1950s and 1960s, public concerns about conditions in state hospitals, the momentum of similar reforms in the developmental disability system, and the expectations of long-term benefits of the newly discovered antipsychotic drugs. In 1955, Congress had established the Joint Commission on Mental Illness and Mental Health, whose 1961 report became the basis of the Community Mental Health Act of 1963. The 1963 act set up the fiscal and regulatory infrastructure for community mental health centers, expected to serve the historical institutional population. The Surgeon General's and New Freedom Commission's historical analyses acknowledge the role of deinstitutionalization in creating a social context that was necessary for recovery to take on its current meanings (for repeated analyses of deinstitutionalization as it progressed, see Bachrach 1978, 1982, 1983; Lamb and Bachrach 2001).

In retrospect, deinstitutionalization involved a number of inaccurate and contradictory ideas about the nature of SMI. On one hand, the sociological and psychological studies showing the toxic effects of institutional environments gave the impression that simply escaping those environments would foster normal personal and social functioning. On the other hand, the belief that antipsychotic drugs would normalize functioning reflected a reductionist biomedical perspective, insensitive to social factors, and anathema to the contemporary recovery movement. Neither of the ideas were completely wrong, but by the 1980s it was clear that suppression of psychotic symptoms with drugs seldom leads to broader normalization. Instead of being absorbed into community life, formerly institutionalized people gravitated to "mental health ghettos" of substandard housing, exploitative landlords, minimal social services, high crime rates, and abject poverty. Ironically, the expectation that people could reintegrate in the community, if simply given access to medication and the conventional psychotherapy of the time, contradicted the persistent, widespread belief that SMI is an incurable, irreversible, and disabling disease. A "trans-institutionalization" process began, with an explosive increase in the representation of people with SMI in prisons and jails that continues as of this writing, although it may have peaked some time before 2010. (Deinstitutionalization itself was not necessarily the sole factor in the increase of people with SMI in prisons and jails, and may be secondary to the differential impact on the SMI population of the overall increase in incarceration rates associated with the "zero tolerance" politics of the late twentieth century.)

Both successes and failures of deinstitutionalization set the stage for the recovery movement. The state hospital population was reduced by some 90 % nationwide, over the subsequent decades. However, less than half of the envisioned mental health centers were actually built, and none were funded sufficiently to serve the population. Of those that survived, most became more like publicly subsidized public practices, serving indigent populations with conventional mental health needs, not the historical institutional population. It was a foreshadowing of the contemporary "cherry-picking" process by which provider organizations tap into funding streams meant for people with SMI without serving people with SMI. Even when services were available, it became evident that neither medication nor the psychosocial treatment of the time was sufficient to help people in the historical institutional population regain normal functioning or have a decent quality of life. Even in light of the under-funding of the community system, more money alone would not solve the problems. New paradigms were needed.

## Psychiatric Rehabilitation

The limited success of deinstitutionalization stimulated research to find more effective methods of treatment. William Anthony, a psychologist with a background in rehabilitation of physical disabilities, provided an organizing concept for much of this work in his landmark translation of rehabilitation psychology into the psychiatric context (Anthony 1979). At the conceptual level, the most revolutionary idea in psychiatric rehabilitation was that SMI must be seen not as a disease to be cured, but as a disability to be overcome. It was an idea that effectively competed with the reductionist expectation (gradually devolving to a fantasy) that eventually an SMI "wonder drug" would be discovered, and also with the public's stereotype of people with SMI. Rehabilitation had gained respectful public attention in the aftermath of World War II, as wounded and disabled war heroes successfully returned to civilian life. It made sense to people that SMI is in important ways more like paralysis from a spinal injury than an infectious disease, and recovering from disability is different from curing an illness. Most importantly, it was obvious in physical rehabilitation that overcoming disability requires not only biomedical treatment, but psychological and socio-environmental levels of intervention as well. Hope, acceptance, determination, and support are critical for success.

The theoretical framework of rehabilitation psychology was social learning theory, the same set of ideas that had propelled the earlier work on token economy. In addition to its sensitivity to the social--interpersonal context of behavior, social learning theory provided a powerful new idea about treatment: virtually everything that we do can be understood as exercising a *skill* that we have *learned*. Social roles are essentially sets of skills that we apply in the course of performing those roles. Accordingly, any "impairment" or "deficit" or "failure" in personal or social functioning can be understood as the absence of a needed skill set. People can overcome disabilities by learning new skills. Rehabilitation is a learning process. The learner is a student, not a patient.

Psychiatric rehabilitation prolifically generated new social learning-based treatment approaches and adapted others for use with SMI. The early principles of token economies were developed into more versatile and sophisticated approaches for community settings (e.g., Heinssen et al. 1995; Heinssen 2002; Liberman et al. 1976; Wong et al. 1986). The basic idea of skill training as a type of therapy led to *social skills training*, a structured approach to recovering interpersonal functioning (Corrigan et al. 1992; Liberman et al. 1975). Skill training led to other applications, including the skills required to self-manage one's own psychiatric condition (Eckman et al. 1990, 1992; Liberman et al. 1986; Lukoff et al. 1986) and skills families could use to reduce conflict and effectively support their members with SMI (Mueser and Glynn 1995). *Cognitive behavioral therapy* (CBT), an individual psychotherapy approach based on social learning theory, which had proved effective for problems with anxiety, depression, and substance abuse in other populations, was adapted for SMI, and extended to include problems unique to SMI, such as delusions and hallucinations (Barrowclough et al. 2001; Haddock et al. 1998). The cognitive impairments of schizophrenia became targets for specialized treatment (Silverstein et al. 2009; Spaulding et al. 1999). *Motivational interviewing*, another individual therapy modality combining nondirective and CBT principles, was adapted to help stimulate hope and engage people with SMI and their families in the rehabilitation enterprise (Sherman et al. 2009). Comprehensive textbooks educated new practitioners as the approach evolved (Liberman 2008; Pratt et al. 2014; Spaulding et al. 2003). As the treatment array expanded and diversified, the idea of recovery remained an organizing principle and superordinate outcome goal. Psychiatric rehabilitation became a "tool kit" for pursuing individuals' recovery goals.

Psychiatric rehabilitation is sometimes confused with *psychosocial rehabilitation*. There is considerable overlap, especially in fundamental principles related to recovery. Both eschew traditional biomedical assumptions about recovery and the primacy of medical treatment, and both emphasize the importance of functional dimensions such as social affiliation and work, in both subjective and objective domains. Psychosocial rehabilitation is historically associated with two organizations, Fountain House and Thresholds, in New York City and Chicago, respectively. Both organizations developed the *clubhouse model*, a living and working arrangement wherein groups of people help each other identify and pursue personal recovery goals (Macias et al. 1999). A version of a clubhouse model of psychosocial rehabilitation was developed in the Veterans Administration healthcare system, known as the Fairweather model after its founder George Fairweather (Fairweather et al. 1969). The psychosocial rehabilitation model predated psychiatric rehabilitation. By the time recovery was explicitly recognized as the key element in psychiatric rehabilitation (Anthony 1993), it had been so in psychosocial rehabilitation for over 40 years. Over time the particular principles and practices of psychosocial rehabilitation, including the centrality of recovery, became completely subsumed by the psychiatric rehabilitation rubric. In 1995, the pioneering Psychosocial Rehabilitation Journal was renamed Psychiatric Rehabilitation Journal. By 2005, the professional organization International Association of Psychosocial Rehabilitation Services had spawned national affiliates, with the American one named United States Psychiatric Rehabilitation Association.

## Locus and Focus

As the idea of recovery evolved in the late twentieth century, debates arose over some of its critical features. One such debate was about whether recovery could occur in institutional settings, and by implication, whether psychiatric rehabilitation could legitimately be provided there. In commenting on the debate of where rehabilitation and recovery can occur, William Anthony is said to have quipped, "It's the focus, not the locus."

There was never any debate about whether the coercion and loss of liberty in psychiatric institutions are incompatible with the values of recovery, but as deinstitutionalization progressed it became increasingly evident that state hospitals were not completely disappearing. In 2014, there were 207 state operated psychiatric hospitals nationwide, housing some 40,600 people (Haupt 2014). Deinstitutionalization did, for the most part, reduce the state hospital population to people who are consigned there through criminal courts (adjudicated "not guilty by reason of insanity") or civil processes (civil commitment), but it did not eliminate those populations. The recovery-oriented psychiatric rehabilitation tool kit provides the most effective means of achieving discharge from a state hospital. Most individuals in state hospitals would endorse discharge as a high-priority personal recovery goal. Under these circumstances, denying the propriety of recovery-oriented services in institutions becomes abandonment of the remaining institutional population.

This debate had been mostly resolved by the end of the twentieth century, at least in the scholarly mental health community (Spaulding 1999), with the realization that recovery-oriented psychiatric rehabilitation transforms the role, mission, and processes of state institutions. Today the momentum of the discourse has shifted to the importance of the asylum role (Sisti et al. 2015), as opposed to the dubious presumption that the medical accouterments of a "hospital" provide anything other than a secure environment. Psychiatric rehabilitation has known effectiveness for helping people move from institution to the community (Silverstein et al. 2006). Nevertheless, dissemination of recovery-oriented practices in state institutions is still agonizingly slow, and the canard that "rehabilitation and recovery can only happen in the community" still appears as a gambit to preserve the unaccountability and sinecure of vested institutional interests (Spaulding et al. 2010), to the detriment of the mental health service system and its clientele (Tarasenko et al. 2013).

Psychiatric rehabilitation in long-term institutions or state hospitals is a different issue from treatment of SMI in acute or short-term "inpatient" settings. The inpatient time frame is too short for meaningful rehabilitation or recovery, but acute hospitalization may be a key starting point for both. Also, the context of short-term hospitalization can be made recovery-oriented. Research continues on maximizing the recovery orientation of hospital settings (Chen et al. 2013; Tsai et al. 2010).

## Recovery Science: Objective and Subjective Domains

Recovery from SMI occurs in individual people, who subjectively experience the joys and sorrows of being empowered or disempowered, hopeful or hopeless, engaged or disengaged community members. People with SMI (and everybody else) also have very objective goals, e.g., living outside an institution, having friends, maintaining employment, being independent without a guardian, or conservator. Achievement of objective goals is both impacted by and impacts people's experience of empowerment, hopefulness, and engagement. Current research on recovery addresses both objective and subjective dimensions.

Closely related to the objective/subjective distinction is that between recovery as outcome versus process (Silverstein and Bellack 2008). Earlier in the evolution of recovery some saw this as two competing perspectives, the former of the scientific community and the latter of the consumer community. The Surgeon General report emphasized the need for services that produce better outcomes, and the New Freedom Commission characterized recovery as a journey. Contemporary research tends not to reflect a presumption of incompatibility, and both are assumed to be important, even "two sides of the same coin." Nevertheless, recovery is complicated, and separate consideration of its objective and subjective processes and outcomes is necessary for heuristic manageability.

## Prevalence of Recovery, Objectively Defined

A series of long-term outcome studies on people with serious mental illness was instrumental in the New Freedom Commission's announcement that *recovery happens*. Generally, approximately 20–25 % of people show a return to essentially premorbid functioning levels, another 50–60 % of people achieve a substantial reduction in symptomatology and significant improvement in functioning levels, while approximately 20–25 % of people maintain significant symptoms and functional deficits (Silverstein and Bellack 2008). Some estimates put the percentage of people with "good" long-term outcomes at around 50 % (Bellack 2006).

The majority of the studies establishing prevalence rates of recovery were cross-sectional in nature. Harrow et al. (2005) conducted a 15-year longitudinal study in which they assessed participants at three-year intervals. Their results indicated that recovery is not linear, which is consistent with the episodic nature of serious mental illness. At least 41 % of their participants met their definition of "recovered" for at least one time point; however, very few met the criteria on multiple occasions. Overall, the presence of symptoms was negatively associated with functional recovery.

Considering the episodic nature of serious mental illness and recovery as an outcome, the value of concurrent research on more subjective components of recovery is clear. Theoretically, including a view of recovery as a process or journey, in which an individual becomes increasingly empowered to live a meaningful life while overcoming the challenges presented by mental illness, can mitigate the negative impact of symptom relapse or loss of objectively-defined "recovered" status. Furthermore, empowering mental health policies, such as shared decision-making or psychiatric advance directives, can help protect an individual's progress by sustaining the recovery process even when objectively defined recovery suffers a setback.

## Research on Personal and Environment Factors Impacting Recovery as an Outcome

When recovery is defined as an outcome, several domains are typically included (Bellack 2006). Symptom remission, as measured by the Brief Psychiatric Rating Score, the Global Assessment Scale, or being unable to meet diagnostic criteria, is typically one domain. Occupational functioning is typically another domain, represented through employment, both procurement of employment and often a threshold of hours per week required. The psychosocial functioning domain is evaluated through engagement in social relationships or participation in one's community. Residential status and independent functioning in areas like money management are also considered domains, and evaluated as inpatient or institutional, supported living, or independent living. Finally, all of these domains must be maintained sufficiently for a period of time before recovery as an outcome is typically considered achieved. Time frames typically vary from a year to five years.

There is a significant amount of research investigating links between personal or environmental factors and the domains typically comprising the definitions of recovery as an outcome. While most environmental factors are identified through consensus as face valid (e.g.Silverstein and Bellack 2008; Onken et al. 2002; Young et al. 2000; Styron et al. 2005), there are a few that have been empirically supported. Access to comprehensive, coordinated, and continuous treatment, as well as a social network of supportive individuals who promote realistic expectations while supporting incremental progress, have been empirically supported as linked to better recovery outcomes (Silverstein and Bellack 2008; Kopelowicz et al. 2005; Liberman et al. 2002).

Chen et al (2013) developed a mental health staff competency profile, through interviews with consumers, family members, staff, and providersand amalgamated with information from a literature review resulting in a list of key competencies necessary for the provision of recovery-oriented services. Eight competency areas were identified: reducing environmental tensions (e.g., maintaining a therapeutic environment in an ordered inpatient setting), reducing personal tensions (e.g., empowering consumers to find ways to manage their health in their preferred ways), reducing providers' own tensions (e.g., facilitating practitioners in their efforts to demonstrate a recovery orientation in daily practice), setting goals, and planning with consumers individually, engaging consumers in decision-making, fostering a positive recovery cycle, promoting recovery, and providing transitional services.

An alternative list of mental health staff behaviors was created based on their conceptual link to facilitating recovery in consumers, including developing a therapeutic relationship, conducting reliable symptom assessments and diagnostic evaluations, providing access to medical evaluation and treatment, completing functional assessments, empowering the individual, integrating psychopharmacology and psychosocial treatments, providing social skills training and family education, encouraging family involvement in treatment, providing access to transitional and supported employment, conducting clinical case management, and teaching consumers self-help and advocacy (Coursey et al. 2000a, b; Silverstein and Bellack 2008).

Brekke (2007) posited three environmental factors that are necessary for functional outcomes to improve, namely, opportunity, support, and enhancements. These were defined as options for functional capacity to flower into functional outcomes (e.g., affordable housing options to enable more independent living), a social support network of family, friends, peers, and staff promoting adaptive changes, and access to appropriate treatment and services that facilitate improved functional outcomes, respectively. All these socio-environmental factors had been operationalized in Paul and Lentz' (1977) outcome study (discussed in the previous section of this chapter), and quantitatively measured by systematic observation of staff-patient interactions.

Another body of research has addressed personal factors that are linked to changes in the likelihood of achieving recovery as an outcome. Anxiety (Harrow et al. 2006) and a history of poor functioning (Schimming and Harvey 2004) are negatively related to recovery, and the latter is also specifically predictive of a worsening of negative symptoms over time (Schimming and Harvey 2004). Other individual factors related to more positive recovery outcomes include a shorter duration of untreated psychosis, good initial response to neuroleptics, adherence to treatment, supportive therapy with a collaborative therapeutic alliance, preserved executive cognitive functioning, verbal fluency, and verbal memory abilities, and a good premorbid history (Silverstein and Bellack 2008; Kopelowicz et al. 2005; Liberman et al. 2002). Early treatment is also significantly positively associated with better functional outcomes (Gearing et al. 2009).

Neurocognition is a more robust predictor of recovery outcomes than the presence or severity of positive or negative symptoms (Brekke and Nakagami 2010). Multiple deficits in neurocognition, including problems with memory, attention, language, and executive function, are found among the SMI population. Individual functioning can be divided into three levels: (1) functional capacity, defined as one's ability to perform basic, daily tasks, (2) functional performance, defined as one's actual performance of basic, daily tasks in the real world, and (3) functional outcomes, e.g., income and independence. Of these three levels, functional capacity seems to be most strongly influenced by cognitive functioning, while functional performance and functional outcomes are highly impacted by environmental factors. Social functioning is impacted by cognitive deficits in attention, memory, and verbal learning, while occupational functioning is impacted by cognitive deficits in memory, verbal learning, and processing speed, primarily. Independent living skills are most impacted by executive functioning deficits, as well as memory and verbal learning deficits.

Social cognition also has a significant impact on recovery outcomes (Brekke and Nakagami 2010). People with schizophrenia show multiple areas of impairment in social cognition, including social perception, social knowledge, theory of mind, attributional style, and perception of emotion, with the last being typically considered as the domain with the most impairment, on average. Deficits in social perception are associated with reduced functioning in social problem solving, social behavior, community functioning, and occupational functioning. Additionally, there may be an interaction between neurocognition and social cognition, so that while they both impact functional outcomes, their influence may not be entirely independent. For instance, early visual processing, verbal recognition memory, vigilance, executive functioning, and sensorimotor gating are related to perception of emotion and social perception.

Finally, another personal factor impacting recovery outcomes is motivation level. Negative symptoms of schizophrenia can impact motivation levels significantly through an individual's experience of anhedonia, avolition, or amotivation. These three are demonstrated mediators between an individual's symptoms and their recovery outcomes (Yamada et al. 2010). Additionally, other studies suggest that intrinsic motivation specifically is a mediator between cognitive deficits and recovery outcomes (Brekke and Nakagami 2010).

## Research on Objective Recovery-Focused Outcomes

While a comprehensive review of the research on improving each domain typically included in a definition of recovery as an outcome could be compiled into its own book, a very brief review of relevant literature is included here, primarily to serve as an overview and a starting place for further study. Factors that predict symptomatic relapse include use of alcohol or drugs (Maslin 2003; Kopelowicz et al. 2005; Liberman et al. 2002), discontinuation of antipsychotic medications (Gitlin et al. 2001; Robinson et al. 1999), poor premorbid psychosocial function (Robinson et al. 1999), major life stressors, and an emotionally charged family environment (Butzlaff & Hooley 1998). Additionally, the development of group-based programs like Illness Management and Recovery (Mueser et al. 2002; Mueser et al. 2006), along with individual therapy, can be used to educate consumers on ways to manage symptoms and reduce the likelihood of symptomatic relapse while accommodating individual goals and encouraging empowerment (Bond et al. 2004).

There is a strong relationship between psychosocial functioning and the experiential process of recovery. Consumers report higher levels of engagement in their recovery process when they also have higher levels of social support and increased engagement in activities (Hendryx et al. 2009). The nature of the activity (e.g., social, physical, outside of the home, etc.) is not as important as the actual engagement in it, especially for those with lower levels of social support.

Employment is an objective outcome of substantial interest in the recovery movement, often studied in the context of *supported employment*, a psychiatric rehabilitation modality (Mueser et al. 2004). In supported employment, individuals with serious mental illness whose level of functioning would typically render them ineligible for traditional approaches to vocational rehabilitation (e.g., skill training or job counseling), are placed as regular employees in integrated settings where they work for pay but with ongoing support (Mueser et al. 1997).

In a project known as the "Hartford Study," over two hundred clients with serious mental illness were randomly assigned to standard services, a supported employment model, or a psychosocial rehabilitation program using a more traditional approach to vocational functioning (Mueser et al. 2004). Participants in the supported employment condition had significantly better outcomes than clients in the other two settings, by being more likely to procure competitive work (73.9 %, compared to 18.2 % in the traditional rehabilitation condition or 27.5 % in the standard services condition) and more likely to procure any paying work (73.9 %, compared to 34.8 % in the psychosocial program or 53.6 % in the standard services condition). The results from thirteen studies showed similar findings, where 40–60 % of the participants did not find competitive employment, while less than 20 % of their counterparts did (Bond 2004).

While supported employment produces the objective outcome of vocational functioning, there are limitations. Although it is effective in creating access to desirable paid employment, it does not necessarily normalize vocational functioning (Mueser et al. 2004). In the Hartford study, only 33.8 % of participants in the supported employment condition eventually worked more than twenty hours a week. The average number of weeks worked per job was relatively low, the average amount earned was low, and half of the people who obtained jobs had lost them by the six month follow-up time point. Furthermore, it is currently unclear whether improved vocational functioning impacts the subjective experience of recovery. Some studies indicate that supported employment does not improve self-ratings of mood, life satisfaction, or self-esteem, while some indicate that it does (Silverstein and Bellack 2008). There is no evidence of a direct link between supported employment and better outcomes in other domains of recovery, such as symptom remission or social functioning (Bond 2004). Links between domains of objective and subjective recovery cannot be taken for granted.

Additional work has continued to improve the impact of supported employment. Several barriers have been identified including cognitive impairment, low educational attainment, depression, lack of self-confidence, and financial disincentives against increased income (e.g., disability pensions) (McGurk and Mueser 2006; McGurk et al. 2007). Outcome improved when supported employment was combined with occupational skills training (Wallace and Liberman 2004) or neurocognitive therapy (McGurk et al. 2007).

While reducing cognitive impairment is not often explicitly listed as a recovery outcome, cognitive functioning is strongly related to functioning in the areas that are explicitly listed (Kopelowicz et al. 2005; McGurk and Mueser 2006; Smith et al. 2004). Service intensity is predictive of functional improvement, but only when complimented by neurocognitive improvement (Brekke et al. 2009). Improvement of social cognition can improve the therapeutic alliance, which is related to both recovery as an outcome and as a process (Deegan 1996).

Neurocognitive therapy, aka *cognitive remediation*, produces objective recovery outcomes. A meta-analysis of cognitive remediation found that its addition to other rehabilitation interventions improve cognitive and functional outcomes (McGurk et al. 2007). Other meta-analyses of cognitive remediation showed improvement in global neurocognition, as well as neurocognitive domains, such as verbal working memory (Brekke and Nakagami 2010).

Finally, there are a variety of assessment tools available to clinicians seeking to evaluate these levels of functional recovery in consumers (Mausbach et al. 2009). The assessments include topics such as social skills, medication management, independent living, and global functioning. They include clinician administered, self-report, and skill performance data gathering methods. These tools can be used to supplement the more facially valid outcome measures (e.g., maintenance of a job) to aid clinicians in assessing client progress towards recovery as an outcome.

## Research on Subjective Dimensions of Recovery

Even when outcome research is inconclusive, social values must be incorporated into treatment design, and research shows negative outcomes when these values are neglected (Silverstein and Bellack 2008).

The Recovery Assessment Scale was originally developed from the narratives of consumers (Corrigan et al. 1999). A total of 41 items were produced for the measure, which provides a single score of recovery. The scale was then piloted on 35 individuals with a severe mental illness diagnosis and displayed test–retest reliability and internal consistency. The Recovery Assessment Scale was positively correlated with measures of social support, quality of life, self-esteem, and self-orientation to empowerment, and negatively correlated to psychiatric symptoms and age. A factor analysis was later conducted which revealed five factors, with 24 total items: (1) personal confidence and hope, (2) willingness to ask for help, (3) not dominated by symptoms, (4) goal and success orientation, and (5) ability to rely on others (Corrigan et al. 2004).

A similar instrument is the Mental Health Recovery Measure (Young and Ensing 1999; Ralph et al. 2000). This tool is based on six aspects of recovery: (1) overcoming "stuckness," (2) discovering and fostering self-empowerment, (3) learning and self-redefinition, (4) return to basic functioning, (5) striving to attain overall wellbeing, and (6) striving to reach new potentials. These six aspects of recovery are put into a model with three stages: stage one involves the first aspect of recovery, stage two involves the second, third, and fourth aspects of recovery, and stage three involves the last two aspects of recovery. This measure is comprised of 41 total items that break down into six subscales that match the six aspects of recovery. There is excellent internal consistency for the total scale and a range of fair to good internal consistency for the subscales. The measures demonstrate convergent validity with the Community Living Skills Scales (Smith and Ford 1990) and with a measure of empowerment.

An alternative stage model of recovery, Stages of Recovery, is based on four themes: (1) finding and maintaining hope, (2) re-establishing a positive identity, (3) finding meaning in life, and (4) taking responsibility for one's life (Andresen et al. 2003). These four themes are maintained across proposed five stages of recovery: (1) moratorium—a time of withdrawal characterized by a profound sense of loss and hopelessness, (2) awareness—a realization that not all is lost and that a fulfilling life is possible, (3) preparation—measuring strengths and weaknesses for recovery and beginning work on recovery skill development, (4) rebuilding—setting meaningful goals and taking control of one's life, moving towards a positive identity, and (5) growth—living a full and meaningful life, characterized by self-management of the illness, resilience, and a positive sense of self. In this conceptualization of recovery stages, the fifth and final stage is also where an objective outcome of recovery is realized. The stages are intended to be sequential, but not necessarily linear or tied to specific timeframes to reflect the episodic nature of serious mental illness. A symptomatic relapse can occur at any stage without necessitating a return to an earlier stage, encouraging a resilient response.

The Stages of Recovery Instrument (STORI) measures movement through the proposed stages (Andresen et al. 2006). Ten themes were identified and then a conceptually valid item for each theme in each stage was developed, for a measure with a total of fifty items, with five stage subscales. Each item can be answered by selecting a response on a six point Likert scale, from "Not true at all now" to "Completely true now." A mean score is calculated for each of the five stage subscales, and stage of recovery is determined by the highest mean score, with a tie going to the higher stage. There is also a positively correlated companion brief stage measure that allows consumers to self-identify their stage of recovery, Self-Identified Stage of Recovery (SISR). This scale is a single-item measure that has five sentences, one for each stage of recovery, and participants select the item they feel best corresponds to their stage of recovery. This SISR is positively correlated with the Recovery Assessment Scale, but negatively correlated with a self-report measure of psychological distress (Kessler-10, Andrews and Slade 2001) and with a clinician-rated report of psychiatric symptoms (Health of a Nation Outcome Scale, Wing et al. 1998). The STORI is positively correlated with time elapsed since last inpatient treatment, as well as mental health variables, including psychological wellbeing, hope, resilience, and the Recovery Assessment Scale.

While these tools are available to measure the subjective experience of recovery as a whole, there is a significant amount of research showing the independent importance of the common themes found in these subjective descriptions. One theme consistently present among descriptions of the recovery process is that of empowerment. People with schizophrenia often discuss their lives in terms indicating they do not feel a sense of agency (Lysaker et al. 2003). One component of a successful recovery process is being able to develop a narrative, attributing agency to themselves and interpreting life events in the context of a recovery process (Silverstein and Bellack 2008). Increasing the internality of perceived control over life events has been positively associated with recovery in schizophrenia (Harrow et al. 2009). At the very least, consumers reported that when empowerment was incorporated into the provision of mental health care, their motivation to be actively involved improved and their recovery progress increased (Cruce et al. 2012).

The idea of empowerment has many similarities to the idea of recovery. Neither has one single operational definition and both can be viewed as an outcome and a process (Swift and Levin 1987). Empowerment also often incorporates several of the other themes commonly identified as crucial aspects of recovery as a process, such as self-direction, individualized care, hope, holistic care, and strengths-based approaches (Rappaport 1981), as well as touching on the psychosocial domain of recovery as an outcome by encouraging community participation (Rappaport 1987). Measurements of empowerment are positively correlated with measurements of recovery orientation, and negatively correlated with internalized stigmatization of mental illness measures (Boyd et al. 2014).

One way in which empowerment is implemented is through the practice of shared decision-making. Shared decision-making involves the client using their knowledge about their lived experience with mental illness while the provider uses their knowledge about mental illness and its treatments to collaboratively develop, implement, and evaluate an individualized treatment plan (Deegan and Drake 2006; Corrigan et al. 2012). It moves beyond treatment adherence or compliance maximizing approaches to foster a truly mutual decision-making process. As such, shared decision-making is consistent with several of the recovery process themes often identified, such as individualized and self-directed care, self-responsibility, and holistic care (SAMHSA 2004). Shared decision-making can be used not only for medication management (Deegan and Drake 2006), but for the wide variety of decisions relevant to an individual's mental health (Corrigan et al. 2012). Consumers involved in shared decision-making report higher levels of satisfaction with their treatment plan and providers, improved communication with treatment providers, increased perceived involvement in decision-making, and increased knowledge (Corrigan et al. 2012; Drake et al. 2009). Use of shared decision-making does increase later compliance with the treatment plan, although it may not directly change health decisions or behaviors of consumers (Corrigan et al. 2012).

*Self-esteem*, or some variation thereof, is also a common theme among definitions of recovery as a process. Self-esteem was directly related to subjective reports of recovery progress (Bell and Zito 2005) and self-esteem changes one year after hospital discharge predicted symptomatic severity (Roe 2003). However, some research indicates that if interventions solely target self-esteem, to the neglect of behavioral change, they do not have the desired outcome (Silverstein and Bellack 2008). This may be because self-esteem is generated through behavioral change, resulting in personal effectiveness (Silverstein and Bellack 2008).

However, response to behavioral change interventions may be improved by attending to self-esteem (Swann et al. 2007) and self-efficacy (Silverstein et al. 2006). This may be because self-efficacy is associated with more adaptive coping strategies (Ventura et al. 2004), while use of avoidant coping strategies can reduce self-efficacy (Vauth et al. 2007). Avoidant coping styles are also positively associated with symptomology (Wickett et al. 2006).

*Strengths-based* approaches have also been included as a common theme in recovery process definitions (SAMHSA 2004). Currently, there are some studies showing a strengths-based service delivery model may have some promise (Rapp and Goscha 2011). Although studies tend to lack an operationalized description of the intervention, there are some consistent aspects: service delivery is collaboratively developed and individualized to consumer strengths, primarily using existing community resources, and it takes place in the community. A recent meta-analysis of the relatively few available experimental or quasi-experimental designs testing this service delivery model revealed no significant differences for participants' level of functioning or quality of life, but a significant preference for other service delivery models for improvement in psychiatric symptoms (Ibrahim et al. 2014).

*Peer support* is defined as the mutual support between consumers to encourage each other in recovery and bring about desired social or personal change (Solomon 2004; SAMHSA 2004). It can take a variety of forms, including peer advocacy, peer clubhouses, peer employment, or self-help groups (Armstrong et al. 1995; Roberts et al. 1999). One particularly interesting development from the peer support movement is the use of WRAP, or Wellness and Recovery Action Plans (Copeland 2002). WRAP is an illness self-management program that facilitates consumers developing an individualized plan to respond to their mental health symptoms, using personal resources based on their preferences (Jonikas et al. 2013). WRAP sessions are typically conducted by peers who are in recovery from serious mental illness and specially trained in WRAP (Cook et al. 2011, 2014a, b). Consumers utilizing WRAP reported increased hopefulness, recovery, self-advocacy, and physical health, with a decrease in psychiatric symptoms; these changes were more pronounced for participants with higher engagement in the WRAP intervention (Cook et al. 2011, 2014a; Jonikas et al. 2013). Consumers also reported lower levels of anxiety and depression symptoms (Cook et al. 2014b). Additionally, implementation of WRAP was associated with a decrease in perceived need for behavioral health services, as well as a decrease in utilization of those services (Cook et al. 2013). It is not yet clear whether WRAP confers benefits comparable to or beyond those conferred by similar illness management skill training modalities designed for delivery by professionals.

Peer support is also often utilized in the form of case management. Randomized controlled trials have supported the proposition that there are no major differences in outcomes when case management services are provided by peers, as opposed to non-peers (Davidson et al. 2006); in fact, one study resulted in lower hospitalization rates when these services were provided by a peer (Clarke et al. 2000). Peer-support programs aimed at improving physical health behaviors to decrease comorbidity and mortality in this high-risk population have also shown promise (Druss et al. 2010). This may be because some peer support providers are better positioned to encourage treatment engagement than traditional case managers (Sells et al. 2006). However, consumers who become peer counselors are more likely to have had premorbid and mental illness characteristics that are predictive of good long-term outcomes, in contrast to the individuals who are in long-term care, who are more likely to have had premorbid and mental illness characteristics that are predictive of poor long-term outcomes (Silverstein and Bellack 2008). This dissymmetry may make it more difficult for peer counselors to relate to their clients. Arguably though, this would be no more difficult than it is for a counselor with no lived experience of mental illness to relate to consumers.

There is also support for the inclusion of at least some structured training for peer counselors, rather than relying solely on their lived experience. Some group participants in groups led by peer counselors display a high number of "bizarre and inappropriate behaviors" while group leaders sometimes display less than ideal group management styles (Bellamy et al. 2006).

## Practice Models of Recovery

We now turn to a focused analysis of two models of recovery-oriented practice and will discuss how these models can be integrated into services today.

## Evidence-Based Practice (EBP)

EBP, in its broadest sense, is a model of clinical decision-making that involves integrating the strongest research evidence, clinical expertise, and client characteristics, values and preferences (APA 2006; see Fig. 1.4). The American Psychological Association's definition of EBP was originally derived from the Institute of Medicine's definition of Evidence-Based Medicine (EBM; Sackett et al. 1996), which in turn evolved from an evidence-based practice movement in the medical community (Guyatt et al. 1992). EBP in psychology, although similar to EBM, emphasizes client factors and clinician experience as equally important to research evidence since research for specific disorders or clinical problems may be scarce (American Psychological Assocation Presidential Task Force on Evidence-based Practice, 2006). Thus, when implemented as intended, EBP in psychology is the *balanced* integration of these three sources of knowledge, hence its nickname, the "three-legged stool of EBP."

The practice of using the best available research evidence involves the clinician drawing knowledge of a hierarchy of empirical findings from a range of research methods (APA 2006; see Fig. 1.5). In this research hierarchy, findings from meta-analytic, single-case design, and randomized controlled trial (RCT) studies lie at the very apex to reflect their high quality, methodological rigor. Quasi-experimental designs and naturalistic studies fall in the middle and often are useful in demonstrating the external validity of findings from well-controlled research. Qualitative, correlational, observational, or systematic case studies form the base of the hierarchy, and represent the foundation of the beginnings of research—novel hypothesis generation.

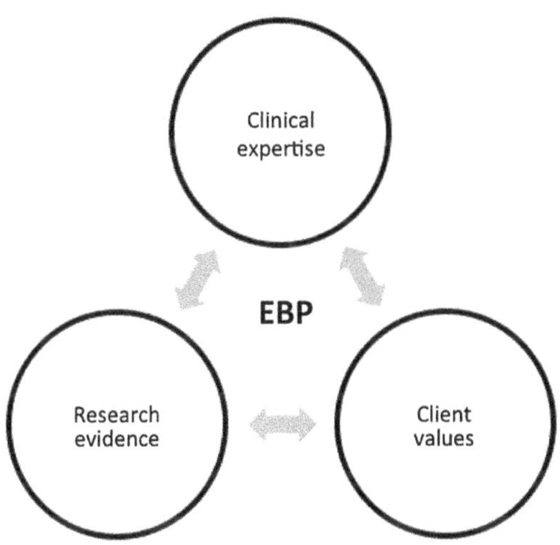


**Fig. 1.4** Graphic representation of the EBP model

## Empirically Supported Treatments

Related to the empirical evidence aspect of EBP is the concept of *Empirically Supported Treatments* (ESTs). ESTs are clearly defined psychological treatments demonstrated to be efficacious for treating a specific problem in a delineated population (Chambless and Hollon 1998). ESTs are often established after they are rigorously tested in well-controlled experimental research using randomized controlled trials. A treatment receives a designation of "well established" after two independent research teams replicate its efficaciousness for a specific problem and after the treatment shows superiority to placebo control conditions or a bona fide treatment (Chambless and Hollon 1998; Chambless and Ollendick 2001). Meta-analytic studies, although not necessary in defining a treatment as an EST, do provide additional confidence in the efficacy of a treatment due to its ability to aggregate research findings and create pooled treatment effect sizes.

For nearly 20 years, the Schizophrenia Patient Outcomes Research Team (PORT) has played an important role in evaluating the quality of treatment research and recommending ESTs for schizophrenia spectrum disorders (Lehman and Steinwachs 1998; Lehman et al. 2004). The PORT workgroup's most recent update (Kreyenbuhl et al. 2010) consisted of a review of 600 psychosocial and pharmacological research studies published between 2002 and 2008. An expert panel of 39 consumers, researchers, and practitioners recommended a total of eight psychosocial treatments previously discussed in our

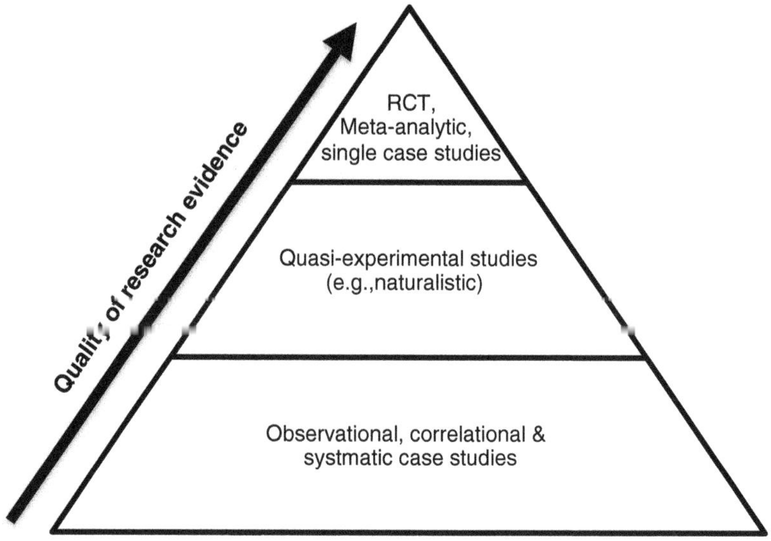


**Fig. 1.5** Graphic representation of the hierarchy of evidence

review, including assertive community treatment (ACT), social skills training (SST), behavioral family therapy (BFT) supported employment (SE), cognitive behavioral therapy for psychosis (CBTp). (Strictly speaking, ACT is an organizational scheme, not a treatment modality. It was originally based on the typical staffing structure of state hospitals, extended to community settings, stimulating the nickname "hospital without walls." ACT programs include variable amounts of psychiatric rehabilitation modalities. Without such modalities, ACT recovery outcomes are limited to reduced hospitalization.)

The American Psychological Association's Society of Clinical Psychology (Division 12) maintains a list of ESTs on their website. This list is intended to provide practitioners the research knowledge to provide research-supported treatments for specific disorders. A similar APA document focused on recovery from SMI is accessible at http://www.apa.org/practice/resources/ grid/.

ESTs are an important aspect of mental health practice, but EBP cannot be reduced to rigid implementation of manualized ESTs, especially in the context of care for people with SMI. First, while RCTs are considered the "gold-standard" for treatment development research, their findings may have limited applicability to community treatment seeking individuals with SMI because of strict exclusion criteria in their designs. SMI populations are extremely heterogeneous at all levels, from molecular to molar levels of systemic functioning (Spaulding et al. 2003), to pathogenesis (Heinssen et al. 2003) and treatment response (Peer and Spaulding 2007; Peer et al. 2008). Consequently, the external validity of RCT findings may not be generalized to individuals with SMI in the community. Second, there are also no stand-alone ESTs that address the complex array of clinical problems and diverse needs of SMI to date. In order to provide the most comprehensive care to consumers, practitioners must rely on assessing functional relationships between symptoms and problems (MacDonald-Wilson et al. 2002), selecting the most appropriate treatment or pack of treatments, then modifying treatment or adding adjunctive treatments to meet the individual needs and goals of the client (e.g., McGurk et al. 2005). These practices are reflective of thoughtful clinical decision-making not captured by EST procedure manuals.

## Client Values, Preferences, and Characteristics

EBP also involves integrated knowledge about client characteristics, values, and preferences to guide treatment decision-making and planning

(APA 2006). *Client characteristics* include factors proximal to treatment outcomes such as symptoms, functioning, readiness to change, insight, and social support. Client characteristics also include a range of factors distal from treatment, including developmental, social, cultural, and environmental characteristics. The concept of *client preferences* typically refers to the client's desired treatment decisions, but also may include preferences regarding type of provider or treatment setting, therapist-client match, therapist-client interaction style, treatment-team coordination, level of self-disclosure, occupational activities, and much more. Lastly, *client values* include personal, social, and cultural beliefs that concern how people live and what people consider moral, ethical, important, or personally meaningful. Values include key beliefs or convictions that often underlie or guide how people respond to situations in their day-to-day lives. People of various cultural or social groups may differentially subscribe to the values and customs of their self-identified group. Therefore, clinicians should always assess values and preferences at the individual level prior to making broad assumptions (La Roche and Maxie 2003).

There is an important distinction between values and subjective experience, although both are important in recovery, and both tend to be neglected in the medical model (Farkas 2005). Values are by definition a matter of personal choice, not subject to validation by scientific methods. Subjective experience can be studied scientifically, and we can sensibly ask scientific questions about what environmental conditions influence what subjective experiences. Recovery is, among other things, an array of subjective experiences, e.g., of well-being, satisfaction, affiliation, and hope. Farkas (2005) points out that subjective indicators of recovery are as least important as objective indicators, but are underused as outcome criteria, both for specific EVPs and for service programs. Empirical research can tell us what modalities and conditions are most conducive to subjective recovery. Values have a different role in recovery-oriented services.

Understanding client values, preferences, and characteristics is also essential to a service delivery competency known as *personalization of treatment*. Personalization of treatment is the practice of tailoring treatment plans to individual people to address specific treatment needs, meet personal goals, and aid the individual in acquiring skills and supports necessary to overcome barriers to recovery. Personalization of treatment has recently gained much recognition by the National Institutes of Mental Health (NIMH) as a strategic plan to improve mental health care and research on mental illness (Insel 2010). Personalizing treatments to individuals, rather than clinical problems or symptoms, requires a deep understanding of how the client's individual strengths, assets, and history interact with the presenting problem (Persons and Tompkins 1997). This deep understanding is most often achieved using two important clinical competencies: *clinical assessment* and *case conceptualization*.

In order for treatment to be personalized, the clinician must first gather assessment data to identify all relevant factors related to treatment, as well as to elucidate potential barriers to treatment. A number of approaches can be harnessed for gathering a wealth of information on client characteristics, values, and preferences. For instance, clinical interviews, intelligence, behavioral and neuropsychological tests, global rating scales, and self-report measures are all formal assessment methods useful for gathering information regarding client mental, social, emotional, and global functioning (Kazdin 2003). Nondirective psychotherapy, also known as person-centered therapy, is a less formal approach to assessment that involves clarifying values using Rogerian techniques directly in therapy. Spaulding et al. (2003) propose that both formal assessment approaches and nondirective psychotherapy can aid in the identification of treatment targets, exploration of client goals, and preparation for foreseeable barriers to recovery.

Nondirective techniques and specific assessments can provide a wealth of treatment-related information. However, there is little guidance for clinicians using these methods as to what assessment areas should be prioritized and how to select assessments from an abundance of existing batteries. Evidence-Based Assessment (EBA) is one systematic assessment approach closely tied to the EBP model that uses research and theory to inform the assessment process, such as prioritization of areas in need of assessment and selection of assessment instruments (Hunsley and Mash 2010). In addition to selecting tests that are scientifically valid and clinically meaningful, EBA also involves selecting assessments that are personally relevant to and culturally appropriate for the client for the purpose of gathering the best representation of the client's presenting problem, goals, and unique barriers to recovery. The child and adolescent field has embraced EBA because research has shown that mental health diagnosis has little-to-no treatment utility in youth (Pelham et al. 2005). Because of similar limitations with diagnosis in SMI, the theory-driven EBA approach may be applicable to the treatment of complex cases with severe and persistent mental illness (Tandon et al. 2013).

A central limitation of formal assessment methods and assessment in the therapeutic milieu is that the data are often decontextualized by artificial settings and the unnatural manner of collecting assessment data. More recently authors have advocated for the use of technology to enhance the external validity of assessment informative to the treatment of SMI. Technology such as electronic monitoring devices can collect real-time data in naturalistic environments and provide a range of objective information about medication adherence, socialization, and sleep (Granholm et al. 2008; Hofstetter et al. 2005). In addition, computerized clinical decision support systems have the capacity to collect an immense amount of electronic data and organize it efficiently to optimize clinical decision-making and reduce clinician bias when treating people with SMI (Spaulding and Deogun 2011).

The current best practices for SMI include a range of assessments, such as personality, functional, symptom, disability, risk, neurocognitive and social cognitive assessments, as well as structured clinical interviews (APA 2009). The APA Task Force on Serious Mental Illness and Severe Emotional Disturbance selected these assessment domains based off of an abundance of research capturing the complex interaction between symptoms, clinical problems, and functioning notable in SMI. While diverse assessment and use of technology are important in case formulation and treatment planning, clinicians must also actively monitor for client changes in clinical characteristics, treatment response, and recovery goals—as these factors are known to change over the course of treatment (Spaulding et al. 2003).

The second clinical competency for personalization of treatment involves synthesizing the assessment data into a unified case-level conceptualization, also known as a *case formulation* (Persons and Tompkins 1996). The case formulation involves identifying the client's presenting problem, origins of the presenting problem, strengths and assets, present functioning, and related external events and situations. The clinician then generates a series of working hypotheses that explain the relationship between these factors and identifies *key mechanisms* hypothesized to influence the individual's presenting problem (Persons et al. 2013). The case conceptualization is shared with the client and then modified to fit the client's perception of the interrelationships. After therapist and client develop the conceptualization, they work together in outlining treatment needs and desired goals. Research has shown that collaborative case formulation enhances the effectiveness of manualized treatments when working with clients who have complex psychopathology with multiple comorbidities (Persons et al. 2006), and thus has special importance for SMI.

Spaulding et al. (2003) provided a biosystemic case formulation approach specifically developed for recovery-oriented treatment and rehabilitation of SMI. This approach is accompanied by thorough clinical assessment of the recovering person's preferences, values, social relationships, community characteristics, and barriers to recovery. The approach thus organizes an abundance of information, including physiological, cognitive, interpersonal, behavioral, and environmental, leading to selection of specific interventions and other avenues for individuals to pursue goals related to recovery.

The client-values aspect of EBP is important because all clinical decisions cannot be solely informed by research. However, assessing client characteristics, values, and preferences is also an ethical imperative as much as it is a practical necessity for a number of reasons. First, assessing and engaging client values and preferences in treatment is important in selecting treatments, enhancing informed consent to treatment, and promoting shared decision-making throughout the treatment process (Drake et al. 2009; Drake and Deegan 2009). Second, gathering data on client values may prevent individuals from being subjected to treatments that are counter to individual or cultural values. Third, an assessment of each person's unique strengths, limitations, and needs may also reduce the probability of subjecting the client to unnecessary treatment or treatments that involve high probability of failure. Lastly, selecting an individualized, person-conscious treatment approach is expected to avoid potential conflict between client and provider, and increase adherence (Kim et al. 2005; Kreyenbuhl et al. 2009).

## Clinician Knowledge, Skills, and Experience

Clinical expertise involves the clinician reflecting upon existing skills and past experiences, and using knowledge generated from this process to inform and enhance treatment. Clinical expertise is often cultivated through self-reflection, continuous education, and experience. Integral to this aspect of EBP is also self-awareness of the limitations of clinical judgment, including biases, heuristics, and overgeneralizations (APA 2006). Routine self-reflective practice is important in the context of treatment and rehabilitation of SMI because there are few guidelines for practicing with severe mental illness and supervised training experiences are rare (Buck and Lysaker 2010). In addition, to reduce professionals' own stigmatizing views of people with mental illness (Rüsch et al. 2005; Schulze and Angermeyer 2003), they should routinely engage in self-reflection and seek out resources (e.g., consultation, research, assessment data) as needed when conducting clinical activities for the purposes of reducing bias and providing better services.

Despite great enthusiasm, efforts to ground recovery on a scientific foundation, as in the case of EBP, have met challenges and criticism over the last decade. The first challenge to the EBP model is about how researchers define "evidence." The privileging of objective empirical data over subjective personal accounts is contradictory to recovery values (Anthony 2001; Farkas et al. 2005). The lived experience of recovery in the eyes of consumers is undeniably important (Deegan 1988), but it is not easy to operationalize and measure, as it is an individually unique dynamic process. A related criticism of the EBP model of recovery is whether the objective outcomes defined in ESTs are relevant and of interest to consumers. Importantly, published recovery outcomes often do not coincide with outcomes that consumers associate with recovery and subjective outcomes are often not reported in published research (Anthony 2001).

The feasibility and dissemination of EBPs are often overlooked, but necessary for steps for service change. A study of 211 psychology, psychiatry, and social work programs identified barriers to early trainee exposure to evidence-based treatments (EBTs) in 2004 (Weissman et al. 2006). The top three barriers to EBT exposure for trainees included (1) a lack of trainee interest in EBT, (2) difficulty teaching EBT, and (3) lack of qualified faculty to teach EBT. In addition, other researchers have pointed out that while psychometric instruments assessing recovery concepts have been developed, these measures have not been widely adopted in practice (Silverstein et al. 2006).

## Values-Based Practices and Recovery

Values-Based Practice (VBP) is described as the "twin concept" to evidence-based approaches (Farkas 2006). In VBP, recovery-oriented values are entrenched in every level of program operation to demonstrate organizational commitment to recovery (Farkas et al. 2005). VBP can be thought of as a model of *program-level* decision-making and is unique from EBP model of *clinician-level* decision-making in several ways. The values of recovery differ from principles of the so-called *medical model*, the prevailing paradigm of healthcare, and this creates special challenges to development of recovery-oriented services (Farkas et al. 2005). VBP is essentially an operational elaboration of the recovery values described in the preceding sections of this chapter.

The first recovery value is the *person-orientation*, which can be broadly thought of as a perspective that views consumers as people, first and foremost. The person-orientation is not merely a perspective, but also a methodological approach that requires the program to gather an understanding of each individual's strengths, limitations, talents, supports, and interests. It is also dynamic in that individual characteristics are likely to change over time with novel, life-altering experiences. Under the person-orientation framework, mental health professionals and services strive to actively monitor and engage each person's unique strengths and limitations related to all aspects of living, not just illness-related aspects.

In contrast to the person-oriented perspective is the *patient-orientation* (Davidson and Strauss 1992), the prevailing orientation of the medical model. Personally meaningful individual differences are undervalued in this framework because of its exclusive focus on disease, rather than persons. In the medical model, patients are only offered standard medical care, rather than personalized treatment. Standard medical care consists of a professional determining the patient's diagnosis and then selecting an intervention based off of professional's understanding of medicine, clinician guidelines, and the *disease*. Disease and illness are distinct in that disease defines a pathophysiological process, whereas an illness refers the unique experience of the disease pathology and how disease interacts with the individual's physical, psychological, and social environments (Green et al. 2002). Consequentially, programs that subscribe to patient-orientation do not afford consumers opportunities to engage in non-patient social roles, e.g., the role of an artist, leader, sibling, partner, advocate, friend, or mentor (Schulze et al. 2003).

*Personal involvement* is the second value associated with the recovery process that extends the person-orientation to a standard of practice in psychiatric rehabilitation and mental health more broadly. Personal involvement is simply the process of providing consumers opportunities to participate in all aspects of treatment and recovery planning. This value is a practice-related extension of the person-orientation in that *people* have preferences about their level of participation in treatment decision-making (Jacobson and Greenley 2001).

In the medical model, the expected role of the patient is to comply with the professional's prescribed treatment while the physician continues to systematically follow standard medical care. Patients that do not adhere to treatment recommendations were formerly labeled as "treatment noncompliant," a term later discouraged in professional discourse because of its paternalistic and derogatory connotations. In contrast to personal involvement, the provider-directed patient compliance model does not always consider client preferences, interests, or rights.

*Self-determination* is a recovery value that involves providing consumers the opportunity to make choices about their lives and treatment. Choice is afforded to the consumer despite what is convenient or favored by the professional. This recovery value is deeply rooted in the person-oriented philosophy in that it is viewed as a basic *human right* for a person to make autonomous choices about wellbeing and living. Self-determination is as much about making decisions to *disengage* in services or activities, as it is to engage in services or activities. Self-determinism has been rapidly adopted in care settings due to arguments that it is an ethical imperative to provide consumers choice and participation in treatment decision-making (Drake and Deegan 2009).

In the medical model, the physician assumes the authority to make treatment decisions on the patient's behalf. The physician acts as the chief decision-making authority due to the assumption that the patient has no expertise in disease knowledge, and thus no place in treatment decision-making (i.e., since treatment decision-making is solely based on medical knowledge).

*Growth potential* is the final core recovery-promoting value that involves openness to and maintenance of future change. This recovery value involves adapting services to promote personal growth, as well as recognizing the person's existing progress towards recovery. Growth potential is underscored by notion of hope—that any individual has the capacity to experience meaningful positive change while living with psychiatric disability.

The medical model, in contrast, has viewed long-term prognosis of people with severe and persistent mental illness as bleak. The medical narrative of people with schizophrenia often involved a description of progressive functional deterioration, symptom exacerbation, and treatment resistance (Frese et al. 2009). Because of these assumptions, many mental health professionals still believe today that people with SMI cannot recover, despite research indicating otherwise. The medical community and pharmaceutical industry still promote schizophrenia and other SMI as "brain diseases" (see Corrigan and Watson 2004).

## Values-Based Program Operation

Farkas et al. (2005) outline a number of organizational practices consistent with VBP. As stated previously, VBP has been fundamentally discussed as program and organizational practices to promote recovery. Here we will summarize VBPs in the context of their associated program dimensions noted in Farkas et al. (2005).

Written aspects of program organization, such as the program mission statement, client records, and organizational policies, can engage recovery-oriented values in a number of ways. Language that communicates respect for consumers (*person orientation*) and instills hope for recovery (*growth potential*) can enhance program mission statements. Policies may also be written to convey recovery-oriented values, such as by writing policies so that they do not unfairly exclude or penalize people who choose to selectively enroll in services (*self-determination*). For individuals whose symptoms or functional difficulties interfere with their participation in conditional services, policies can be adapted to provide accommodation so that a person interested in a service can participate (*personal involvement*). Lastly, policies regarding program services, quality assurance practices, and other practices can routinely survey consumer input and solicit recommendations.

The practices previously described are also consistent with the APA taskforce on SMI (2009) proficiencies in ideology and attitudes when working with SMI. These attitudes and ideologies broadly include sensitivity and respect to people with SMI, as communicated through provider (1) attitudes that recovery is possible, (2) recognition that mental illness is subjective, (3) use of non-stigmatizing people first language, and (4) flexibility in treatment and service provisions. The ideology and attitudes, often conveyed in written aspects of program organization, are important in that they most closely reflect the organizational culture of the setting. Programs striving to promote a recovery-oriented culture, by definition in VBP, must have mission statements and written policies engage recovery-oriented values and goals.

Procedural aspects of program operation can be tailored to recovery-oriented values. Program procedures are important in that they provide a clear series of steps for how a policy will be implemented in practice. Program policies regarding client complaints or grievances, for instance, outline the steps that occur when a consumer chooses to file a complaint or grievance, as well as who is involved in each step of the process. Program procedures provide additional opportunities for organizations to demonstrate their commitment to recovery-oriented policies and missions. Procedures that include steps related to gathering to client input and engaging personal choice reflect program commitment to *self-determination* and *personal involvement* recovery values.

Consumer input can inform organizational practices like quality assurance and record keeping in a number of ways. Farkas et al. (2005) note the consumer input is not limited to solely providing a response to quality assurance surveys, but also in what measures are used and what program dimensions should be assessed to determine program strengths and limitations. Program quality assurance practices can also share program data with consumers (*personal involvement*) to demonstrate program-level progress and needed areas of improvement (*growth potential*). Record keeping is a personalized form of quality assurance that allows the client to monitor his or her own progress and evaluate treatment goals. Record keeping can be written and stored so that the information is most accessible to clients for their own use (*personal involvement*). In addition, client records should include information regarding all aspects of the person, including strengths, limitations, talents, interests, and clinical and personal goals (*person orientation*).

These program practices also coincide with the SMI Task Force's recommendations for systems and service-related knowledge and skills. Proficiency in evaluating programs, collaborating with staff and consumers, and providing systematic guidelines for program operation are all requisite skills for SMI treatment. Recovery-oriented practices like the ones previously described may potentially encourage engagement in treatment and shared decision-making due to the transparency and emphasis on the positive role of consumer input at individual and program levels.

*Physical environment* can directly impact mental and physical wellbeing of people in recovery. Much like program practices, the physical environment of the program conveys the values and interests of the organization. Hospital settings are often sterile, uninviting, and impersonal experiences. VBP applications to physical settings include making spaces (e.g., waiting rooms, bathrooms) shared spaces in order to promote parity between clients and providers (*person orientation*). Much like in other aspects of program operation, consumers should have opportunities to provide their input on the physical environment, make choices about their physical environment (*self-determination*), as well as volunteer to use their skills (e.g., art, music, decorating, crafting, etc.) to personalize their physical environment (*personal involvement*).

Lastly, VBP can also be applied to progress staff selection, training, and supervision in a number of ways. Staff selection practice can include surveying candidates on their recovery knowledge, skills, and attitudes to ensure that consumers are treated consistently and respectfully by all members of the treatment team (*person orientation*). Consumers can also be surveyed about what qualities or skills they would like to see in their staff and these qualities can be considered when making hiring decisions, or during staff training and supervision (*personal involvement*). Organizations should also make efforts to assess recovery attitudes of their current staff, and provide information or exposure to clients who have met recovery goals when staff attitudes are incompatible with the recovery values of the program (*growth potential*).

We should expect empirical research to confirm that adherence to recovery values, by providers and others, stimulates subjective and objective recovery in those receiving their services. Such research has barely begun. One mixed qualitative and quantitative longitudinal study, known as STARS (Study of Transitions and Recovery Strategies) found that recovery-oriented and person-directed programs were associated with recovery outcomes. On the other hand, specific practices thought to reflect recovery orientation, such as "strength-based" assessment (Ibrahim et al. 2014), may not contribute as expected. Relationships between values, practices, subjective recovery, and objective recovery outcomes will be a key focus of research in the foreseeable future.

To summarize, evidence-based and values-bed practice models of recovery have evolved from different movements. Their differences largely reflect the interests of their respective movements

**Table 1.1** Differences between medical, evidence-based, and values-based practices

| Medical | Evidence-based | Values-based |
|---|---|---|
| *Philosophy* | | |
| Value-free | Value-conscious | Value-centered |
| Authoritarian | Person-conscious | Person-centered |
| *Knowledge base* | | |
| Disease and research knowledge | Client, clinician, and research knowledge | Person values and preferences |
| *Practices are ...* | | |
| Standard medical treatment | Individually-tailored treatment | Person-centered care |
| Prescriptive decision-making | Collaborative decision-making | Autonomous decision-making |
| *Recovery is ...* | | |
| An outcome | An outcome | A Process |
| Symptom remission | Psychosocial improvement | Disability management |
| Return to normalcy | Functional improvement | Personal growth |

and stakeholders. Practitioners and service programs have an ethical responsibility to offer evidence-based approaches (APA 2006) to consumers, yet EBP must respect the interests and goals of consumers (Drake et al. 2009; Drake and Deegan 2009). There is no inherent conflict between EBP and VBP, but effective integration is a social and technological challenge. There may be conflict between VBP and particular models of healthcare. Table 1.1 summarizes differences between medical, evidence-based recovery, and values-based recovery models.

## Conclusion

The idea of recovery pervades contemporary research, clinical practice and policy in mental health. It is a protean and nuanced idea, still subject to debate (Drake and Whitley 2014). It expresses itself in different ways, different contexts, and different people. It has both objective and subjective dimensions. It is both process and outcome. We can scientifically evaluate the degree to which specific policies and practices are associated with recovery processes and outcomes. Although science cannot evaluate social values associated with recovery, we can assess the degree to which adherence to social values facilitates recovery. The contemporary era of research on recovery is barely a decade old. We should expect it to continue in the foreseeable future, and to have a formative effect on our pursuit of mental health.

## References

American Psychological Association Presidential Task Force on Evidence-based Practice (2006). Evidence-based practice in psychology. *American Psychologist, 61*(4), 271–285. doi: 10.1037/0003-066X.61.4.271.

Andresen, R., Caputi, P., & Oades, L. (2006). Stages of recovery instrument: Development of a measure of recovery from serious mental illness. *Australian and New Zealand Journal of Psychiatry, 40*(11–12), 972–980.

Andresen, R., Oades, L., & Caputi, P. (2003). The experience of recovery from schizophrenia: Towards an empirically validated stage model. *Australian and New Zealand Journal of Psychiatry, 37*(5), 586–594.

Andrews, G., & Slade, T. (2001). Interpreting scores on the Kessler psychological distress scale (K10). *Australian and New Zealand Journal of Public Health, 25* (6), 494–497.

Anthony, W. (1979). *Principles of psychiatric rehabilitation*. Baltimore: University Park Press.

Anthony, W. (1993). Recovery from mental illness: The guiding vision of the mental health service system in the 1990s. *Psychosocial Rehabilitation Journal, 16*, 11–23.

Anthony, W. A. (2001). A vision for psychiatric rehabilitation research. *Psychiatric Rehabilitation Journal, 25*(1), 1–2. doi: 10.1037/h0095057.

Anthony, W., & Liberman, R. P. (1986). The practice of psychiatric rehabilitation: Historical, conceptual, and research base. *Schizophrenia Bulletin, 12*(4), 542–559.

Anthony, W., Rogers, E. S., & Farkas, M. (2003). Research on evidence-based practices: Future directions in an era of recovery. *Community Mental Health Journal, 39*(2), 101–114.

APA Task Force on Serious Mental Illness and Severe Emotional Disturbance. (2009). Assessment and treatment of serious mental illness. Retrieved from http://www.apa.org/practice/resources/treatment-mental.aspx

Armstrong, M. L., Korba, A. M., & Emard, R. (1995). Of mutual benefit: The reciprocal relationship between consumer volunteers and the clients they serve. *Psychiatric Rehabilitation Journal, 19*(2), 45–49.

Ayllon, T., & Azrin, N. H. (1968). *The token economy*. New York: Appleton-Century-Crofts.

Bachrach, L. L. (1978). A conceptual approach to deinstitutionalization. *Psychiatric Services, 29*(9), 573–578.

Bachrach, L. L. (1982). Assessment of outcomes in community support systems: Results, problems, and limitations. *Schizophrenia Bulletin, 8*(1), 39–61.

Bachrach, L. L. (1983). Evaluating the consequences of deinstitutionalization. *Hospital & Community Psychiatry, 34*(2), 105.

Barrowclough, C., Haddock, G., Tarrier, N., Lewis, S. W., Moring, J., O'Brien, R., et al. (2001). Randomized controlled trial of motivational interviewing, cognitive behavior therapy, and family intervention for patients with comorbid schizophrenia and substance use disorders. *American Journal of Psychiatry, 15*, 1706–1713.

Bell, M. D., & Zito, W. (2005). Integrated versus sealed-over recovery in schizophrenia: BORRTI and executive function. *Journal of Nervous and Mental Disease, 193*, 3–8.

Bellack, A. S. (2006). Scientific and consumer models of recovery in schizophrenia: Concordance, contrasts, and implications. *Schizophrenia Bulletin, 32*, 432–442.

Bellamy, C. D., Garvin, C., Macfarlane, P., Mowbray, O. P., Mowbray, C. T., & Holter, M. C. (2006). An analysis of groups in consumer-centered programs. *American Journal of Psychiatric Rehabilitation, 9*(3), 219–240. doi:10.1080/15487760600962152

Bond, G. R. (2004). Supported employment: Evidence for an evidence-based practice. *Psychiatric Rehabilitation Journal, 27*(4), 345–359.

Bond, G. R., Salyers, M. P., Rollins, A. L., Rapp, C. A., & Zipple, A. M. (2004). How evidence-based practices contribute to community integration. *Community Mental Health Journal, 40*(6), 569–588.

Boyd, J. E., Otilingam, P. G., & DeForge, B. R. (2014). Brief version of the internalized stigma of mental illness (ISMI) scale: Psychometric properties and relationship to depression, self esteem, recovery orientation, empowerment, and perceived devaluation and discrimination. *Psychiatric Rehabilitation Journal, 37*(1), 17.

Braginsky, B., Braginsky, D., & Ring, K. (1969). *Methods of madness: The mental hospital as a last resort*. New York: Holt, Rhinehart & Winston.

Brekke, J. (2007). The relationship between cognitive and environmental determinants of the functional dimensions in schizophrenia. Invited presentation to NIMH-sponsored conference, Measurement and Treatment Research to Improve Cognition in Schizophrenia (MATRICS-CT). Bethesda, August 21–22, 2007.

Brekke, J. S., & Nakagami, E. (2010). The relevance of neurocognition and social cognition for outcome and recovery in schizophrenia. In V. Roder & A. Medalia (Eds.), *Neurocognition and social cognition in schizophrenia patients: Basic concepts and treatment* (Vol. 177). Basel: Karger Medical and Scientific Publishers.

Brekke, J. S., Phillips, E., Pancake, L., Anne, O., & Duke, J. (2009). Implementation practice and implementation research: A report from the field. *Research on Social Work Practice, 19*(5), 592–601.

Buck, K. D., & Lysaker, P. H. (2010). Clinical supervision for the treatment of adults with severe mental illness: Pertinent issues when assisting graduate nursing students. *Perspectives in Psychiatric Care, 46*(3), 234–243.

Burnam, M. A., & Watkins, K. E. (2006). Substance abuse with mental disorders: Specialized public systems and integrated care. *Health Affairs, 25*(3), 648–658.

Butzlaff, R. L., & Hooley, J. M. (1998). Expressed emotion and psychiatric relapse. *Archives of General Psychiatry, 55*(6), 547–552. doi: 10.1001/archpsyc.55.6.547.

Chambless, D. L., & Hollon, S. D. (1998). Defining empirically supported therapies. *Journal of Consulting and Clinical Psychology, 66*(1), 7–18.

Chambless, D. L., & Ollendick, T. H. (2001). Empirically supported psychological interventions: Controversies and evidence. *Annual Review Psychology, 52*(1), 685–716. doi:10.1146/annurev.psych.52.1.685

Chen, S.-P., Krupa, T., Lysaght, R., McCay, E., & Piat, M. (2013). The development of recovery competencies for in-patient mental health providers working with people with serious mental illness. *Administration and Policy in Mental Health and Mental Health Services Research, 40*(2), 96–116. doi:10.1007/s10488-011-0380-x

Clarke, G., Herincks, H., Kinney, R., Paulson, R., Cutler, D., Lewis, K., & Oxman, E. (2000). Psychiatric hospitalizations, arrests, emergency room visits, and homelessness of clients with serious and persistent mental illness: Findings from a randomized trial of two ACT programs vs. usual care. *Mental Health Service Research, 2*(3), 155–164.

Cook, J. A., Copeland, M. E., Floyd, C. B., Jonikas, J. A., Hamilton, M. M., Razzano, L., et al. (2014a). A randomized controlled trial of effects of wellness recovery action planning on depression, anxiety, and recovery. *Psychiatric Services, 63*(6), 541–547.

Cook, J. A., Copeland, M. E., Floyd, C. B., Jonikas, J. A., Hamilton, M. M., Razzano, L., et al. (2014b). A randomized controlled trial of effects of wellness recovery action planning on depression, anxiety, and recovery. *Psychiatric Services, 60*(2), 246–249.

Cook, J. A., Copeland, M. E., Jonikas, J. A., Hamilton, M. M., Razzano, L. A., Grey, D. D., et al. (2011). Results of a randomized controlled trial of mental illness self-management using wellness recovery action planning. *Schizophrenia Bulletin, 38*(4), 881–891.

Cook, J. A., Jonikas, J. A., Hamilton, M. M., Goldrick, V., Steigman, P. J., Grey, D. D., et al. (2013). Impact of wellness recovery action planning on service utilization and need in a randomized controlled trial. *Psychiatric Rehabilitation Journal, 36*(4), 250.

Copeland, M. E. (2002). *Wellness recovery action plan*. West Dummerston, VT: Peach Press.

Corrigan, P., Angell, B., Davidson, L., Marcus, S., Salzer, M., Kottsieper, P., et al. (2012). From adherence to self-determination: Evolution of a treatment paradigm for people with serious mental illnesses. *Psychiatric Services, 63*(2), 169–173.

Corrigan, P. W., Giffort, D., Rashid, F., & Leary, M. (1999). Recovery as a psychological construct. *Community Mental Health Journal, 35*(3), 231–239. doi:10.1023/A:1018741302682

Corrigan, P. W., Salzer, M., & Ralph, R. O. (2004). Examining the factor structure of the recovery assessment scale. *Schizophrenia Research, 30*(4), 1035–1041.

Corrigan, P. W., Schade, M. L., & Liberman, R. P. (1992). Social skills training. In R. P. Liberman (Ed.), *Handbook of psychiatric rehabilitation* (pp. 95–126). New York: Macmillan.

Corrigan, P. W., Steiner, L., McCracken, S. G., Blaser, B., & Barr, M. (2001). Strategies for disseminating evidence-based practices to staff who treat people with serious mental illness. *Psychiatric Services, 52* (12), 1598–1606.

Corrigan, P. W., & Watson, A. C. (2004). At issue: Stop the stigma: Call mental illness a brain disease. *Schizophrenia Bulletin, 30*(3), 477.

Coursey, R. D., Curtis, L., Marsh, D. T., Campbell, J., Harding, C. M., Spaniol, L., et al. (2000a). Competencies for direct service staff members who work with adults with severe mental illnesses: Specific knowledge, attitudes, skills, and bibliography. *Psychiatric Rehabilitation Journal, 23*(4), 378–392.

Coursey, R. D., Curtis, L., Marsh, D. T., Campbell, J., Harding, C. M., Spaniol, L., et al. (2000b). Competencies for direct service staff members who work with adults with severe mental illnesses in outpatient public mental health/managed care systems. *Psychiatric Rehabilitation Journal, 23*(4), 370–377.

Cruce, G., Öjehagen, A., & Nordström, M. (2012). Recovery-promoting care as experienced by persons with severe mental illness and substance misuse. *International Journal of Mental Health and Addiction, 10*(5), 660–669. doi:10.1007/s11469-011-9363-0

Davidson, L., Chinman, M., Sells, D., & Rowe, M. (2006). Peer support among adults with serious mental illness: A report from the field. *Schizophrenia Bulletin, 32*(3), 443.

Davidson, L., & Strauss, J. S. (1992). Sense of self in recovery from severe mental illness. *British Journal of Medical Psychology, 65*(2), 131–145. doi:10.1111/j.2044-8341.1992.tb01693.x

Deacon, B., & Baird, G. (2009). The chemical imbalance explanation of depression: Reducing blame at what cost? *Journal of Social and Clinical Psychology, 28* (4), 415–435.

Deacon, B. J., & Lickel, J. J. (2009). On the brain disease model of mental disorders. *The Behavior Therapist, 32* (6), 113–118.

Deegan, P. E. (1988). Recovery: The lived experience of rehabilitation. *Psychosocial Rehabilitation Journal, 11* (4), 11.

Deegan, P. (1996). Recovery as a journey of the heart. *Psychiatric Rehabilitation Journal, 19*(3), 91.

Deegan, P. E., & Drake, R. E. (2006). Shared decision making and medication management in the recovery process. *Psychiatric Services, 57*(11), 1636–1639.

Drake, R., Cimpean, D., & Torrey, W. (2009). Shared decision making in mental health: Propsects for personalized medicine. *Dialogues in Clinical Neuroscience, 11*, 455–463.

Drake, R. E., & Deegan, P. E. (2009). Shared decision making is an ethical imperative. *Psychiatric Services, 60*(8), 1007.

Drake, R. E., Mueser, K. T., Brunette, M. F., & McHugo, G. J. (2004). A review of treatments for people with severe mental illnesses and co-occurring substance use disorders. *Psychiatric Rehabilitation Journal, 27*(4), 360–374.

Drake, R. E., & Whitley, R. (2014). Recovery and severe mental illness: Description and analysis. *Canadian Journal of Psychiatry. Revue Canadienne de Psychiatrie, 59*(5), 236–242.

Druss, B. G., Zhao, L., Silke, A., Bona, J. R., Fricks, L., Jenkins-Tucker, S., et al. (2010). The health and recovery peer (HARP) program: A peer-led intervention to improve medical self-management for persons with serious mental illness. *Schizophrenia Research, 118*(1), 264–270.

Eckman, T. A., Liberman, R. P., Phipps, C. C., & Blair, K. E. (1990). Teaching medication management skills to schizophrenic patients. *Journal of Clinical Psychopharmacology, 10*, 33–38.

Eckman, T., Wirshing, W., Marder, S., Liberman, R., Johnston-Cronk, K., Zimmerman, K., & Mintz, J. (1992). Techniques for training schizophrenic patients in illness self-management: A controlled trial. *American Journal of Psychiatry, 149*(11), 1549–1555.

Fairweather, G., Sanders, D., Maynard, H., & Cressler, D. (1969). *Community life for the mentally ill: An alternative to institutional care*. Chicago: Aldine.

Farkas, M. (2007). The vision of recovery today: What it is and what it means for services. *World Psychiatry, 6* (2), 68.

Farkas, M., Gagne, C., & Anthony, W. (2005). Implementing recovery oriented evidence based programs: Identifying the critical dimensions. *Community Mental Health Journal, 41*(2), 141–158.

Foucault, M. (1961/2006). *History of madness* (J. Khalfa & J. Murphy, Trans. J. Khalfa Ed.). New York: Routledge.

Frese, F. J., Knight, E. L., & Saks, E. (2009). Recovery from schizophrenia: With views of psychiatrists, psychologists, and others diagnosed with this disorder. *Schizophrenia Bulletin, 35*(2), 370–380.

Gearing, R. E., Mian, I., Sholonsky, A., Barber, J., Nicholas, D., Lewis, R., et al. (2009). Developing a risk-model of time to first relapse for children and adolescents diagnosed with psychotic disorders or mood disorders with psychotic features. *Journal of Nervous and Mental Disease, 197*(1), 6–14.

Gelfand, D. M., Gelfand, S., & Dobson, W. R. (1967). Unprogrammed reinforcement of patients' behavior in a mental hospital. *Behaviour Research and Therapy, 5* (3), 201–207.

Gitlin, M., Nuechterlein, K., Subotnik, K. L., Ventura, J., Mintz, J., Fogelson, D. L., et al. (2001). Clinical outcome following neuroleptic discontinuation in patients with remitted recent-onset schizophrenia. *American Journal of Psychiatry, 158*, 1835–1842.

Goffman, E. (1961). *Asylums*. Garden City, NY: Doubleday, Anchor Books.

Granholm, E., Loh, C., & Swendsen, J. (2008). Feasibility and validity of computerized ecological momentary assessment in schizophrenia. *Schizophrenia Bulletin, 34*(3), 507–514. doi:10.1093/schbul/sbm113

Green, A. R., Carrillo, J. E., & Betancourt, J. R. (2002). Why the disease-based model of medicine fails our patients. *Western Journal of Medicine, 176*(2), 141.

Guyatt, G., Cairns, J., Churchill, D., Cook, D., Haynes, B., Hirsh, J., et al. (1992). Evidence-based medicine: A new approach to teaching the practice of medicine. *Journal of the American Medical Association, 268* (17), 2420–2425.

Haddock, G., Tarrier, N., Spaulding, W., Yusupoff, L., Kinney, C., & McCarthy, E. (1998). Individual cognitive-behavior therapy in the treatment of hallucinations and delusions: A review. *Clinical Psychology Review, 18*(7), 821–838.

Hamm, J. A., Hasson-Ohayon, I., Kukla, M., & Lysaker, P. H. (2013). Individual psychotherapy for schizophrenia: Trends and developments in the wake of the recovery movement. *Psychology Research and Behavior Management, 6*, 45–54.

Harrow, M., Grossman, L. S., Jobe, T. H., & Faull, R. (2006, April). *Do patients with schizophrenia show periods of complete recovery? A 20 year follow-up*. Paper presented at the Annual Meeting of American Psychiatric Association, New York City.

Harrow, M., Grossman, L. S., Jobe, T. H., & Herbener, E. S. (2005). Do patients with schizophrenia every show periods of recovery? A 15 year multi-follow-up study. *Schizophrenia Bulletin, 31*(3), 723–734.

Harrow, M., Hansford, B. G., & Astrachan-Fletcher, E. B. (2009). Locus of control: Relation to schizophrenia, to recovery, and to depression and psychosis—A 15-year longitudinal study. *Psychiatry Research, 168*(3), 186–192. doi: 10.1016/j.psychres.2008.06.002.

Haupt, M. (2014). *The vital role of state psychiatric hospitals: NASMHPD Medical Directors Council Technical Report*. National Association of State Mental Health Program Directors. Retrieved from http://www.nasmhpd.org/content/vital-role-state-psychiatric-hospitals-nasmhpd-medical-directors-council-technical-report

Heinssen, R. K. (2002). Improving medication compliance of a patient with schizophrenia through collaborative behavioral therapy. *Psychiatric Services, 53* (3), 255–257.

Heinssen, R. K., Cuthbert, B. N., Breiling, J., Colpe, L. J., & Dolan-Sewell, R. (2003). Overcoming barriers to research in early serious mental illness: Issues for future collaboration. *Schizophrenia Bulletin, 29*(4), 737–745.

Heinssen, R., Levendusky, P., & Hunter, R. (1995). Client as colleague: Therapeutic contracting with the seriously mentally ill. *American Psychologist, 50*(7), 522–532.

Hendryx, M., Green, C. A., & Perrin, N. A. (2009). Social support, activities, and recovery from serious mental illness: STARS study findings. *The Journal of Behavioral Health Services & Research, 36*(3), 320–329. doi: 10.1007/s11414-008-9151-1.

Hofstetter, J. R., Lysaker, P. H., & Mayeda, A. R. (2005). Quality of sleep in patients with schizophrenia is associated with quality of life and coping. *BMC psychiatry, 5*(1), 13.

Hunsley, J., & Mash, E. (2010). *The role of assessment in evidence-based practice. The Oxford handbook of clinical psychology*. London: Oxford Press.

Ibrahim, N., Michail, M., & Callaghan, P. (2014). The strengths based approach as a service delivery model for severe mental illness: A meta-analysis of clinical trials. *BMC Psychiatry, 14*(1), 243–254. doi:10.1186/s12888-014-0243-6

Insel, T. R. (2010). Rethinking schizophrenia. *Nature, 468*(7321), 187–193. doi: 10.1038/nature09552.

Insel, T. (2013). *Getting serious about mental illnesses*. [Director's Blog]. Retrieved from http://www.nimh.nih.gov/about/director/2013/getting-serious-about-mental-illnesses.shtml

Jacobson, N., & Greenley, D. (2001). What is recovery? A conceptual model and explication. *Psychiatric Services, 52*(4), 482–485.

Jonikas, J. A., Grey, D. D., Copeland, M. E., Razzano, L. A., Hamilton, M. M., Floyd, C. B., et al. (2013). Improving propensity for patient self-advocacy through wellness recovery action planning: Results of a randomized controlled trial. *Community Mental Health Journal, 49*(3), 260–269.

Kazdin, Alan. (2003). *Research design in clinical psychology* (4th ed.). Needham Heights, MA: Allyn & Bacon.

Kim, B. S., Ng, G. F., & Ahn, A. J. (2005). Effects of client expectation for counseling success, client-counselor worldview match, and client adherence to Asian and European American cultural values on counseling process with Asian Americans. *Journal of Counseling Psychology, 52*(1), 67.

Kopelowicz, A., Liberman, R. P., Ventura, J., Zarate, R., & Mintz, J. (2005). Neurocognitive correlates of recovery from schizophrenia. *Psychological Medicine, 35*(8), 1165–1173.

Kreyenbuhl, J., Buchanan, R. W., Dickerson, F. B., & Dixon, L. B. (2010). The schizophrenia patient outcomes research team (PORT): Updated treatment recommendations 2009. *Schizophrenia Bulletin, 36*(1), 94–103.

Kreyenbuhl, J., Nossel, I. R., & Dixon, L. B. (2009). Disengagement from mental health treatment among individuals with schizophrenia and strategies for facilitating connections to care: A review of the literature. *Schizophrenia Bulletin, 35*(4), 696–703.

Kuhn, T. (1962). *The structure of scientific revolutions*. Chicago: University of Chicago Press.

Kutchins, H., & Kirk, S. (1997). *Making us crazy: The psychiatric bible and the creation of psychiatric disorders*. New York: Free Press.

Laib, K. (2015). *Services for people with serioius mental illness: The impact of national, state and local policy and practice*. Doctoral dissertation, University of Nebraska - Lincoln, Lincoln NE.

La Roche, M. J., & Maxie, A. (2003). Ten considerations in addressing cultural differences in psychotherapy. *Professional Psychology: Research and Practice, 34* (2), 180.

Lamb, H. R., & Bachrach, L. L. (2001). Some perspectives on deinstitutionalization. *Psychiatric Services, 52* (8), 1039–1045.

Lehman, A. F., Kreyenbuhl, J., Buchanan, R. W., Dickerson, F. B., Dixon, L. B., Goldberg, R., et al. (2004). The schizophrenia patient outcomes research team (PORT): Updated treatment recommendations 2003. *Schizophrenia Bulletin, 30*(2), 193–217.

Lehman, A. F., & Steinwachs, D. M. (1998). Translating research into practice: The Schizophrenia patient outcomes research team (PORT) treatment recommendations. *Schizophrenia Bulletin, 24*(1), 1–10.

Liberman, R. P. (2008). *Recovery from disability: Manual of psychiatric rehabilitation*. Washington, DC: American Psychiatric Press.

Liberman, R. P., King, L. W., & Derisi, W. J. (1975). *Personal effectiveness: Guiding patients to improve their social skills*. Champaign, IL: Research Press.

Liberman, R., King, L., & DeRisi, W. (1976). Behavior analysis and modification in community mental health. In H. Leitnberg (Ed.), *Handbook of behavior therapy and behavior modification* (pp. 566–603). Englewood Cliffs, NJ: Prentice-Hall.

Liberman, R. P., Kopelowicz, A., Ventura, J., & Gutkind, D. (2002). Operational criteria and factors related to recovery from schizophrenia. *International Review of Psychiatry, 14*(4), 256–272.

Liberman, R. P., Mueser, K. T., Wallace, C. J., Jacobs, H. E., Eckman, T., & Massel, H. K. (1986). Training skills in the psychiatrically disabled: Learning coping and competence. *Schizophrenia Bulletin, 12*(4), 631–647.

Lukoff, D., Wallace, C. J., Liberman, R. P., & Burke, K. (1986). A holistic program for chronic schizophrenic patients. *Schizophrenia Bulletin, 12*(2), 274–282.

Lysaker, P. H., Wickett, A. M., Wilke, N., & Lysaker, J. (2003). Narrative incoherence in schizophrenia: The absent agent-protagonist and the collapse of internal dialogue. *American Journal of Psychotherapy, 57*(2), 153–166.

MacDonald-Wilson, K. L., Nemec, P. B., Anthony, W. A., & Cohen, M. R. (2002). *Assessment in psychiatric rehabilitation. Handbook of measurement and evaluation in rehabilitation*. Baltimore: Paul Brookes.

Macias, C., Jackson, R., Schroeder, C., & Wang, Q. (1999). What is a clubhouse? Report on the ICCD 1996 survey of USA Clubhouses. *Community Mental Health Journal, 35*(2), 181–190. doi:10.1023/A:1018776815886

Magaro, P., Gripp, R., McDowell, D., & Miller, I. (1978). *The mental health industry: A cultural phenomenon*. New York: Wiley.

Maslin, J. (2003). Substance misuse in psychosis: Contextual issues. In H. L. Graham, A. Copello, M. J. Birchwood, & K. T. Mueser (Eds.), *Substance misuse in psychosis: Approaches to treatment and service delivery* (pp. 3–23). West Sussex, England: Wiley.

Mausbach, B. T., Moore, R., Bowie, C., Cardenas, V., & Patterson, T. L. (2009). A review of instruments for measuring functional recovery in those diagnosed with psychosis. *Schizophrenia Bulletin, 35*(2), 307–318.

McGurk, S. R., & Mueser, K. T. (2006). Strategies for coping with cognitive impairments of clients in supported employment. *Psychiatric Services, 57*(10), 1421–1429.

McGurk, S. R., Mueser, K. T., Feldman, K., Wolfe, R., & Pascaris, A. (2007). Cognitive training for supported employment: 2–3 year outcomes of a randomized controlled trial. *American Journal of Psychiatry, 164* (3), 437–441.

McGurk, S. R., Mueser, K. T., & Pascaris, A. (2005). Cognitive training and supported employment for persons with severe mental illness: One-year results from a randomized controlled trial. *Schizophrenia Bulletin, 31*(4), 898–909.

Mueser, K. T., Clark, R. E., Haines, M., Drake, R. E., McHugo, G. J., Bond, G. R., et al. (2004a). The Hartford study of supported employment for persons with severe mental illness. *Journal of Consulting and Clinical Psychology, 72*(3), 479–490.

Mueser, K. T., Corrigan, P. W., Hilton, D. W., Tanzman, B., Schaub, A., Gingerich, S., et al. (2002). Illness management and recovery: A review of the research. *Psychiatric Services, 53*(10), 1272–1284.

Mueser, K. T., Drake, R. E., & Bond, G. R. (1997). Recent advances in psychiatric rehabilitation for

patients with severe mental illness. *Harvard Review of Psychiatry, 5*(3), 123–137.
Mueser, K., & Glynn, S. (1995). *Behavioral family therapy for psychiatric disorders*. Boston: Allyn & Bacon.
Mueser, K. T., Meyer, P. S., Penn, D. L., Clancy, R., Clancy, D. M., & Salyers, M. P. (2006). The illness management and recovery program: Rationale, development, and preliminary findings. *Schizophrenia Bulletin, 32*(suppl 1), S32–S43.
Mueser, K. T., Salyers, M. P., Rosenberg, S. D., Goodman, L. A., Essock, S. M., Osher, F. C., et al. (2004b). Interpersonal trauma and posttraumatic stress disorder in patients with severe mental illness: Demographic, clinical, and health correlates. *Schizophrenia Bulletin, 30*, 45–57.
Onken, S. J., Dumont, J. M., Ridgway, P., Dornan, D. H., & Ralph, R. O. (2002, October). Mental health recovery: What helps and what hinders? A national research project for the development of recovery facilitating system performance indicators. *Phase one research report: A national study of consumer perspectives on what helps and hinders mental health recovery.* Alexandria, VA: National Association of State Mental Health Program Directors (NASMHPD) National Technical Assistance Center (NTAC).
Paul, G. L., & Lentz, R. J. (1977). *Psychosocial treatment of chronic mental patients: Milieu vs. social learning programs*. Cambridge: Harvard University Press.
Peer, J. E., & Spaulding, W. D. (2007). Heterogeneity in recovery of psychosocial functioning during psychiatric rehabilitation: an exploratory study using latent growth mixture modeling. *Schizophr Research, 93*(1–3), 186–193.
Peer, J., Strachan, E., & Spaulding, W. (2008). Heterogeneity in behavioral treatment response in severe mental illness. *Journal of Nervous and Mental Disease, 196*, 198–206.
Pelham, W. E., Fabiano, G. A., & Massetti, G. M. (2005). Evidence-based assessment of attention deficit hyperactivity disorder in children and adolescents. *Journal of Clinical Child and Adolescent Psychology, 34*(3), 449–476.
Persons, J. B., Beckner, V. L., & Tompkins, M. A. (2013). Testing case formulation hypotheses in psychotherapy: Two case examples. *Cognitive and Behavioral Practice, 20*(4), 399–409.
Persons, J. B., Roberts, N. A., Zalecki, C. A., & Brechwald, W. A. (2006). Naturalistic outcome of case formulation-driven cognitive-behavior therapy for anxious depressed outpatients. *Behaviour Research and Therapy, 44*(7), 1041–1051.
Persons, J. B., & Tompkins, M. A. (1997). Cognitive-behavioral case formulation. *Handbook of psychotherapy case formulation*, 314–339.
Pratt, C., Gill, K., Barrett, N., & Roberts, M. (2014). *Psychiatric rehabilitation* (3rd ed.). New York: Academic Press.
President's New Freedom Commission on Mental Health (2003), *Achieving the Promise: Transforming Mental Health Care in America*. Rockville MD: SAMSHA. Retrieved from https://store.samhsa.gov/shin/content/SMA03-3831/SMA03-3831.pdf
Ralph, R. O., Kidder, K., & Phillips, D. (2000). *Can we measure recovery? A compendium of recovery and recovery-related instruments*. The Human Services Research Institute (HSRI) Evaluation Center. Retrieved from http://www.tecathsri.org/pub_pickup/pn/pn-43.pdf
Rapp, C. A., & Goscha, R. J. (2011). *The strengths model: A recovery-oriented approach to mental health services*. New York: Oxford University Press.
Rappaport, J. (1981). In praise of paradox: A social policy of empowerment over prevention. *American Journal of Community Psychology, 9*(1), 1–25.
Rappaport, J. (1987). Terms of empowerment/exemplars of prevention: Toward a theory for community psychology. *American Journal of Community Psychology, 15*(2), 121–148.
Roberts, L., Salem, D., Rappaport, J., Toro, P., Luke, D., & Seidman, E. (1999). Giving and receiving help: Interpersonal transactions in mutual-help meetings and psychosocial adjustment of members. *American Journal of Community Psychiatry, 27*(6), 841–868.
Robinson, D., Woerner, M. G., Alvir, J. M. J., Bilder, R., Goldman, R., Geisler, S., et al. (1999). Predictors of relapse following response from a first episode of schizophrenia or schizoaffective disorder. *Archives of General Psychiatry, 56*(3), 241–247.
Roe, D. (2003). A prospective study on the relationship between self-esteem and functioning during the first year after being hospitalized for psychosis. *The Journal of Nervous and Mental Disease, 191*(1), 45–49.
Rüsch, N., Angermeyer, M. C., & Corrigan, P. W. (2005). Mental illness stigma: Concepts, consequences, and initiatives to reduce stigma. *European Psychiatry, 20* (8), 529–539.
Sackett, D. L., Rosenberg, W., Gray, J. A., Haynes, R., & Richardson, W. (1996). Evidence-based medicine: What it is and what it isn't. *BMJ, 312*, 71–72.
Schimming, C., & Harvey, P. D. (2004). Disability reduction in elderly patients with schizophrenia. *Journal of Psychiatric Practice, 10*(5), 283–295.
Schulze, B., & Angermeyer, M. C. (2003). Subjective experiences of stigma. A focus group study of schizophrenic patients, their relatives and mental health professionals. *Social Science and Medicine, 56*(2), 299–312.
Sells, D., Davidson, L., Jewell, C., Falzer, P., & Rowe, M. (2006). The treatment relationship in peer-based and regular case management for clients with severe mental illness. *Psychiatric Services, 57*(8), 1179–1184.
Sheedy, C., & Whitter, M. (2009). *Guiding principles and elements of recovery-oriented systems of care: What do we know from the research?* HHS Publication No. (SMA) 09-4439; Rockville, MD: Center for Substance Abuse Treatment, Substance Abuse and Mental Health Services Administration

Sherman, M. D., Fischer, E., Bowling, U. B., Dixon, L., Ridener, L., & Harrison, D. (2009). A new engagement strategy in a VA-based family psychoeducation program. *Psychiatric Services, 60*(2), 254–257. doi:10.1176/appi.ps.60.2.254

Silverstein, S. M., & Bellack, A. S. (2008). A scientific agenda for the concept of recovery as it applies to schizophrenia. *Clinical Psychology Review, 28*(7), 1108–1124. doi:10.1016/j.cpr.2008.03.004

Silverstein, S., Hatashita-Wong, M., Wilkniss, S. M., Blcoh, A., Smith, T., Savitz, A., & Terkelsen, K. (2006). Behavioral rehabilitation of the treatment-refractory schizophrenia patient: Conceptual foundations, interventions and outcome data. *Psychological Services, 3*, 145–169.

Silverstein, S. M., Spaulding, W. D., Menditto, A. A., Savitz, A., Liberman, R. P., Berten, S., & Starobin, H. (2009). Attention shaping: A reward-based learning method to enhance skills training outcomes in schizophrenia. *Schizophrenia Bulletin, 35*(1), 222–232.

Sisti, D. A., Segal, A. G., & Emanuel, E. J. (2015). Improving long-term psychiatric care: Bring back the asylum. *Journal of the American Medical Association, 313*(3), 243–244. doi:10.1001/jama.2014.16088

Smith, M. K., & Ford, J. (1990). A client-developed functional level scale: The community living skills scale (CLSS). *Journal of Social Service Research, 13*(3), 61–84.

Smith, T. E., Hull, J. W., Huppert, J. D., Silverstein, S. M., Anthony, D. T., & McClough, J. F. (2004). Insight and recovery from psychosis in chronic schizophrenia and schizoaffective disorder patients. *Journal of Psychiatric Research, 38*(2), 169–176.

Solomon, P. (2004). Peer support/peer provided services underlying processes, benefits, and critical ingredients. *Psychiatric Rehabilitation Journal, 27*(4), 392–401.

Spaulding, W. (Ed.). (1999). *The role of the state hospital in the 21st century* (Vol. 84). San Francisco: Jossey-Bass.

Spaulding, W., & Deogun, J. (2011). A pathway to personalization of integrated treatment: Informatics and decision science in psychiatric rehabilitation. *Schizophrenia Bulletin, 37*(suppl. 2), S129–S137.

Spaulding, W., Reed, D., Sullivan, M., Richardson, C., & Weiler, M. (1999). Effects of cognitive treatment in psychiatric rehabilitation. *Schizophrenia Bulletin, 25*(4), 657–676.

Spaulding, W., Sullivan, M., & Poland, J. (2003). *Treatment and rehabilitation of severe mental illness*. New York: Guilford.

Spaulding, W. D., Sullivan, M. E., Poland, J. S., & Ritchie, A. J. (2010). State psychiatric institutions and the left-behinds of mental health reform. *American Journal of Orthopsychiatry, 80*(3), 327–333.

Styron, T. H., Shaw, M., McDuffie, E., & Hoge, M. A. (2005). Curriculum resources for training direct care providers in public sector mental health. *Administration and Policy In Mental Health, 32*(5–6), 633–649.

Substance Abuse and Mental Health Services Administration. (2014). *Recovery and recovery support*. Retrieved from http://www.samhsa.gov/

Swann, W. B., Chang-Schneider, C., & McClarty, K. L. (2007). Do people's self-views matter? *American Psychologist, 62*(2), 84–94.

Swift, C., & Levin, G. (1987). Empowerment: An emerging mental health technology. *Journal of Primary Prevention, 8*(1–2), 71–94.

Tandon, R., Bruijnzeel, D., & Rankupalli, B. (2013). Does change in definition of psychotic symptoms in diagnosis of schizophrenia in DSM-5 affect caseness? *Asian Journal of Psychiatry, 6*(4), 330–332. doi: 10.1016/j.ajp.2013.05.011.

Tarasenko, M., Sullivan, M., Ritchie, A., & Spaulding, W. (2013). The effects of eliminating psychiatric rehabilitation from the secure levels of a psychiatric service system. *Psychological Services, 10*, 442–451.

Torrey, E. F. (2015). Bungling the job on substance abuse and mental health. *The Wall Street Journal*. Retirved from http://www.wsj.com/articles/e-fuller-torrey-bungling-the-job-on-substance-abuse-and-mental-health-1428099529

Tsai, J., Salyers, M. P., & Lobb, A. L. (2010). Recovery-oriented training and staff attitudes over time in two state hospitals. *Psychiatric Quarterly, 81*(4), 335–347. doi:10.1007/s11126-010-9142-2

U.S. Government Accountability Office. (2014). MENTAL HEALTH: HHS leadership needed to coordinate federal efforts related to serious mental illness. Retrieved from http://www.gao.gov/assets/670/667644.pdf

U.S. Surgeon General. (1999). *Mental health: A report of the Surgeon General*. Rockville MD: National Institutes of Health, DHHS. Retrieved from http://profiles.nlm.nih.gov/ps/retrieve/ResourceMetadata/NNBBHS

Vauth, R., Kleim, B., Wirtz, M., & Corrigan, P. W. (2007). Self-efficacy and empowerment as outcomes of self-stigmatizing and coping in schizophrenia. *Psychiatry Research, 150*(1), 71–80.

Ventura, J., Nuechterlein, K. H., Subotnick, K. L., Green, M. F., & Gitlin, M. J. (2004). Self-efficacy and neurocognition may be related to coping responses in recent onset schizophrenia. *Schizophrenia Research, 69*(2), 343–352.

Wallace, C. J., & Liberman, R. P. (2004). Supplementing supported employment with the workplace fundamentals module. *Psychiatric Services, 55*, 513–515.

Weissman, M. M., Verdeli, H., Gameroff, M. J., Bledsoe, S. E., Betts, K., Mufson, L., et al. (2006). National survey of psychotherapy training in psychiatry, psychology, and social work. *Archives of General Psychiatry, 63*(8), 925–934.

Wickett, A., Essman, W., Beck-Jennings, J., Davis, L., McIlvried, J., & Lysaker, P. H. (2006). Cluster B and C personality traits, symptom correlates, and treatment utilization in postacute schizophrenia. *The Journal of Nervous and Mental Disease, 194*(9), 650–653.

Wikipedia. (2015). *Recovery approach*. Retrieved from https://en.wikipedia.org/wiki/Recovery_approach

Wing, J. K., Beevor, A. S., Curtis, R. H., Park, S. B., Hadden, S., & Burns, A. (1998). Health of the nation outcome scales (HoNOS). Research and development. *The British Journal of Psychiatry, 172*(1), 11–18.

Wong, S., Massel, H., Mosk, M., & Liberman, R. (1986). Behavioral approaches to the treatment of schizophrenia. In G. Burroughs, T. Norman, & G. Rubenstein (Eds.), *Handbook of studies on schizophrenia* (pp. 79–100). Amsterdam: Elsevier Science Publishers.

Yamada, A., Lee, K. K., Dinh, T. Q., Barrio, C., & Brekke, J. S. (2010). Intrinsic motivation as a mediator of relationships between symptoms and functioning among individuals with schizophrenia spectrum disorders in a diverse urban community. *Journal of Nervous and Mental Disease, 198*(1), 28–34. doi:10.1097/NMD.0b013e3181c8aa71

Young, S. L., & Ensing, D. S. (1999). Exploring recovery from the perspective of people with psychiatric disabilities. *Psychiatric Rehabilitation Journal, 22*(3), 219.

Young, A. S., Forquer, S. L., Tran, A., Starzynski, M., & Shatkin, J. (2000). Identifying clinical competencies that support rehabilitation and empowerment in individuals with severe mental illness. *Journal of Behavioral Health Services and Research, 27*(3), 321–333

# 2 Principles for Recovery-Oriented Inpatient Care

Larry Davidson, Erika Carr, Chyrell Bellamy, Janis Tondora, Ellie Fossey, Thomas Styron, Maryanne Davidson and Shady Elsamra

## Introduction

The statements below represent two ends of a continuum describing adoption of a recovery orientation in inpatient settings:

> Recovery has no place in the hospital. How can you talk to patients about recovery when they're acutely psychotic?
>
> —Hospital Director

> Recovery has enabled us to reclaim nursing.
>
> —Psychiatric Nursing Leader

The first instance expresses fairly common views in the early days of the recovery movement, when many mental health professionals found the very notion of "recovery" foreign to their way of thinking about serious mental illnesses and their treatment. They typically viewed recovery as something that happens—if it happens at all—outside of the hospital setting, with no relevance to what and how care is provided in inpatient and other acute care settings. As evident in this Hospital Director's statement, many professionals also saw the implications of adopting recovery as the overall aim of mental health care [as stipulated both in the U.S. Surgeon General's *Report on Mental Health* (DHHS 1999) and in *Achieving the Promise*, the final report of the U. S. President's New Freedom Commission on Mental Health (DHHS 2003)] as being limited to discussing the concept of recovery with persons experiencing serious mental illnesses. As we discuss in this chapter, this is only one of many implications of shifting to a recovery paradigm in transforming inpatient care, the vast majority of which have little to do with using the term "recovery" in our discussions with our patients.

At the other end of the continuum we find a national nursing leader declaring that adoption of a recovery vision in inpatient care empowers psychiatric nurses to reclaim their profession. As she explained further, recovery brings nurses back to the philosophical and historical roots of nursing as a profession in order to reestablish a central, caring role in what had become a highly medicalized milieu devoted to risk assessment and management, prevention of medication errors, and the proliferation of paperwork (cf., Seed and Torkelson 2012). While we agree that many principles of the recovery vision—which we describe below—are consistent with the founding principles not only of nursing, but also of medicine, psychology, social work, and occupational therapy, we caution that there also are new elements to recovery that we will not be

L. Davidson (✉) · E. Carr · C. Bellamy
J. Tondora · T. Styron · S. Elsamra
Department of Psychiatry,
Yale University School of Medicine,
New Haven, CT, USA
e-mail: larry.davidson@yale.edu

E. Fossey
Department of Occupational Therapy,
Monash University, Melbourne, Australia

M. Davidson
College of Nursing, Sacred Heart University,
Fairfield, CT, USA



N.N. Singh et al. (eds.), *Handbook of Recovery in Inpatient Psychiatry*,
Evidence-Based Practices in Behavioral Health, DOI 10.1007/978-3-319-40537-7_2

able to grasp or implement if we only look backwards. There is much work to do in moving the field forward instead and, as a recent, thoughtful review on recovery and inpatient care conducted by Kidd et al. (2014b) pointed out, this remains an area of modest effort when compared to the amount of work being done to implement the recovery vision in outpatient and community settings. Briefly stated, we really do not know what recovery-oriented inpatient care will eventually look like a generation or so down the road. This book constitutes an important step in that direction, but it also reflects the fact that this work is just at the beginning stage.

Most efforts to date have focused on eliciting patients' views on what may be helpful and not so helpful in inpatient care (Jaeger et al. 2015; Repper 2000; Siu et al. 2012; Tee et al. 2007; Walsh and Boyle 2009), training inpatient staff and patients about recovery (Chen et al. 2011, 2014; Knutson et al. 2013), including with persons in recovery serving as trainers (Hillbrand et al. 2008; Kidd et al. 2014a), reducing the use of restraint and seclusion (Barton et al. 2009; Bennington-Davis and Murphy 2005; Fisher 2003; Wale et al. 2011; Wieman et al. 2014), making inpatient care more responsive to the histories of trauma so prevalent among persons with serious mental illnesses (Chandler 2008; Muskett 2014), and reconsidering issues of power and control more broadly (Tee et al. 2007; Walsh et al. 2008). Nursing, in particular, has produced two new models for acute care that emphasize relationships and the eliciting and understanding of patient narratives as key foci (Barker and Buchanan-Barker 2010, 2011; Shanley and Jubb-Shanley 2007), and there have been attempts to develop recovery-oriented forensic units, primarily in the United Kingdom (Davies et al. 2014; McKenna et al. 2014a, b). On the whole, however, hospitals have been the most reluctant to embrace transformation, for a variety of reasons, including the social control, safety, and supervision functions they serve and the common perception, described above, that recovery is only relevant to persons who are no longer acutely ill.

In this chapter, we step back from the more operational issues that might be involved in transformation to reflect, first, on the guiding principles of recovery and recovery-oriented practice and the implications they have for inpatient care. We may mention specific practices (e.g., advance directives, Wellness Recovery Action Planning, positive behavioral supports), but these will be offered primarily as examples of the kinds of interventions that would follow from and be consistent with the principles we describe. We also will address the respective roles of each of the professions typically involved in inpatient care, but again from the perspective of how these various roles embody different aspects of core recovery principles. The remainder of this volume will offer much grist for further discussion once these principles and roles have been delineated.

## Guiding Principles for Recovery-Oriented Care

There have been numerous attempts to identify and articulate core values and guiding principles for recovery and recovery-oriented practice, including the consensus statement on behavioral health recovery issued by the U.S. Substance Abuse and Mental Health Services Administration (SAMHSA) in 2011. This statement, which integrated two previous, separate statements about recovery in mental health and recovery in addiction, listed the following ten shared principles: Recovery (1) emerges from hope, (2) is person-driven, (3) occurs via many pathways, (4) is holistic, (5) is supported by peers and allies, (6) is supported through relationship and social networks, (7) is culturally-based and influenced, (8) is supported by addressing trauma, (9) involves individual, family, and community strengths and responsibility, and (10) is based on respect (SAMHSA 2011). While familiar with this list of principles—some of which we will come back to below—as well as with other attempts to break down the concept of recovery into its constituent parts (Leamy et al.

2011; Le Boutillier et al. 2011), we have chosen to offer a different set of principles that we suggest are especially relevant to the inpatient setting. This list is not in any way in contradiction to the SAMHSA vision described above, or at odds with any of the attempts we have seen in the nursing literature, in particular, with nurses having produced the most literature to date on the interface of recovery and inpatient care. We hope, however, that this list will be more directly and concretely applicable to inpatient care than previous efforts.

We also feel a need to clarify one of several areas of confusion related to recovery prior to launching into the principles per se. This has to do with the difference between recovery and recovery-oriented care, which, as different as they may sound on the surface, are often confused, as in the SAMSHA list above. Some of the SAMHSA principles, such as emerging from hope, being person-driven, and being holistic, appear to be referring to the phenomenon of recovery itself. These are concepts that apply to the person who is living with a mental illness, who is a whole person (mind, body, and spirit), who needs to have hope, and who is the driver of his or her own recovery. Other principles appear to refer to recovery-oriented practice instead, which via many pathways, is supported by addressing trauma and is based on respect. One sees this kind of confusion in mental health settings when staff says things like, "We do recovery here" or "we're doing recovery now." This same confusion is evident in such statements as: "My client won't cooperate with his recovery" or "The patient's recovery goal is to reach a level 4 before discharge."

We offer, therefore, the following division of labor as a way of parsing these related (but not synonymous) concepts; a distinction we suggest is particularly important for thinking through how recovery-oriented care (rather than "recovery") can be implemented in inpatient settings.

*Recovery* is what a *person* with a mental illness does to manage his or her condition and reclaim his or her life from the distress and wreckage the illness, and the stigma and discrimination associated with having the illness, may have caused. For some people, this process of recovery leads to a complete, enduring elimination of all symptoms and an amelioration of any deficits or dysfunctions associated with the disorder. These people are said to have achieved a "clinical recovery" or to have recover*ed* from a mental illness. Other people, however, engage in and pursue the process of recovery in the face of an ongoing mental illness; a form of recovery referred to as "personal recovery" or being "in" recovery; a notion inspired in part by the self-help philosophies in addiction and chronic illness management (e.g., being in cancer recovery; Davidison and Roe 2007; Slade 2009). Early in the process, it may not be possible to tell whether someone is recovering *from* a mental illness or figuring out how to live a full and meaningful life *with* a mental illness. Over 200 years of experience tells us, though, that few if any people recovered from a serious mental illness by putting their lives on hold. Since the 1970s, accumulating new evidence suggests that many people may, however, find the illness becoming less and less disruptive as they learn how to manage it in the context of their daily lives (Davidison and Roe 2007).

*Recovery-oriented care*, on the other hand, is what *health care providers* offer in support of the person's own efforts toward recovery and includes enhancing the person's access to opportunities to learn how to manage his or her condition while pursuing "a meaningful life in the community" (DHHS 2003). Health care providers cannot "do" recovery for someone else, and recovery is not something they can do to people either. A similar distinction underlies educational philosophy and practice: while the teacher can teach, only the student can learn. The teacher cannot learn *for* the student, and there is little that teachers can do to students to make them learn against their wishes. Learning, like recovery, happens all the time without the person's explicit intention, though; it is not necessarily a willful or deliberate process. But it is a process in which the person or student is engaged nonetheless. While recovery, much like learning, is the primary task of the individual, there is still much that caring others can do to facilitate this process through both formal (i.e., health care providers) and informal (e.g., family, friends, employers) roles. It is within this arena that we see the great potential of recovery-oriented care as this approach—one based on mutual respect and a willingness to adapt based on each patient's own lived experiences and preferences—has increasingly been recognized as a powerful determinant in recovery outcomes among persons living with serious mental illnesses (Coulter et al. 2013).

With this central distinction in place, we can now begin to discuss what these principles mean for transforming inpatient care to a recovery orientation. We begin with what perhaps is the most crucial, but also most challenging principle when it comes to the inpatient milieu, as inpatient staff is under considerable pressure to do things to people in a safe, timely, efficient, and effective manner. By the time the person arrives at the hospital, he or she will have become overwhelmed by the illness, lost some degree of control over his or her life, and have had some capacities and decision-making abilities compromised. From an inpatient staff member's point of view, the effects of the illness and the wreckage it has brought may be much more obvious or prominent than the person to whom this onslaught has occurred. Under such circumstances, it may be very difficult for staff to connect with the person behind or underneath the effects of the illness. Recovery-oriented care is based on the premise that doing so is not only possible, but also a necessary foundation for almost everything else the staff might attempt to do.

## Principle #1: It is, first and foremost, the person's recovery

In Western democracies, like the U.S., recovery-oriented care for many adults is person-centered and respectful of the value of autonomy, while for some persons from ethnic or cultural minority communities, as well as in more collectivist societies, recovery-oriented care may be family-centered and respectful of the core values of these cultures (such as social harmony in China). Recovery-oriented care thus makes space for individual variation based on a person's cultural identification and preferences. Resilience-$_{\text{oriented}}$ care for children and youth is similarly family-centered. But, as a matter of law, adults in the U.S. retain their rights to make their own decisions, both in health care and in life in general, unless, until, and then only for as long as they may pose serious, imminent risks to self or others, are gravely disabled, or have been determined not competent to take care of themselves by a judge. Why is this important, the reader may wonder, when people are typically only admitted for inpatient care when they meet one or more of these criteria? It is important to lay this legal and philosophical/ethical foundation for our insistence on autonomy and choice for at least two essential reasons.

First, regardless of the shape the person is in when he or she is admitted, the vast majority of people leaving inpatient care return to a community in which they retain their right to self-determination. No matter how restrictive the inpatient milieu may be, most people will resume making their own decisions, both about their mental health care and their lives, soon after they leave the unit. Rather than simply ignore this important fact, or become frustrated about the patients who continue to make poor choices or bad decisions after discharge, planning for how people will make key decisions for themselves once they leave the hospital could and should be a major concern of inpatient staff (Repper 2000). It is not enough to reduce symptoms or stabilize someone clinically, focusing solely on the present stay. It is equally important to identify reasons or precipitants for the admission (the past) and to ensure that the person has the inspiration, information, and tools needed to take care of him or herself once back in the community (the future). The vast majority of persons with serious mental illnesses no longer live in hospitals. Having a serious mental illness therefore is no longer an adequate reason for being hospitalized, nor is it adequate for staff to focus only on stabilizing the illness. In other words, it is not a person's mental illness alone that brings him or her to the hospital. It is how that illness was being managed or not, and/or the life circumstances in which the person with the illness was living (e.g., a sudden loss) that brings him or her to the hospital.

Second, recognizing that most people will resume responsibility for their self-care and recovery upon discharge has substantial implications for what and how care should be delivered on the unit. Rather than primarily treating the illness, it becomes incumbent on the staff to inform, educate, and role model self-care strategies for the person, that is, to encourage and equip the patient to take care of him or herself upon discharge (Caldwell et al. 2010; Davidson 2005; Seed and Torkelson 2012); to encourage patients to make the shift, for example, from simply taking medication because the doctor told them to, to using medication as a tool in their recovery (Baker et al. 2013). In order to do so, many people in general, and many people with serious mental illnesses more specifically, require a certain amount of self-confidence in their abilities to take on this challenge. If there is nothing I can do on my own behalf to better manage my condition or improve my overall life (which is how we can talk to people about recovery without using the term "recovery"), then why should I bother trying (Corrigan 2004; Schmutte et al. 2009). In addition to providing information, education, and some encouragement, staff may need to assess the degree to which each person views him or herself as being in control and in charge of his or her life. Should the requisite degree of a sense of agency and efficacy needed for self-care be lacking, this provides an important focus for intervention.

But how can inpatient staff assist people in developing a sense of agency, efficacy, confidence, and control? First, by separating the person from the illness, staff play a central role in helping the person to see that he or she is not the illness itself (e.g., consistently using, and reminding the individual to use, "person-first" language rather than referring to the person as "a schizophrenic" or "a bipolar") and that he or she can learn to battle back against and manage the illness over time (Davidson 2003). As described eloquently by Amy Johnson, a woman diagnosed with schizophrenia in her teens who is now well along in her own recovery:

> If I am my illness, instead of I am a person who an illness happens to, then I can never get better. Because I can't pull the illness off of me if *I am* the illness. If the illness and I are the same thing, then there ain't nothin' I can do. I can't change me, I can't… The forest and the tree are the same thing. But if you separate the two, suddenly I find strength. I ask myself: Where? How do you find it? I find it in the separation. If we are not the same thing, if I am not the illness, then I can beat it, I can trick it, I can out maneuver it, I can go to the library and read about how to navigate around it… If I am not the illness, then the hope that I can maybe beat it springs forth… hope then, comes from splitting off the illness from the person.

Within this context, the staff might in fact find it useful to talk with the person about how recovery is possible—whether or not that exact word is used—no matter how acutely psychotic the person might be. Everyone needs hope, and people who are in desperation need hope desperately. As a result, inpatient units need to be hopeful places where people can be inspired and encouraged to be hopeful about their prospects for having a better life.

That better life can even begin on the unit itself should the staff view assisting their patients to develop a sense of agency, efficacy, confidence, and control as a central part of their role. In addition to separating the person from the illness, there are several things staff can do to elicit and promote these essential resources. Adopting a "strength-based" perspective is crucial to recovery-oriented practice and precisely for this (as well as other) reasons. Through both formal assessments and informal conversations, staff can help patients identify their existing internal and external strengths (what they have and are good at) as well as cultivate new ones by taking an active interest in them as people. These include interests, aptitudes, meaningful activities, and connections to others. Staff can elicit and honor patients' preferences for how they would like to be addressed and what options they would like to be offered if and when they are having particular difficulties on the unit (e.g., developing a Personalized Safety Plan that may note a person's preference to take time out in a comfort room, to sit quietly with a staff member, or to have a cup of tea). Staff can maximize the degree to which patients can exercise their own autonomy while on the unit, respecting the fact that they are adults both by limiting restrictions to those that are necessary for safety and creating opportunities for people to have and make choices in terms of how they spend their time, who they spend their time with, and what activities, services, and supports they engage in. In this way, to the degree possible, a hospital stay for a psychiatric illness should resemble a hospital stay for a chronic medical condition (e.g., asthma, cardiovascular disease), interfering with the person's ongoing life only when necessary for monitoring and treating the person's health condition, but otherwise respecting his or her autonomy in all matters.

It is quite possible that some persons with serious mental illnesses may seem at first to have few, if any, interests, preferences, connections, or meaningful activities in their lives and, when asked, may suggest that they have no strengths or goals. Whether this presentation is due to depression, the negative symptoms of schizophrenia, or a history of demoralization and prior treatment experiences that have socialized the person into a passive and hopeless role, it becomes incumbent upon inpatient staff to work patiently and persistently with patients to assist them in rediscovering things that were important to them in the past or things that might be of interest to them in the future. Strategies for doing so include acknowledging long-term recovery goals on recovery plans, even if such goals may seem unrealistic or are not to be pursued directly within the context of the current admission; maximizing the use of peer specialists, whether individually or in groups, to inspire hope and role model the possibility of recovery; having other people's recovery narratives widely accessible in diverse multimedia formats including print and video; exposing the person to new activities or resources with which he or she may be unfamiliar; and finding opportunities for people to make valued contributions to others (a form of "giving back" that many people will take up prior to turning to their own self-care).

Once identified, it is then important to initiate referrals to community-based rehabilitation and recovery supports that will enable the person to continue these activities so that these connections are in motion prior to the individual leaving the hospital (e.g., arranging for a ride to Sunday services at the person's church in addition to ensuring that she has a week's supply of medications and a follow-up appointment at the community mental health center).

## Principle #2: Recovery-oriented care is person/family-centered and culturally responsive

In addition to exploring patients' interests, strengths, and aspirations as a way of activating them for self-care, such discussions will be important in helping to frame and develop a person and/or family-centered care or recovery plan that will guide both their inpatient stay and their discharge plan. Person-centered recovery plans (Tondora et al. 2014) are not only tailored to the unique needs, preferences, values, and cultural affinities of each person, but are also oriented toward enabling that person to determine and pursue his or her own interests, meaningful activities, and life goals. It is not only a treatment plan that identifies what treatments will be provided by whom to reduce which symptoms or ameliorate which deficits or dysfunctions, but it is also a plan for how the person, his or her health care providers, and his or her natural supports (i.e., family, friends, employers, faith leaders, landlords) will work together to support the person in achieving the kind of life he or she will have reason to value (Sen 1999).

Inpatient recovery plans should include a statement about a person's hopes and dreams for the future as such long term goals can be a critical source of hope and motivation for the individual even if they are not actively addressed in the current inpatient admission. In addition, discharge plans should attend not only to the immediate clinical needs of an individual (e.g. being released with a week's worth of meds and an appointment with their outpatient therapist), but also to the types of meaningful activities which will help to sustain their recovery in the community (e.g., an intake at the Vocational Rehabilitation Center and a ride to Sunday services).

Such person-centered care plans obviously cannot be developed without substantial input from the person him or herself (which may mean the person requires up-front education and preparation regarding treatment planning and their role within it) and/or from those people whom the patient most trusts and/or who know the person best (which may mean helping people to map their network of supporters and identify who they might like to involve and then remaining flexible regarding the scheduling of treatment planning meetings to ensure their participation).

As noted in our discussion of the first principle, not every person presenting for hospitalization will want to be the primary decision-maker in his or her own care. In addition to considering his or her psychiatric condition and competence to do so when acutely ill, staff will need to explore and understand the person's cultural affinities and values in relation to decision-making. Even in Western democracies, persons from different cultural backgrounds may have different preferences for who should make what decisions about his or her care and life in general. Persons from different cultural backgrounds may also have different perceptions, and expectations of the roles of doctors, nurses, and other staff. These preferences and expectations are to be explored and understood as much as possible so that the care provided can be offered in as much of a person- and family-centered fashion as possible, not only out of respect for each person but also because the care is then more likely to be effective and its effects more enduring over the longer-term.

As just one example, a person will be much less likely to take prescribed medication after discharge if (1) the family he or she lives with does not support the use of medication, (2) the clergy or elders in his or her faith community do not accept that the person has an illness or approve of psychiatric medication, or (3) the person's daily routine has not been structured in such a way as to maximize the likelihood that he or she will either remember or be reminded to take the medication at certain times (e.g., to take it with meals, before leaving the apartment for class, and so on). Intimate knowledge of these kinds of details of the person's life can be instrumental in ensuring the success of discharge plans. On the other hand, the most carefully crafted discharge plan may be doomed to fail should the staff not see these kinds of considerations as central to their role. We have seen discharge plans, for instance, that have required patients to take several different medications on several different schedules, resulting in one person being expected to take one or more pills every hour over the course of a single day, leaving little if any time for anything else.

Person-centered recovery plans also provide the foundation for implementing a number of specific strategies for further tailoring care to the unique needs, preferences, and challenges of each patient. Should a psychiatric advance directive or Wellness Recovery Action Plan (WRAP) have already been developed prior to admission, honoring this plan or directive enables the staff to abide by the person's preferences and wishes even when he or she has been rendered temporarily incapable of expressing them directly. Should the person not have an advance directive or WRAP when admitted, developing one prior to discharge will prepare and equip both the person and the staff to make more safe, efficient, and effective use of any future readmissions, should they become necessary. In the absence of an advance directive, staff can use preference assessments on admission to determine how to best care for patients should they become more distressed, agitated, or isolative during the admission. Simple questions about what has worked well for the person in the past when he or she has been upset, confused, or withdrawn minimize the need for guess work or staff having to make stabs in the dark in trying to maintain a safe, welcoming, and supportive milieu. For individuals who may feel overwhelmed in responding to such open-ended questions, it can also be helpful for staff to develop simple "comfort profiles" or "safety inventories" in which an individual can review a wide variety of self-soothing and staff-supported strategies and simply check off those that can be offered/encouraged when they are having a difficult time on the unit.

Finally, person-centered recovery plans provide a framework for the design and use of positive behavioral supports tailored to the needs of each person as a recovery-oriented alternative to generic, dehumanizing level or privilege systems that are inappropriate for adults. These systems, in which patients have to "earn" certain opportunities, activities, or resources by demonstrating "good behavior," arose over 200 years ago in the British retreats developed during the era of "moral treatment" (cf., Davidson et al. 2010). The underlying premise of this approach was expressed by one of its founders, Tuke (1813) as: "There is much analogy between the judicious treatment of children and that of insane persons" (p. 150). In other words, persons with serious mental illnesses were viewed as analogous to misbehaving children and thereby needed to be resocialized within a supportive and structured family-like community. Within this community, the superintendent of the retreat functioned as a stern but judicious father, rewarding good, and punishing bad, behaviors. It was up to the superintendent to correct the patients' "erroneous views" and teach them to control their "wayward propensities" (p. 133). This was to be accomplished through a combination of instilling fear of punishment for unwanted behaviors and incentivizing good behavior by offering rewards, such as increased freedom and access to opportunities to socialize with people who were not fellow patients (e.g., retreat staff, family, and friends).

We must simply raise the question of whether such level systems are used on any other units within general hospitals to call into question the appropriateness of their use on a recovery-oriented inpatient unit. Are privilege systems or punishments used on any other units? Does someone who has had a heart attack or an asthma attack have to work his or her way up through a level system in order to be discharged? Does someone whose diabetes has not been well controlled have to earn privileges while in the hospital in order to visit the gift shop or take a walk in the garden? While to some readers these questions may initially seem silly, they are precisely the kinds of questions we need to ask when implementing a recovery orientation.

Mental illnesses are *illnesses*; they do not represent or result from faulty parenting, ignorance, limited intelligence, or "wayward propensities." John Nash, the Nobel Prize winning mathematician who taught at Princeton (and was the subject of the book and film *A Beautiful Mind*) had a psychotic disorder (Nasar 1998), as has Saks (2007), an Associate Dean of the Law School at the University of Southern California and winner of a MacArthur Fellowship, and Jamison (1995), a professor of psychiatry at Johns Hopkins University and noted author, among many others. The major difference between these accomplished people and other persons who have been hospitalized is not the nature of their illness; having a psychotic disorder does not render an adult child-like. Rather than perpetuating these stereotypes, recovery-oriented practices—whether on inpatient units or in community settings—need to combat discrimination and promote empowerment, self-determination, respect, and the intrinsic equality of individuals in recovery.

But if we are not to continue to use level systems, how are we to manage the unit, ensuring the safety of patients and staff and engaging patients in therapeutic activities? Through the use of individualized recovery plans that, when necessary (but *only* when necessary), include the design and use of positive behavioral support. Positive behavioral support is a strength-based method of behavioral analysis that has been shown to be effective in increasing prosocial behaviors and decreasing behaviors of concern without resorting to coercion (Carr et al. 2002). This method is congruent with recovery-oriented care as it (1) focuses on skill development based on the unique needs and strengths of each individual, and (2) promotes ecological changes on inpatient units (and in the broader community) to improve person/environment fit in order to support people in using more effective and prosocial means of communication that decrease the need for behaviors of concern.

Positive behavioral support also involves equipping staff with new skills such as de-escalation techniques and other ways of avoiding the use of coercive measures for dealing with behaviors of concern such as seclusion and restraint (Carr et al. 2002; LeBel et al. 2004). These behavioral methods have been shown to reduce the use of seclusion and restraint and are now considered the preferred methods of intervention for behaviors that in the past would have led to such measures (Donat 2005). In addition to allowing for unit management without resorting to punishment, these methods are also recognized for producing other benefits. There is hope, for example, that should persons perceive inpatient care as less infantilizing and aversive, they may be more prone to access hospitalization earlier on when needed (e.g., in the case of an ensuing crisis) rather than as a last resort or involuntarily (Kidd et al. 2014b).

**Principle #3: Anticipate, and welcome, trauma survivors**

Although we still have significant challenges to address, restraint and seclusion use has been reduced significantly since passage of the 1999 Dodd-Lieberman Act, which was initially developed in response to numerous deaths that occurred while patients were in restraints. Training staff in how not to provoke aggression in the first place by avoiding unnecessary power struggles, in the use of de-escalation techniques for persons who appear to be becoming agitated, and in the use of comfort rooms have all contributed to these reductions. We suggest, however, that these approaches are most effective, and most likely to be sustained, on units that undergo a more extensive transformation of their organizational culture to one that anticipates, and is welcoming and responsive to, the history of trauma the majority of persons with serious mental illnesses have experienced.

Research suggests that up to 80 % of such persons will have experienced some trauma prior to the onset of their psychotic symptoms (Cusack et al. 2004; Mueser et al. 2002). It only seems reasonable to assume that for the remaining 20 %, the process of being hospitalized on a psychiatric unit will represent a traumatic experience in and of itself (Priebe et al. 1998; Robins et al. 2005). As a result, it is important for staff to understand that people entering the unit will most likely be bearing the burden, and effects, of trauma; they will, in effect, be seeking respite from some battle that has been raging in their mind, in their home, and/or in their community. To begin the process of implementing a trauma-responsive unit culture, staff needs to shift their view of patients from being the embodiments of illness (e.g., bipolars and borderlines) to being wounded warriors, fresh from the battlefield and suffering the effects of what has been done to them and/or what they have witnessed. Trauma-informed care proponents capture this shift in their suggestion that staff stop asking patients (implicitly) the question: "What is wrong with you?" and start asking them explicitly instead: "What has happened to you?" to be followed by the question: "And how can I be of most help?" (Fallot and Harris 2008).

This shift in perspective, and the extensive staff training required to accomplish it, has not only led to reductions or the total elimination of the use of restraints and seclusion (Azeem et al. 2011; Barton et al. 2009; Bennington-Davis and Murphy 2005; Bowers et al. 2006; Gaskin et al. 2007; Greene et al. 2006; LeBel et al. 2004; Master et al. 2002; Schreiner et al. 2004; Smith et al. 2005; Sullivan et al. 2004; Wale et al. 2011; Wieman et al. 2014), but to reductions in the use of so-called chemical restraints as well (the use of PRN or "as needed" sedating medications; Barton et al. 2009; Donat 2005). Patients are encouraged to take on active roles in their own care, are empowered and activated to take care of themselves, and to work collaboratively with staff to understand the effects of the trauma, and to plan and work accordingly toward preventing any abuses or retraumatization that might occur unintentionally (Chandler 2008; Huckshorn 2004; Muskett 2014; Robins et al. 2005). Equipping staff for these roles requires education on the neurobehavioral effects of trauma, including Posttraumatic Stress Disorder, in the lives of adults, including the previously overlooked but potentially disabling effects they may have on self-care and functioning in social, familial, educational, and occupational domains.

Other key features of trauma-informed care include increasing feelings of safety for both patients and staff through the cultivation of respectful, collaborative, and genuinely caring relationships (Polacek et al. 2015) and the use of personal safety plans; transforming the unit's physical environment to be less institutional and more home-like, including the use of comfort rooms, increasing patient choices in relation to food, activities, and treatment options, and reframing symptoms as possibly representing meaningful attempts to cope with awful and overwhelming experiences (Chandler 2008; Huckshorn 2004; Muskett 2014). One example of what this looks like in practice is the woman who specified in her Personal Safety Plan that staff should avoid telling her to "be quiet" or obscuring her vision during periods when restraint might become necessary as she had been exposed to years of sexual abuse as a child, during which she had been blindfolded and instructed to "be quiet." As a result, if staff triggered her traumatic memories inadvertently by recreating either of these experiences, her situation would further deteriorate rather than improve.

As trauma always occurs within the context of a person's life, shifting to trauma-informed care also requires more of an incorporation of the person's cultural identity and background, in terms of understanding both the context for the traumatic events and the person's culturally-based ways of responding to and trying to manage the trauma and its effects. Faith and other community leaders may be extremely valuable guides in helping staff explore these issues in a manner that demonstrates respect and appreciation for the key role spirituality plays in the lives of many persons with serious mental illnesses.

## Principle #4: Expand the interdisciplinary team

Whether on an inpatient unit or in community settings, recovery-oriented care is provided through an interdisciplinary team that includes at least the person in recovery, one or more mental health practitioners, and those people in the person's life outside of formal mental health services who significantly support the person's self-care efforts (otherwise referred to as natural supports; Tondora and Davidson 2006). Although, within the hospital setting, the term interdisciplinary team has historically referred to inpatient staff from various professional disciplines (e.g., psychiatry, nursing, social work), a final principle for recovery-oriented practice within this setting is that this notion of a team needs to be expanded to include both the parties described above and the outpatient and community-based staff who worked with the person prior to admission and/or will be working with the person following discharge. In addition to adding the person in recovery, his or her natural supports, and community providers, it is important that the power that has traditionally resided with the physician be distributed across this team to create a more collaborative and person/family-centered process.

An increasing number of tools are becoming available to assist practitioners in operationalizing this principle in terms of how such teams are convened and managed in developing recovery plans (e.g., Tondora et al. 2014) and utilizing shared decision-making tools (e.g., SAMHSA 2014), and will not be described here. What we will do is to describe briefly the role of each member of this team so as to offer a map of the territory to be covered. As roles invariably overlap, we limit our discussion to those aspects of each role that are more specific to that practitioner or stakeholder group.

*The role of the person in recovery*. Each path to recovery is as unique as is each individual, and only the person who is experiencing the illness first-hand will know all of the ins and outs of what has and has not worked along his or her journey. In appreciation of this lived experience, the person in recovery should be seen as possessing valuable expertise and his or her active participation and empowerment should be encouraged across all aspects of inpatient care. Supporting self-determination, wherein an individual has as much control as possible over his or her own treatment and life-defining decisions, is both expected within a recovery-oriented system and endorsed by our country's laws. This is not to discredit or disregard the knowledge and experience clinicians and other professionals on the team may bring, but rather to encourage the team to listen and learn from the person in terms of how they can best assist and support each unique individual's recovery.

We recognize that this role may not come naturally to many service users who have prior experiences with mental health services in which being "treatment compliant" has often been valued above all else. In contrast, person-centered recovery planning is most effective when the person fully understands and participates in all steps of the plan development, documentation, and implementation. Some individuals will naturally take the reins and engage in this process immediately. Others will find person-centered planning to be a new and even uncomfortable experience. In such cases, formal and informal group or individual educational interventions (frequently delivered by peer staff or members of the rehabilitation department) can help a person to develop concrete skills which allow him or her to more actively partner in the development of his or her own recovery plan. It may take time to empower people to learn from and trust their experiences, but this will prove to be an invaluable and worthwhile endeavor.

*The role of the family and other natural supports.* Family, friends, and other community members considered a part of the person's circle of support outside of the traditional medical/mental health system are known as "natural supporters" and can arguably prove to be some of the most influential and supportive individuals in a person's recovery (Tondora et al. 2014). These people are often part of a person's family and may also include, but are not limited to, friends, religious community leaders and members, neighbors, and coworkers. Each of us has natural supporters in our lives and our relationships with each of them are different. While a recovery-oriented system strives to build a supportive network of people beyond the mental health system, the final decision to include such people in one's care while in the hospital lies in the hands of the person receiving services (Tondora et al. 2014).

When a person decides to actively involve natural supporters in the planning process, these people need orientation to what role they've been invited to play and information about what to expect from the process. A friend or family member may have learned much in supporting his or her loved one through years of illness and recovery and this experience should be respected and welcomed in the dialogue. However, it should be clear to natural supporters that the person holds the ultimate decision-making power and the intention of the meeting is not to give the team an opportunity to collectively coerce or convince the person to do something against his or her will. First and foremost, natural supporters are encouraged to be positive, respectful, and supportive of the person in recovery and his or her identified needs, values, and preferences. Specific activities may include helping the person to think about priorities and goals ahead of time, asking him or her what kinds of support would be helpful, assisting the person in advocating for him or herself, or following through on specific action steps on the plan to help the person in recovery to achieve identified life goals (Tondora et al. 2014). Having supports, above and beyond the traditional paid roles of mental health staff, especially when a person is transitioning from an inpatient unit back to the community, can prove a valuable resource.

*The role of community-based practitioners.* People served in inpatient settings frequently work with a variety of community-based providers both prior to admission and are anticipated to on discharge. For instance, a person engaged in services at a local community mental health center might have both a primary clinician as well as a care coordinator. If taking medication, he or she would also have routine contact with a psychiatrist or nurse practitioner. If also meeting with a peer specialist, or working with a benefits coordinator, the team of providers within the community-based network grows to include numerous people, serving a variety of functions based on their specific training and expertise.

What exactly is the role of such community-based practitioners during hospitalization? And how does thinking through a recovery lens impact the interface between inpatient and outpatient service providers?

It is not uncommon for hospital admissions to be treated as discrete treatment episodes with limited continuity of care maintained with the primary outpatient providers. The minimal contact and collaboration that does occur tends to be restricted to the moments of admission and discharge with many missed opportunities in between. When an individual requires an inpatient level of care, it is critical to coordinate efforts with this outpatient network of providers as they may have a wealth of information both about what precipitated the individual's admission and how the team can work together in the future to avoid another episode. This requires adequate exchange of necessary information as well as a shared understanding of recovery goals that continue to be relevant across levels of care.

This type of care coordination and information exchange is sometimes achieved by a generic outpatient representative, often referred to as a local or regional "hospital liaison" whose primary function is to participate in discharge planning to promote continuity of care. While this may be a step in the right direction, it is often woefully inadequate in the eyes of service users as it fails to appreciate the importance of the human connections and real relationships they may have with their primary community providers. It is critical to ask the individual: Who knows you best from your team in the community? Who do you trust and feel most comfortable with? Who can help us plan for what you need/want—both here in the hospital and upon discharge? And upon learning the answer, do we do everything possible to ensure that individual's ongoing involvement (in person or via phone or video conference)? There is no substitute for this authentic human relationship. People do not want to be yet another "case" to be managed by a generic hospital liaison. Whether they are living in their apartment or being treated in the hospital, they want to know that they matter and the presence of a preferred outpatient provider is a powerful reminder that someone truly cares about them and their wellbeing.

*The role of the psychiatrist.* Psychiatrists have the opportunity to play a highly influential role both in the creation of a recovery-oriented and trauma-responsive culture on the unit and in the delivery of person/family-centered, recovery-oriented care within that context. Psychiatrists are at the heart of medical decision-making and can set a collaborative and inclusive tone that values the contributions of all parties, with the aim of educating and empowering patients to exercise their responsibility for self-care. Notably, as some persons may not believe or acknowledge having a mental illness or addiction, and/or may not want to take medication, psychiatrists can also play an important role in modeling for staff how to explore respectfully the person's and family's own understanding of their situation in order to identify potential junctures or opportunities for education and intervention. A combination of motivational interviewing, inviting the person and family to consider other perspectives, and offering education regarding medication benefits and costs/side effects should be incorporated to respect the individual's or family's autonomy while enhancing their capabilities for decision-making.

Psychiatrists elicit patient preferences, honor advance directives, and assume that people are capable of making their own decisions unless there is persuasive evidence to the contrary. In the case that a person's decisional capacity is being compromised by illness, psychiatrists seek the input of substitutive decision-makers, whether they have accepted this role formally by law or are identified by the patient as someone who knows the patient well and has his or her trust. Psychiatrists assess for risk, with a focus on safety planning both on the unit and in preparing for discharge, involving family and natural supports to the degree that is possible based on the patient's consent. If chairing the recovery planning team meetings, psychiatrists ensure the meaningful participation of all parties, seek out and consider alternative perspectives, and maintain a collaborative stance throughout the process. They are informed by the practitioners who were working with the person prior to his or her admission and plan for discharge in collaboration with those practitioners who will be working with him or her upon returning to the community. Finally, psychiatrists consider acute admissions to represent crises that offer opportunities for enhancing the person's senses of autonomy, responsibility, and self-efficacy through learning new lessons about processes and pathways of recovery.

*The role of the psychiatric nurse.* Inpatient psychiatric nurses have responsibility for the overall, twenty-four hour monitoring of physical safety, and planning and implementation of nursing focused recovery-oriented care for patients in the hospital setting. Nurses are key in setting the standards of recovery-oriented care, including through demonstrating respect and maintaining a collaborative stance within all patient and staff interactions and relationships. In particular, nurses are role models for all other staff in how to avoid getting into power struggles with patients and how to implement de-escalation techniques when patients begin to become distressed.

In conventional inpatient environments, nursing plans of care are often predesigned based on institution safety requirements, patients' documented medical needs, symptoms, and behaviors of concern. These plans of care have typically assumed that the nurse is in the best position to plan care based on his or her expertise and experience. Patients, on the other hand, may have "received" care with little input into its design, implementation, or outcome. In contrast, recovery-driven nursing care supports the belief that patients are also experts, especially with respect to their own strengths, preferences, and needs and are most intimately familiar with the ins and outs of the illness(es) they have. They, therefore, should also participate, to the best of their ability, in designing the plan of care. In addition to working in collaboration with their patients in developing, implementing, and evaluating plans of care, nurses are role models and educators related to other components of person-centered care. Given their historical role in managing the unit milieu, nursing influence is especially important in advancing the recovery orientation of the structure and functioning of the milieu and the overall unit culture. Nurses must be involved in designing and supporting policies that increase patient independence and eliminate punitive, negative policies based on fear rather than on evidenced-based practice. Inpatient policies such as denial of computer and phone access, staff-selected or screened visitors lists, denial of personal clothing, and limitation of access to foods and beverages, are but a few of the policies nursing can directly impact to bring care into the recovery era.

*The role of the social worker.* Social workers as a profession are guided by values, which are fundamental to a recovery orientation, such as recognizing "the dignity and worth of a person" and "the importance of human relationships" (National Association of Social Workers 2014). Training and education is strength-based and work involves exploring individuals' needs and wants while keeping in context the individuals' relationships with families and communities. Social workers bring this skill set of working with the "whole person" to interdisciplinary inpatient care teams. Too often social workers have been misunderstood in teams as simply discharge planners, without other professionals fully understanding what that means and the level of skill that is inherent in this work. Effective discharge planning by a social worker involves recovery-oriented care, having a skill to connect with patients and get to know them upon admission, to listen to and find out their needs and preferences, to explore their circumstances within the family and community system, and to plan for how each person can live successfully once he or she returns home to family and community.

In many cases, social workers find themselves advocating for patients when on inpatient units where patients' dignity and self-worth appears not to be recognized or valued. This can easily and unintentionally occur within a quick-paced system of care in which there are constantly moving parts. As a result of their philosophical grounding in a social justice framework, social workers may thus find themselves at times called to serve as the conscience or watchdog for their colleagues from other professions.

Social workers provide a connection to community and community resources for patients as well as for the other professionals on interdisciplinary teams. They have knowledge of services and supports available to individuals, families, and communities and serve as advocates and brokers so patients and families obtain the supports they need and prefer. Educating others on the values and ethics of social work and discussing how these values are consistent with recovery-oriented principles is important for new and well-seasoned social workers and also for other professionals.

*The role of the psychologist.* The role of the psychologist in recovery-oriented inpatient care may be multifaceted. Psychologists who are in leadership positions may play a major role in creating a culture of recovery that is responsive to trauma, for example. They can use their understanding of organizational and system dynamics to help foster a recovery mission for staff that views patients as people first, fosters hope, builds on strengths, and partners with patients in building autonomy, self-determination, and lives of meaning and purpose. Creating such a culture involves providing training and education on trauma and its effects, on person/ family- centered care planning and the involvement of the person and his or her natural supports as part of the interdisciplinary team, and on discharge planning within a social inclusion framework (Repper 2000). In terms of direct care, psychologists can offer group and individual psychological and social interventions including strength-based assessments, evidence-based psychotherapies, and skills training approaches that can best meet patient needs, and are responsive to patient preferences, goals, and choices. Psychologists are best positioned to provide such interventions as they typically have advanced clinical training, are highly skilled in the provision of psychotherapy, and are well versed in the provision of evidence-based approaches.

Psychologists also are most qualified to contribute their expertise in two focal areas. First is in relation to the importance of a sense of agency, efficacy, and self-confidence in promoting self-care among persons receiving care on inpatient units. As these are psychological concepts, psychologists are in the best position to assess for and promote these often-diminished capacities in persons with serious mental illnesses. They can suggest ways to promote the development of these capacities on the unit, as well as identify ways to support their development while accommodating their absence in community settings following discharge. For example, one woman who had been maintained for weeks on 1:1 observation due to severe self-injury finally came to be able to participate safely in her own care once the unit psychologist discovered that she was an avid reader who used getting caught up in books as a temporary escape from her trauma. Not only did she find reading books on the unit to be self-soothing, but she also was coaxed by the psychologist to volunteer to sort and reshelf books in the hospital library—an activity which was then incorporated into her discharge plan and continued in the community.

Secondly, many psychologists also will have received specialized training in behavioral analysis and the provision of positive behavioral supports. When indicated, they can bring this expertise to the interdisciplinary team, developing and implementing this aspect of a person's recovery plan in promoting strengths, increasing skills, and improving person/environment fit while mitigating the likelihood of the need for coercive measures. Integrating positive behavioral supports will likely have ongoing impact on fostering a culture of a recovery as well, with units becoming more hopeful and supportive, and less traumatizing and punitive, places as patients become hopeful, build on their own strengths, enhance their self-care, work towards achieving personal goals, and ultimately build a life of meaning and purpose.

*The role of the occupational therapist.* The major focus of occupational therapy is directed toward creating opportunities for participation; enabling skill development; collaborative problem-solving and use of strategies to make environmental adjustments, with the intended outcome of enabling participation in activity patterns that support recovery, health, well-being, and social connectedness (Kielhofner 2009; Krupa et al. 2010). As referred to here, occupation is inclusive of the range of paid and unpaid ways in which we may look ourselves, connect with others, find enjoyment, learn, and contribute in communities socially and economically (Townsend and Polatajko 2007). It also involves everyday tasks that may sometimes be taken for granted, but bring rhythm to daily life, allow assumption of valued roles, develop abilities and capacities, and define who we are in the social world (Hammell 2004; Kielhofner 2009). Occupational therapists undertake varied roles to implement recovery principles in acute care settings, using their knowledge of occupation and how to enable participation. Broadly, these roles are likely to include directly working with individuals to understand their occupational experiences and challenges, enabling individual and group participation in occupations, and environment-level practices with a focus on altering acute care environments to promote recovery.

At an individual level, occupational therapists work directly alongside people to assist and support their recovery through attending to the varied ways in which daily life may have been disrupted by experiencing mental health issues and being in a hospital environment. Perhaps the most obvious is that not being in one's usual surroundings that support familiar activities and routines can add to or exacerbate the person's distress. In such a case, tools and opportunities for involvement in ordinary activities can provide important grounding experiences amid the turmoil that a person may be experiencing whilst in acute care. Occupational therapists also have available to them frameworks and tools to support listening and learning about person's lived experiences of occupations, patterns of activity engagement, interests and choices, how disruptions or difficulties in occupation might be experienced, what factors might be contributing, and how these might be addressed. In turn, this means occupational therapists can contribute to the team's understanding of individuals as persons with everyday life contexts (including occupations, community involvement, relationships, aspirations, and so forth). In addition, through the analysis of actions and skills underlying performance, occupational therapists may also contribute to understanding individuals' strengths and difficulties in doing, and how their strengths, skills, and environments can best be utilized to support them in pursuing those occupations in which they seek to participate (Krupa et al. 2010).

Occupational therapists' approaches to working alongside persons in recovery tend to be participatory and action-oriented, frequently using processes such as guiding, coaching, information-sharing, prompting, consulting, and reflecting to support individuals to try out and discover interests; to learn, use, and practice skills; to find practical solutions to problems of everyday living; to clarify occupational choices; and to develop strategies for participating congruent with their values, preferences, aspirations, and circumstances (McDermott et al. 2012). Similarly, occupational therapy group work in inpatient settings typically has goals more focused on *doing* than those of verbal groups. These usually include opportunities for direct experiences of doing and collaborating with others; supporting information exchange, storytelling, giving and receiving feedback and assistance; and aiming to positively influence participants' experiences of engagement, social connection, peer support, and satisfaction (Kielhofner 2009). Choices about whether and how to be involved are important for enabling participation and supporting recovery. Recognizing that group participation can seem difficult or even overwhelming initially, occupational therapists who facilitate groups in acute care may encourage simply being in a group as a first step towards joining in as and when a person chooses, rather than requiring participation.

At an environmental level, occupational therapists also use their knowledge of factors external to individuals that influence participation (e.g., social, physical, cultural, and institutional factors) to attend to the extent to which inpatient and other acute care programs focus on, create, and develop opportunities to engage in meaningful and satisfying occupations (Krupa et al. 2010). One example of this environment-level practice is that occupational therapists often play a lead role in advocating for and organizing activity programming in inpatient settings. The primary purpose of activity programming has sometimes been understood within services as to relieve boredom, or fill in time on inpatient units while treatment is taking place. Yet, in recovery-oriented inpatient care, opportunities to engage in ordinary activities and experiences can be catalysts for several key recovery processes. For instance, they create opportunities to exercise choice and control; to stay connected or reconnect with activities, interests, and a sense of self beyond being defined by illness; to use existing strengths or discover new strengths; to explore different ways of dealing with symptoms, distress, and effects of trauma; and to explore possibilities for rebuilding a meaningful and satisfying life in the world beyond hospital. However, to maximize the recovery-promoting potential of acute care environments requires more than opportunities for activity engagement; it also requires attention to how these environments are experienced. Here, using their skills and tools for analyzing environments, occupational therapists may work collaboratively with peer providers and other team members to consider "what is it like to be and spend time here", and to identify ways in which acute care environments may be altered to create more welcoming spaces, as well as spaces that address other needs such as those for privacy, calm and quietude, socializing with others, and activity engagement.

*The role of the peer support staff*. Peer support staffs are individuals that identify as people in recovery from mental illness and/or substance use, trained and hired to provide supports to others with similar lived experiences. Peers hired on inpatient units provide hope to patients in these settings, particularly when they have a shared story of hospitalization or institutionalization. Peers are trained in the foundations of recovery-oriented care, thus guided by "meeting an individual where they are at" and assisting an individual, instead of "doing for" as he or she walks their own individuated recovery journeys. While there are many skills that peers bring to their work on inpatient units, two will be briefly discussed: sharing of their own lived experiences to model one path of recovery and learning to work within a behavioral health system in where they are open about their own mental health history.

The first skill of sharing and modeling recovery is a skill that can be developed over time by peers. Learning to share in a way that promotes the growth and dignity of others is key. Sharing indiscriminately is not appropriate. Instead, stories are used as examples of how challenges were faced in their own recovery journeys. In some cases, the peer may not have similar or shared lived experiences, the "we" story becomes important so that the stories are about collective ways in which individuals recover not focused solely on the peer's own experiences. Developing the skill of disclosure is not a simple task, though there are some peer staff who appear to do it naturally. Supervisors, ideally persons with lived experience themselves, should provide supervision that incorporates the learning and development of disclosure.

The second skill involves learning to work in an environment in which they were once served. It has only been recently that we have seen the expansion of peers working within the traditional behavioral health workforce. Unfortunately, it is a system that only too recently believed that people were not capable of "recovery" (unfortunately some staff may continue to believe this because of societal stigmas of mental illness and addictions). Peers working in these settings often find themselves advocating for themselves on teams as well as for those they serve. Supervisors and other staff in inpatient settings should serve as allies to promote a culture that values the work of the peers.

In some inpatient settings, peers are assigned to be on interdisciplinary teams and do not have a recognized department. In fact, some find themselves as the only peer on the unit or in the psychiatric hospital. It is highly advisable, though, for peers to be able to learn from other peers and have the opportunity to reflect on the work they are doing with others that do it. Hiring more than one peer therefore is recommended. Other inpatient settings have developed a peer department that is free standing and provides services to individuals or providers requesting peer support. There are pros and cons to each model; however, developing a culture that believes in the evidence of peer services and values the principles and ethics of peer support is necessary in promoting recovery-oriented care.

Finally, peers are also trained in providing assistance with individuals to connect them back to their communities. Again, "having been there" is important; however, learning ways that have worked for others as well as learning about peer modalities will be useful to doing this work successfully (i.e., Wellness Recovery Action Planning, person-centered care planning). Being in an inpatient psychiatric unit can be scary and challenging as well as awfully lonely. Even more difficult is transitioning back to community, to work, to family, to school. Peers can prepare and serve as a bridge from the time people walk into the hospital until they are discharged. They can provide linkages to peers working in outpatient settings and/or to other self-help and/or community programs. Peers working in inpatient settings signify that people do recover, people do return to work, and that people should be involved in their own care. This in and of itself may help patients/individuals alleviate internalized stigma of mental illness, to see beyond the engulfment of their mental illness, and to visualize that recovery can and does work.

## Conclusion

This chapter has presented guiding principles for the implementation of recovery-oriented practices in inpatient settings and described the respective roles of staff from the various disciplines as well as the patient him or herself, his or her natural supports, and community-based practitioners in developing and implementing person/family-centered recovery plans. We offer these principles and roles as a useful framework for rethinking many of the more operational and practical issues faced in delivering inpatient care to persons in acute distress, who are significantly disabled by a mental illness, and/or who pose risks to themselves or others. Preliminary results of implementing some recovery-oriented and trauma-informed practices—such as de-escalation techniques, preference assessments, positive behavioral support, and advance directives—have been promising, but much work remains to be done in creating welcoming, supportive, strength-based, and person/family-centered milieu that are truly respectful of and responsive to the dignity, autonomy, and tremendous suffering of the people they are intended to serve.

## References


Azeem, M. W., Aujla, A., Rammerth, M., Binsfeld, G., & Jones, R. B. (2011). Effectiveness of six core strategies based on trauma informed care in reducing seclusions and restraints at a child and adolescent psychiatric hospital. *Journal of Child and Adolescent Psychiatric Nursing, 24*(1), 11–15.

Baker, E., Fee, J., Bovington, L., Campbell, T., Hewis, E., Lewis, D., et al. (2013). From taking to using medication: Recovery-focused prescribing and medicines management. *Advances in Psychiatric Treatment, 19*, 2–10.

Barker, P. J., & Buchanan-Barker, P. (2011). Mental health nursing and the politics of recovery: A global reflection. *Archives of Psychiatric Nursing, 25*(5), 350–358.

Barker, P., & Buchanan-Barker, P. (2010). The tidal model of mental health recovery and reclamation: Application in acute care settings. *Issues in Mental Health Nursing, 31*(3), 171–180.

Barton, S. A., Johnson, M. R., & Price, L. V. (2009). Achieving restraint-free on an inpatient behavioral health unit. *Journal of Psychosocial Nursing, 47*(1), 34–40.

Bennington-Davis, M., & Murphy, T. (2005). *Restraint and seclusion: The model for eliminating use in healthcare*. Oregon: HCPro Inc.

Bowers, L., Brennan, G., Flood, C., Lipang, M., & Oadapol, P. (2006). Preliminary outcomes of a trial to reduce conflict and containment on acute psychiatric wards: City nurses. *Journal of Psychiatric and Mental Health Nursing, 13*, 165–172.

Caldwell, B. A., Sclafani, M., Swarbrick, M., & Piren, K. (2010). Psychiatric nursing practice and the recovery model of care. *Journal of Psychosocial Nursing, 48* (7), 42–48.

Carr, E. G., Dunlap, G., Horner, R. H., Koegel, R. L., Turnbull, A. P., Sailor, W., et al. (2002). Positive behavior support evolution of an applied science. *Journal of Positive Behavior Interventions, 4*(1), 4–16.

Chandler, G. (2008). From traditional inpatient to trauma-informed treatment: Transferring control from staff to patient. *Journal of the American Psychiatric Nurses Association, 14*, 363–371.

Chen, S.-P., Krupa, T., Lysaght, R., McCay, E., & Piat, M. (2011). The development of recovery competencies for inpatient mental health providers working with people with serious mental illness. *Administration and Policy in Mental Health, 40*(2), 96–116.

Chen, S.-P., Krupa, T., Lysaght, R., McCay, E., & Piat, M. (2014). Development of a recovery education program for inpatient mental health providers. *Psychiatric Rehabilitation Journal, 37*(4), 329–332.

Corrigan, P. (2004). How stigma interferes with mental health care. *American Psychologist, 59*(7), 614–625.

Coulter, A., Entwistle, V. A., Eccles, A., Ryan, S., Shepperd, S., & Perera, R. (2013). *Personalized care planning for adults with chronic or long-term health conditions*. Issue: The Cochrane Library. 5.

Cusack, K. J., Frueh, B. C., & Brady, K. T. (2004). Trauma history screening in a community mental health center. *Psychiatric Services, 55*, 157–162.

Davidson, L. (2003). *Living outside mental illness: Qualitative studies of recovery in schizophrenia*. New York: New York University Press.

Davidson, L. (2005). Recovery, self-management, and the expert patient: Changing the culture of mental health from a UK perspective. *Journal of Mental Health, 14* (1), 25–35.

Davidison, L., & Roe, D. (2007). Recovery from versus recovery in serious mental illness: One strategy for lessening confusion plaguing recovery. *Journal of Mental Health, 16*(4), 1–12.

Davidson, L., Rakfeldt, J., & Strauss, J. S. (2010). *The roots of the recovery movement: Lessons learned*. London: Wiley-Blackwell.

Davies, J., Maggs, R. G., & Lewis, R. (2014). The development of a UK low secure service: Philosophy, training, supervision, and evaluation. *International Journal of Forensic Mental Health, 9*(4), 334–342.

DHHS. (1999). *Mental health: A report of the Surgeon General*. Rockville, MD: Substance Abuse and Mental Health Services Administration.

DHHS. (2003). *Achieving the promise: Transforming mental health care in America*. Rockville, MD: Substance Abuse and Mental Health Services Administration.

Donat, D. C. (2005). Encouraging alternatives to seclusion, restraint, and reliance on PRN drugs in a public psychiatric hospital. *Psychiatric Services, 56*(9), 1105–1108.

Fallot, R. D., & Harris, M. (2008). Trauma-informed approaches to systems of care. *Trauma Psychology Newsletter, 3*(1), 6–7.

Fisher, W. (2003). Elements of successful restraint and seclusion reduction programs and their application in a large, urban, state psychiatric hospital. *Journal of Psychiatric Practice, 9*(1), 7–15.

Gaskin, C. J., Elsom, S. J., & Happell, B. (2007). Interventions for reducing the use of seclusion in psychiatric facilities: Review of the literature. *The British Journal of Psychiatry, 191*(4), 298–303.

Greene, R. W., Ablon, J. S., & Martin, A. (2006). Use of collaborative problem solving to reduce seclusion and restraint in child and adolescent inpatient units. *Psychiatric Services, 57*, 610–612.

Hammell, K. W. (2004). Dimensions of meaning in the occupations of daily life. *Canadian Journal of Occupational Therapy, 71*(5), 296–305.

Hillbrand, M., Hawkins, D., Howe, D. M., & Stayner, D. (2008). Through the eyes of another: Improving the skills of forensic providers using a consumer-informed role-play procedure. *Psychiatric Rehabilitation Journal, 31*(3), 239–242.

Huckshorn, K. A. (2004). Non-abusive psychological and physical intervention for a safer workplace. NAPPI International Training Program. Held on March 8–10, 2004. Augusta, ME: NAPPI, Inc.

Jaeger, M., Konrad, A., Rueegg, S., & Rabenschlag, F. (2015). Patients' subjective perspective on recovery orientation on an acute psychiatric unit. *Nordic Journal of Psychiatry, 69*(3), 188–195.

Jamison, K. R. (1995). *An unquiet mind: A memoir of moods and madness*. New York, NY: Vintage.

Kidd, S., McKenzie, K. J., Collins, A., Clark, C., Costa, L., Mihalakakos, G., & Paterson, J. (2014a). Advancing the recovery orientation of hospital care through staff engagement with former clients of inpatient units. *Psychiatric Services, 65*(2), 221–225.

Kidd, S., McKenzie, K. J., & Virdee, G. (2014b). Mental health reform at a system level: Widening the lens on recovery-oriented care. *Canadian Journal of Psychiatry, 59*(5), 243–249.

Kielhofner, G. (2009). *Conceptual foundations of occupational therapy* (4th ed.). Philadelphia: F.A. Davis.

Knutson, M. B., Newberry, S., & Schaper, A. (2013). Recovery education: A tool for psychiatric nurses. *Journal of Psychiatric and Mental Health Nursing, 20*, 874–881.

Krupa, T., Fossey, E., Anthony, W., Brown, C., & Pitts, D. (2010). Doing daily life: How occupational therapy can inform psychiatric rehabilitation practice. *Psychiatric Rehabilitation Journal, 32*(3), 155–161.

Leamy, M., Bird, V., Le Boutillier, C., Williams, J., & Slade, M. (2011). Conceptual framework for personal recovery in mental health: Systematic review and narrative synthesis. *The British Journal of Psychiatry, 199*(6), 445–452.

LeBel, J., Stromberg, N., Duckworth, K., Kerzner, J., Goldstein, R., Weeks, M., et al. (2004). Child and adolescent inpatient restraint reduction: A state initiative to promote strength-based care. *Journal of the American Academy of Child and Adolescent Psychiatry, 43*, 37–45.

Le Boutillier, C., Leamy, M., Bird, V. J., Davidson, L., Williams, J., & Slade, M. (2011). What does recovery mean in practice? A qualitative analysis of international recovery-oriented practice guidance. *Psychiatric Services, 62*, 1470–1476.

McDermott, F., Hupert, D., Blashki, G., Stone, L., Epstein, M., Olsen, A., et al. (2012). Active participants in mental health services. In G. Meadows, J. Farhall, E. Fossey, M. Grigg, F. McDermott, & B. Singh (Eds.), *Mental health in Australia: A collaborative community practice* (3rd ed., pp. 267–319). Melbourne, Australia: Oxford University Press.

McKenna, B., Furness, T., Dhital, D., Ennis, G., Houghton, J., Lupson, C., et al. (2014a). Recovery-oriented care in acute inpatient mental health settings: An exploratory study. *Issues in Mental Health Nursing, 35*, 526–532.

McKenna, B., Furness, T., Dhital, D., Park, M., & Connolly, F. (2014b). The transformation from custodial to recovery-oriented care: A paradigm shift that needed to happen. *Journal of Forensic Nursing, 10*(4), 226–233.

Master, K. J., Bellonci, C., & Bernet, W. (2002). Practice parameter for the prevention and management of aggressive behavior in child and adolescent psychiatric institutions, with special reference to seclusion and restraint. *Journal of the American Academy of Child and Adolescent Psychiatry, 41*(Suppl. 2), 4S–25S.

Mueser, K. T., Rosenberg, S. D., Goodman, L. A., & Trumbetta, S. L. (2002). Trauma, PTSD, and the course of severe mental illness: An interactive model. *Schizophrenia Research, 53*(1), 123–143.

Muskett, C. (2014). Trauma-informed care in inpatient mental health settings: A review of the literature. *International Journal of Mental Health Nursing, 23* (1), 51–59.

Nasar, S. (1998). *A beautiful mind: A biography of John Forbes Nash*. Jr: Simon & Schuster.

National Association of Social Workers. (2014). *Code of ethics of the National Association of Social Workers*. Approved by the 1996 NASW Delegate Assembly and revised by the 2008 NASW Delegate Assembly. http://www.naswdc.org/pubs/code/code.asp

Polacek, M. J., Allen, D. E., Damin-Moss, R. S., Schwartz, A. J. A., Sharp, D., Shattell, M., et al. (2015). Engagement as an element of safe inpatient psychiatric environments. *Journal of the American Psychiatric Nurses Association, 21*(3), 181–190.

Priebe, S., Bröker, M., & Gunkel, S. (1998). Involuntary admission and posttraumatic stress disorder symptoms in schizophrenia patients. *Comprehensive Psychiatry, 39*, 220–224.

Repper, J. (2000). Adjusting the focus of mental health nursing: Incorporating service users' experiences of recovery. *Journal of Mental Health, 9*(6), 575–587.

Robins, C. S., Sauvageot, J. A., Cusack, K. J., Suffoletta-Maierle, S., & Frueh, B. C. (2005). Consumers' perceptions of negative experiences and "sanctuary harm" in psychiatric settings. *Psychiatric Services, 56*, 1134–1138.

Saks, E. (2007). *The center cannot hold. My journey through madness*. New York: Hyperion Books.

SAMHSA. (2011). *Consensus definition of recovery in behavioral health*. http://blog.samhsa.gov/2011/12/22/samhsa%E2%80%99s-definition-and-guiding-principles-of-recovery. Accessed February 1, 2015.

SAMHSA. (2014). http://archive.samhsa.gov/BRSS-TACS-Decision-Tool/. Accessed August 4, 2015.

Schmutte, T., Flanagan, E., Bedregal, L., Ridgway, P., Sells, D., Styron, T., & Davidson, L. (2009). Self-efficacy and self-care: Missing ingredients in health and healthcare among adults with serious mental illnesses. *Psychiatric Quarterly, 80*, 1–8.

Schreiner, G. M., Crafton, C. G., & Sevin, J. A. (2004). Decreasing the use of mechanical restraints and locked seclusion. *Administration and Policy in Mental Health, 31*, 449–463.

Seed, M. S., & Torkelson, D. J. (2012). Beginning the recovery journey in acute psychiatric care: Using concepts from Orem's self-care deficit nursing theory. *Issues in Mental Health Nursing, 33*, 394–398.

Sen, A. (1999). *Development as freedom*. New York, NY: Oxford University Press.

Shanley, E., & Jubb-Shanley, M. (2007). The recovery alliance theory of mental health nursing. *Journal of Psychiatric and Mental Health Nursing, 14*(8), 734–743.

Siu, B. W. M., Ng, B. F. L., Li, V. C. K., Yeung, Y. M., Lee, M. K. L., & Leung, A. Y. H. (2012). Mental health recovery for psychiatric inpatient services: Perceived importance of the elements of recovery. *East Asian Archives of Psychiatry, 22*(2), 39–48.

Slade, M. (2009). *Personal recovery and mental illness: A guide for mental health professionals*. Cambridge: Cambridge University Press.

Smith, G. M., Davis, R. H., Bixler, E. O., Lin, H. M., Altenor, A., Altenor, R. J., et al. (2005). Pennsylvania State Hospital system's seclusion and restraint reduction program. *Psychiatric Services, 56*, 1115–1122.

Sullivan, D., Wallis, M., & Lloyd, C. (2004). Effects of patient-focused care on seclusion in a psychiatric intensive care unit. *International Journal of Therapy and Rehabilitation, 11*, 503–508.

Tee, S., Lathlean, J., Herbert, L., Coldham, T., East, B., & Johnson, T. J. (2007). User participation in mental health nurse decision-making: A co-operative enquiry. *Journal of Advanced Nursing, 60*(2), 135–145.

Tondora, J. & Davidson, L. (2006). *Practice guidelines for recovery-oriented behavioral health care*. Connecticut Department of Mental Health and Addiction Services.

Tondora, J., Miller, R., Slade, M., & Davidson, L. (2014). *Partnering for recovery in mental health: A practical guide to person-centered planning*. London: Wiley-Blackwell.

Townsend, E. A., & Polatajko, H. J. (2007). *Enabling occupation II: Advancing an occupational therapy vision for health, wellbeing and justice through occupation*. Ottawa: CAOT Publications ACE.

Tuke, S. (1813). *A description of the retreat, an institution near York, for insane persons of the Society of Friends*. York, England: W. Alexander.

Wale, J. B., Belkin, G. S., & Moon, R. (2011). Reducing the use of seclusion and restraint in psychiatric emergency and adult inpatient services: Improving patient-centered care. *The Permanente Journal, 15*(2), 57–62.

Walsh, J., & Boyle, J. (2009). Improving acute psychiatric hospital services according to inpatient experiences. A user-led piece of research as a means to empowerment. *Issues in Mental Health Nursing, 30*(1), 31–38.

Walsh, J., Stevenson, C., Cutcliffe, J., & Zinck, K. (2008). Creating a space for recovery-focused psychiatric nursing care. *Nursing Inquiry, 15*(3), 251–259.

Wieman, D. A., Camacho-Gonsalves, T., Huckshorn, K. A., & Leff, S. (2014). Multisite study of an evidence-based practice to reduce seclusion and restraint in psychiatric inpatient facilities. *Psychiatric Services, 65*(3), 345–351.

# 3 Sexuality and Sexual Health

Kristin M. Hunter and Anthony O. Ahmed

## Introduction

Practitioners in inpatient psychiatric settings are periodically faced with the question of how to address issues of sexuality and sexual health among inpatient psychiatric patients. The question—should hospitalized patients be allowed to express themselves sexually in socially acceptable ways?—is one that elicits knee-jerk responses among practitioners, patients, and consumer advocates. Whereas, many providers in inpatient settings may not be inclined to allow patients to engage in intercourse, there may be less resistance to other forms of sexual expression. In contrast, patients and consumer advocates have argued that restrictions inpatient settings place on the expression of sexual interest and behavior of patients reflect a general propensity of traditional care settings to limit the rights of hospitalized patients. They argue that the normal expression of sexuality is a civil rights issue.

Deegan (1999) best encapsulated the consumer and consumer advocate view when she wrote, "Like all people, we [people with mental illness] experience the need for love, companionship, solitude, and intimacy. Like all people, we want to feel loved, valued, and desired by others…" (p. 21). Of course, for practitioners, allowing the free expression of sexuality may raise issues of risk, liability, and even practicality. Where does a practitioner draw the line between what represents culturally acceptable sexual expression versus clinically significant sexual behavior? If patients are allowed to have sex on the unit, what challenges does that place on the unit in terms of accommodations for privacy, consent, sexual health, and birth control?

The convention has been for mental health practitioners to ignore issues of sexuality among hospitalized psychiatric patients (Barr 1912; Brown et al. 2014; Collins 2001; Quinn et al. 2011). This has been to the peril of the mental health system as it contributes to evidence that traditional care is poorly responsive to the wishes of patients. The sexuality of psychiatric patients, whether one believes it should be ignored as a potential distraction to treatment (a view

K.M. Hunter
Department of Counseling and Human Development Services, University of Georgia, Athens, USA

A.O. Ahmed (✉)
Department of Psychiatry, Weill Cornell Medical College, New York, USA
e-mail: aoa9001@med.cornell.edu



N.N. Singh et al. (eds.), *Handbook of Recovery in Inpatient Psychiatry*, Evidence-Based Practices in Behavioral Health, DOI 10.1007/978-3-319-40537-7_3

espoused by many care providers) or embraced as part of holistic approach to treatment, remains an important yet divisive topic within the psychiatric inpatient literature (Perlin et al. 2009).

## A Clash of Perspectives

The following case vignettes provide a snapshot of the tensions that exist between the practitioner and patient perspectives on sexual expression on the inpatient unit.

### Case Vignette #1

Patient A is a 55-year-old, married, Caucasian male who was admitted to the Chronic Mental Health Unit of SMI Psychiatric Hospital 22 months ago. He had first been admitted to the Acute Unit of the hospital 24 months ago after he attempted suicide by overdosing on over-the-counter medication during a depressive episode. Patient A was first diagnosed with Schizoaffective Disorder when he was in his early 20s, and he has a longstanding history of psychiatric readmissions due to his medication nonadherence. Over the past two weeks, nursing staff have caught him twice pretending to take his prescribed medication (i.e. cheeking his medications). During his weekly individual psychotherapy session, the patient revealed that he and his wife are planning on having sexual relations during their next visit in two weeks. In preparation for this visit, the patient reported that he has stopped taking his antidepressant medication for the last two days, as one of the side effects of this medication is his difficulty achieving and maintaining an erection.

The patient's interdisciplinary treatment team is informed of the patient's medication nonadherence and intent to have sexual relations with his wife during their private visit. As a result, the treatment team informs the patient that he will not be allowed to meet with his wife privately for the next several visits, as the hospital has a firm policy restricting patient's sexual activity, regardless of the marital status of the patient. In addition, the patient will now have to take his antidepressant medication in front of nursing staff in order to prevent him from not adhering to his medication regimen. Nursing staff will check under his tongue and in his cheeks to ensure that he is not "cheeking" his medication. If patient continues to not adhere to his medication, he will be given intramuscular (IM) injections of Oral Dispersible Tablets (ODT) alternatives to ensure his treatment adherence.

### Case Vignette #2

Patient B is a 23-year-old, reportedly engaged, African-American female who was admitted to the Acute Unit of the SMI Psychiatric Hospital three weeks ago after she walked into the middle of a busy highway. When queried about why she had engaged in this dangerous behavior, Patient B reported that she had been attempting to use her superhuman powers to "stop cars in the highway by looking at them directly." Following a comprehensive psychiatric evaluation, Patient B was diagnosed with schizophrenia. During the course of her admission, Patient B attended psychoeducational and group psychotherapy classes at the hospital's day treatment center. After two weeks of consistent medication adherence, nursing staff alerted the patient's interdisciplinary team when Patient B refused to take her prescribed antipsychotic medication for two consecutive days. Patient B informed the treatment team that an angel had told her in a dream that antipsychotic medications would harm her fetus, and she stated that she had decided not to take her medication since she and her fiancé were actively trying to start a family. Her treatment team is uncertain about her reality testing capacity and some staff members question whether she really has a fiancé. Despite the treatment team's recommendation that Patient B focus on her recovery before starting a family, the patient stated that she would not willingly take psychotropic medication until the birth of her first child.

## Case Vignette #3

When Dr. Allen took over the administrative responsibilities of a state hospital, he envisioned a program that would be informed by the recovery model and sensitive to the civil rights of patients. After consulting with his state Department of Behavioral Health, relevant state laws and statues, lawyers, and several colleagues, he developed a plan to reform the hospital's policy with regard to patients and sexual expression. He also restructured his hospital units to allow patients to schedule and have conjugal visits. Dating and relationships was now allowed among patients and consensual sex among patients was allowed under a set of conditions—documentation of consent by parties involved, psychoeducation about sexual behavior and communication, and safe sex.

Dr. Allen ensured that training was provided to staff with regard to the implementation of the new policy. On the hospital units, greater accommodation was provided to patients to allow them to have more privacy. Patients generally received the policy shift gladly, whereas many staff members were very concerned about the risks involved in the policy shift and the challenges of protecting vulnerable patients from sexual coercion. At one year, following the implementation of the hospital's new policy, it was clear that patient satisfaction was increased. Some staff members also felt that some patients benefited with regard to increased opportunities to work on their social and interpersonal skills. Several challenges were, however, apparent. Staff members often grappled with the issue of whether particular patients should be "allowed" to consent and many suggested that such issues should be reviewed by the treatment team. There were concerns that certain dating/relationship contexts such as breakups often affected the progress of treatment for some patients. Many psychiatrists continued to raise issues of liability, particularly with a few situations in which vulnerable patients were involved. Some staff members expressed concerns that some patients were not practicing safe sex and were at increased risk of sexually transmitted diseases. Others noted that many patients often demanded to be taken of medications so they could have sex regardless off its impact on their psychiatric symptoms.

It is clear from all three vignettes that there exist tensions between practitioner goals for patients and what patients deem as important. Whereas, practitioners underscore the need for the patient to remain fairly compensated through medication and treatment adherence, patients' interests and degree of treatment adherence may be influenced by non-clinical factors (Deegan and Drake 2006). Criteria such as their desire to engage in valued social roles such as a parent, husband, wife, or sexual partner, may drive patient's own decision to engage in sexual relationships. The third case vignette is an illustration of some of the challenges of a more open and responsive approach to sexuality in inpatient settings.

This chapter will cover the history of sexuality within the context of the psychiatric unit and legislation and current rulings pertinent to sexual health on the inpatient unit. Existing tensions between staff attitudes toward inpatient sexuality, current hospital policies, and risks associated with sexual autonomy on the inpatient unit will be discussed. We will highlight several issues germane to sexual expression in people with mental illnesses. These include normal expressions of human sexuality and the impact of psychiatric symptoms, substance use, and psychotropic medication on sexuality. Within the discussion of normal sexual expression among people with serious mental illnesses, the chapter will highlight the psychosocial aspects of sexuality, sexual and reproductive health, and family planning in individuals admitted to an inpatient unit.

## Historical Background and Relevant Legislation

Until relatively recently, sexuality has been viewed as a cause of symptoms of psychopathy (Deegan 1999). As such, the sexuality of patients on the psychiatric inpatient unit or ward has been considered either as a potential sign of "deviancy" that requires close monitoring and restrictive parameters, or a topic to be ignored in its entirety unless forced by circumstances (Brown et al. 2013; Doak 2000; Quinn et al. 2011). A historical turning point occurred with the 1972 Wyatt v. Stickney case, which subsequently led to the District Court of Alabama mandating minimum standards of care for individuals with mental illness and mental retardation (Perlin 2008). A full listing of "The Wyatt Standards" can be viewed in Table 3.1. The Wyatt Standards underscored a range of civil rights for psychiatric patients including adequate care and provisions that guaranteed heterosocial interactions. The Wyatt standards informed the subsequent patient bill of rights that many states adopted. Although, many states adopted the Wyatt Standards but few actually adopted the provision relevant to heterosocial interactions. Rather, many state hospitals operate with gender-segregated units.

Several other litigations were filed related to the sexual rights of people with psychiatric disabilities since the landmark Wyatt case, but a review of litigation history is beyond the scope of this section. A 1983 landmark case, however, warrants comment. Foy v. Greenblott, involved a former psychiatrically hospitalized patient in California who sued her former care provider for not preventing her from having sex while she was hospitalized. The plaintiff had gotten pregnant and gave birth during her hospital tenure. She claimed that her care provider failed to provide adequate supervision to prevent her from having sex and failed to provide her with contraceptives and reproductive education. The California court in this case ruled against the former patient. The court opined that as a patient, she had a right to engage in voluntary sexual relationships:

> A conservatee or other institutionalized mental health patient enjoys the "same rights and responsibilities guaranteed all other persons" except those which are specifically denied by law (medically contraindicated) or court order (declaration *of* lack of capacity to consent). Every institutionalized person *is* entitled to individualized treatment under the "least restrictive" conditions feasible – the institution should minimize interference with a patient's individual autonomy, including her" "personal privacy" and "social interaction", which includes the freedom to engage in consensual sexual relations." Foy v. Greenblott (1983) 141 Cal.App.3d

The court invoked the provision of "least restrictive condition" as necessary to provide

**Table 3.1** The Wyatt standards

| Category |
|---|
| Physical living environment and custodial care |
| Personal liberties |
| Treatment and record keeping |
| Medical care |
| Use and administration of psychotropic medications |
| Protection from harm and physical safety |
| Adequate staffing and staff supervision |
| High risk or unusually restrictive treatment |
| Seclusion and restraint |
| Treatment in the least restrictive environment appropriate and transitional services |
| Children's services |

ample opportunities for mental health patients to engage in heterosocial interactions. The court also underscored that contrary to the plaintiff's claim of "wrongful birth," her child had not been affected because mental health patients do not give birth to inferior children. The court, however, opined that the defendant denied the patient's right of reproductive choice by not providing contraception and sex-related counseling.

Given the absence of laws or litigation that protects the rights of people with physical and psychiatric disabilities in many countries, the United Nations recently convened the Convention on the Rights of Persons with Disabilities. The mandate of the convention was to collaborate with representatives from all of the countries represented at the convention to define the rights of people with disabilities and develop a plan to seek legislation and reform that is responsive to those rights. The United Nations Convention on the Rights of Persons with Disabilities proposed in Article 25 of its 39-point articles of convention adopted on December 13, 2006 that "nations provide persons with disabilities with the same range, quality, standard of free or affordable health care and programs as provided to other persons, including in the area of sexual and reproductive health and population-based public health programmes" (UN General Assembly 2007, p. 18).

In summary, existing legal precedent appears to favor hospital decisions/policies that allow psychiatric inpatients to exercise their autonomy and preference with regard to their sexuality. It also appears that legally, fostering an environment that supports the free exercise of sexual preference requires that certain accommodations and protections be put in place in the treatment milieu. These legal precedents have thus far done little to change the current practices in inpatient settings as units that allow sexual relationships among hospitalized patients are very rare. Several other pressures appear to exert more of an effect on the expression of sexuality among inpatients.

## Staff Attitudes Toward the Sexual Autonomy of Patients

Practitioners' and other staff members' own attitudes about people with mental illness may influence the degree to which patients' expression of sexuality is encouraged. Evidence suggests that negative attitudes about people with mental illnesses are prevalent among mental health practitioners although in degrees lower than that of the general population (Stuber et al. 2014). Such attitudes include beliefs about the competence and dangerousness of mental health patients and desires for social distance from mental health patients. To the degree that staff members view psychiatric patients as incompetent, they may be less inclined to support policies that encourage sexual autonomy. Similarly, some staff members' fears about the possibility of sexual coercion may be fueled by exaggerated notions about the dangerousness of many psychiatric patients. Staff members' attitudes and resistance to the possibility of sexual autonomy on the psychiatric unit may be similarly consolidated by isolated incidents of challenging sexual behavior that they have witnessed on the unit. Interestingly, these isolated or anecdotal reports of sexual discretion often form the bases for broad generalizations about the sexuality of others with mental illnesses.

As illustrated in the third case vignette, practitioners and other unit staff members do harbor concerns about the clinical implications and potential logistical challenges posed as a result of sexual interactions between patients. A number of studies have documented such concerns including—questions about the decisional capacity of some patients to consent to sexual activity and the potential risk of transmission of sexually transmitted diseases (Brown et al. 2014; Carey et al. 1997; Cole et al. 2003; Mandarelli et al. 2010; Mossman et al. 1997). Decisional capacity in the context of sexual consent remains to be standardized or operationalized; as such, it remains in the purview and discretion of hospital staff members to express their own impressions.

Treatment teams on psychiatric units have differing perspectives about the level of sexual autonomy that should be allowed on a unit. Whereas, some staff members may believe that the potential liability issues that may arise overrides the petition for patient sexual autonomy presents; other staff members subscribe to a level of "responsible risk taking" (McCann 2000). It is our impression that whereas many in the medical disciplines may be inclined to err on the side of safety, many of the rehabilitative disciplines (e.g., social work, peer support) may be more likely to view the expression of sexuality in the context of the individual's aspirations, valued social roles, and recovery context.

In a qualitative study of 14 psychiatric nurses, Quinn et al. (2011) identified four themes around which mental health nurses viewed the sexual health of their patients and their job roles. Specifically, mental health nurses indicated that despite the acknowledgment of the importance of sexuality: (1) discussions of sexuality were avoided unless the patient indicated that they were experiencing a sexual problem; (2) nurses felt that talking about sexuality was not a part of their job description; (3) some nurses felt that sexuality was not a priority for mental health services; and (4) some nurses felt that sexuality of patients was poorly addressed by other mental health practitioners. Earlier research studies similarly suggested that other mental health professionals might incorrectly assume that individuals with diagnoses such as schizophrenia are asexual, are incapable of maintaining meaningful relationships, or that sexual activity would worsen their symptoms (Buckley 1999).

The clinical repercussions of the active avoidance of discourse around issues of sexuality are unclear. In the absence of a discussion about the patient's own sex/relationship goals, practitioners lose an opportunity to give due consideration to how medication effects (including sexual dysfunction, weight gain) may impact those sex/relationship goals. Moreover, such discussions may have provided an opportunity for the provider to elicit the patient's "buy-in" through negotiation and shared decision-making. Thus, the high prevalence of treatment disengagement including medication nonadherence among psychiatric patients (Kreyenbuhl et al. 2009) may be at least partly understood in the context of care providers who are unresponsive to the patient perspective.

Mental health professionals may not be solely responsible for this silence. Maurice and Yule (2010) postulate that the absence of frank discussions with patients about their sexual health results from the "conspiracy of silence" (p. 470) between the professional and patient. This conspiracy of silence refers to the mutual decision between professional and patient to not broach a sensitive topic such as sexuality and sexual health. The conspiracy of silence appears to be particularly prominent in patients without recognized partners, as mental health professionals may not believe that the topic of sexuality is relevant for such patients. Brown et al. (2014) suggested that the absence of frank discussions with patients about their sexual health coupled with the lack of sexual autonomy experienced by patients on the inpatient unit results in a new type of "amputated sexuality" (p. 250). Amputating the sexuality of psychiatric inpatients is convenient for the unit staff striving to maintain order on the unit. On discharge, however, amputating sexuality may attenuate the degree to which patients are able to form intimate relationships after discharge.

## Hospital Policies

Current hospital policies play a large role in the management of sexual expression on the inpatient unit in the United States and abroad. In 1996, the Royal College of Psychiatrists recommended that psychiatric facilities in the United Kingdom develop policies about sexual expression and recommended that these policies have an individualized approach for each institution (Bartlett et al. 2010). More specifically, the Royal College of Psychiatrists (1996) reported, "sexuality and sexual issues are considered a part of individual care plans" (p. 2). Despite the recommendation that psychiatric facilities use an individualized approach to hospital policies about sexuality and emotional relationships, Bartlett et al. (2010) found that most hospitals in the United Kingdom prohibited or actively discouraged the expression of sexuality.

Although most institutions in the UK are prohibitive toward sexual expression, actual written policies varied widely among psychiatric institutions with regard to conjugal visits, expressions of affection, and contraception. For example, some facilities viewed conjugal visits as permissible with the consent of the multidisciplinary team, while other facilities disallowed even physical expressions of affection such as handholding or hugging (Bartlett et al. 2010). Likewise, some facilities allowed patients to obtain condoms with the approval of the treating practitioner, while other facilities viewed condoms as contraband. For the most part, longer term units tended to be more open to patient intimacy than acute units (Apfel and Handel 1993).

One of the first policies ever adopted in the attempt to balance the sexual rights of patients with the logistical and clinical concerns of sexual autonomy was the revised policy of the Riverview Hospital in British Columbia (Welch and Clements 1993). The stated mission of this policy was to equitably balance patients' rights with the duties of the hospital. As such, the policy is broken down into different emphases to help maintain this balance. The first and fourth parts of the policy underscore patients' right to sexual intimacy in a private and dignified setting. These include access to private suites for masturbation or sexual intimacy, sexual health education, counseling, birth control, protection, and erotic materials. The second and third parts of the policy delineate the infrastructure necessary to implement the aforementioned parts of the policy (e.g., privacy suites, access to condoms) and the orientation, treatment, assessment, and treatment protocol for patients experiencing sexual issues (Welch and Clements 1993).

The outcome of this new hospital policy was reviewed following its implementation (Welch et al. 1999). This review identified steps that could be helpful to future hospitals in implementing a similar policy, as well as strategies that would help improve the current policy at Riverview Hospital. Specifically, the strategies suggest that staff should be provided with information about the policy and its implementation in order to reduce resistance from staff. This information dissemination would explicitly explain how the policy would prevent harm to patients by providing safe areas for sexual relations and the assessment of the sexual needs of each patient, and utilizing behavioral techniques (i.e., reinforcement) to be motivated to attend sex education classes (1999).

Although the Riverview Hospital policy was one of the first sexually "less restrictive" policies of its kind to be implemented, the pursuit of sexual autonomy for psychiatric inpatients goes back about four decades. In the 1970s, there were sexual training workshops created to help guide rather than restrict sexuality in inpatients. Research was geared to guide policy formation on the management of sexual relationships between adults with mental illness in residential care were in vogue (Wilson and Baldwin 1976; Torkelson and Dobal 1999). Other policies that have been developed, but not implemented, bear striking similarities to the policy implemented at Riverview Hospital in British Columbia. All of these policies share overarching principles that include: (1) a summary of patient rights; (2) the capacity to provide consent; (3) provision of sex education; (4) specific logistical considerations for masturbation; and (5) the rights of privacy and dignity within consensual sexual relations (Mossman et al. 1997).

The subculture of an institution may have as great an impact on sexual activity on an inpatient unit as the restrictiveness or permissiveness of hospital policies (Buckley et al. 1999). The subculture of each hospital is affected not only by the official hospital policy, but also by factors such as the acuteness and types of mental illness on the unit. Specifically, acute units are more likely to prohibit sexual expression as compared to longer term units. The overall type of unit also appears to have a significant effect on the sexual expression seen on a unit. For example, sexual intercourse between males is most often seen on all male units and masturbation is the most common form of sexual expression on geriatric units (1999). One commonality among all units is the propensity for sexual bartering by patients for items such as food or cigarettes (Buckley et al. 1999).

## Risks Related to Sexual Autonomy on the Inpatient Unit

Common to all of these aforementioned policies is the need to balance patient's rights with the duties of the hospital. Hospitals must balance patients' right to sexual autonomy with the increased risk for sexually transmitted diseases (Carey et al. 1997; Henning et al. 2012), the risk of sexual assault (Barlow and Wolfson 1997; Cole et al. 2003), the ability to consent to sexual activity (Mandarelli et al. 2014), and the clinical impact of sexual activity on an inpatient unit (Bartlett et al. 2010). A summary table of the risks related to sexual autonomy can be seen in Table 3.2.

Unfortunately, individuals with severe and persistent mental illness are at greater risk for sexually transmitted diseases than individuals without psychiatric diagnoses (Lagios and Deane 2007). As with all sexual activity, the potential for the transmission of sexually transmitted diseases remains an area of great concern on an inpatient psychiatric unit. Infection with the human immunodeficiency virus (HIV) in individuals with severe and persistent mental illness has been found to be 10–76 times greater than rates found in the general population (Carey et al. 1997). In addition, syphilis, which may cause or aggravate symptoms of psychiatric disorders, has well-established comorbidity with HIV (Henning et al. 2012). Both the potential for sexual assault and the aforementioned life-changing diseases can further exacerbate psychiatric symptoms, as well as leave the hospital vulnerable to possible litigation if the assault or infection occurs within the inpatient hospital (Farago v. Sacred Heart General Hospital 1989).

The prospects of sexual assault within inpatient psychiatric units, is also perceived by many staff members to potentially increase with the allowance of consensual sexual relationships on an inpatient unit. For example, Cole et al. (2003) surveyed nursing and medical staff members of an adult psychiatric hospital with regard to their perceptions and concerns about sexually active inpatients. Results from this study indicated that 16.7 % of doctors and 28.2 % of nurses were concerned that they would possibly be blamed for an assault. Moreover, there remains the possibility that female patients who form sexual relationships on the unit would be vulnerable to abuse and exploitation (Cole et al. 2003). Of course concerns about sexual assault, abuse, or exploitation are well founded. For example, Barlow and Woflson (1997) found that approximately 56 % of female inpatients surveyed had been sexually harassed or assaulted during their psychiatric hospitalization. Given that the survey had been completed in one hospital in the UK, it is unclear how much unit-specific characteristics, such as staffing levels and unit structure, might have contributed to the rates reported. Moreover, there was no evidence that the program had specific policies regarding sexuality. Notwithstanding the generalizability of the study findings, any loosening of restrictions among patients on psychiatric units should include protections against assault, abuse, and exploitation.

**Table 3.2** Risks related to sexual autonomy on the inpatient unit

| Type of risk | Supporting research |
|---|---|
| Increased risk for sexually transmitted disease | Carey et al. (1997), Henning et al. (2012) |
| Increased risk of sexual assault | Cole et al. (2003), Barlow and Wolfson (1997) |
| Concern about the ability to consent to sexual activity | Mandarelli et al. (2014) |
| Clinical impact of sexual activity on the inpatient unit | Bartlett et al. (2010) |

One protection against the risk of sexual exploitation and abuse is the development of executable guidelines for determining if prospective sexual partners have capacity to consent. Unfortunately, there is no consensus definition or criteria established to determine competence to consent to sexual activity (Mandarelli et al. 2014). Existing capacity determination guidelines have focused on determining capacity to consent to treatment or participate in research. With little emphasis on sexual activity competency determination, no validated instruments have been developed to aid sexual consent capacity determination in psychiatric inpatient settings (Mandarelli et al. 2014). Similar to capacity determination for research and treatment, one may conjecture that factors such as the severity of psychopathology or neurocognitive impairments may be contributors to impaired capacity.

A related question relates to the putative components or areas of consent capacity, which should arguably extend beyond the ability to consent to sexual relations. For example, Noffsinger (1999) indicated that five areas of competencies and consent must be evaluated regarding the patient's capacity: (1) to participate in sexual activity; (2) to give consent for birth control; (3) to consent for abortion; (4) to be considered competent as a parent; and (5) to be considered competent to relinquish parental rights. To our knowledge, there are no established standards or criteria to ascertain the absence of sex-related decisional impairment in inpatients. Should possible contributors like severity of psychiatric symptoms and degree of neurocognitive impairments factor into the positive ascertainment of decisional capacity? Further, should decisional competence for sex be a clinical decision or legal adjudication?

Last, some mental health professionals hold reservations about sexual relationships and other forms of sexual expression on psychiatric units due to therapeutic concerns (Bartlett et al. 2010). Providers may, for example, be concerned that some patients with histories of sexual abuse may be revictimized or possibly become perpetrators of abuse should there be less restrictions on sexual activity on the unit. Some providers may also be concerned that allowing sexual relationships between patients might be counter-therapeutic if such relationships become a source of psychosocial stress (e.g., a break-up, heartache). Such concerns may be founded in some cases, but providing adequate psychotherapy/counseling, psychoeducation, and decision support services may be potential safeguards in sexual decision-making. Moreover, consumers and consumer advocates have criticized such benevolent paternalism as fostering of dependence and disability. From the consumer perspective (e.g., Deegan 1996), people with psychiatric illnesses should be afforded the "dignity of risk" and "the right to fail" much like adults without mental illness, many of whom have engaged in high-risk sexual behaviors, one night stands, experienced heartache, or made decisions about their sexuality and relationships they later regretted.

## Sexuality and Serious Mental Illness

Research focused upon sexuality and mental illness has identified the need for the inclusion of sexuality into the case conceptualization and overall treatment for psychiatric patients, particularly for individuals diagnosed with certain disorders such as anorexia nervosa, schizophrenia, and posttraumatic stress disorder (PTSD) (Garte 1989; Kelly and Conley 2004; Leon et al. 1985). Within the past 10–15 years, some researchers have begun to focus upon the limited expression of sexuality within the inpatient unit and the repercussions of this restriction (i.e. limited relationship skills) following discharge as a result of the paucity of research upon this topic (Brown et al. 2014; McCann 1999; Quinn et al. 2011). In a study conducted with 58 outpatients diagnosed with schizophrenia, 63.3 % of these individuals considered sexuality to be an important aspect of their life (Martin et al. 2003). Moreover, psychiatric patients were found to have sexual experiences close to the general population, except for a higher engagement in riskier sexual behavior, such as decreased condom usage and higher rates of sexually transmitted diseases (Gonzalez-Torres et al. 2010).

Leon et al. (1985) suggested that sexuality and concerns related to interpersonal relationships might be an important aspect of treatment for individuals diagnosed with anorexia nervosa. In addition to overall treatment, sex education and other programs focused upon sexual health may be relevant to such patients due to the changes in body image that may result for treatment-induced weight gain. Moreover, other sex-related changes such as the potential for pregnancy even without the resumption of menstruation may be necessary to cover in sex-related psychoeducation (Balakrishna and Crisp 1998).

A similar emphasis on the inclusion of sexual health programs and treatment options is relevant to the care of people with PTSD. For example, Garte (1989) developed a treatment protocol for Vietnam veterans diagnosed with PTSD that addresses sexual health and intimacy during treatment. The author's rationale was that a core aspect of psychopathology in veterans with PTSD may be incomplete resolution of the Eriksonian psychosocial stage of intimacy versus isolation. Moreover, the author determined that veterans were experiencing significantly more difficulties with sexuality and intimacy than the comparison group. A more recent research study conducted by Sautter et al. (2011) introduced the treatment approach of Structured Approach Therapy, which the researchers conceptualized as a couples-based treatment for PTSD that underscores empathic communication training, stress inoculation procedures, and an overall return to intimacy for OEF/OIF veterans and their partners.

Studies suggest that patients with other psychiatric disorders would similarly benefit from holistic treatment plans that address sexual health (McCandless and Sladen 2003; Ostman and Bjorkman 2013). Although some individuals with schizophrenia may exhibit diminished sexual desire as a result of symptoms of the illness or side effects of medication, individuals with schizophrenia are not sexless as previously thought (Van Sant et al. 2012). Regrettably, some symptoms of schizophrenia do adversely affect both sexuality and intimacy. Positive symptoms of schizophrenia can contribute to difficulty forming intimate relationships due to problems in communicating or interpreting interactions with other people (Hirschberg 1985). Negative symptoms may also affect an individual's relational ability as a result of symptoms such as avolition, social anhedonia, poverty of speech, or isolation (Chapman and Chapman 1973).

Despite these barriers, in a study conducted with individuals diagnosed with schizophrenia, the majority of participants indicated that they were prepared to discuss sexual issues and wanted to engage in counseling that focused upon intimate relationships (Kelly and Conley 2004). Not only does it appear that individuals diagnosed with schizophrenia want psychosocial aspects of their health to be incorporated into their treatment, but approximately 50 % of participants reported that they never or infrequently spoke about their sexual functioning with a mental health provider (Rosenberg et al. 2003).

There is a clear need to address the sexual health of people with schizophrenia and other serious mental illnesses. People diagnosed with serious mental illnesses demonstrate suboptimal sexual health due to a history of sexual abuse, long-term sexual abstinence, poor communication with their mental health provider, and a lack of awareness about sexual health (Matevosyan 2010). They also demonstrate high rates of sexual dysfunction with rates as high as 50 % in men and women with schizophrenia (Dossenbach et al. 2005). Interestingly, there appears to be great discordance between patient and psychiatrist estimations of the prevalence of sexual dysfunction. Psychiatrists overall tend to underestimate the prevalence of sexual dysfunction among schizophrenia patients.

Specific impairments in sexual functioning appear to be associated with the type of mental illness experienced by the individual. Women diagnosed with schizophrenia, depression, and anxiety were likely to endorse low satisfaction from sex, while women with depression reported that they experienced symptoms such as decreased pleasure from the sexual experience and difficulty achieving orgasm (Avellanet et al. 2008). Incidents of physical symptoms associated with sexual dysfunction such as dyspareunia, vaginal dryness, and bleeding after intercourse were most highly rated by women diagnosed with PTSD (Schnurr et al. 2009). For all women with serious mental illness, body mass index appears to partly mediate the effect of psychopathology on impaired sexual functioning. This is because women with serious mental illness are more likely to be overweight or obese than individuals in the general population (Matevosyan 2010).

## Sexual Health and Substance Use

The impact of substance use upon sexual health and sexuality is an important facet of the inpatient care of individuals with serious mental illness. Substance use is particularly problematic, as the rates of substance use are higher in individuals with serious mental illness than individuals in the general population (Bahorik et al. 2013). Moreover, for people with mental illness, substance use is associated with a worsening of their mental health, relapse, and an overall poorer recovery (Bahorik et al. 2013).

The use of alcohol and illicit substances has been linked to sexual dysfunction including inhibited orgasm and painful sexual experiences in general population samples (Johnson et al. 2004; Smith et al. 1984). The rates of illicit substance use-related sexual dysfunction have yet to be, however, documented in mental health populations. One would expect higher rates of substance-related sexual dysfunction in mental health samples relative to the general population given their higher rates of illicit substance use. In a community sample, Johnson et al. (2004) found that 37 % of respondents had used illicit substances or heavily used alcohol, and 26 % of participants reported experiencing sexual dysfunction. These rates may be considered lower limits for rates in mental health samples.

Both individuals in the general population and in the psychiatric population are affected differently based upon the type of substance used. Although alcohol is often perceived by users to be an effective aphrodisiac and sexual facilitator, alcohol actually impairs sexual response (e.g., achieving and maintaining an erection, delayed orgasm). Chronic use of alcohol is associated with testicular atrophy and inhibition of testosterone production and spermatogenesis in men, as well as menstrual irregularities and dyspareunia in women (Pacheco and Esteves 2008; Shamloul and Ghanem 2013).

Much like alcohol, cannabis is perceived by users to have beneficial effects on sex as seen in the perceived increase of sexual pleasure and enhanced orgasm; however, inhibited orgasm is related to the use of cannabis (Smith et al. 2010). Likewise, opioid use has the perceived benefits of delayed ejaculation, but episodes of hypersexuality and premature ejaculation are often observed during opioid withdrawal. In addition, sexual side effects such as delayed ejaculation in men and delayed orgasm in women tend to occur with amphetamine and ecstasy use (Bang-Ping 2009; Peugh and Belenko 2001).

In addition to the effects of substances upon functioning, the sexual health and intimate relationships of individuals who abuse drugs are also affected by substance use. Women who use drugs are more likely to have a sexual partner who also uses drugs, although this same relationship is not seen in men (Pacheco and Esteves 2008). Risky sexual behavior, such as prostitution and decreased condom usage with new sexual partners, occur in higher rates in individuals who use substances (Loxley 1998; Mugisha and Zulu 2004). The use of substances by people with psychiatric illnesses impacts their sexual health and their intimate relationships. Moreover, substance users may demonstrate deficits in social skills necessary to build and maintain positive relationships (Pacheco and Esteves 2008).

In addition to their difficulty in maintaining social relationships and the greater tendency to engage in risky sexual behaviors, individuals who use substances are at greater risk for sexual victimization. Women in particular are at particular risk for sexual victimization, as research indicates that 54–60 % of women seeking substance abuse treatment report having been raped at some point in their lifetime (Dansky et al. 1995). This percentage of victimization is significantly higher than seen in adult women in the general population, as the National Survey of Violence Against Women indicates that approximately 18 % of women in the general population report having experiencing rape at some point in their life (Tjaden and Thoennes 2000).

Women are not the only ones at risk for sexual victimization, as men who use substances are also at greater risk. Specifically, while there is a prevalence rate of male sexual victimization between 3 and 7 % in the general population, research indicates that approximately 16 % of male substance users in an inpatient sample had experienced sexual assault during their lifetime (Bullock and Beckson 2011). Moreover, the risk behaviors of illicit drug use and sexual activity have been found to lead to higher rates of HIV infection in individuals who use substances. Both women and men who use substances are more likely to engage in HIV risk behaviors and to use substances following a diagnosis of HIV (Baum et al. 2009; Keen et al. 2014).

## Sexual Health and Psychotropic Medication

Unfortunately, substance use is not the only factor that impacts the sexual health of individuals with serious mental illness. For many psychiatric patients, their sexual health is negatively affected by both their disorder and the very medication prescribed to treat this disorder (Cutler 2003; Rosenberg et al. 2003). Research has focused heavily upon the role of psychotropic medication and sexual dysfunction due to its association with medication noncompliance, potential reproductive concerns, and overall impact on quality of life (Cutler 2003; Hellewell 2000; McCandless and Sladen 2003; Rosenberg et al. 2003). Sexual dysfunction from medication, whether negatively impacting an individual in one or multiple areas (i.e. libido, arousal, and orgasm), can impair quality of life, cause stigma, poor adherence to medication, physical morbidity, and possibly fatal consequences (Haddad and Sharma 2007).

In particular, many patients taking antipsychotic medications report symptoms associated with sexual dysfunction. Antipsychotics like risperidone act at D2 receptors and their blocking action at these receptors induces hyperprolactinemia. This increased prolactin expression in men subsequently causes decreased libido, erectile dysfunction, and potentially galactorrhea. In women, risperidone may also contribute to sexual dysfunction, infertility, and gynecomastia. Indirectly related to sexual dysfunction, patients taking risperidone are at a greater risk for acute extrapyramidal symptoms, and patients compliant with clozapine and olanzapine are at greater risk for weight gain (Haddad and Sharma 2007).

The awareness of potential side effects of psychotropic medication is important for reducing the rate of medication noncompliance, given that sexual dysfunction occurs as a side effect of treatment with conventional antipsychotics in approximately 50 % of patients diagnosed with schizophrenia (Kelly and Conley 2004). Sexual dysfunction is also one of most commonly cited reasons for medication noncompliance. Rosenberg et al. (2003) found that 43 % of participants diagnosed with schizophrenia reported that they had considered stopping their medication due to sexual dysfunction, while 27.5 % of participants actually had stopped taking their prescribed medication due to perceived sexual side effects. Therefore, patients diagnosed with schizophrenia may not be adherent with their medication regimen despite the effectiveness of atypical antipsychotics in acute schizophrenia and in preventing relapse (Gibson et al. 2013; Haddad and Sharma 2007). Unfortunately, it appears that many mental health nurses and other mental health professionals infrequently inquire about possibly medication-induced sexual dysfunction. This may be due to concerns that the patient would be embarrassed talking about sexual problems or concerns that the knowledge itself of the association between psychotropic medications and sexual dysfunctions may cause medication noncompliance (Haddad and Sharma 2007).

Much like conventional and atypical antipsychotic medications, antidepressants have also been shown to have sexual side effects, with estimates of prevalence of sexual dysfunction in depression ranging from 30–50 % in patients prescribed antidepressant medications (Schweitzer and Chee 2009). The percentages may underestimate the actual proportion of patients who experience antidepressant-induced sexual dysfunction. Selective serotonin reuptake inhibitors (SSRIs) may differ with regard to the degree of sexual dysfunction. For example, paroxetine is more likely to be associated with sexual dysfunction, while fluvoxamine is less likely to be associated with sexual dysfunction (Montejo-Gonzalez et al. 1997; Westenburg and Sandner 2006).

Mood stabilizers and anticonvulsants are commonly used in the treatment of manic episodes and depressive polarity without the exacerbation of other mood episodes (Freeman and Gelenberg 2005). During manic episodes, people with bipolar disorder may be at increased risk for sexual health problems due to impulsivity which drives increased sexual risk taking. High-risk sexual behavior during such episodes could pose potentially devastating consequences on the physical and emotional health of these individuals (McCandless and Sladen 2003). Freeman and Gelenberg (2005) postulated that the rates of unplanned pregnancy may be higher in women diagnosed with bipolar disorder than the rest of the general population. This issue is further complicated by the risk all mood stabilizers carry with pregnancy and delivery, such as the risk of fetal malformation, perinatal complications, and poorer long-term child developmental outcomes (Galbally et al. 2010).

## Influence of Sexual Orientation and Gender in Individuals with Severe and Persistent Mental Illness

Identity plays an important role in the recovery and community reintegration of individuals with severe and persistent mental illnesses after discharge (Martin et al. 2011). Many identities of an individual (i.e. sexual orientation, ethnicity) may influence the treatment received in an inpatient setting as well as the social support received upon reintegration into the community. Salient identities such as being diagnosed with a mental illness, being a member of an ethnic minority group, being of a non-heterosexual orientation, or being a women may elicit stigma that may impact the overall well-being of psychiatric patients (Collins et al. 2008).

Studies with sexual minorities—individuals who self-identify as being of a sexual orientation other than heterosexual— suggest that they may face barriers to treatment or recovery as a result of their sexual identity (Hall 2013; Singer 2004). The first is the limited availability of gay-affirmative mental health services (Singer 2004). This finding is particularly disconcerting as there are high rates of homosexual activity among people with serious mental illness (Perry and Wright 2006). There is indeed a need for more affirmative programs due to the particular vulnerabilities faced by Lesbian/Gay/Bisexual/Transsexual/Questioning (LGBTQ) patients such as harassment or homophobia. Further, treatment should address the interaction between their minority status and mental illness in order to achieve more integrated care (Singer 2004). Many patients choose not to disclose their sexual identity for fear of experiencing rejection or discrimination from staff and/or other patients. Some have suggested that full mental health recovery may be elusive in the absence of a safe environment for the full disclosure of sexual identity (Hall 2013). Transgender patients in particular, face additional barriers to treatment and recovery from serious mental illness due to potential encounters with transphobia during treatment, lack of access to health insurance, and increased rates of suicide, self-harm, and trauma (Mizock and Fleming 2011).

In addition to sexual orientation, other identities may also influence psychiatric patients' full engagement in treatment and their overall recovery. In research conducted with married women on an inpatient unit, participants identified that their marital relationship was strained by stress from sexual difficulties (Martin et al. 2011). Moreover, sexual difficulties experienced by married women was also associated with hostility from friends and family, which may further decrease the social support that plays such a significant role in a successful recovery.

An individual's identity as a woman is also associated with risks and vulnerabilities that are not associated with men (Lyon and Parker 2003). Risks for women with serious and persistent mental illness include a higher risk for assault and sexual trauma. In particular, women with severe mental illness are more likely than women in the general population to have experienced sexual abuse, as rates in the former population range from 34–51 % (Harris 1997). In a study of female inpatients, women with a history of abuse were more likely than women without a history of abuse to exhibit psychotic symptoms, to be diagnosed with borderline personality disorder, and to experience suicidal ideation (Harris 1997).

## Intimacy and Family Life

From the recovery perspective, people with severe mental illnesses are entitled to the pursuit of intimacy, family life, and other valued social roles (Ahmed et al. 2011, 2016). The domains of sexuality and intimacy are often rated by patients to be the lowest in satisfaction of all life domains, listed below work, finance, social relations, leisure, living situation, security, family relations, psychological well-being, and general life satisfaction (Ostman 2014). Psychiatric patients tend to face significant difficulty in finding and maintaining an intimate partner relationship due to poor access to sexual partners, sexual dysfunction, social skills deficits, social anhedonia, dysfunctional attitudes, and difficulty forming relationships (Wright et al. 2007). Although studies have shown that cohabitation is positively associated with satisfaction with sexual relationships; most of the relationships that people with severe mental illness form tend to not lead to either cohabitation or marriage (Eklund and Ostman 2009; Perry and Wright 2006). The relationships of people with serious mental illness are usually considered to be less intimate, in addition to having less commitment (Perry and Wright 2006). Partners of individuals diagnosed with a severe mental illness often take on more responsibility within the relationship and face potential conflicts regarding hospitalization and the acceptance of the presence of a mental illness by their diagnosed partner (Crowe 2004). As such, Crowe recommended that within the mental health community, practitioners address the needs of partners of individuals with mental illness and consider the stability of the relationship as part of the treatment plan.

The stress of mental illness on the partner or family of the individual diagnosed with schizophrenia can influence the patient's prognosis and outcome. In a study conducted with the family members of individuals diagnosed with schizophrenia, approximately 52 % of the families were categorized as having High Expressed Emotion (EE; Miura et al. 2004). High Expressed Emotion in families has been associated with a patient's risk for relapse, as approximately 48 % of patients with schizophrenia who reside within high EE families will relapse as opposed to 21 % of patients in families with low EE (Kavanagh et al. 1997). Therefore, treatment that focuses on assisting family members or partners of individuals diagnosed with schizophrenia is beneficial to both the family and the diagnosed individual.

Most of the services and treatments offered on sexuality for psychiatric patients have focused on risk management as opposed to teaching patients how to work toward positive sexual relationships and emotional intimacy. For example, most sexuality-related interventions have focused upon providing information about prevention regarding sexually transmitted diseases and different contraception methods (Kopelowicz et al. 1999). In other words, treatments have tended to emphasize the behavioral and biological aspects of sexuality rather than the psychosocial aspects of a patient's sexual needs. Perry and Wright (2006) have called for a paradigm shift in how mental health providers view the sexuality of people with serious mental illness by practitioners providing psychosocial rehabilitation to help patients gain skills for both platonic and romantic relationships.

Modern psychosocial treatment interventions provide the opportunity to rehabilitate social skills deficits that are germane to sexual behavior in individuals diagnosed with severe mental illness. These include modules with specific emphasis upon the establishment and maintenance of romantic relationships and intimacy. The UCLA Clinical Research Center for Schizophrenia and Psychiatric Rehabilitation modules help patients learn social and independent living skills (Kopelowicz et al. 1999). The friendship, dating, and sexuality module is particularly salient in its focus on providing individuals with knowledge about sexuality and sexual decision-making. The module targets sexual communication skills such as sharing information with a partner about sexuality, verbal and nonverbal communication before sexual activity, communication after sexual activity, and talking about sexual problems. Similarly, Bellack et al.'s (2004) social skills training manual includes modules for the acquisition and performance of dating skills including asking someone for a date, giving or receiving compliments, refusing unwanted sexual advances, and assertively communicating the need for safe sex. These modules are examples of how sexual health and intimacy can be incorporated into treatment at an inpatient psychiatric hospital by providing practical tools and skills for learning about sexuality and intimacy.

## Reproductive Health and Family Planning

Reproductive health, pregnancy, and family planning are of particular importance in the lives of some patients diagnosed with psychiatric illnesses and their experience of recovery. People with psychiatric illness, however, experience challenges that detract from their reproductive goals. Women with psychiatric illnesses are more likely to experience obstetric complications and other negative obstetrics characteristics during pregnancy, such as a higher rate of unwanted pregnancies, abortions, and miscarriages (Howard et al. 2002). Within mental illnesses, the prevalence of these problems tends to vary based upon the type of disorder. For example, the prevalence of abortions tends to be highest in individuals diagnosed with schizophrenia rather than individuals diagnosed with bipolar disorders, while individuals with bipolar disorder are more likely to have an unplanned pregnancy than individuals with schizophrenia (Ozcan et al. 2014). Women with schizophrenia and other disorders may also experience higher rates of obstetric complications due to lower socioeconomic status (Miller 1997). Perinatal risks have also been identified that are related to lifestyle factors such as illicit drug use, smoking, and alcohol use during pregnancy (Hauck et al. 2008). During pregnancy, patients and their treating physicians must weigh the risk of withholding medication with the risk of prescribing medication during pregnancy. Following delivery, there is an increased risk of an exacerbation of psychotic symptoms in women with schizophrenia during the postpartum period (Green et al. 2008; Miller 1997).

Compared to the general population, people with schizophrenia and other mental illnesses are less likely to be married. Marriage rates among men with schizophrenia are even lower compared to those of women with schizophrenia (Apfel and Handel 1993; Tang et al. 2007). Women with schizophrenia are more likely to be childless than the general population and men with schizophrenia have even higher rates of childlessness (Harley et al. 2010; Haverkamp et al. 1982). Men and women with mental illness may lack dating and relationship skills are necessary to attract prospective sexual partners and negotiate the complexities of sexual relationships. Pregnant women on an inpatient psychiatric unit not only have to deal with these barriers, but may also have to contend with staff perceptions of their pregnancy. For instance, a pregnant woman may be reproached by staff members who hold the view that she should not be a mother, or that her baby should automatically be taken away from her upon birth (Apfel and Handel 1993).

From a comprehensive literature review on the reproductive health of women with serious mental illnesses, Matevosyan (2009) concluded that patients with schizophrenia and mood disorders were more likely to experience reduced fertility and have more lifetime sexual partners. They were also more likely to elicit risky sexual behaviors such as lower rates of contraceptive usage, parenting difficulties, have unwanted pregnancies and abortions, and be at greater risk for the loss of child custody. Higher rates of unwanted pregnancies and abortions seem to be linked to the lower rate of contraceptive usage, as women with serious mental illness tend to experience difficulties using barrier (e.g., condom) and hormonal (e.g., synthetic estrogen and progestins) contraception methods. Due to the lack of compliance and improper use of some contraceptive devices, it has been suggested that implants and long-acting progestins may be the most effective forms of contraception for women with severe mental illness (Matevosyan 2009).

A meta-analysis of the literature on motherhood for women with severe mental illness identified several prominent themes related to their illness, their identity/role, and their child (Dolman et al. 2013). Several themes emerged from the meta-analysis: stigma of being a parent diagnosed with a mental illness, fear of custody loss, and concern over the impact of the mother's mental illness on the child (i.e., genetic risk, environmental, and secondary stigma). Moreover, the research literature identified themes of feelings of isolation, coping with dual identities, and the centrality of motherhood within mothers diagnosed with severe mental illness. From this meta-analysis, it was recommended that there was an increased need for education for mothers about their psychiatric disorder as well as general parenting education. Furthermore, integrated services were seen as necessary for the optimal care of both mother and child in order to address the concerns identified in the aforementioned themes (Dolman et al. 2013).

Pregnancy and motherhood are not the only considerations during the treatment of a woman of reproductive age on an inpatient unit. Studies have examined the effects of the female reproductive cycle upon chronic mental illness and found differences regarding the prevalence of menstrual irregularities, as well as differences in symptom severity based upon the stage of the menstrual cycle (Apfel and Handel 1993; Lande and Karamchadani 2002; Sit et al. 2011). One type of menstrual irregularity, amenorrhea, is thought to be strongly affected by psychosis as approximately 27 % of psychiatric patients experience this condition as compared to approximately 5 % of women in the general population (Apfel and Handel 1993). This menstrual abnormality was found to be higher in women with psychosis prior to the introduction of antipsychotic medication (Bargiota et al. 2013).

The menstrual cycle appears to also influence the mental health of women with severe mental illness. For example, some women may experience more severe psychotic symptoms during certain stages of their menstrual cycle, and their menstrual cycle in general may be affected by electroconvulsive therapy and psychotropic medications (Apfel and Handel 1993). Regular menstruation in a female who had previously experienced an irregular menstrual cycle during her admission on an inpatient unit may be an indicator of potential improvement in her overall symptomology. Postmenopausal women may also require higher doses of antipsychotic medication, as medication levels can vary based upon the menstrual phases or the lack of menstruation (Apfel and Handel 1993). Overall, recovery-based inpatient psychiatric care must be sensitive to issues of gender identity, as well as the desires of the patient for parenthood.

## Conclusion

Human sexuality and sexual health are fundamental rights of all individuals regardless of physical or mental disability. This is the view espoused by proponents of the recovery model. With the advancement of the recovery perspective, there is a need to reexamine current psychiatric practices, which have traditionally been prohibitive of sexual contact among patients.

Recent court rulings and legislation lend credence to a recovery-focused perspective and provide legal precedents to adopt less restrictive policies (Hungerford and Kench 2013).

The adoption of less restrictive policies would signal a shift in focus from pathology and risk management to recovery and patient's rights. However, complications and barriers to sexual autonomy for patients remain a prominent concern. The absolute prohibition of sexuality or physical intimacy mainly appears to occur due to concerns about liability, the risk to patients and staff, logistical concerns about the implementation of a new policy, and therapeutic concerns about the effect of consensual sex upon the hospital milieu (Brown et al. 2014; Carey et al. 1997; Cole et al. 2003; Mandarelli et al. 2010). However, progressive ventures into sexual autonomy have occurred, as seen through less restrictive hospital policies (e.g., Riverside Hospital) and more comprehensive sexual education programs focused on personal sexuality, intimacy, and relationships (e.g., UCLA Friendship, Dating, and Sexuality Module). Once less restrictive policies are in place, hospitals should provide education on sexual health on the inpatient unit as part of a program of psychosocial rehabilitation. Such efforts should include teaching patients about the prevention of sexually transmitted diseases, contraception, family planning, and education about mental health and pregnancy.

Future studies may help to frame better understanding of the impact of severe mental illness on reproductive health. These research studies should be on a larger scale and provide more detailed information through the use of control groups and male patients (Bowers et al. 2014; Ozcan et al. 2013). In addition, more information about how mental health professionals discuss sexuality with their patients will help to further identify barriers and hindrances to the provision of holistic care (Quinn et al. 2011).

## References


Ahmed, A. O., Mabe, P. A., & Buckley, P. F. (2011). Recovery in schizophrenia: Perspectives, evidence, and implications. In M.S. Ritsner (Ed.), *Handbook of schizophrenia spectrum disorders (Vol. III): therapeutic approaches comorbidity and outcomes* (pp. 1–22). New York: Springer.

Ahmed, A. O., Marino, B. A., Rosenthal, E., Buckner, A., Hunter, K. M., Mabe, P. A. et al. (2016). Recovery in schizophrenia: what consumers know and do not know. *Psychiatric Clinics of North America, 39*(2), 313–330.

Apfel, R., & Handel, M. (1993). *Madness and loss of motherhood: Sexuality, reproduction, and long-term mental illness*. Washington, D.C.: American Psychiatric Press Inc.

Avellanet, Y., Ortiz, A., Pando, J., & Romaguera, J. (2008). Relationship between loss of libido and signs and symptoms of depression in a sample of Puerto Rican middle-aged women. *Puerto Rico Health Sciences Journal, 27*(1), 85–91.

Bahorik, A., Newhill, C., & Eack, S. (2013). Characterizing the longitudinal patterns of substance use among individuals diagnosed with serious mental illness after psychiatric hospitalization. *Addiction, 108*, 1259–1269.

Balakrishna, J., & Crisp, A. (1998). A pilot programme of sex education for inpatients with anorexia nervosa. *European Eating Disorders Review, 6*, 136–142.

Bang-Ping, J. (2009). Sexual dysfunction in men who abuse illicit drugs: a preliminary report. *The Journal of Sexual Medicine, 6*(4), 1072–1080.

Bargiota, S., Bonotis, K., Messinis, E., & Angelopoulos, N. (2013). The effects of antipsychotics on prolactin levels and women's menstruation. *Schizophrenia Research and Treatment*, 1–10. doi:10.1155/2013/502697

Barlow, F., & Wolfson, P. (1997). Safety and security. A survey of female psychiatric inpatients. *Psychiatry Bulletin, 21*, 270–272.

Barr, M. (1912). The asexualization of the unfit. The duty of the hour. *Alienist and Neurologist, 33*, 1–9.

Bartlett, P., Mantovani, N., Cratsley, K., Dillon, C., & Eastman, N. (2010). You may kiss the bride, but you may not open your mouth when you do so: Policies concerning sex, marriage, and relationships in English forensic psychiatric facilities. *Liverpool Law Review, 31*, 155–176.

Baum, M., Rafie, C., Lair, S., Page, B., & Campa, A. (2009). Crack-cocaine use accelerates HIV disease progression in a cohort of HIV-positive drug users. *Epidemiology and Social Science, 50*, 93–99.

Bellack, A., Mueser, K., Gingerich, S., & Agresta, J. (2004). *Social skills training for schizophrenia: A step-by-step guide*. New York: The Guilford Press.

Bowers, L., Ross, J., Cutting, P., & Stewart, D. (2014). Sexual behaviors on acute inpatient psychiatric units. *Journal of Psychiatric and Mental Health Nursing, 21*, 271–279.

Brown, S., Reavey, P., Kanyeredzi, A., & Betty, R. (2013). Transformations of self and sexuality: psychologically modified experiences in the context of forensic mental health. *Health, 18*(3), 240–260.

Brown, S., Reavey, P., Kanyeredzi, A., & Batty, R. (2014). Transformations of sex and sexuality: Psychologically modified experiences in the context of forensic mental health. *Health, 18*, 240–260.

Buckley, P. (1999). *Sexuality and serious mental illness*. Amsterdam: Harwood Academics.

Buckley, P., Hogan, M., Svendsen, D., & Gintoli, G. (1999). Dilemmas of managing sexual activity among psychiatric patients. In P. Buckley (Ed.), *Sexuality and serious mental illness* (pp. 21–33). Amsterdam: Harwood Academics.

Bullock, C., & Beckson, M. (2011). Male victims of sexual assault: Phenomology, psychology, physiology. *Journal of the American Academy of Psychiatry and the Law, 39*, 197–205.

Carey, M., Carey, K., Weinhardt, L., & Gordon, C. (1997). Behavioral risks for HIV infection among adults with a severe and persistent mental illness: Patterns and psychological antecedents. *Community Mental Health Journal, 33*(2), 133–142.

Chapman, L., & Chapman, J. (1973). *Disordered thought in schizophrenia*. Englewood Cliffs: Prentice-Hall.

Cole, M., Baldwin, D., & Thomas, P. (2003). Sexual assault on wards: Staff actions and reactions. *International Journal of Psychiatry in Clinical Practice, 7*, 239–242.

Collins, P. (2001). Dual taboos: Sexuality and women with severe mental illness in South Africa. Perceptions of mental health care providers. *AIDS and Behavior, 5* (2), 151–161.

Collins, P., von Unger, H., & Armbrister, A. (2008). Church ladies, good girls, and loss: Stigma and the intersection of gender, ethnicity, mental illness, and sexuality in relation to HIV risk. *Social Science and Medicine, 67*, 389–397.

Crowe, M. (2004). Couples and mental illness. *Sexual and Relationship Therapy, 19*(3), 309–318.

Cutler, A. (2003). Sexual dysfunction and antipsychotic treatment. *Psychoneuroendocrinology, 28*, 69–82.

Dansky, B., Saladin, M., Brady, K., Kilpatrick, D., & Resnick, H. (1995). Prevalence of victimization and posttraumatic stress disorder among women with substance use disorders: Comparison of telephone and in-person assessment samples. *International Journal of Addictions, 30*(9), 1079–1099.

Deegan, P. (1996). Recovery as a Journey of the Heart. *Psychiatric Rehabilitation Journal*, 91–97.

Deegan, P. (1999). Human sexuality and mental illness: Consumer viewpoints and recovery principles. In P. Buckley (Ed.), *Sexuality and serious mental illness* (pp. 21–33). Amsterdam: Harwood Academics.

Deegan, P. & Drake, R. (2006). Shared decision making and medication management in the recovery process. *Psychiatric Services, 57*(11), 1636–1639.

Doak, M. (2000). 'She will never get well while doing anything unnatural': Women's sexual deviance and institutional psychiatry in New York City, 1890–1920. *Dissertation Abstracts International Section A: Humanities and Social Science, 60*(8-A).

Dossenbach, M., Hodge, A., Anders, M., Molnar, B., Peciukaitiene, D., Krupka-Matuszczyk, I. et al. (2005). Prevalance of sexual dysfunction in patients with schizophrenia: International variations and underestimation. *Journal of Neuropsychopharmacology, 8*(2), 195–201.

Dolman, C., Jones, I., & Howard, L. (2013). Pre-conception to parenting: A systematic review and meta-synthesis of the qualitative literature on motherhood for women with severe mental illness. *Archives of Women's Mental Health, 16*, 173–196.

Eklund, M., & Ostman, M. (2009). Belonging and doing: Important factors for satisfaction with sexual relations as perceived by people with persistent mental illness. *International Journal of Social Psychiatry, 56*(4), 336–347.

Farago v. Sacred Heart General Hospital. (1989). 562 A 2d 300 (Penn. 1989).

Foy v. Greenblott (1983) 141 Cal. App. 3d, Court of Appeals of California. Retrieved December 22, 2014 http://law.justia.com/cases/california/court-of-appeal/3d/141/1.html

Freeman, M., & Gelenberg, M. (2005). Bipolar disorder in women: Reproductive events and treatment considerations. *Acta Psychiatrica Scandinavica, 112*, 88–96.

Galbally, M., Roberts, M., & Buist, A. (2010). Mood stabilizers in pregnancy: A systematic review. *The Australian and New Zealand Journal of Psychiatry, 44*, 967–977.

Garte, S. (1989). Sexuality and intimacy in Vietnam veterans with post traumatic stress disorder. *Psychotherapy in Private Practice, 7*(2), 103–112.

Gibson, S., Brand, S., Burt, S., Boden, Z., & Benson, O. (2013). Understanding treatment non-adherence in schizophrenia and bipolar disorder: A survey of what service users do and why. *BMC Psychiatry, 13*(1), 1–12.

Gonzalez-Torres, M., Salazar, M., Inchausti, L., Ibanez, B., Pastor, J., Gonzalez, G., et al. (2010). Lifetime sexual behavior of psychiatric inpatients. *International Society for Sexual Medicine, 7*, 3045–3056.

Green, L., Elliot, S., Anwar, L., Best, E., Tero, M., Sarkar, A., et al. (2008). An audit of pregnant women with severe mental illness referred during the first two years of a new perinatal mental health service. *Archives of Women's Mental Health, 11*, 149–158.

Haddad, P., & Sharma, S. (2007). Adverse effects of atypical antipsychotics: Differential risk of clinical implications. *CNS Drugs, 21*(11), 911–936.
Hall, R. (2013). Working with LGBTQ psychiatric inpatients: A spiritual resource guide. *Dissertation Abstracts International, 73*, 10AE.
Harley, E., Boardman, J., & Craig, T. (2010). Sexual problems in schizophrenia: Prevalence and characteristics. A cross sectional survey. *Social Psychiatry and Psychiatric Epidemiology, 45*, 759–766.
Harris, M. (1997). Modifications in service delivery for women diagnosed with serious mental illness who are also the survivors of sexual abuse trauma. In M. Harris & C. Landis (Eds.), *Sexual abuse in the lives of women diagnosed with serious mental illness* (pp. 3–20). Amsterdam: Overseas Publishers Association.
Hauck, Y., Rock, D., Jackiewicz, T., & Jablensky, A. (2008). Healthy babies for mothers with serious mental illness: A case management framework for mental health practitioners. *International Journal of Mental Health Nursing, 17*, 383–391.
Haverkamp, F., Propping, P., & Hilger, T. (1982). Is there an increase of reproductive rates in schizophrenics? Critical review of the literature. *Archiv fur Psychiatric und Nervenkrankenheiten, 232*, 432–450.
Hellewell, J. (2000). *Tolerability and patient satisfaction as determinants of treatment choice in schizophrenia: A multi-national study of the attitudes and perceptions of psychiatrists toward novel and conventional antipsychotics (poster)*. Presented at the 13th European College of Neuropsychopharmacology Congress, Munich, Germany.
Henning, M., Kruger, C., & Fletcher, L. (2012). Syphilis sero-positivity in recently admitted and long-term psychiatric inpatients: Screening, prevalence, and diagnostic profile. *South African Journal of Psychology, 18*(4), 171–175.
Hirschberg, W. (1985). Social Isolation among schizophrenic out-patients. *Social Psychiatry, 20*(4), 171–178.
Howard, L., Kumar, C., Leese, M., & Thornicroft, G. (2002). The general fertility rate in women with psychiatric disorders. *The American Journal of Psychiatry, 159*, 991–997.
Hungerford, C., & Kench, P. (2013). The perceptions of health professionals of the implementation of Recovery-oriented health services: a case study analysis. *Journal of Mental Health Training, Education, and Practice, 8*(4), 208–218.
Johnson, S., Phelps, D., & Cottler, L. (2004). The association of sexual dysfunction and substance use among a community epidemiological sample. *Archives of Sexual Behavior, 33*(1), 55–63.
Kavanagh, D., O'Halloran, P., Manicavasagar, V., Clark, D., Piatkowska, O., & Tennant, C. (1997). The family attitude scale: Reliability and validity of a new scale for measuring the emotional climate of families. *Psychiatry Research, 70*, 185–195.
Keen, L., Dyer, T., Whitehead, N., & Latimer, W. (2014). Binge drinking, stimulant use and HIV risk in a sample of illicit drug using heterosexual Black men. *Addictive Behaviors, 39*(9), 1342–1345.
Kelly, D., & Conley, R. (2004). Sexuality and schizophrenia: A review. *Schizophrenia Bulletin, 30*(4), 767–779.
Kopelowicz, A., Mangano, R., & Caine, M. (1999). Teaching individuals with serious mental illness about friendship, dating, and sexuality. In P. Buckley (Ed.), *Sexuality and serious mental illness* (pp. 21–33). Amsterdam: Harwood Academics.
Kreyenbuhl, J., Nossel, I. R., & Dixon, L. B. (2009). Disengagement from mental health treatment among individuals with schizophrenia and strategies for facilitating connections to care: A review of the literature. *Schizophrenia Bulletin, 35*(4), 696–703.
Lagios, K., & Deane, F. (2007). Severe mental illness is a new risk marker for blood-borne viruses and sexually transmitted infections. *Australian and New Zealand Journal of Public Health, 31*(6), 562–566.
Lande, R., & Karamchadani, V. (2002). Chronic mental illness and the menstrual cycle. *Journal of the American Osteopathic Association, 102*(12), 655–659.
Leon, G., Lucas, A., Colligan, R., Ferdinand, R., & Kamp, J. (1985). Sexual, body image and personality attitudes in anorexia nervosa. *Journal of Abnormal Child Psychology, 13*, 245–258.
Loxley, W. (1998). *Young injecting users and the risk of HIV/aids: Psychosocial and environmental constraints on safer drug using and sexual behavior.* Perth, Australia: National Centre for Research into the Prevention of Drug Abuse, Curtain University of Technology.
Lyon, D., & Parker, D. (2003). Gender-related concerns of rural women with serious and persistent mental illnesses. *Archives of Psychiatric Nursing, 27*(1), 27–32.
Mandarelli, G., Parmigiani, G., Tarsitani, L, Polselli, G., Biondi, M., & Ferracuti, S. (2010). Competence to give informed consent in acute psychiatric hospitalizations. Preliminary results for a case-control study. *European Psychiatry, 25*, 691–691.
Mandarelli, G., Zangaro, S., Raja, M., Azzoni, A., Tatarelli, R., & Ferracuti, S. (2014). Competence to consent to sexual activity in bipolar disorder and schizophrenia spectrum disorders. *Archives of Sexual Behavior, 41*, 507–515.
Martin, N., Vega, F., & Montejo, A. (2003). Sexualidad y salud mental. In A. Montejo (Ed.), *Sexualidad y salud mental* (pp. 117–127). Barcelona: Glosa.
Martin, L., Perlman, C., & Hirdes, J. (2011). Social relationships and activities among married psychiatric inpatients with sexual difficulties. *Journal of Sex and Marital Therapy, 37*, 307–322.
Matevosyan, N. (2009). Reproductive health in women with serious mental illnesses: A review. *Sexuality and Disability, 27*, 109–118.

Matevosyan, N. (2010). Evaluation of perceived sexual functioning in women with serious mental illnesses. *Sexuality and Disability, 28*, 233–243.

Maurice, W., & Yule, M. (2010). Sex and chronic mental illness. In S. Levine (Ed.), *Handbook of clinical sexuality for mental health professionals* (2nd ed., pp. 469–481). New York: Routledge.

McCann, E. (1999). The expression of sexuality in people with psychosis: breaking the taboos. *Journal of Advanced Nursing, 32*, 132–138.

McCandless, F., & Sladen, C. (2003). Sexual health and women with bipolar disorder. *Journal of Advanced Nursing, 44*(1), 42–48.

McCann, E. (2000). The expression of sexuality in people with psychosis: Breaking the taboos. *Journal of Advanced Nursing, 32*(1), 132–138.

Miller, L. (1997). Sexuality, reproduction, and family planning in women with schizophrenia. *Schizophrenia Bulletin, 23*(4), 623–635.

Miura, Y., Mizuno, M., Yamashita, C., Watanabe, K., & Murakami, M. (2004). Expressed emotion and social functioning in chronic schizophrenia. *Comprehensive Psychiatry, 45*(6), 469–474.

Mizock, L., & Fleming, M. (2011). Transgender and gender variant populations with mental illness: implications for clinical care. *Professional Psychology: Research and Practice, 42*(2), 208–213.

Montejo-Gonzalez, A., Llorca, G., & Izquierdo, J. (1997). SSRI-induced sexual dysfunction: Fluoxetine, paroxetine, sertraline, and fluvoxamine in a prospective, multicenter and descriptive clinical study of 344 patients. *Journal of Sex and Marital Therapy, 23*, 176–194.

Mossman, D., Perlin, M., & Dorfman, D. (1997). Sex on the wards: Conundra for practitioners. *Journal of the American Academy of Psychiatry and the Law, 25*(4), 441–460.

Mugisha, F., & Zulu, M. (2004). High prevalence of high-risk behavior and the identification of predictors for sharing injecting materials among young drug users in Prague, Czech Republic. *Central European Journal of Public Health, 4*, 228–235.

Noffsinger, S. (1999). Sex and mental illness: Legal considerations. In P. Buckley (Ed.), *Sexuality and serious mental illness* (pp. 21–33). Amsterdam: Harwood Academics.

Ostman, M. (2014). Low satisfaction with sex life among people with severe mental illness living in a community. *Psychiatry Research, 216*, 340–345.

Ostman, M., & Bjorkman, A. (2013). Schizophrenia and relationships: The effect of mental illness on sexuality. *Clinical Schizophrenia and Related Psychoses, 7*(1), 20–24.

Ozcan, N., Boyacioglu, N., Enginkaya, S., Dinc, H., & Bilgin, H. (2013). Reproductive health in women with serious mental illness. *Journal of Clinical Nursing, 23*, 1283–1291.

Ozcan, N, Boyacioglu, N., Enginkayas, S., Dinc, H., & Bilgin, H. (2014). Reproductive health in women with serious mental illnesses. *Journal of Clinical Nursing, 23*(9/10), 1283–1291.

Pacheco, P., & Esteves, M. (2008). Drugs of abuse and sexual functioning. In E. Balon (Ed.), *Sexual dysfunction: The brain-body connection* (pp. 131–149). Switzerland: Karger.

Perlin, M. (2008). Everybody is making love/or else expecting rain: Considering the sexual autonomy rights of persons institutionalized because of mental disability in forensic hospitals and in Asia. *Washington Law Review, 83*(4), 481–512.

Perlin, M., Birgden, A., & Gledhill, K. (2009). 'The witness who swore he left little doubt': a comparative consideration of expert testimony in mental disability law cases in common and civil law systems. *Journal of Investigative Psychology and Offender Profiling, 6*(1), 59–88.

Perry, B., & Wright, E. (2006). The sexual relationships of people with serious mental illness. *Journal of Sex Research, 43*(2), 174–181.

Peugh, M., & Belenko, S. (2001). Alcohol, drugs, and sexual function: A review. *Journal of Psychoactive Drugs, 33*, 223–232.

Quinn, C., Happell, B., & Browne, G. (2011). Talking or avoiding: Mental health nurses' views about discussing sexual health with consumers. *International Journal of Mental Health Nursing, 20*, 21–28, 150–161.

Rosenberg, K., Bleiburg, K., Koscis, J., & Gross, C. (2003). A survey of sexual side effects among severely mentally ill patients taking psychotropic medication: Impact on compliance. *Journal of Sex and Marital Therapy, 29*(4), 289–296.

Royal College of Psychiatrists. (1996). *Sexual abuse and harassment in psychiatric settings*. London: Royal College of Psychiatrists.

Sautter, F., Armelie, A., Glynn, S., & Wielt, D. (2011). The development of a couple-based treatment for PTSD in returning veterans. *Professional Psychology: Research and Practice, 42*(1), 63–69.

Schnurr, P., Lunney, C., Fordshay, E., Thurston, V., Chow, B., Resick, P., et al. (2009). Sexual function outcomes in women treated for posttraumatic stress disorder. *Journal of Women's Health, 10*, 1549–1557.

Schweitzer, K., & Chee, N. (2009). Sexual side-effects of contemporary anti-depressants: Review. *The Australian and New Zealand Journal of Psychiatry, 43*(9), 795–808.

Shamloul, R., & Ghanem, H. (2013). Erectile dysfunction. *The Lancet, 381*(9861), 153–165.

Singer, M. (2004). Being gay and mentally ill: The case study of a gay man with schizophrenia treated at a community mental health facility. *Journal of Gay and Lesbian Psychotherapy, 8*(3/4), 115–125.

Sit, D., Seltman, H., & Wisner, K. (2011). Menstrual effects on mood symptoms in treated women with bipolar disorder. *Bipolar Disorders, 13*, 310–317.

Smith, D. E., Wesson, D. R., & Apter-Marsh, M. (1984). Cocaine and alcohol-induced sexual dysfunction in patients with addictive diseases. *Journal of Psychoactive Drugs, 16*(4), 359–361.

Smith, A. M. A., Ferris, J. A., Simpson, J. M., Shelley, J., Pitts, M. K., & Richters, J. (2010). Cannabis use and sexual health. *The Journal of Sexual Medicine, 7* (2pt1), 787–793.

Stuber, J., Rocha, A., Christian, A., & Link, B. (2014). Conceptions of mental illness: attitudes of mental health professionals and the general public. *Psychiatric Services, 65*(4), 490–497.

Tang, Y., Gillespie, C., Epstein, M., Mao, P., Jiang, F., Chen, Q., et al. (2007). Gender differences in 542 Chinese inpatients with schizophrenia. *Schizophrenia Research, 97*(1–3), 88–96.

Tjaden, P., & Thoennes, N. (2000). *Extent, nature, and consequences of intimate partner violence: Findings from the National Violence Against Women Survey*. Washington, D.C: National Institute of Justice.

Torkelson, D., & Dobal, M. (1999). Sexual rights of people with serious and persistent mental illness: Gathering evidence for decision making. *Journal of the American Psychiatric Nurses Association, 5*(5), 150–161.

UN General Assembly. (2007). *Convention on the rights of persons with disabilities: Resolution/adopted by the General Assembly*, January 24, 2007, A/RES/61/106. Available at: http://www.un.org/disabilities/convention/conventionfull.shtml. Accessed July 5, 2014.

Van Sant, S., Ahmed, A., & Buckley, P. (2012). Schizophrenia, sexuality, and recovery. *Journal of Ethics in Mental Health, 7*, 1–5.

Welch, S., & Clements, G. (1993). Development of a policy on sexuality for hospitalized chronic psychiatry patients. *Canadian Journal of Psychiatry, 41*, 273–279.

Welch, S., Clements, G., & Moreau, M. (1999). Developing and implementing a policy for consensual sex between patients. In P. Buckley (Ed.), *Sexuality among patients with serious mental illness*. Amsterdam: Harwood Academic Publishers.

Westenburg, H., & Sandner, C. (2006). Tolerability and safety of fluvoxamine and other antidepressants. *International Journal of Clinical Practice, 60*, 482–491.

Wilson, R., & Baldwin, B. (1976). A pilot sexuality training workshop for staff at an institution for the mentally retarded. *American Public Health Association, 66*(1), 77–78.

Wright, E., Wright, D., Perry, B., & Foote-Ardah, C. (2007). Stigma and the sexual isolation of people with serious mental illness. *Social Problems, 54*(1), 78–98.

# 4 Teaching Clinicians the Practice of Recovery-Oriented Care

P. Alex Mabe, Michael Rollock and Gina N. Duncan

## Introduction

Since the 1990s, the advocacy of recovery-oriented practices in mental health care has been gaining considerable traction worldwide. In contrast to the traditional model of mental health care that focuses on reduction of symptoms and restoration of individuals to premorbid levels of functioning, this emerging model of care places the emphasis on recovery as a restoration of individuals to meaningful lives regardless of the ongoing presence of mental illness (Davidson et al. 2009; Davidson and Roe 2007). This new recovery model, often referred to as personal recovery, acknowledges and attends to the suffering related to mental illness, but contextualizes clinical symptoms within the larger picture of what it means to be human. That is, it emphasizes the wholeness, strengths, cultural identity, and striving for meaning that individuals with mental illness share in common with their peers in the population as a whole. Within the past 10 years, virtually every mental health professional and advocacy organization in the United States has endorsed the recovery model of mental health care.

The adoption of this new model of mental health care has been a primary mission of the Substance Abuse and Mental Health Services Administration (SAMHSA). In 2009, the Center for Mental Health Services (CMHS), Office of the Associate Director for Consumer Affairs within SAMHSA, contracted with Developmental Services Group, Inc. (DSG) to launch a 5-year Recovery to Practice (RTP) initiative to translate the vision of recovery into the practice of mental health professionals of all disciplines (Davidson and Dain 2010). In 2004, the Department of Veterans Affairs initiated a 5-year action plan for the transformation of the Veterans Administration mental health services into recovery-oriented services (Greenberg and Rosenheck 2009). The enthusiasm that has been driving the ascendance of the recovery movement appears to focus its emphasis on: (1) broader treatment goals and measures of success that extend beyond symptom reduction (e.g., hope, empowerment, and life satisfaction); (2) a truly collaborative relationship between the clinician and the consumer of services; and (3) the inclusion of individuals with mental illness, their family members, and advocacy groups as members of the treatment team (Peebles et al. 2007).

Supported by national policies, professional organization endorsements, and mental health advocacy groups the push to explicitly train the mental health workforce in recovery-oriented approaches has certainly been gaining momentum. As a consequence, several training initiatives

P. Alex Mabe (✉) · M. Rollock · G.N. Duncan
Department of Psychiatry and Health Behavior, Medical College of Georgia, Augusta University, 997 St. Sebastian Way, Augusta, GA 30912, USA
e-mail: amabe@gru.edu



N.N. Singh et al. (eds.), *Handbook of Recovery in Inpatient Psychiatry*, Evidence-Based Practices in Behavioral Health, DOI 10.1007/978-3-319-40537-7_4

have been developed to bring about mental health care system transformation. Most of these initiatives, however, have focused on broad organizational and procedural changes as well as hospital and clinic staff development. Unfortunately, in the promotion of recovery-oriented care relatively little attention has been focused on the training of clinicians. Consequently, it is not surprising that surveys of the key providers of mental health services including psychiatrists, psychologists, and social workers suggest that they have little familiarity with the recovery literature and hold mixed beliefs regarding the feasibility and utility of recovery-oriented practice (e.g., Hardiman and Hodges 2008). It is proposed that if recovery-oriented care is to be effectively implemented, as proposed by recent national policies and endorsements, the clinicians engaged in such work need to be taught the key principles, processes, and practices of recovery-oriented care.

This chapter addresses the formidable challenge by first examining recent reports of efforts to teach recovery-oriented care and then presenting a conceptual model based on the theoretical and empirical literature pertaining to effective methods of teaching and implementing changes in patient care practices. It should be noted that the conceptual model for teaching recovery-oriented care was borne out of the efforts of Project Georgia Recovery-based Educational Approach to Treatment (GREAT) that represents a 7-year programmatic initiative to transform the Department of Psychiatry and Health Behavior at the Augusta University (formerly the Medical College of Georgia) into a department that fully embraces the recovery orientation to mental health care. Similar to the initiatives of the Recovery Education in the Academy Program (REAP) at the University of Illinois, Chicago (Razzano et al. 2010), Project GREAT aspired to influence the education and practice of a diverse array of trainees and practitioners including clinical staff and faculty, medical students, nursing students, psychiatry residents, psychology predoctoral interns, and postdoctoral fellows. The primary focus of Project GREAT as well as the focus of this chapter, however, has been to develop strategies to shape the recovery knowledge, attitudes, and practices of clinicians in the fields of psychiatry and psychology.

While there is no overarching blueprint for recovery-oriented care, there appears to be an emerging consensus regarding the fundamental nature of personal recovery and the processes that clinicians can facilitate to support recovery in both outpatient and inpatient settings. Thus, it is believed that the processes and methods that are proposed to teach recovery-oriented care to clinicians have a broad applicability to the various clinical contexts in which psychiatric care is provided.

## Outcome Studies of Recovery Training for Clinicians

Published reports regarding the impact of recovery training for clinicians have been extremely limited and have primarily entailed survey studies and prepost quasi-experimental design studies. Survey studies regarding the impact of any recovery training experiences on mental health staff have generally reported positive outcomes of recovery training that have included: (1) improved optimism regarding patient outcomes (Tsai et al. 2010, 2011); (2) higher overall personal optimism (Tsai et al. 2011); (3) greater sense of agency recovery attitudes (Tsai et al. 2010, 2011); and (4) higher levels of recovery-oriented competencies when more in-depth training was provided (Stuber et al. 2014a). Though details regarding the types of trainings examined in these survey studies were lacking, Tsai et al. (2010) reported in their survey of staff in two-state psychiatric hospitals that those who received specific, practical training as opposed to more general, inspirational training had a greater increase in agency recovery attitudes.

A limited number of examinations of recovery-oriented workshops have been reported that have ranged from 2–4 days of recovery-oriented care training. The content of these recovery workshops has been remarkably similar in their inclusion of teaching the participants recovery principles, promoting attitudes that support recovery-oriented care (e.g., eliminating stigmatizing views of individuals with mental illness, viewing patients as equal partners in their care), and introducing recovery-oriented practices such as self-directed goal-setting, identifying patients' strengths, and methods for instilling hope. The format and techniques utilized were also found to cut across several of the training programs examined and included group discussion and problem solving, demonstrations, role play/skill building exercises, and the sharing of recovery narratives. Most of the workshops included participation by individuals with a lived experience of mental illness as trainers; a strategy bolstered by the core message of empowerment advocated in recovery-oriented care and research findings that have indicated the benefits of using consumer trainers (e.g., Cook et al. 1995).

Overall, the outcome findings for recovery workshops have consistently demonstrated that improved knowledge of recovery principles and practices are quite achievable (Crowe et al. 2006; Gilburt et al. 2013; Meehan and Glover 2009; Peebles et al. 2009; Salgado et al. 2010; Wilrycx et al. 2012). In addition, findings support the position that beliefs and attitudes supportive of recovery-oriented care can be measurably enhanced through workshop trainings. These include attitudes of general hopefulness and optimism regarding recovery (Salgado et al. 2010), the belief that individuals with mental illness have skills and competence and are capable of participating in their own care (Peebles et al. 2009), and beliefs that individuals with mental illness are capable of setting and achieving goals even if symptoms are present (Crowe et al. 2006). It is noteworthy, however, that in their examination of a two-day recovery workshop, Peebles et al. (2009) indicated that while attitudes of hopefulness regarding recovery and beliefs about individuals' ability to participate actively in their own care did increase, more stigmatizing attitudes such as beliefs that patients should be feared, pitied, and/or avoided, were not impacted by the workshop. This suggests that further work needs to be done to explore techniques or approaches that impact both positive and negative recovery attitudes.

In their examination of a four-day recovery workshop and an in-team half-day session on supporting recovery, Gilburt et al. (2013) found that providers' knowledge, attitudes, and preliminary clinical practices were all positively impacted. Specifically, this workshop included the topic of assessment and care planning from service users' perspective, and in an audit of the care plans of 700 patients, it was reported that the clinicians who participated in the workshop made significantly more changes to their plans consistent with service users' perspectives than clinicians who did not participate in the workshop. Gilburt et al. (2013) further described qualitative findings pertaining to the impact of recovery workshops on the participants. They conducted 16 team leader interviews following their four-day workshops and an in-team session on supporting recovery. In these interviews, the training was highly rated with over half of the interviewees favoring mandated recovery training. Most viewed the training as leading to staff consideration of areas of care that emphasized improvement more so than just maintaining the patients' current mental status. Also in a positive direction were attitudes that hope was a universally positive value that was integral to mental health care. There were, however, problematic reactions to the training experience. For example, following the training there continued to be confusion about what recovery meant, and many members of the staff believed that they "already did recovery." Furthermore, following the training, many framed recovery as something primarily driven by staff, failing to appreciate the role of service users. While multidisciplinary services were considered a valuable aspect of recovery-oriented care, a prevailing attitude was that when physicians were not on-board, they could be barriers to recovery-oriented care. Many interviewees noted that recovery-oriented care was often seen as conflicting with, rather than complementing, the overarching roles of the service agency (e.g., "moving people on"). Finally, interviewees expressed doubts concerning the availability of resources to actually implement recovery-oriented care.

Efforts to successfully transfer or incorporate training into practice have been a longtime aspiration of those who seek to bring about the sustained implementation and application of new knowledge, skills, and attitudes in clinicians. Yet, trainers have often been left feeling disappointed about the degree of integration of the principles and practices in various settings. In regard to recovery-oriented care training, Uppal et al. (2010) examined the transfer of training impact of an initial two-day recovery training workshop, followed by one-day booster sessions between 6 and 12 months later. A core aspect of the recovery training was the use of collaborative goal-setting and collaborative homework assignments. In chart audits conducted six months after the individual training, approximately 37 % of the trained clinicians participating in the study were found to be implementing collaborative goal-setting and collaborative homework assignments in clinical practice. Moreover, the average time taken to implement these recovery practices was 5.6 months following training. Thus, it was concluded that transfer of recovery training in the form of recovery workshops followed by booster sessions may be difficult to achieve in clinical practice.

Deanne et al. (2014) examined the benefits of adding individual coaching for a 12-month period following the initial workshop trainings. The study compared the results of monthly coaching consisting of either an emphasis on skills acquisition training or transformational coaching that focused on clinicians' personal values versus promotion of personal growth and/or professional development. Chart audits examining the use of collaborative goal-setting indicated that coaching in general, even though the study implementation only achieved coaching sessions approximately every two months, was able to improve transfer of training over workshops alone. There was some trend that the transformational coaching was somewhat superior in achieving clinicians' use of care planning than the skills acquisition coaching.

The empirical study of recovery training is clearly in its infancy. Of the few published reports, the content and teaching techniques used to teach recovery-oriented care have been quite similar, but often lacked detail in regard to rationale and theory. The studies that do report outcomes of efforts to train clinicians in recovery-oriented care have generally reported positive results in terms of gains in recovery knowledge and attitudes, and initial steps toward recovery-oriented practice. It should be pointed out that this initially positive view of recovery-oriented training needs to be tempered by the relative absence of strong methodological designs used to study recovery training outcomes and initial findings that effective transfer of training to practice should not be assumed.

These initial studies also suggest that barriers to the adoption of recovery-oriented practice are evident and include clinician confusion about the principles and practice of recovery-oriented care as well as institutional issues, such as lack of resources, and an agenda that may not be compatible with recovery-oriented care (e.g., "moving people on"). In this early phase of "research and design" of recovery training, the unavoidable conclusion is that there is, as yet, no empirically based implementation strategy specific to training clinicians in effective applications of the recovery model. Nevertheless, there is valuable research and conceptual literature pertaining to effective methods of teaching and implementing changes in patient care practices that can be readily applied to the development of recovery-oriented care training.

## Designing a Recovery-Oriented Care Training Model

As suggested by Stuart et al. (2004), education and training in health care is best viewed as a teaching-learning process, and in our consideration of this process we will now examine: (1) the content that need to be taught; (2) the characteristics of the targeted learners that would influence the teaching-learning process; (3) the characteristics of the training providers that would best facilitate desired outcomes; and (4) general teaching strategies designed to promote adoption of recovery-oriented care.

## The Content that Needs to be Taught

***Knowledge of Recovery***. It is uncontroversial to suggest that any recovery-oriented training ought to teach the foundational principles of recovery. More controversial, however, is just what those foundational principles are. Since the inception of recovery-oriented care, there have been numerous disparate attempts to conceptualize, categorize, and define what is meant by recovery. Historically, the concept of recovery emanated from two distinct forces (Davidson and Roe 2007). One argument for rethinking traditional views of mental health care has been based on the accumulating evidence that the course of even serious mental illness is not inevitably negative. In fact, many people with serious mental illness can and do recover to levels that allow them to resume productive and meaningful lives even in the presence of enduring symptoms (Davidson et al. 2009). Moreover, these recoveries are not always brought about by traditional forms of mental health care, but often entail efforts independent of standard forms of treatment such as medications or psychotherapy (Davidson et al. 2009). From this clinical focus on people's illness and dysfunction, there has been an emphasis on recovery being related to traditional clinical outcomes of amelioration or remission of symptoms.

A second argument pertains to the fundamental dissatisfaction with what consumers of mental health care characterize as paternalistic and stigmatizing care. Beginning in the late 1980s, a consumer movement arose in opposition to traditional mental health care and proposed that the emphasis on illness and dysfunction generated feelings of helplessness and hopelessness (Bellack 2006). In addition, it was argued that traditional care often placed patients in highly dependent roles in which personal choice and strengths were often overlooked. In response to these assertions against traditional mental health care, the concept of recovery became associated with processes that emphasized an empowerment approach to care that acknowledges the right to individual choice, equal partnership in care, and the pursuit of meaningful lives even in the context of illness. Slade (2009) differentiated between these two perspectives of recovery, with the former representing *clinical recovery* and the latter representing *personal recovery*. The teaching of recovery may benefit from the adoption of both of these ostensibly contrasting views of recovery. From an educational perspective, two arguments can be made for the use of both clinical and personal recovery concepts. First, adult learners come to learner situations with pre-existing knowledge and experiences that frame their expectations and influence their facility in learning new information. When there is an interaction between existing knowledge and new knowledge or skills, training success tends to be more likely (Lyon et al. 2011). In the context of training clinicians, it can be anticipated that teaching the concept of clinical recovery as a component of recovery-oriented care would validate their prior knowledge and skill, and make them more comfortable in expanding their view of recovery. Second, learners are more likely to be motivated to learn new knowledge or skills when it becomes clear that existing practices are inadequate (Lyon et al. 2011). By presenting both clinical and personal recovery concepts, the learner begins with the familiar understanding of recovery, but then can begin to see the insufficiency of clinical recovery in contrast to personal recovery that promotes a focus on the process of recovery (e.g., a way of living a satisfying, hopeful and meaningful life even with the limitations imposed by illness). Davidson et al. (2009) described this complementary approach to the concept of recovery and noted that the addition of recovery in a personal sense highlights that people do recover from mental illness and many more find meaning in the face of enduring illness.

A commonly used definition of recovery comes from SAMHSA (2006), initially defining mental health recovery as "a journey of healing and transformation enabling a person with a mental health problem to live a meaningful life in a community of his or her choice while striving to achieve his or her full potential." Along with this definition, SAMHSA listed ten fundamental components of recovery: self-direction, individualized and person-centered, empowerment, holistic, nonlinear, strengths based, peer support, respect, responsibility, and hope. In 2012, SAMHSA offered a new working definition of recovery from mental disorders and/or substance use disorders, emphasizing that recovery is "[a] process of change through which individuals improve their health and wellness, live a self-directed life, and strive to reach their full potential (Paragraph 5)." In this updated definition of recovery, SAMHSA further delineated four dimensions that support recovery: health, home, purpose, and community. Though efforts to comprehensively define and elucidate the multiple pathways, processes, outcomes, and characteristics of a life in recovery are both necessary and laudable, it is the very breadth and heterogeneity of this construct that pose significant challenges to those who seek to educate about the principles and resulting practices associated with recovery. Specifically, critical reviews of the educational research that informs the teaching of clinicians have indicated that in terms of content, "Less is more" (Stuart et al. 2004; Van der Vleuten et al. 2000). That is, the less complex and more concise the material being taught, the more that will be attained and applied to clinical practice. For example, even a basic change, such as attempting to get health care providers to practice proper standards of hand washing, has proven to be quite difficult (Grol and Grimshaw 2003). Therefore, effective teaching of recovery-oriented practice must incorporate this "less is more" educational principle.

Leamy et al. (2011) provided a systematic review of 366 papers that explicitly described or developed a conceptualization of personal recovery. In so doing, they arrived at a narrative synthesis that sought to define the overarching processes of personal recovery, the acronym of which is CHIME: **C**onnectedness (e.g., being a part of a community, having relationships, receiving support from others); **H**ope and optimism about the future; **I**dentity (e.g., rebuilding/redefining positive sense of identity, overcoming stigma); **M**eaning in life (e.g., meaningful life goals and social roles, quality of life); and **E**mpowerment (e.g., personal responsibility, control over life, and focusing on strengths).

We believe that these recovery processes are sufficiently representative of the domain of personal recovery while also being succinct thus making them a teachable model of recovery that can readily inform clinical practice.

***Attitudes***. Attitudes generally reflect a mental disposition and readiness that, for clinicians, can significantly influence reactions to and actions with individual with mental illness. Many leaders in the field contend that the concept of recovery fundamentally reflects an attitude about people with mental illness (e.g., Davidson et al. 2009; Resnick et al. 2005). Clinicians who hold positive attitudes toward recovery are more likely to promote empowerment and encourage an optimistic approach to the treatment of mental illness (Corrigan 2002). Thus, implementing recovery-oriented care requires clinician attitudes that support patient rights and empowerment. Through our examination of conceptual writing in the extant literature on recovery, as well as commonly used measures of recovery-oriented attitudes, the following attitudes emerge as key targets for recovery teaching efforts:

1. Recovery is a civil right of the individual to access and join in those elements of community life that the person chooses and to be in control of his or her own life, including making choices about one's own health care.
2. Stigma toward individuals with mental illness is a significant part of the illness experience and thus should be addressed by clinicians as it exists in the community and within the system of mental health care.
3. Individuals with mental illness are capable of being full partners in their own mental health care and they should be empowered to achieve their own recovery.
4. Recovery can be difficult and its course will vary among people.
5. Risk taking is an inevitable part of recovery processes and willingness to take risks is an essential aspect of empowering people to take control of their lives.

6. Recovery is possible. It should be emphasized that a general sense of hopefulness about recovery being possible is an essential attitude to be held by clinicians and to be fostered in individuals collaborating in their care.

***Clinician Competencies***. While knowledge of recovery principles and processes along with attitudes supportive of recovery are foundational, recovery-oriented care will not take root unless clinicians change their practice in some fashion. In the absence of evidence-based recovery practices, the current state of the field is represented by various attempts to define clinician competencies that are necessary for recovery-oriented care. Lakeman (2010) conducted an online Delphi survey of experts in mental health recovery and identified 18 top-ranked recovery competencies of which the top five were (p. 62):

1. A competent mental health worker recognizes and supports the personal resourcefulness of people with mental illness.
2. To work in a recovery-focused way, mental health workers need to reflect a belief that recovery is possible.
3. To work in a recovery-focused way, mental health workers need to be able to listen to what service users are actually saying and respect their views.
4. To work in a recovery-focused way, mental health workers need to reflect respect for the expertise and unique knowledge gained as a result of having experienced mental health problems.
5. A competent mental health worker helps persons in recovery to develop belief in themselves, thereby promoting their ability to help themselves.

Le Boutillier et al. (2011) conducted a qualitative analysis of international recovery-oriented practice guidelines and found 16 dominant themes within the following four practice domains (p. 1474):

1. Promote citizenship—support individuals with mental illness to reintegrate into society and live as equal citizens.
2. Organizational commitment—organizational commitment to ensure that there is a work environment and service structure that promotes recovery-oriented practice.
3. Support personally defined recovery—there is a focus on supporting personally defined recovery and viewing recovery as the heart of clinical practice.
4. Working relationship—clinician interactions demonstrate a genuine desire to support individuals and their families to fulfill their potential and shape their own future.

We view both of these aggregating efforts to establish practice competencies as meaningful at the broad policy and organizational level, though generally lacking in the specificity needed for the clinician in the field who is attempting to translate knowledge of recovery processes into competencies that they can learn to support recovery. Also, these proposed general competencies do not meet the educational principle of "less is more" and thus will likely be viewed by clinicians as too complex and time-consuming to be adopted in any meaningful way. In order to effectively teach recovery-oriented practice to clinicians, the competencies to be taught should meet the following criteria: (1) the competency conceptually links to one of the five core processes described in the CHIME model of personal recovery (see Leamy et al. 2011); (2) the competency can be readily integrated with the tasks generally focused on in clinical as opposed to personal recovery; and (3) the competency can be practiced within the usual time constraints of patient encounters.

As outlined in Table 4.1, we provide the competencies chosen by Project GREAT to be taught as an illustration of how these criteria may be applied. The competencies provided are not intended to be comprehensive or necessarily reflective of an optimal list of competencies for all mental health care settings. We contend, however, that the list of competencies suggested is sufficiently parsimonious, teachable, and adaptable to a variety of clinical contexts, from inpatient psychiatric settings to outpatient community clinics. Through our iterative efforts to disseminate and enhance recovery knowledge, attitudes, and practices via Project GREAT, we have discovered that even our own competency

**Table 4.1** Clinician recovery-oriented competencies to be taught

| Recovery process (Leamy et al. 2011) | Competency to be taught |
|---|---|
| Connectedness (e.g., being a part of a community, having relationships, receiving support from others) | 1. Conducting social support assessments<br>2. Making referral to and working with peer support specialists |
| Hope and optimism about the future | 1. Teaching recovery as a nonlinear process<br>2. Using hope inducing strategies (see Snyder et al. 2000) |
| Identity (e.g., rebuilding/redefining positive sense of identity, overcoming stigma) | 1. Conducting whole person assessments<br>2. Promoting advocacy |
| Meaning in life (e.g., meaningful life goals and social roles, quality of life) | 1. Conducting ongoing life goal assessments that inform treatment goals and care plans<br>2. Using quality of life measures for treatment monitoring |
| Empowerment (e.g., personal responsibility, control over life, and focusing on strengths) | 1. Conducting ongoing strengths assessments<br>2. Routinely engaging in shared decision-making |

recommendations pose instructional challenges that require significant time, effort, feedback, and consistently honed teaching skills to execute training effectively. It is our hope that the proposals that we advance in this chapter will be of benefit to those seeking to impact learners in a personally meaningful manner that brings about sustained change in their recovery-oriented practices.

## Characteristics of the Targeted Learners

Recovery-oriented care requires a fundamental shift in how clinicians address mental health care. Analysis of the targeted learners suggests three core features of clinicians that would need to be addressed to effectively teach them recovery-oriented care.

***Indoctrinated in Traditional Views of Illness and Mental Health Care***. Most clinicians hold core beliefs about mental illness and its treatment that are likely to be hindrances to the adoption of the transformative model of recovery. In traditional conceptualizations of mental illness, it is the clinician that is "the expert" and thus has primary responsibility for defining and "curing" illness. The focus on intervention begins with an accurate diagnosis formed by an assessment of symptoms and concludes with interventions designed to cure or ameliorate symptoms associated with the underlying illness.

From a recovery orientation, however, such a myopic view of mental illness neglects to consider that healing can entail more than the elimination or reduction of symptoms, and can touch on such profound issues as finding purpose and meaning in life even while experiencing the demands and stresses of mental illness. Traditional models of care maintain that the "nature of healing" lies in scientifically derived interventions designed and implemented by the expert to address the underlying etiology of mental illness. Though collaboration may be emphasized as an important component of the clinical strategy, the clinical recovery lens leans heavily on adherence to the prescribed treatment devised by the expert. Inevitably, this view of mental health care makes it difficult for clinicians to connect with other realties such as the importance of patients' sense of ownership about their own recovery, their strengths, their resources, and healing actions that they might take that lie outside those prescribed by the clinician.

As is readily apparent, the teaching of clinicians in recovery-oriented care must necessarily encourage an expansion beyond traditional views of illness and associated treatments to fully embrace the possibility that satisfying and meaningful lives entail more than just the reduction or elimination of symptoms. Moreover, the practice of mental health care must acknowledge that there truly are two experts in the room that can and should share the responsibility for defining problems and devising pathways to recovery.

Finally, it is important to note that the traditional model of mental health care has been founded on the clinicians' sense of duty to reduce risks for their patients. For example, the Hippocratic oath compels doctors to avoid doing harm to their patients, and medical risk management strategists advise against any practice that might risk an increase in symptoms or risk for relapse. Playing safe and avoiding risks are routinely taught and practiced in traditional models of care. Initial introductions to recovery-oriented care are often met with concerns by clinicians that the risks are too great to allow patients to make decisions about their own care when their judgment is impaired. They express fears associated with the possible risks to their patients' wellbeing and their own professional liability should "bad" decisions be made. In contrast, recovery-oriented care must encourage clinicians to view self-determination and choice as patient rights that are an integral pathway to recovery. Moreover, individuals should be encouraged to take risks in the service of seeking opportunities for a life with greater purpose and meaning, even though making such efforts might result in an increase in stress and symptoms (see Davidson et al. 2006).

***Stigmatizing Attitudes***. Attitudinal surveys have suggested that clinicians have greater support for the civil rights of their patients and generally more positive attitudes toward individuals with mental illness than the general public. Yet, many clinicians also hold stigmatizing attitudes such as beliefs that individuals with mental illness are more dangerous and less capable than those without mental illness (Schulze 2007; Stuber et al. 2014b; Wahl and Aroesty-Cohen 2010). Moreover, clinicians commonly appear to be quite similar to the general public in regard to a "them versus us" attitude in which they view individuals with mental illness as socially undesirable and people to be avoided (Schulze 2007; Stuber et al. 2014b; Wahl and Aroesty-Cohen 2010). Unfortunately, such negative beliefs are likely to make it quite difficult for clinicians to fully engage with their patients as equal partners and have hopeful attitudes of achieving clinical or personal recovery.

The implications for the educator attempting to instill recovery-oriented principles and practices in clinicians are that stigmatizing attitudes must be identified and targeted for intervention. Based on research findings (e.g., Corrigan 2004; Corrigan et al. 2012; Rüsch et al. 2005; Wood and Wahl 2006), we propose the following efforts to diminish problems of stigma among clinicians: (1) education that identifies stigmatizing attitudes and provides information that counters misunderstandings regarding individuals with mental illness; (2) self-reflection and perspective taking that increase understanding for and empathy with individuals with mental illness; and (3) contacts with individuals with mental illness in contexts in which their competencies and general social desirability are manifest. At the very least, consumers should play active roles in recovery instruction of clinicians.

***Adult Learners***. Educational theory and research has pointed out that methods in teaching adults need to take into account their unique characteristics that distinguish them from children or adolescent learners. Based on representative theory and research in the field of health professional training (Bowen 2006; Bussema and Nemec 2006; Davies 2000; Stuart et al. 2004; Zisook et al. 2005), the following instructional strategies are advised in teaching clinicians recovery-oriented care:

1. Adults have a foundation of life experiences and knowledge, and by drawing out connections of this existing data bank to the new knowledge, attitudes, and skills to be learned, adoption of the new material is facilitated. For example, the skills developed by clinicians in the context of developing treatment goals would be quite relevant for learning the skills required in developing life goals. More specifically, assessment of life goals and treatment goals require steps to turn general

ideas into actions and behaviors, and both require specification of goals that can be addressed in the short-term as well as the long-term.
2. Adults are relevancy oriented and thus they will need to see the reason for learning something. For example, the teaching of the nonlinear nature of recovery is more likely to be perceived as relevant by clinicians when the presentation of this concept includes clinical vignettes that illustrate problems of symptom relapse that may lead to premature termination of treatment by their patients.
3. Adults are goal-directed, and thus instruction must show participants how the learning experience will help them attain their goals. For the clinician who is trained with a focus on clinical recovery, the complementary nature of clinical recovery and personal recovery could be emphasized. Considering relapse problems, clinicians will be more inclined to embrace the teaching of the nonlinear when it is emphasized that patients that are better informed about the ups and downs of recovery are more likely to sustain treatment efforts and bounce back from relapses of symptoms.
4. Adults tend to be autonomous and self-directed in their learning style, and thus respond better to active learning. Consequently, clinicians are more likely to be engaged in learning recovery-oriented practices when there is a sense of challenge and active learning through Socratic questions, clinical vignettes are presented that pose problems to be solved, and skill practice are components of instruction.

## The Characteristics of the Instructors

Learning recovery-oriented care entails more than merely transferring knowledge about recovery principles and practices. Integral to the practice of recovery-oriented care are the emotions and attitudes that have been compelling forces in the recovery movement. Therefore, the effectiveness of teaching recovery-oriented practice requires careful attention to the characteristics of the messenger and not just the message.

***Provider-Driven Training*.** Educational research has consistently demonstrated that effective teachers are knowledgeable, establish clear goals of the instruction, and are able to present key information in an organized fashion using familiar and understandable language (Sutkin et al. 2008; Towler and Dipboye 2001). Moreover, effective teachers are generally approachable, open-minded, show patience and respect for students, care about students' success and are fair, show enthusiasm and humor, and intentionally engage with their students to establish rapport (Benson et al. 2005; Sutkin et al. 2008).

In clinical contexts, the experience and expertise of the instructor play important roles in eliciting the attention of learners and helping them learn and retain knowledge and skills obtained during instruction (Burke and Hutchins 2008; Sutkin et al. 2008). Research has yet to be conducted on those characteristics of instructors that may effectively teach recovery-oriented care. On conceptual grounds, and based on Project GREAT's experience in disseminating recovery-oriented care training over the past seven years, we propose the following additional characteristics of effective instructors:

1. It is important to have instructors with similar educational and clinical experiences as those of the learners in order to maximize the relevance of the instruction being provided. Instructors with doctoral training in the mental health field and practical experience in the provision of mental health care have the advantage of familiarity with the existing knowledge, beliefs, attitudes, and practices of the learners targeted. With this knowledge of the learners, the content can be presented in an effective manner.
2. Clinical teaching in general is demanding, and those who do it well have passion for their work as well as a high level of technical skill (Bussema and Nemec 2006; Irby and Papadakis 2001; Stuart et al. 2004). Likewise, the effective teaching of recovery-oriented

care requires passion to convey the emotions and attitudes that are the compelling force behind the recovery movement. Therefore, to train others in recovery-oriented care, the instructor must possess a strong conviction of its worth and have the ability to stimulate serious contemplation of the fallibilities of traditional models of mental health care, while inspiring a heartfelt desire to do more for those facing the challenges of mental illness. The outcome of the recovery instruction will rely heavily on the ability of the instructor to passionately convey the message and to share inspiring stories that move clinicians toward recovery-oriented care.

3. Finally, instructors who have personally experienced the process of transformation from a traditional model of mental health care to a recovery-based one are more likely to be more persuasive models of and advocates for recovery-oriented care. With this personal experience of professional practice change, the instructor would have the advantage of having a greater appreciation for the challenges involved in systems and practice change, and thus could better direct the learner in addressing these challenges. Moreover, a coping model of a clinician/instructor who has actively engaged in and succeeded in transforming his or her practice into a recovery model can be a valuable change agent.

***Consumer-Driven Training***. Recovery-oriented care champions the individuality of the lived experience and the ownership of the recovery process (Oades et al. 2005). Individuals with a lived experience of mental illness have valuable insights that can contribute to the development of curriculum and influence presentation of the recovery process (Young et al. 2005). Research has suggested that by involving consumers in mental health education both positive knowledge and attitude change can be enhanced (Happell et al. 2014; Wood and Wahl 2006). In addressing diverse problems with stigma/prejudice/discrimination, there is accumulating evidence that exposure to the stigmatized group can reduce adverse attitudinal and social responding problems (Wood and Wahl 2006).

Individuals with a lived experience of mental illness are not only helpful in teaching clinicians principles and practices of recovery, but also absolutely essential in addressing matters of attitude (e.g., perceptions of consumer competence and social desirability). By presenting competent consumers articulately telling their recovery stories, clinicians will begin to form more positive impressions of consumers and their ability to collaborate in their care. Moreover, by encouraging consumer educators to contrast their traditional psychiatric care experiences with recovery care experiences, clinicians would have "real" examples of the potential value of the recovery-oriented care. Consumer involvement in the education of clinicians can also better ensure that the curriculum content is responsive to the needs and goals of those individuals who use mental health services.

The use of consumer-driven education is not without some potential problems. For example, if consumers have limited teaching roles then they may experience a sense of tokenism in the educational enterprise and likewise clinician participants may devalue the consumer's potential contributions while maintaining a "them versus us" attitude. Moreover, if presentations by individuals with mental illness are adversarial toward mental health professionals and/or reflect poor communication skills, then attitudes toward recovery-oriented care with its emphasis on collaborative care would be adversely affected. Therefore, we would propose the following qualifications and preparations to maximize the contribution of consumer-driven training:

1. Consumer educators must have meaningful lived experiences with mental illness so that insights regarding the impact of mental illness and associated interventions can be shared with clinicians in an effective manner. Communication regarding these experiences may include negative experiences with clinicians, but these negative experiences should not be the sole message. In other words, consumer educators should be encouraged to convey a

positive message of hope regarding recovery-oriented care as opposed to merely taking the opportunity to be critical of past encounters with clinicians.

2. Consumer educators must also have meaningful recovery stories that they can effectively articulate in a manner that demonstrates how embracing recovery processes can lead to positive life outcomes. They certainly do not emphasize stories of clinical recovery and, in fact, consumer educators may be even more effective in their message when they present not as "expert models" but as "coping models" who continue to be challenged by mental illness, but demonstrate the courage and competence to achieve personal recovery.
3. Consumer educators and professional instructors need to model a collaborative approach to the teaching of recovery-oriented care such that the learners can appreciate the reality that there are "two experts in the room," and both appreciate and use the expertise of the other.
4. As is the case with instructors, the effectiveness of consumer educators will rely heavily on their skills in gaining rapport with the learner, technical competence in teaching, and passion for recovery-oriented care. However, merely being an individual with a compelling recovery story is insufficient for the broader enterprise of teaching recovery-oriented care. Consumer educators also need to learn to appreciate the challenges that clinicians face, to recognize how clinicians think, to develop patience and diplomacy with those clinicians who have difficulty understanding and adopting recovery principles and practices, and to learn effective strategies for influencing clinicians' attitudes and behaviors.

## General Teaching Strategies

Attempting to achieve the transformative changes in clinicians' knowledge, attitudes, and clinical practice behavior as advocated by the recovery approach to mental health care is a daunting enterprise. As Bussema and Nemec (2006, p. 315) stated, "… making lasting changes in the behavior of mental health practitioners is astoundingly difficult, and implementing new practices in mental health systems is painfully slow." Moreover, there is no empirically based general teaching strategy specific to recovery-oriented care training. There is, however, valuable research literature pertaining to effective methods of teaching and implementing changes in patient care practices that can be applied to the teaching of recovery-oriented care. In examining original studies and systematic reviews regarding interventions to change medical practices across disciplines, the most robust and consistent finding has been that single teaching strategies are ineffective in changing practice behaviors (Grol and Grimshaw 2003; Lyon et al. 2011). Instead, changes in medical practice are more likely when multiple strategies are implemented (Chow et al. 2009; Grol and Grimshaw 2003). On the basis of a narrative review of the effectiveness of various teaching strategies in changing clinical practice as well as consideration of the resource and time feasibility of implementing teaching strategies within traditional mental health settings, we propose the following five general strategies for teaching recovery-oriented care.

***Workshops and Courses***. Despite evidence of its modest effectiveness, direct instruction of recovery-oriented practice through workshops or courses likely represents a necessary though insufficient strategy for teaching recovery. Effective recovery workshops and courses should have the following characteristics:

*Content that needs to be taught*. The content of instruction should adhere to the "less is more" principle in which complexity is reduced as much as possible. The concepts of clinical recovery (i.e., "recovery from") and personal recovery (i.e., "recovery in") should be taught as legitimate components of clinical practice, although the insufficiency of sole attention to clinical recovery should be highlighted. In addition to recovery principles and processes, instruction should also explicitly address clinician attitudes and competencies that are needed to support recovery-oriented care.

*Characteristics of the targeted learners.* Indoctrinated in traditional views of mental illness and care, clinicians should be instructed in a more expanded view of care that recognizes the possibility of a satisfying and meaningful life even when patients are experiencing ongoing psychiatric symptoms. Furthermore, the value of and civil right to receive a collaborative model of mental health care should be emphasized. Clinicians should be challenged to recognize and directly address their own stigmatizing views of the individuals that they serve. In the endeavor to teach adult learners, recovery instruction should acknowledge and use clinicians' existing knowledge and experiences, make the case for the clinical relevance of recovery processes and practices, link recovery instruction with clearly articulate clinician goals, and employ active learning strategies such as discussion questions, problem solving around case vignettes, and skill practice.

*Characteristics of the instructors.* Both clinicians and individuals with lived experience with mental illness and its treatment best deliver instruction in recovery. In addition to having skills in engaging with and teaching adult learners, both professional instructors and consumer educators need to be knowledgeable, experienced, and passionate regarding recovery-oriented care. Furthermore, the professional instructors and consumer educators need to be able to effectively model respect for one another and a collaborative partnership in the teaching endeavor.

***Coaching.*** As previously noted, one of the few empirical findings regarding efforts to train clinicians in recovery-oriented care demonstrated that the addition of individual coaching enhanced the transfer of recovery knowledge into practice (Deane et al. 2014). In this strategy, the instructor meets with the individual clinician in the work setting and offers feedback and instruction directly related to the clinician's attitudes and behavior. Thus, coaching not only provides more specific and direct feedback to the learner, but also it extends the time of instruction and provides instruction within the highly relevant context of actual clinical practice (Lyon et al. 2011). In addition, coaching provides an opportunity for the instructor to address the clinician's questions and ambivalence about adopting new clinical practices and supporting the clinician's morale and engagement in the adoption of recovery-oriented practice (Lyon et al. 2011).

***Reminders/Prompts.*** Research has indicated that prompts to engage in recommended practice habits can be effective in implementing clinical care changes (Grol and Grimshaw 2003; Lyon et al. 2011; Stuart et al. 2004). Point-of-care reminders or prompts are provided in the context of routine practice and can be issued in the form of written or electronic communications. For example, Project GREAT has used worksheets provided to patients that inquire about their life goals and strengths that are to be shared with their clinicians. Thus, clinicians are reminded by their patients of the importance of obtaining and using such information that is vital to recovery-oriented care. Project GREAT also embedded prompts for recovery-oriented care in the electronic health care record so that all documentation of care templates includes recovery-relevant information. Of course, the most effective reminders or prompts require a response from the clinician (e.g., acknowledging a receipt of information or documenting that a certain practice was performed) and, with the increasing use electronic records, the technology is available to insure that clinicians are at least responding to recovery-oriented care reminders/prompts.

***Audit and Feedback.*** This strategy entails periodic audits of clinician's professional practice along with feedback offered to the clinician with accompanying benchmarks or peer comparisons. The feedback may or may not include practice recommendations to guide the clinician's future behavior. Research has suggested that audit and feedback may be most effective when there is significant room for improvement, the person responsible for the audit and feedback is a supervisor or colleague, the process is repeatedly provided, feedback is provided in both verbal and written forms, and feedback includes clear targets for action (Ivers et al. 2012). As an example of how this might be applied to the teaching of recovery-oriented care, Project GREAT took advantage of the audit and feedback system within the institution which consisted of a routinely administered patient satisfaction survey. Specifically, we have been able to revise the departmental patient satisfaction measure to better assess recovery-oriented care by including the five-item Empowerment subscale of the Recovery-Promoting Relationship Scale (Russinova et al. 2006). Patient satisfaction information can be used as a training tool for individual clinicians as well as used as a metric for monitoring overall progress in the implementation of recovery-oriented care in the department.

***Mass Media Communications in the Form of Newsletters/Pamphlets***. Mass media campaigns have been used to modify health knowledge, attitudes, and behaviors in the general population using a variety of social marketing strategies. These efforts have realized promising outcomes in changing clinician behaviors as well (Grol and Grimshaw 2003). For example, mass media campaigns have had positive impact in reducing excessive antibiotic dispensing (Butler et al. 2012). From the perspective of training clinicians, the premise is that broad efforts to change patients' behavior can result in changes in clinicians' behavior. In the context of recovery-oriented care, transformation of knowledge, attitudes, and behaviors in clinicians can be greatly enhanced by changes in individuals that they serve. That is, by teaching the consumer about the processes of personal recovery, the manner in which they relate to their clinicians and their positive engagement in their own care could be quite influential on the practice of clinicians.

SAMHSA's Recovery to Practice initiative provides an excellent example of a program that broadly disseminates recovery-oriented information through an online centralized information center that has the potential to impact how clinician's use recovery processes and practices in their care as well as how consumers of mental health services participate in their care. Project GREAT has employed two teaching strategies along this line. First, a newsletter entitled "Taking Flight" is broadly distributed to patients and clinicians providing a recovery story as well as instruction on recovery processes and practices. Second, a patient pamphlet is distributed at the time of the initial appointment entitled, "Making the Most of Your Care." This pamphlet provides basic information about the clinic and the services available, and also instructs patients on an active and collaborative approach to their own care.

## Conclusion

Despite the broad advocacy for recovery-oriented care, there are significant challenges to the teaching and implementation of a recovery orientation to mental health care. In addition to the challenges imposed by the complexities of defining recovery-oriented care, the traditional views of mental illness and treatment as well as ongoing stigmatizing attitudes of clinicians, there are practice stresses that will likely limit the efforts of teaching recovery-oriented care. For example, time with the doctor is limited and has been steadily decreasing over the past 20 years across all of medicine and specifically in psychiatric care (Olfson et al. 1999). For the most part, there is an insufficient workforce to provide the mental health care that is needed for our society today, and thus caseloads of existing mental health workers are quite high, limiting the time needed for training in recovery-oriented care.

Moreover, it is not surprising that psychiatric practice appears to be drifting toward primarily psychopharmacological management with precious little time available to address such recovery matters as identifying life goals relevant for treatment or identification and utilization of consumer strengths and supports to achieve life goals. That "health care comes at a price," has also been increasing over the past 20 years (Rowan et al. 2013). Though mental health care is more than just a commodity that responds predictably to market pressures, the reality is that the financial price tag for recovery-oriented care must be addressed.

Systems adopting the recovery model of care have to consider how to pay for the training and how to get reimbursement for what, at present, does not fall into the traditional forms of psychiatric care (e.g., peer specialist services and psychoeducational training in wellness activities versus traditional services that are reimbursed—

diagnostic assessments, medication management, and psychotherapy). In addition, the mental health care system has been persistently "underfunded and undermanned" (Appelbaum 2002) and, as a result, the mental health system has by and large become focused on crisis stabilization and does not aspire to longer term goals that are the focus of recovery. Unfortunately, this crisis stabilization focus likely perpetuates and at times exacerbates the deteriorating patterns of more frequent and more severe relapses, further driving the focus of care toward symptom reduction rather than the development of sustained efforts to develop and build upon the broader goals of developing a life of meaning and purpose.

Overcoming these challenges to the teaching and implementation of recovery-oriented care will require administrative leadership and support. Written policies that promote recovery-oriented practice and even the hiring of peer specialists can represent only token measures that ultimately fail to achieve the cultural changes needed. Instead, there will need to be administrative leadership that promotes an organizational mission and vision that truly embraces recovery and commits the necessary capital to recovery-oriented training and practice. Administrative leadership will also be needed to build a consensus among the clinicians in a system of care that values recovery and believes that the goals of recovery can be achieved. Essential will be administrative steps to integrate consumers as full partners in the education of clinicians including roles of designing recovery-oriented curricula and providing teaching to clinicians. Finally, administrative leadership is needed to balance the organization's need to reduce risk and contain cost with the higher calling of giving individuals, facing the challenges of mental illness the hope that a recovery journey can be achieved that offers worth and meaningful connections with others.

We have learned through Project GREAT that exposure to recovery stories can be a powerful tool in overcoming the challenges facing recovery-oriented care. While we embrace the value of using empirical evidence to support the design and implementation of teaching strategies to support the adoption of recovery-oriented care, we have learned that personal recovery stories can inspire genuine change in clinicians' attitudes and practice behaviors. Inherent in these recovery stories are a deeper understanding of the lived experiences of those facing the challenges of mental illness. Inherent in their telling is an authenticity that recovery is "real" and not just an aspiration drawn from the more abstract principles of recovery. Moreover, recovery stories convey struggles and emotions that stir up affect in the learner that can more effectively influence beliefs, attitudes, and behaviors than mere presentation of recovery principles. And, for clinicians and patients alike, recovery stories provide vivid pictures of coping models that did not easily provide recovery-oriented care or overcome the challenges of mental illness. And yet in those stories can be found partners in care who had the courage and determination to endure hardships and setbacks in order to achieve lives of purpose and meaning.

## References


Appelbaum, P. S. (2002). Starving in the midst of plenty: The mental health care crisis in America. *Psychiatric Services, 53*(10), 1247–1248.

Bellack, A. S. (2006). Scientific and consumer models of recovery in schizophrenia: Concordance, contrasts, and implications. *Schizophrenia Bulletin, 32*(3), 432–442.

Benson, T. A., Cohen, A. L., Buskist, W., Gurung, R. A., Cann, A., Marek, P., et al. (2005). Faculty forum. *Teaching of Psychology, 32*(4), 237–270.

Bowen, J. L. (2006). Educational strategies to promote clinical diagnostic reasoning. *New England Journal of Medicine, 355*(21), 2217–2225.

Burke, L. A., & Hutchins, H. M. (2008). A study of best practices in training transfer and proposed model of transfer. *Human Resource Development Quarterly, 19* (2), 107–128.

Bussema, E., & Nemec, P. (2006). Effective teaching. *Psychiatric Rehabilitation Journal, 29*(4), 315–317.

Butler, C. C., Simpson, S. A., Dunstan, F., Rollnick, S., Cohen, D., Gillespie, D., & Evans, M. R. (2012). Effectiveness of multifaceted educational programme to reduce antibiotic dispensing in primary care: Practice based randomised controlled trial. *British Medical Journal, 344*, d8173.

Chow, C., Cichocki, B., & Leff, H. S. (2009). The support for evidence-based training strategies. *Psychiatric Rehabilitation Journal, 33*(2), 156–159.

Cook, J. A., Jonikas, M. J. A., & Razzano, L. (1995). A randomized evaluation of consumer versus nonconsumer training of state mental health service providers. *Community Mental Health Journal, 31*(3), 229–238.

Corrigan, P. (2004). How stigma interferes with mental health care. *The American Psychologist, 59*(7), 614–625.

Corrigan, P. W. (2002). Empowerment and serious mental illness: Treatment partnerships and community opportunities. *Psychiatric Quarterly, 73*(3), 217–228.

Corrigan, P. W., Morris, S. B., Michaels, P. J., Rafacz, J. D., & Rüsch, N. (2012). Challenging the public stigma of mental illness: A meta-analysis of outcome studies. *Psychiatric Services, 63*(10), 963–973.

Crowe, T., Deane, F., Oades, L., Caputi, P., & Morland, K. (2006). Effectiveness of a collaborative recovery training program in Australia in promoting positive views about recovery. *Psychiatric Services, 57*(10), 1497–1500.

Davidson, L., & Dain, D. (2010). *Recovery to practice—Project overview*. Retrieved November 16, 2011, from http://www2.dsgonline.com/rtp/webinar_materials/Handout%201.6.8.10.pdf

Davidson, L., Drake, R. E., Schmutte, T., Dinzeo, T., & Andres-Hyman, R. (2009). Oil and water or oil and vinegar? Evidence-based medicine meets recovery. *Community Mental Health Journal, 45*(5), 323–332.

Davidson, L., O'Connell, M., Tondora, J., Styron, T., & Kangas, K. (2006). The top ten concerns about recovery encountered in mental health system transformation. *Psychiatric Services, 57*(5), 640–645.

Davidson, L., & Roe, D. (2007). Recovery from versus recovery in serious mental illness: One strategy for lessening confusion plaguing recovery. *Journal of Mental Health, 16*(4), 459–470.

Davies, P. (2000). Approaches to evidence-based teaching. *Medical Teacher, 22*(1), 14–21.

Deane, F. P., Andresen, R., Crowe, T. P., Oades, L. G., Ciarrochi, J., & Williams, V. (2014). A comparison of two coaching approaches to enhance implementation of a recovery-oriented service model. *Administration and Policy in Mental Health and Mental Health Services Research, 41*, 660–667.

Gilburt, H., Slade, M., Bird, V., Oduola, S., & Craig, T. K. (2013). Promoting recovery-oriented practice in mental health services: A quasi-experimental mixed-methods study. *BMC Psychiatry, 13*, 167–178.

Greenberg, G. A., & Rosenheck, R. A. (2009). An evaluation of an initiative to improve Veterans Health Administration Mental Health Services: Broad impacts of the VHAs mental health strategic plan. *Military Medicine, 174*(12), 1263–1269.

Grol, R., & Grimshaw, J. (2003). From best evidence to best practice: Effective implementation of change in patients' care. *The Lancet, 362*(9391), 1225–1230.

Happell, B., Byrne, L., McAllister, M., Lampshire, D., Roper, C., Gaskin, C. J., & Lakeman, R. (2014). Consumer involvement in the tertiary-level education of mental health professionals: A systematic review. *International Journal of Mental Health Nursing, 23* (1), 3–16.

Hardiman, E., & Hodges, J. (2008). Professional differences in attitudes toward and utilization of psychiatric recovery. *Families in Society, 89*(2), 220–227.

Irby, D. M., & Papadakis, M. (2001). Does good clinical teaching really make a difference? *The American Journal of Medicine, 110*(3), 231–232.

Ivers, N., Jamtvedt, G., Flottorp, S., Young, J. M., Odgaard-Jensen, J., French, S. D., et al. (2012). Audit and feedback: Effects on professional practice and healthcare outcomes. *Cochrane Database Systematic Review, 6*.

Lakeman, R. (2010). Mental health recovery competencies for mental health workers: A delphi study. *Journal of Mental Health, 19*(1), 62–74.

Le Boutillier, C., Leamy, M., Bird, V. J., Davidson, L., Williams, J., & Slade, M. (2011). What does recovery mean in practice? A qualitative analysis of international recovery-oriented practice guidance. *Psychiatric Services, 62*(12), 1470–1476.

Leamy, M., Bird, V., Le Boutillier, C., Williams, J., & Slade, M. (2011). Conceptual framework for personal recovery in mental health: Systematic review and narrative synthesis. *The British Journal of Psychiatry, 199*(6), 445–452.

Lyon, A. R., Stirman, S. W., Kerns, S. E., & Bruns, E. J. (2011). Developing the mental health workforce: Review and application of training approaches from multiple disciplines. *Administration and Policy in Mental Health and Mental Health Services Research, 38*(4), 238–253.

Meehan, T., & Glover, H. (2009). Using the Recovery Knowledge Inventory (RKI) to assess the effectiveness of a consumer-led recovery training program for service providers. *Psychiatric Rehabilitation Journal, 32*(3), 223–226.

Oades, L., Deane, F., Crowe, T., Lambert, W. G., Kavanagh, D., & Lloyd, C. (2005). Collaborative recovery: an integrative model for working with individuals who experience chronic and recurring mental illness. *Australasian Psychiatry, 13*(3), 279–284.

Olfson, M., Marcus, S. C., & Pincus, H. A. (1999). Trends in office-based psychiatric practice. *American Journal of Psychiatry, 156*(3), 451–457.

Peebles, S. A., Mabe, P. A., Davidson, L., Fricks, L., Buckley, P. F., & Fenley, G. (2007). Recovery and systems transformation for schizophrenia. *The Psychiatric Clinics of North America, 30*(3), 567–583.

Peebles, S. A., Mabe, P. A., Fenley, G., Buckley, P. F., Bruce, T. O., Narasimhan, M., & Williams, E. (2009). Immersing practitioners in the recovery model: An educational program evaluation. *Community Mental Health Journal, 45*(4), 239–245.

Razzano, L. A., Jonikas, J. A., Goelitz, M. A., Hamilton, M. M., Marvin, R., Jones-Martinez, N., & Cook, J. A. (2010). The recovery education in the academy program: Transforming academic curricula with the principles of recovery and self-determination. *Psychiatric Rehabilitation Journal, 34*(2), 130–136.

Resnick, S. G., Fontana, A., Lehman, A. F., & Rosenheck, R. A. (2005). An empirical conceptualization of the recovery orientation. *Schizophrenia Research, 75* (1), 119–128.

Rowan, K., McAlpine, D. D., & Blewett, L. A. (2013). Access and cost barriers to mental health care, by insurance status, 1999–2010. *Health Affairs, 32*(10), 1723–1730.

Rüsch, N., Angermeyer, M. C., & Corrigan, P. W. (2005). Mental illness stigma: Concepts, consequences, and initiatives to reduce stigma. *European Psychiatry, 20* (8), 529–539.

Russinova, Z., Rogers, E. S., & Ellison, M. L. (2006). *RPRS manual: Recovery promoting relationships scale*. Bostob, MA: Boston University, Center for Psychiatric Rehabilitation.

Salgado, J. D., Deane, F. P., Crowe, T. P., & Oades, L. G. (2010). Hope and improvements in mental health service providers' recovery attitudes following training. *Journal of Mental Health, 19*(3), 243–248.

Schulze, B. (2007). Stigma and mental health professionals: a review of the evidence on an intricate relationship. *International Review of Psychiatry (Abingdon, England), 19*(2), 137–155.

Slade, M. (2009). The contribution of mental health services to recovery. *Journal of Mental Health, 18*(5), 367–371.

Snyder, C. R., Ilardi, S. S., Cheavens, J., Michael, S. T., Yamhure, L., & Sympson, S. (2000). The role of hope in cognitive-behavior therapies. *Cognitive Therapy and Research, 24*(6), 747–762.

Stuart, G., Tondora, J., & Hoge, M. (2004). Evidence-based teaching practice: Implications for behavioral health. *Administration and Policy in Mental Health and Mental Health Services Research, 32* (2), 107–130.

Stuber, J., Rocha, A., Christian, A., & Johnson, D. (2014a). Predictors of recovery-oriented competencies among mental health professionals in one community mental health system. *Community Mental Health Journal, 50*, 909–914.

Stuber, J. P., Rocha, A., Christian, A., & Link, B. G. (2014b). Conceptions of mental illness: Attitudes of mental health professionals and the general public. *Psychiatric Services, 65*(4), 490–497.

Substance Abuse and Mental Health Services Administration. (2006). *National consensus statement on mental health recovery*. Rockville, MD: U.S. Department of Health and Human Services. Retrieved from http://mentalhealth.samhsa.gov/publications/allpubs/SMA05-4129/

Substance Abuse and Mental Health Services Administration. (2012). *SAMHSA's working definition of recovery*. Rockville, MD: U.S. Department of Health and Human Services, U.S.

Sutkin, G., Wagner, E., Harris, I., & Schiffer, R. (2008). What makes a good clinical teacher in medicine? A review of the literature. *Academic Medicine, 83*(5), 452–466.

Towler, A. J., & Dipboye, R. L. (2001). Effects of trainer expressiveness, organization, and trainee goal orientation on training outcomes. *Journal of Applied Psychology, 86*(4), 664–673.

Tsai, J., Salyers, M. P., & Lobb, A. L. (2010). Recovery-oriented training and staff attitudes over time in two state hospitals. *Psychiatric Quarterly, 81* (4), 335–347.

Tsai, J., Salyers, M. P., & McGuire, A. B. (2011). A cross-sectional study of recovery training and staff attitudes in four community mental health centers. *Psychiatric Rehabilitation Journal, 34*(3), 186–193.

Uppal, S., Oades, L. G., Crowe, T. P., & Deane, F. P. (2010). Barriers to transfer of collaborative recovery training into Australian mental health services: Implications for the development of evidence-based services. *Journal of Evaluation in Clinical Practice, 16*(3), 451–455.

Van der Vleuten, C. P. M. V. D., Dolmans, D. H. J. M., & Scherpbier, A. J. J. A. (2000). The need for evidence in education. *Medical Teacher, 22*(3), 246–250.

Wahl, O., & Aroesty-Cohen, E. (2010). Attitudes of mental health professionals about mental illness: A review of the recent literature. *Journal of Community Psychology, 38*(1), 49–62.

Wilrycx, G., Croon, M., van den Broek, A., & Van Nieuwenhuizen, C. (2012). Mental health recovery: Evaluation of a recovery-oriented training program. *The Scientific World Journal*. doi:10.1100/2012/820846. (ID: 820846).

Wood, A. L., & Wahl, O. F. (2006). Evaluating the effectiveness of a consumer-provided mental health recovery education presentation. *Psychiatric Rehabilitation Journal, 30*(1), 46–53.

Young, A. S., Chinman, M., Forquer, S. L., Knight, E. L., Vogel, H., Miller, A., & Mintz, J. (2005). Use of a consumer-led intervention to improve provider competencies. *Psychiatric Services, 56*(8), 967–975.

Zisook, S., Benjamin, S., Balon, R., Glick, I., Louie, A., Moutier, C., & Servis, M. (2005). Alternate methods of teaching psychopharmacology. *Academic Psychiatry, 29*(2), 141–154.

# Shared Decision-Making

# 5

Gina N. Duncan, Anthony O. Ahmed, P. Alex Mabe, Brian Anderson, Gareth Fenley and Michael Rollock

## Introduction

Providing treatment to people with severe mental illnesses on an inpatient unit is fraught with challenges. Many patients are acutely ill and may be experiencing very severe symptoms that coexist with poor insight, emotional dysregulation, impulsivity, aggression, and severe disability. Moreover, many patients are involuntarily hospitalized and may be less cooperative with inpatient treatment. Some civilly committed patients may view their hospital tenure as needlessly lengthy and forced medications as impinging on their civil rights, while longing for less restrictive environments. For many practitioners, these are clinical challenges that adversely impact treatment adherence and ultimately positive treatment outcomes. Patients that are seemingly resistant to treatment are viewed as uncooperative and less ready for discharge, leading to longer hospital tenure for such individuals. This line of reasoning may represent the mainstream, prevailing view of treatment disengagement and nonadherence. The recovery model, in contrast, makes starkly different assumptions about treatment disengagement in psychiatric practice. It deemphasizes a process in which practitioners insist on adherence and underscores the participation of the patient. This chapter presents the practice of shared decision-making as a means of enhancing patient engagement in clinical care.

## Clinical Decision-Making

Clinical decisions on the inpatient unit demand careful treatment planning and coordination across several disciplines and levels of care. Some treatment decisions may involve high risk, such as complex medication management and monitoring, determinations of levels of supervision to ensure safety during the patient's tenure, and discharge readiness. Other decisions may involve less risk-taking, such as the timing or frequency of appointments, setting a treatment group schedule, completing a referral for neuropsychological testing, or scheduling independent activities. For psychiatrists and other mental health professionals, care decisions may be classified into two forms: (1) when there is clearly a best option, and (2) when there is less certainty regarding the best course of action to

G.N. Duncan (✉) · P.A. Mabe · B. Anderson · M. Rollock
Department of Psychiatry and Health Behavior, Medical College of Georgia, Augusta University, 997 St. Sebastian Way, Augusta, GA, USA
e-mail: gduncan@eastpsych.com

A.O. Ahmed
Department of Psychiatry, Weill Cornell Medical College, Cornell University, 21 Bloomingdale Road, White Plains, NY, USA

G. Fenley
College of Social Work, University of South Carolina, 902 Sumter Street, Columbia, SC, USA

 
N.N. Singh et al. (eds.), *Handbook of Recovery in Inpatient Psychiatry*, Evidence-Based Practices in Behavioral Health, DOI 10.1007/978-3-319-40537-7_5

take because there is likely more than one viable option.

Quite rare in psychiatric care are those decisions made when only one choice/option is available to the practitioner. Most decisional contexts in psychiatric care are characterized by the availability of options. These contexts include several medication options for the management of many psychiatric symptoms, increasing options for neuromodulatory interventions [e.g., electroconvulsive therapy (ECT), repeated transcranial magnetic stimulation, transcranial direct current stimulation], multiple psychosocial treatments, behavior intervention plans, and community placements options. It can be argued that the availability of more than one reasonable choice or option to the practitioner provides room for flexibility and creativity in clinical decision-making. It may also allow practitioners' final clinical decision to be informed by more factors and decisional criteria that may influence treatment success. For example, the extent to which care recipients "buy-in" to treatment decisions and engage in their own care may mitigate the effectiveness of most clinical decisions. The availability of options creates an opportunity to enhance the engagement and commitment of care recipients by sharing some care-related decisions. To understand the rationale and potential benefits of such an approach to decision making, however, it is important to begin by reexamining its alternatives. For the purpose of discussion in this chapter, we will contrast three decision-making alternatives: the Traditional Compliance Model, the Informed Choice Model, and the Shared Decision-Making Model.

## The Traditional Compliance Model

The first is the conventional approach to care decision making in psychiatry that we have called a traditional compliance model because of one of its central assumptions about compliance as necessary (although insufficient) for decision effectiveness. In the traditional compliance model, the practitioner assumes the role of the sole expert in the provider-patient dyad in a way that encourages a top-down, one-directional transfer of information. The practitioner is solely responsible for gathering information germane to treatment decision-making including the identification of treatment targets, symptom ratings, and review of history. The practitioner independently decides what information is relevant to the final treatment decision, what treatment options should be considered, and the decisional criteria to be considered in making the decision. Grounded in the traditional medical model, psychopharmacological treatment decisions are informed by general consensus regarding the neurobiological basis of most psychiatric syndromes. To prescribers, this mechanistic view of psychopathology translates to clear objective criteria that should guide prescription practice.

For example, the involvement of hypersensitive dopamine receptors in the mesolimbic pathway in the phenomenology of positive symptoms potentiates the use of compounds with DRD2 blocking capacity. Guided by such objective criteria, the practitioner chooses a treatment option to which the patient is asked to assent. Important objectives in traditional medication management include ensuring that the care recipient is taking the medications as prescribed by the *expert* provider, completing necessary blood work and other periodic medical monitoring activities (e.g., vital signs, electrolyte levels), and reporting periodically on medication side effects. The success of all of these objectives is predicated on the care recipient adhering to the prescriber's recommendations. To varying degrees, other disciplines in mental health have also adopted the traditional compliance model. Common psychotherapies follow structured treatment formats that expect success when the psychotherapist provides treatment as directed in the manual and the care recipient engages by attending sessions, completing homework, and participating as directed by the psychotherapist.

Again, it should be emphasized that the traditional compliance model appears to lean heavily on the compliance of care recipients for treatment objectives to be accomplished. An examination of the literature, however, demonstrates that psychiatric care is characterized by high rates of noncompliance, medication nonadherence, dropouts, and overall treatment disengagement (Fenton et al. 1997; Kreyenbuhl et al. 2009). Poor treatment compliance may explain why improvement rates in psychopharmacology and psychotherapy generally do not exceed medium effects (Huhn et al. 2014).

The top-down, one-directional flow of information that is characteristic of the traditional compliance model seems rather unfounded when one considers that treatment effectiveness and positive outcomes may be predicated on the patient's willingness or ability to adhere to the treatment recommendation. One may thus argue that the traditional compliance model is relatively weak because it fails to predict and produce desired outcomes. On the one hand, it fosters a power differential that places all consequential decisions in the hands of the provider while underestimating the care recipient's role in fostering positive outcomes; conversely, it stipulates that positive outcomes depend on the care recipient. Moreover, it is not uncommon for practitioners to negatively evaluate or, in some cases, pathologize instances when care recipients deviate from treatment recommendations as indicative of poor insight, disorganization, intellectual impairment, or resistance. The possibility that the practitioner did not have all of the information necessary to make an optimal clinical decision is less likely to be considered as a reason for poor treatment adherence. Patients, advocates, and many proponents of the recovery model have advanced other criticisms of the traditional compliance model. These include arguments that the traditional compliance model is inherently paternalistic, fosters dependency on the provider, and impugns on the rights of psychiatric patients.

## The Informed Choice Model

An alternative approach to the traditional compliance model, one that some may view as it is opposite, has emerged in response to mounting pressures from the current zeitgeist of consumerism in the United States. These pressures include calls for increased patient autonomy and involvement in medical decisions given the greater access to medical information on the part of patients, increasing treatment options, and the rising cost of medical care (Woolf et al. 2005). Informed choice runs in contrast to the traditional compliance model, in which medical decisions are made solely by the practitioner, who makes recommendations that the care recipient follows. Rather, informed choice places the decision of which option is best solely in the hands of the care recipient. The role of the practitioner in informed choice is that of a technical expert or consultant who provides information about options and choices to the care recipient who makes the final medical decision. Informed choice imposes a new dynamic on the provider-patient dyad with new roles and expectations for the treatment relationship. Practitioners are expected to withhold their preferences, judgments, and recommendations and rather yield to the preferences of the care recipient. The informed choice model presupposes that choices or alternatives exist with regard to medical decisions, and that all alternatives are viable and available. The model also assumes that care recipients are interested, sufficiently informed, and able to make treatment choices when provided with information that is salient to the medical decision.

It is reasonable to assume that choices are available to care recipients in inpatient settings with regard to medications for the management of symptoms. In addition, inpatient treatment programs may provide several psychosocial treatment groups as part of a "treatment mall" or rehabilitation group program in which care recipients are enrolled during their hospital tenure. The informed choice model certainly fosters more patient-centered discussions around the potential benefits and risks of many medication management options. Informed choice also allows care recipients to evaluate the potential impact of decisional preferences on their lives. With regard to psychosocial treatment options, informed choice allows patients to enroll in treatment or psychoeducational groups most consistent with their life goals, wishes, and personal values.

The informed choice model is certainly desirable to the degree that it empowers care recipients and fosters their autonomy and sense of efficacy. The model is, however, not without its limitations when applied in a psychiatric context. Even when care recipients have access to necessary information provided by the practitioner or obtained from other sources, the increased availability of knowledge may not necessarily translate to increased patient involvement. Studies suggest that not all care recipients are interested in absolute control over treatment-related decisions (Benbassat et al. 1998; Robinson and Thomson 2001). Moreover, some care recipients may find the process of vetting several options and alternatives with regard to their merits and disadvantages overwhelming. Informed decision-making may be particularly challenging for acutely symptomatic care recipients and others for whom intellectual deficits impair their decisional capacity. It is doubtful that relinquishing the final treatment decision to an impaired care recipient is viable.

Some may argue that the informed choice model encourages treatment practices that overly deemphasize the expertise of the practitioner, who may need to exercise some clinical judgment informed by experience, but unrepresented in the research literature. Prescribers, for example, often make nuanced and creative decisions about medications depending on how the care recipient is responding. Prescribers may also wish to exercise autonomy in prescribing practices informed by their clinical judgment. As an illustration, many prescribers would be less inclined or may exercise greater caution with prescribing benzodiazepines to care recipients with a history of substance use problems. It may be argued that such situations preclude informed choice (Drake and Deegan 2009).

There remains the question of whether practitioners can or are willing to assess and provide care recipients with accurate information to make informed decisions. Many practitioners may be unwilling to extend themselves to increase the knowledge of their patients given the time constraints experienced by most practitioners. Questions may also abound about literacy and cultural barriers that may impair the capacity of some care recipients to absorb knowledge of their options and express preferences. Despite their limitations, the traditional compliance model and the informed choice model reflect opposing pressures between two forces that ultimately provide a framework for a more viable decision-making model. This more viable model, called shared decision-making, attempts to strike a balance between an absolute reliance on the expertise of practitioners and the consequent paternalism of traditional care, and the rights of care recipients for choice, self-determination, and involvement.

## Shared Decision-Making Model

Shared decision-making is a system of enhancing the active participation of care recipients in treatment decisions in a way that is meaningful and consequential to the treatment by providing them with access to information and alternatives (Adams et al. 2007). In shared decision-making, practitioners (or treatment teams) and care recipients, rather than either party alone, are the participants in and deciders of the course of the treatment decision. The perspectives and preferences of both parties are consequential to each stage of the decision-making process and the final treatment decision.

There are several components to this form of decision making. The first is recognition of the shared expertise of practitioners and care recipients that contributes to a bidirectional information exchange (Charles et al. 1997; Kriston et al. 2010). The practitioners expertise in their discipline—psychiatry, psychology, social work, case management, nursing, etc.—puts them in a position to educate and inform the patient about possible alternatives guided by their training and knowledge of their discipline. The practitioner's role is critical in this vein, as shared decision-making requires diligence on the part of the practitioner to provide and educate patients about alternatives. The degree of information provided to the patient may be predicated on the extent to which the patient wants to be educated about options, the patient's intellectual capacity and education, and the patient's interest in the decision-making process (Makoul and Clayman 2006).

The patient's expertise lies with knowledge of his/her own preferences, values, past response to treatment (e.g., side effects, benefits or lack thereof), and life circumstances that may be impacted by or consequential to treatment decisions (Godolphin 2009). These may include the importance of activities like fasting during Lent or Ramadan, returning to school, a new job, marriage, pregnancy, dieting, or engaging in a new hobby. The patient also assumes a partnership role in investigating treatment options that the patient may then present to the practitioner for discussion. In some cases, the bidirectional flow of information is enhanced by a third party, such as a family member, during hospital visits. Family members may be vital sources of historical information that may inform treatment decisions, particularly when the patient suffers impairments that may limit their shared decision-making capacity. Family members may have ideas, questions, concerns, or expectations about aspects of the patient's care that the provider ascertains and responds to in collaboration with the patient and family members.

The bidirectional exchange of information in shared decision-making increases both parties' awareness of the available treatment options—a necessary condition to the exercise of choice. Next, shared decision-making leads to a deliberation of the identified treatment options in terms of the preferences of both the practitioner and the patient. Both parties evaluate available options in terms of their decision criteria. Criteria important to both the practitioner and the patient are weighted equally and actively for each available option (Kriston et al. 2010). For example, whereas a case manager may prioritize proximity to a day treatment program or other community supports as criteria for an acceptable community residence following discharge, a patient may prioritize proximity to their family members, place of worship, or shopping mall. All of these criteria should, however, be weighted equally in the evaluation of community placement options.

Psychiatrists and psychologists are often interested in weighing the evidence base for available treatment options, and the degree of empirical support for a particular option may be rated as high as a decision criterion. Depending on the patient's preference for information, practitioners may share this information with the patient and express their own preference for evidence-based interventions (Adams and Drake 2006; Barratt 2008). They then endeavor to guide the patient through an evaluation of values, life style, and goals in relation to the empirical support for the treatment options. The selection of the final option is then negotiated between the practitioner and the patient with a goal to identify an option that would be consistent with the patient's values and preferences.

Questions would be raised at this juncture about the possibility of occasions when the practitioner and the patient disagree about the best treatment option. This will be discussed again later in this chapter. Certainly, the implementation of shared decision-making in clinical decisions can result in agreement or disagreement about the best treatment course. Should the practitioner simply acquiesce to the patient's perspective or attempt to persuade the patient to agree the practitioner's preferred treatment option? It may be argued that erring toward acquiescing to the patient's preference is a more recovery-oriented approach and therefore preferred course of action. Some may view attempts at persuading the patient to agree with the practitioner as returning to a traditional compliance model.

The issue of disagreements raises a larger question about the nature of shared decision-making. On the one hand, shared decision-making refers to a process of arriving at a clinical decision that involves two experts engaged in a bidirectional information exchange and evaluation of preferences in light of their decisional criteria. Shared decision-making also involves a mutual acceptance of a treatment choice—a shared decision—that may not necessarily conform to one or either's idea of the best choice, but is agreed upon by both parties as the course of action (Charles et al. 1997). What is, therefore, crucial in shared decision-making is not whether the practitioner acquiesces or tries to persuade the patient, but that the practitioner ensures that there is agreement on the final decision. Although practitioners should not shy away from sharing their preferences about the best course of action, it should be acknowledged that there remains a risk that practitioners may inadvertently impose their preferences on the patient. The inherent power differential that exists between the practitioner and the patient would often lend greater weight to their opinions.

## Case Vignette

Ms. Angela Dixon, a 42-year-old African American woman, was receiving services on an acute inpatient unit. She had been diagnosed with schizophrenia in her late 20s after she reported auditory and visual hallucinations, and endorsed persecutory delusional beliefs. She particularly found her visual hallucinations very distressing, as she would often see malevolent faces emerging from walls, trees, and the floor. She also believed that her home was haunted and that she could hear demons conversing in the basement about her thoughts and actions. Her experiences contributed to significant fearfulness, depression, and irritability.

Ms. Dixon had been hospitalized frequently since her first psychotic episode. She had been treated with several antipsychotics, some of which had produced improvements. However, she had difficulty in maintaining medication adherence due to her discomfort with medication side effects, problems with organization, and some suspiciousness about antipsychotic medications. On one occasion, she had stopped taking her olanzapine because she believed it made her "feel heavy" even though her psychotic and mood symptoms improved. During her current hospitalization, she had refused to take antipsychotic medications and expressed feelings of anger related to being "forced" to take pimozide, which caused her to have hand tremors, and risperidone, to which she believed she was allergic.

Ms. Dixon refused medications frequently and the treatment team began to consider changing hospitalization status from voluntary to involuntary in order to seek a court ruling to provide ECT. The team believed that involuntary treatment was the only course of action left, as it had made efforts to engage Ms. Dixon in her care. Moreover, by that time, Ms. Dixon had been hospitalized for three months and was making little improvement in her psychiatric symptoms. Ms. Dixon had also been refusing to attend groups in the hospital treatment mall. She often sat by herself, but had periodically asked for drawing pads on which she sketched clothing designs. Her treatment team ultimately decided to transfer her to a different hospital unit.

Upon Ms. Dixon's transfer, Dr. Abrams reviewed her history and noticed that she had often responded quickly to many antipsychotic regimens, but that their effectiveness was not sustained in the long term. He learned that Ms. Dixon had very strong resistance to taking medications and had often gotten into arguments with her previous psychiatrists and the nursing staff about her treatment. He was also aware that she had become resistant to attending groups or participating in unit milieu-based activities. In their first meeting together, Ms. Dixon expressed to Dr. Abrams her general frustration with psychiatrists and other mental health professionals due to their unresponsiveness to the concerns she had repeatedly raised about taking medications. Dr. Abrams found that although some of her opinions about her medications were unfounded, Ms. Dixon spoke with some clarity about her medication history and was able to provide information about how she had responded to medications in the past.

Dr. Abrams decided to involve Ms. Dixon in more frequent discussions about her medications. He reasoned that the treatment might benefit from involving Ms. Dixon in discussions that increased her knowledge about her medications and that also allowed her to provide information about her medication history, preferences, and treatment goals to inform medication decision-making.

Consequently, Dr. Abrams learned that Ms. Dixon often assumed that psychiatric medications worked like other medications (i.e. that she could stop taking them after her symptoms subsided). He also learned that she was very sensitive to the side effects of medications. For example, she reported that she had developed an unsightly "bulging stomach" when she started taking olanzapine. She argued that risperidone and other antipsychotics caused her to have skin breakouts although her psychiatric records indicated that this was not apparent under close monitoring.

Dr. Abrams encouraged Ms. Dixon to partner with him in identifying the best treatment course that would allow her to stay out of the hospital and pursue her life goals. He learned that Ms. Dixon loved to knit sweaters and scarfs and that she also enjoyed sketching dresses and had a prior career as a tailor. He also learned about her opinions on all of the antipsychotics she had taken. Dr. Abrams provided information about several possible strategies for medication management to Ms. Dixon, discussing their rationale, side effects, and their potential impact on her life goals. Ultimately, they agreed to try a regimen that conferred a low risk of tardive dyskinesia. Ms. Dixon was committed to the success of the regimen, given that she had effectively influenced the final choice. Both agreed to meet daily to review their collaborative plan. Ms. Dixon experienced significant improvements in her psychotic and mood symptoms. Moreover, the treatment team observed that she began to participate more actively in her own care by taking her medications, attending groups, meeting with her psychiatrist daily, and completing blood work and vital signs. She was subsequently discharged back to the community where she maintained her treatment gains with sustained community tenure at 12 months.

## Is There a Need for Shared Decision-Making?

As the case vignette illustrates, hospital practitioners are often faced with the dilemma of managing occasions when the care recipient is seemingly non-adherent to or skeptical about some or all aspects of psychiatric care. It is not unusual for treatment teams to label such care recipients as "noncompliant," "demanding," "help-rejecting," or "difficult" (Roberts and Dyer 2003). Subsequently, treatment teams may respond by further insisting on treatment recommendations—seen during occasions when adjudication is sought for forced medications—or transferring the care recipient to another treatment setting. In some cases, insisting on treatment recommendations or transferring care may be the appropriate treatment response. It is clear, however, in the above vignette, as in many similar cases that there had been an absence of engagement or "buy-in" on the part of the care recipient. The case is made in the above vignette that shared decision-making is a possible intervention for poor treatment engagement. The state of the evidence for shared decision-making to such end will of course be better supported by systematic studies and this will be subsequently discussed. First, however, we discuss the rationale for incorporating shared decision-making in hospital psychiatric care. This includes an examination of treatment disengagement, consumer rights and the recovery model, and the impact of paternalism on psychiatric care.

## High Rates of Treatment Disengagement in Traditional Compliance Approaches

The case for shared decision-making begins with a consideration of the state of the traditional mental health system, which relies on treatment compliance or adherence as a treatment objective for ensuring and maintaining treatment gains. Indeed, the effectiveness of all forms of medical treatment, including psychiatric interventions, depends on the degree to which the care recipient engages in the treatment plan. For example, high treatment adherence predicts better treatment outcomes among patients receiving medical care (DiMatteo et al. 2002). Among people with schizophrenia, poor adherence to antipsychotics, especially in the early course of illness, contributes to poorer long-term treatment outcome, including greater risks for relapse (Masand et al. 2009). Several studies suggest that psychiatric services are plagued by high rates of nonadherence. The National Schizophrenia Fellowship survey of service recipients in the United Kingdom that had received antipsychotic medications revealed that 12 % had ceased taking prescribed antipsychotics without informing their prescriber (Corry et al. 2001). Remarkably, the fellowship survey also revealed that while the majority of psychiatrists discussed medications with care recipients (70 %), they rarely offered choices to care recipients (40 %). Valenstein et al. (2004) examined pharmacy data from the VA National Psychosis Registry and found over 40 % of care recipients were medication non-adherent—defined as having medication possession ratios (MPR) < 0.80. Medication adherence rates were especially low among African Americans and patients earlier in the course of illness.

One perspective held by former patients and patient advocates is that poor medication adherence rates among psychiatric care recipients may reflect a larger problem of disengagement from psychiatric services. Treatment disengagement is defined here as ceasing or reducing prior contacts with mental health services or care despite the need or clinician recommendation for such services. Indicators of treatment disengagement could include medication nonadherence, missed appointments, lateness to treatment appointments, referral failures from emergency services and other diversionary sources, and noncompliance with aftercare recommendations. In psychiatric inpatient settings, disengagement may be evident in care recipients who "cheek" medications, refuse to complete relevant blood work, refuse to complete routine vital signs and other procedures, refuse to attend treatment groups, remain isolated in their rooms, or refuse to participate in recommended evaluations. It should be acknowledged that for some patients, psychiatric symptoms (e.g., delusions, amotivation) may contribute to the refusal to participate in some aspects of their care. It may be necessary to rule out the role of acute illness and intervene appropriately in such cases. Notwithstanding the impact of symptoms, however, noncompliance often reflects poor engagement.

Several studies suggest that traditional psychiatric care has failed at fostering treatment engagement especially among individuals with severe mental illnesses (Doyle et al. 2014; Kreyenbuhl et al. 2009; Stowkowy et al. 2012). Doyle et al. (2014) reviewed 10 studies and found that the reported rates of disengagement among first-episode psychosis patients ranged from 20.5 % to as high as 50 %, with most studies reporting rates that exceeded 30 %. Interestingly, people with a lower baseline severity of illness were found to be more likely to disengage from treatment (Conus et al. 2010; Stowkowy et al. 2012). Individuals with high illness severity were more likely to have been encouraged by family members to continue to receive services.

Several factors have been identified as likely contributors to treatment disengagement in care recipients. These include demographic factors—male, young, low socioeconomic status, unmarried, ethnic minority status, clinical factors such as illness severity, insight, and illness stage, and treatment factors such as poor therapeutic alliance (Kreyenbuhl et al. 2009). Some studies have sought the perspective of care recipients to illuminate causes of treatment disengagement. Commonly cited reasons have included dissatisfaction with treatment, not being listened to, skepticism about the benefits of the treatment they were receiving, and a desire to maintain one's own independence and sense of control (O'Brien et al. 2009; Priebe et al. 2005; Rossi et al. 2008).

Shared decision-making has been touted as an intervention to enhance engagement given that it directly counters many of the reasons care recipients drop out of treatment. Specifically, it provides a platform that allows the care recipient to be listened to and it encourages the care recipient to share their expertise in their own care. It also encourages the autonomy of the care recipient and empowers the care recipient to contribute to the final decision.

## The Recovery Model and Consumer Rights Versus Paternalism

The recovery model of mental health adds further impetus to incorporate shared decision-making into critical aspects of psychiatric care. The principles of recovery based on the Substance Abuse and Mental Health Service Administration (SAMHSA) definition have been recently distilled psychometrically into four critical domains (Ahmed et al. 2013). These domains—hope, empowerment, self-direction, and strengths—were extracted using latent variable modeling of items from the Maryland Assessment of Recovery for Severe Mental Illnesses (MARS; Drapalski et al. 2012). The recovery domains of empowerment and self-direction are especially relevant to shared decision-making as they underscore the capacity of care recipients to make personal choices, exercise preference, establish goals, and influence the course of their own lives. By implication, treatment programs that aim to be recovery oriented would want to adopt shared decision-making in critical care decisions as it balances the expertise of the practitioner with recognition of the autonomy of care recipients to influence the course of their own lives and empowers recipients to make care decisions. Indeed, shared decision-making is central to recovery-focused psychopharmacology—a recently proposed model of medication management that places recovery as the central focus of medication management (Buckley and Ahmed 2013; Deegan and Drake 2006; Noordsy et al. 2000).

As mental health systems around the world have adopted the recovery model (Ahmed et al. 2012), there has been a growing demand in mental health systems for increased patient involvement in psychiatric treatment decisions. This patient-centered view is advocated internationally by prominent health care and policy organizations including the New Freedom Commission, the National Institute of Health and Care Excellence (NICE) standards, the American Psychiatric Association, the American Psychological Association, the Veterans Affairs Health Care System, and other international guidelines (Hamann et al. 2010). These organizations generally agree that contemporary psychiatric services should aim for partnerships with care recipients and their family members and shared decision-making may provide a framework for such involvement. While it is acknowledged that increased involvement of care recipients and their family members may impact how readily care decisions are made, this has also been argued as an ethical imperative (Drake and Deegan 2009). Moreover, it has been emphasized that the autonomy of the care recipient and the principles of empowerment and self-direction should be weighted heavily when care decisions involve alternatives that are equivocal or situations that are controversial (Mistler and Drake 2008).

In psychiatric inpatient settings, shared decision-making provides an alternative to traditional practices that have been viewed as paternalistic and fostering of dependency and the "sick role." These practices include forced medication, offering rewards to encourage medication compliance, the provision of long-acting injectable alternatives (depots), oral dispersible tablets (ODT), and mouth checks to avoid "cheeking." There is little evidence to suggest that these practices are effective for long-term treatment adherence. For example, a recent study dispelled previously held assumptions by showing that long-acting injectable medications were no better than orals at fostering clinical improvements and preventing relapse in people with schizophrenia (Buckley et al. 2015). Moreover, other practices employed in psychiatric inpatient settings are rarely continued in the community following discharge, therefore many care recipients stop taking medications as soon as they are discharged. The result is a short community tenure and rehospitalization following discharge. Inpatient psychiatric medication management is further fraught with disagreements between care recipients and hospital staff about treatment. Forced medication often results in patients having negative attitudes about the hospital staff and psychiatric treatment overall (Hamann et al. 2009). It is therefore unsurprising that many people who require or could benefit from psychiatric care generally avoid seeking treatment (Kreyenbuhl et al. 2009).

## Shared Decision-Making in Practice

A national survey of health care providers showed that 75 % support shared decision-making. And yet, it is not widely implemented in practice (Patel et al. 2008; Shared Decision-Making in Mental Health Care: Practice, Research, and Future Directions 2010). Why would this be? One reason relates to logistical issues, specifically time and skills training. As discussed above, shared decision-making represents a departure from the traditional, paternalistic model of patient care in which most practitioners have been trained. Thus, from a logistical standpoint, successful implementation of shared decision-making requires changes in the flow of the clinical encounter and the development of new skills.

Another reason for the limited implementation of shared decision-making in mental health care practice relates to provider attitudes. Despite general endorsement of the concept of shared decision-making, mental health care providers also report holding beliefs that serve as barriers to its implementation (Shared Decision-Making in Mental Health Care: Practice, Research, and Future Directions 2010). Chief among these concerns is a misperception of consumer capacity to make treatment decisions (Hamann et al. 2009; Shared Decision-Making in Mental Health Care: Practice, Research, and Future Directions 2010). Other beliefs relate to a lack of research evidence regarding shared decision-making, time limitations for consultations, their own lack of skills in risk communication, mistaking information sharing for decision sharing, consumer reluctance to take decision-making responsibility, consumers' abilities to cope with the stress of decision making, and a lack of technical support (Shared Decision-Making in Mental Health Care: Practice, Research, and Future Directions 2010). To achieve true clinician buy-in and effective implementation of shared decision-making, these barriers must be acknowledged and individually explored.

## Overcoming Barriers to Shared Decision-Making

**Time**. Time constraints represent a systems level barrier that cannot be ignored (Patel et al. 2008). Our clinical environments have become increasingly harried, and face-to-face care is typically delivered in 10–20 min increments. Time constraints as related to the implementation of shared decision-making play a critical role in at least three areas: (1) the amount of face-to-face time available for clinical encounters; (2) in-service time available for clinicians to learn and be trained in new skills; and (3) the amount of time providers have for wellness and self-care. Each of these time-related barriers can be addressed in several key ways.

With regard to face-to-face clinical encounter time, there is evidence that shared decision-making is comparable in time to usual care (Patel et al 2008). A study looking specifically at shared decision-making for inpatients with schizophrenia found that it did not take up more of the physician's time than care as usual (Schauer et al. 2007).

The availability of in-service time for clinicians to be trained in new skills such as shared decision-making also plays a factor. Ensuring the availability of such time takes effort, however, clinical departments and inpatient units can take steps to incorporate trainings into existing in-service sessions such as grand rounds and staff meetings. Residency training programs can incorporate trainings into didactic schedules. Regular reinforcement can occur through followup seminars, consultations, clinical care templates that prompt clinicians to implement shared decision-making, and patient care forms that prompt patients to use shared decision-making skills. Clinicians should also be encouraged to participate in external conferences and workshops where shared decision-making training is provided.

A third area in which time can play a significant role is the time providers who make for practicing wellness and self-care. A lack of both, in conjunction with a stressful work environment, can impact provider attitude, leading to burnout and negatively impacting patient care (Schulze 2007). As practitioners of mental health care, we bring not only our skills but also *ourselves* into the treatment relationship. In order to model and promote wellness and recovery for the persons we serve, it is critical that we attend to these same areas in our own lives. This includes appropriate work-life balance, healthy eating, regular physical activity, meaningful social engagement, and supportive relationships.

**Information sharing versus decision sharing.** Evidence-based medicine is now the standard of medical practice, and most physicians are highly experienced in presenting patients with the risks and benefits of a proposed treatment and obtaining informed consent. It can be easy to view a patient's participation in a discussion of information about a treatment and their subsequent agreement to a treatment plan as actually sharing in the decision-making process. However, information-sharing and treatment decision-making are two distinct goals in the medical encounter (Charles et al. 1997). Participants in the 2007 Center for Mental Health Services' meeting on shared decision-making expressed concern that many providers feel they are already doing shared decision-making when they are not (Shared Decision-Making in Mental Health Care: Practice, Research, and Future Directions 2010).

As an illustration, let us imagine a common inpatient treatment scenario: Ms. Mellen is a young woman in her mid 30s, who has been hospitalized for major depression. As Dr. G., the inpatient attending, reviews Ms. Mellen's chart, she notes that Ms. Mellen's medical history is significant for obesity. She considers four first-line antidepressants that could potentially be prescribed to treat Ms. Mellen's depression: drugs A, B, C, and D. As she prepares to see Ms. Mellen, Dr. G. eliminates drugs B, C, and D from consideration based on her clinical experience and on her greater familiarity with drug A, which has a lower likelihood of weight gain and GI side effects than the others. On rounds, Dr. G. establishes a good rapport with Ms. Mellen, empathizes with her feelings of depression, and presents Drug A as the treatment recommendation. Dr. G. reviews with Ms. Mellen the side effect profile of Drug A, and answers Ms. Mellen's questions regarding the dosing schedule and the expected length of time before the medicine begins to "kick in." Ms. Mellen consents to begin treatment with Drug A.

In this scenario, Dr. G. has delivered standard care—she has considered evidence-based treatment options, taken into account side effect profiles relevant to Ms. Mellen's medical history, established good rapport, and shared with Ms. Mellen the risks and benefits of Drug A. However, by not presenting Drugs B, C, and D, Dr. G. has not allowed Ms. Mellen the opportunity to appraise for herself how Drug A compares to others with regard to her broader goals and values, and to participate in selecting Drug A from among those options. Thus, shared decision-making has not occurred (Charles et al. 1997).

It is important to remember that while physicians have expert technical knowledge, patients are experts in their own preferences (Charles et al. 1997). The sharing of patient preference is a requisite for shared decision-making, and can have a significant impact not only on patient satisfaction but also on the ultimate treatment decision. In one study, in 22 % of cases the psychiatrist indicated that engaging in shared decision-making resulted in a different treatment strategy (Hamann et al. 2006).

Returning to the example above, let us imagine that Ms. Mellen has a goal of taking a new position at work that would result in a pay raise, but require a much earlier start to her shift. While weight gain is a concern to her, of greater concern is her ability to be alert and fully awake on the job. Had she known that Drug B was an option with equivalent antidepressant efficacy and tends to be more activating, her preference would have been to try it instead.

**Research evidence supporting shared decision-making**. Surveys in general medicine have shown that the overwhelming majority of the public (over 70 %) expressed a wish to participate in shared decision-making (Flynn et al. 2006; Levinson et al. 2005). This includes the General Social Survey of 2,765 adults which found that 96 % of respondents wanted to participate in discussions about their care and be provided with treatment choices (Levinson et al. 2005). Similarly, a survey of 5,199 older adults showed that their entire sample preferred a system of "high information exchange" that is characteristic of shared decision-making with their practitioner (Flynn et al. 2006). Further, the majority of their sample (46 %) was classified as "deliberative autonomist"—individuals who preferred to exercise choice after embarking on a discussion of options with their practitioner.

Recent studies among psychiatric patients have demonstrated a similar preference for shared decision-making as seen in general medicine. Adams et al. (2007) surveyed the decisional preferences of 30 people with schizophrenia with regard to psychiatric medications and general medical care. They found that whereas 77 % of their sample preferred shared decision-making for medication decisions, only 23 % preferred shared decision-making for general medical care. Hamann et al. (2010) similarly surveyed the decisional preferences of a larger sample of people with schizophrenia ($N = 300$). They found that the majority of their sample wanted shared decision-making, with only 12 % expressing a preference for a doctor's unilateral decision. They also found that less than 50 % of care recipients who preferred shared decision-making had the opportunity to participate in shared decision-making. Moreover, it also appeared that care recipients who expressed preference for shared decision-making tended to have a poorer working alliance with the treatment team.

One belief expressed by clinicians that serves as a barrier to shared decision-making is a concern that there is a lack of research evidence on shared decision-making feasibility and outcomes in mental health care. It is true that the research base on the feasibility and outcomes of shared decision-making is smaller relative to other areas in mental health. However, this literature base has advanced significantly in the past decade and evidence to date demonstrates that shared decision-making in mental health care is both feasible and effective in achieving positive outcomes, including improved patient satisfaction, self-management, treatment adherence, patient knowledge, decreased long-term rehospitalization rates, and the quality of decisions made as rated by practitioners (Hamann et al. 2007; Hamann et al. 2006; Loh et al. 2006; Malm et al. 2003; Patel et al. 2008; Shared Decision-Making in Mental Health Care: Practice, Research, and Future Directions 2010; Stewart et al. 2003).

**Communication of risk/uncertainty**. Another barrier to shared decision-making reported by providers is a perceived lack of skill in risk communication as well as a "reluctance to change or challenge their perceived role responsibilities to demonstrate authority and provide advice and cure" (Shared Decision-Making in Mental Health Care: Practice, Research, and Future Directions 2010). As discussed by Gordon et al. (2000), medical education has been described as "training for certainty" with overemphasis on unambiguous facts, solvable problems, and correct answers (Gordon et al. 2000). As trainees take on more clinical responsibility, their efforts are aimed at controlling uncertainty (Gordon et al. 2000). Research, however, supports physician communication of uncertainty in the treatment relationship as beneficial. A study by Gordon et al. (2000) demonstrated a link between physician expressions of uncertainty during the clinical encounter and other behaviors that are associated with patient satisfaction. These behaviors—soliciting patients' opinions, facilitating patient conversation, and checking patients' understanding—have been associated with fewer malpractice suits (Gordon et al. 2000). They are also key components of shared decision-making.

## The Role of Provider Hope and Expectations in Shared Decision-Making

A prerequisite for effective engagement in shared decision-making is the belief that both the clinician and the patient have the capacity to work collaboratively to bring about positive/desired outcomes. Providing mental health services can be fulfilling and rewarding, but it can be equally taxing on an emotional level. Clinicians often find themselves trying to make a difference in the lives of the people they serve, while constrained by limited resources in the form of patients' intrinsic coping skills, education, financial stability, social support, and a medical system that affords limited clinical time and provides limited reimbursement. When one's contact with patients occurs in brief encounters in acute settings, such as the inpatient unit, it can be easy to lose sight of the broader picture of recovery.

Mental health care providers have been ascribed the proverbial role of "holding the hope" for the persons we serve when those individuals have lost their own sense of hope for a better future and a meaningful life. Yet holding the hope can be difficult, or nearly impossible, if providers do not have hope themselves (Schrank et al. 2012). Mental health care providers who participated in a series of focus groups conducted by the Recovery to Practice (RTP) Initiative indicated struggling to maintain hope for themselves in the context of seeing poor outcomes despite what research said, feeling excluded or not listened to by the broader medical community, being mistreated or even attacked by patients, and having inadequate time and resources to really succeed with their patients (Association and Psychiatrists 2011). The role of hope cannot be overemphasized, both as a central component in recovery, and as a prerequisite for shared decision-making. For what must we, as providers, hope? Principally, that the work to which we have dedicated ourselves is meaningful and that the persons we serve can get better.

Studies of attitudes and expectations in mental health care have shown that professionals tend to have optimistic expectations of treatment (i.e., the expectation that medication and therapy would be helpful), but were ambivalent as to eventual recovery (Schulze 2007). Another study of mental health professionals' knowledge and attitudes about recovery found that staff members had a good understanding of roles of self-definition and peers in recovery, as well as roles and responsibilities in recovery (Bedregal et al. 2006). However, they were less knowledgeable about how to develop "realistic yet hopeful expectations of their clients with respect to their participation in their own recovery and in their lives in general" (Bedregal et al. 2006).

Hope cannot be constrained by low expectations. Is such hope really hope at all? It is here that the provider must examine him or herself: Do you believe that recovery is possible for your patients? Have you internalized recovery as a nonlinear journey toward self-determination and a meaningful life even in the context of psychiatric illness on which a patient will be for the rest of their life? Viewing recovery as something attainable only through total symptom (and setback) eradication while working with persons experiencing chronic illness is a set-up for a diminished ability to hope.

## Provider Expectations of Patient Decision-Making Capacity

Adopting any new practice perspective requires the provider to be "bought in." Successful shared decision-making requires that the provider go into the encounter with the expectation that the patient is capable of understanding the options presented, weighing those options, and is capable of bringing to the table information of critical relevance to the treatment process. In one large survey, psychiatrists expressed "doubts about whether they can accept patients as competent partners in medical decisions" (Hamann et al. 2009). A provider who considers an individual incapable of making health care decisions is not likely to engage that person in shared decision-making (Schauer et al. 2007). This was also identified by participants in the 2007 Center for Mental Health Services meeting on shared decision-making as a barrier to the promotion of shared decision-making in mental health care (Shared Decision-Making in Mental Health Care: Practice, Research, and Future Directions 2010).

It must be recognized that the vast majority of patients—even those with severe illness—do have the capacity to participate in medical decision-making (Improving the Quality of Health Care for Mental and Substance-Use Conditions: Quality Chasm Series 2006; Shared Decision-Making in Mental Health Care: Practice, Research, and Future Directions 2010). Shared decision-making with patients being treated for depression has been shown to produce positive outcomes, specifically with regard to improved knowledge, improvement in decision stage, greater satisfaction with decision-making, improved involvement, and decreased depression and stress (Shared Decision-Making in Mental Health Care: Practice, Research, and Future Directions 2010)..The use of shared decision-making with individuals in treatment for schizophrenia specifically has also been shown to be feasible and effective, with positive outcomes including improved patient knowledge, social interaction, and satisfaction (Shared Decision-Making in Mental Health Care: Practice, Research, and Future Directions 2010). Bunn et al. (1997) evaluated the ability of 96 people with schizophrenia to participate in decisions to continue/discontinue antipsychotic treatment. They found that their participants were able and often took inventory of the severity of their symptoms and medication side effects in the final decision. In their sample, 87 % of care recipients chose to continue their current regimen, whereas only 3.13 % chose to discontinue.

Hamann et al. (2009) discussed research that has shown patients with schizophrenia often show poorer decisional capacity than persons without any physical or mental conditions. They noted, however, that "this poor performance of patients with schizophrenia…did not reflect an enduring inability. The performance of most patients with schizophrenia was equal to that of persons in the comparison group when they received an additional (educational) intervention that allowed them to review and reflect on the information necessary to consent to treatment" (Hamann et al. 2009). Other tools such as Decisional Aids have also been shown to aid decisional capacity (Deegan et al. 2008).

To the concern expressed by providers that sharing in decisions would be too stressful for patients, the overwhelming majority of care recipients want to participate in health care decisions, and most individuals receiving mental health services prefer shared decision-making (Adams et al. 2007; Flynn et al. 2006; Hamann et al. 2010; Levinson et al. 2005). As illustrated in the case vignette of Ms. Dixon above, even patients in the midst of severe, acute illness may be able to effectively consider their symptoms and potential medication side effects, and contribute in a meaningful way to decisions regarding their treatment (Burns and Kendrick 1997).

## Provider Expectations of Individuals' Desires for and Capability of a Meaningful Life

In addition to the expectation that the individuals they serve are capable of participating in treatment decision-making, providers must also approach the treatment relationship with the expectation that the patient has hopes and desires for a meaningful life beyond their illness. Regardless of whether those hopes have been diminished due to the patient's experience with their illness, the provider must hold the expectation that the patient is capable of experiencing a meaningful life on a holistic level. That is, to experience a life that is about more than the presence, absence, or severity level of illness symptoms and having basic needs met; a life that includes the key dimensions of wellness—satisfying interpersonal relationships, self-direction, optimization of physical health, contribution to others, participation in society, setting, and achieving goals, a place to call home. In other words, providers must believe in personal recovery, which entails more than the amelioration of symptoms or restoration to a premorbid state (Diamond 2006).

## Stigma

Stigma is a powerful factor influencing both provider attitudes and expectations. Stigmatization affects quality of life for people with mental illness with consequences for employment, relationships, self-esteem, and care-seeking behavior as well as disease treatment, progression, and recovery (Hansson et al. 2013; Kingdon et al. 2004). The core cognitive and behavioral features of mental illness stigma include stereotypes (cognitive knowledge structures), prejudice (cognitive and emotional consequence of stereotypes), and discrimination (behavioral consequence of prejudice) (Rüsch et al. 2005). Most providers of mental health care would likely acknowledge experiencing some degree of professional stigma as a result of society's view of mental illness and those who treat it (e.g., references to the professional working with "crazy people"). This has been referred to as "associative stigma" or "stigma by proxy," as mental health professionals work in a discipline and with a patient population that has been less valued than other areas in the health care system (Hansson et al. 2013).

Anti-stigma campaigns directed at the general public have gained support in recent decades and are showing effectiveness in raising awareness of mental illnesses (Schulze 2007). Much less discussed, though, is the role of stigma in mental health care and the fact that contact with mental health care services contributes to feelings of stigmatization among people with mental illness (Hansson et al. 2013; Schulze 2007). In focus groups conducted by SAMHSA's Elimination of Barriers Initiative, mental health consumers reported that "providers of mental health care were among those who most stigmatized mental health clients" (Schauer et al. 2007). The significance of stigma on clinicians' abilities and behavior is also discussed in the Institute of Medicine's 2005 report on *Improving the Quality of Health Care for Mental and Substance Use Conditions* (Schauer et al. 2007). Studies examining clinicians' attitudes toward individuals with mental illness suggest that providers' better knowledge of mental illness symptoms and treatment, exposure to patients in treatment, and even their support for individual rights "do not act as a protective factor against stigma, as they are neither associated with fewer stereotypes nor a greater willingness to closely interact with people with mental illness" outside of the clinical setting (Nordt et al. 2006; Schulze 2007).

This is not surprising because providers of mental health care are not isolated from the influence of the broader society in which they live. "Mental health professionals are…as citizens exposed to early socialization processes that may induce an internalization of stigmatizing attitudes and discriminatory behavior" (Hansson et al. 2013). The media act as powerful disseminators of public sentiments and contribute to the development of collective consciousness with regard to mental illness. One needs only to reflect on the media's coverage of and public response to the horrific mass shootings of the last two decades (e.g., the 2007 Virginia Tech massacre) in which the perpetrators' mental illness has been a central focus. As noted by Nordt et al. (2006), "before mental health professionals can inform and teach the general public about mental illness and thus help to reduce its stigma, they should carefully examine their own attitudes…they should not assume that they themselves have no negative stereotypes or are more willing to closely interact with the affected than anyone else" (Nordt et al. 2006).

An unwillingness or reluctance to closely interact with individuals who have a mental illness can be referred to as a preference for social distance. In studies of attitudes toward people with mental illness, psychiatrists have indeed expressed this preference (Schulze 2007). As described by Link and Phelan (2001), a preference for social distance reflects behavioral intentions ensuing from negative stereotypes. That is, a person may have feelings of empathy toward, and investment in, their individual patients, including optimistic beliefs in the helpfulness of medication and therapy. And yet, that person may simultaneously possess a preference for social distance from the general population of which the patient is a part as a result of negative internal stereotypes ascribed to certain groups with regard to dangerousness, worthiness, intellect, value, and social capital in society.

Social distance has been described by Nordt et al. (2006) as "one of the most significant components of stigmatization." It is critical that mental health care practitioners recognize and take steps to address this, because "persons with a stigmatizing condition like serious mental illness perceive and interpret their condition and the negative responses of others. The collective representations in the form of common stereotypes influence both the responses of others and the interpretation of the stigmatized" (Rüsch et al. 2005).

Working with persons who have, by virtue of their illness, cultural background, socioeconomic status, or combination of all of the above, life experiences that are significantly different from one's own can create an us versus them perspective in and of itself. This perspective is further facilitated by the societal stigma of mental illness; the implicit hierarchy arising from the traditional medical model and other, false, socially derived distinctions based on class, culture, race/ethnicity, education, and economic status.

Hansson et al. (2013) investigated and compared mental health staff to people receiving mental health services with regard to their beliefs about devaluation and discrimination, and their attitudes related to those beliefs. There were several key findings, all of which support the idea that exposure to recovery in action has an impact on provider attitudes and beliefs, and that this can have implications for providers' behavior. One finding related to patient diagnosis (i.e., staff working with patients with psychotic disorders) held more negative beliefs than those treating patients with other diagnoses. Another finding was that younger staff held more negative beliefs than those who had been in practice longer. A third finding related to practice setting—staff working in inpatient settings held more negative beliefs than those working in outpatient settings.

Most differences were found in comparisons between staff in inpatient and outpatient settings. The authors noted that this might be a reflection of the fact that these subgroups of staff to a greater extent have contacts with people with more severe, long-term, and recurrent illness, which might induce attitudes where they think less of people with mental illness and view them as less trustworthy, and less capable of acquiring or maintaining a job. If such negative beliefs of possibilities for people with a severe mental illness to acquire a job are reflected in actual rehabilitation work and in treatment planning, this may reduce ambitions of recovery and work on behalf of the patient and instead induce pessimism and hopelessness in the individual. This may also on a service level prevent the implementation of evidence-based interventions in this field such as supported employment, where several reviews have shown that more than half of patients engaged in this intervention get a job in the open labor market (Bond et al. 2008). Consequently, an implication of negative beliefs in staff may on a more general level be an important obstacle to the implementation of an evidence-based practice in various intervention domains (Hansson et al. 2013).

## Stigmatizing Behaviors

It is universally accepted in the field of mental health that one's thoughts, feelings, and behaviors influence each other. Providers should be aware of several key ways in which their own attitudes can translate into behavior that contributes to feelings of stigmatization among people receiving mental health services. As providers, our body language, verbal communication, and the way in which we structure the clinical encounter all send a powerful message to the consumer as to how valued they are. In studies looking specifically at their experiences of stigma in their relationships with mental health care providers, patients have reported feeling stigmatized in particular by clinicians' lack of interest in them as a person and by the use of psychiatric labels. "In the case of schizophrenia, [psychiatric labeling] has been shown to elicit beliefs that those affected by the illness are dangerous and unpredictable, which, in turn, resulted in negative emotional reactions and an increased desire for social distance" (Angermeyer and Matschinger 2003).

Mental health professionals view those receiving mental health services through a highly trained diagnostic lens. Applying labels to aspects of human suffering they encounter enables mental health care providers to bring forth their expertise to help those in need. "However, if these labels evoke negative outcome expectations in the clinician, this is discouraging for both the patient hoping to get better, and the practitioner him- or herself, who is striving for therapeutic success, while actually not quite believing in it. This negative outlook inherent in the helping relationship has been found to contribute to burnout (Maslach 1982; Schaufeli and Enzmann 1998)—with damaging consequences both for mental health professionals' health and quality of care" (Schulze 2007).

## Overcoming Stigma to Promote Recovery

Mental health care is perhaps most unique among the health professions in the extent to which the provider brings him- or herself into the treatment, using his/her way of being with the patient to facilitate the healing process. Individuals receiving mental health care are often in need of a corrective emotional experience, one in which the person feels validated, heard, accepted, valued, not judged, and encouraged to find their voice and strength. This is what an engaged practitioner should seek to provide. Interactions that are cold, indifferent, and rushed, on the other hand, serve to reinforce the negative experiences and many individuals have had with others in their life and in society at large.

Taking the time to examine how we think and feel about, as well as behave toward the people we serve is imperative as a foundational step to engaging in shared decision-making and promoting recovery-oriented care. But self-examination should be followed by action; one should endeavor to challenge all beliefs and behaviors that are potentially stigmatizing, both in oneself and in others (e.g., tendency toward social distance, use of psychiatric labels), and to engage in behaviors that have been shown to promote recovery. We would argue that a commitment to shared decision-making is a central part of this endeavor.

## Putting Shared Decision-Making into Practice

Simon et al. (2006) have identified the following steps involved in shared decision-making: (1) recognition that a decision needs to be made; (2) identification of partners in the process as equals; (3) statement of the options as equal; (4) exploration of understanding and expectations; (5) identifying preferences; (6) negotiating options/concordance; (7) sharing the decision; and (8) arranging followup to evaluate decision-making outcomes (Shared Decision-Making in Mental Health Care: Practice, Research, and Future Directions 2010; Simon et al. 2006). These do not have to take place in the same encounter, but should occur over the course of arriving at a final decision.

## Shared Decision-Making Competencies

Successful shared decision-making requires that both the provider and the consumer develop specific skills. Towle and Godolphin (1999) have proposed competencies for both providers and patients.

### Provider Competencies

1. The ability to facilitate a partnership relationship.
   This is critical to developing the framework for shared decision-making. The provider must not only communicate caring, but also facilitate sharing through an explicit

discussion about the patient-provider relationship and encourage a sense of mutual responsibility (Cousin et al. 2012).

2. The ability to mutually set the agenda for the clinical encounter.
   "Before patients can decide whether or not to share in decision-making, they must be offered the choice of participation by their physician" (Charles et al. 1997). Mutually setting the agenda allows the provider to communicate interest in the patient's priorities and values. Furthermore, it facilitates effective time management and improves the efficiency of the clinical encounter.

3. The ability to recognize that a decision can or must be made and to hold a position of professional equipoise when there is more than one reasonable treatment approach (Elwyn et al. 2000).
4. The ability to effectively identify and evaluate the possible courses of action, including no treatment if that is relevant or reasonable.
5. The ability to clearly present the problem/illness and the decision to be made to the patient, including an overview of the medical evidence regarding risks and benefits.
6. The ability to engage the patient in a discussion that (a) establishes the patient's preferred role in the decision-making process, (b) covers the existence and nature of any uncertainty about the course of action to take, and (c) helps the patient to reflect on the options in the context of his/her values and lifestyle.
7. It is important that the provider elicit the patient's thoughts, concerns, and opinions using open-ended questions while providing reassurance and encouragement. The provider must be flexible in addressing the patient's response to the issue at hand, recognizing that some patients will have difficulty coming to a decision and may prefer to defer to the provider's opinion.
8. The provider must be able to see to it that an agreement is reached on each of the following: (a) a treatment that is consistent with the patient's value and preferences; (b) a plan of action for implementing the treatment; and (c) a plan for followup.

It is critical that both the individual and provider are clear on the decision that has been made and that an understanding has been reached regarding the plan and what it entails, as well as expectations, roles and responsibilities, and arrangements for followup (Towle and Godolphin 1999). Certified Peer Specialists can play a key role in strengthening provider competencies. Multiple studies have shown this to be the case. Of particular importance is exposure to consumer-led interventions, where "the person is the message" (Boyd et al. 2010; Corrigan et al. 2010; Corrigan et al. 2001; Peebles et al. 2009).

## Patient Competencies

Sharing in decision making requires that individuals receiving services also have specific skills. As described by Towle and Godolphin (1999), competencies for the patient include:

1. Defining for oneself the preferred provider-patient relationship;
2. Finding a provider and developing an effective partnership;
3. Articulating for oneself the problem(s) at hand;
4. Communicating to the provider relevant feelings, beliefs, and expectations;
5. Evaluating the available information in order to participate in making the decision; and
6. Having a willingness to negotiate decisions, give feedback, resolve conflict, and agree on an action plan.

For most individuals, the preference for a particular type of doctor–patient relationship evolves naturally over the course of one's health care experiences. However, it is likely that most do not take the step of formally defining for themselves what that preferred relationship would actually entail. In the psychiatric inpatient setting, patients are most often assigned to a provider on the unit and rarely have the ability to choose their provider. This does not, however, have to preclude the development of an effective partnership in which shared decision-making can take place.

## Strengthening Patient Competencies

Individual's active involvement in their care should be supported and encouraged at all times. Street et al. (2005) have described three forms of communication behaviors that represent active patient participation: asking questions; expressing concerns and negative feelings such as frustration or fear, and being assertive (stating opinions and preferences). Clinicians can facilitate active patient involvement in several key ways, namely: directly soliciting and affirming patients' opinions and feelings (e.g., "What do you think about this plan?" "Tell me more about that."); asking open-ended questions; inquiring regularly about preferences; encouraging the individual to write down questions and concerns before the next encounter; and making use of Decision Aids (DAs) (Street et al. 2005). Such behaviors on the provider's part legitimize the individual's perspective and create expectations and opportunities for the individual to discuss needs and concerns (Street et al. 2005). Individuals who are more hesitant or reluctant to share their opinions and preferences should still be encouraged to participate in the decision-making process. Participating in making even the smallest of decisions about care may serve as a first step to making other decisions (Shared Decision-Making in Mental Health Care: Practice, Research, and Future Directions 2010).

## Challenges in Shared Decision-Making: Managing Disagreement

There are times when, perhaps due to a lack of clear clinical evidence or the existence of strong patient or provider preference, there is disagreement on the course of action to take. In such instances, a decision must be negotiated through open back and forth communication until the conflict is resolved. Disagreement that persists despite efforts at negotiation may reflect factors such as differing cultural perspectives, the individual's educational background, or emotional distress associated with the clinical situation. With the exception of cases in which a delay in the implementation of treatment would clearly result in imminent harm to the individual or others, tabling the discussion with a plan to followup at a specified time in the near future may be most appropriate. Providing the individual with a DA to review prior to the next encounter and involving their loved ones or other members of the health care team may be helpful strategies to move toward a shared decision in such situations.

## Using DAs

Psychiatric decisions frequently require weighing benefits against lifestyle-impacting side effects, whether from medications (e.g., sexual dysfunction, weight gain, tardive dyskinesia), somatic therapies, (e.g., short-term memory impairment from ECT), or psychosocial interventions (e.g., group home placement). In these situations, DAs can be powerful facilitators of shared decision-making, helping individuals deliberate about the personal value of the benefits and harms of the treatment options available and to understand and clarify their choices and preferences (O'Connor 2001; Shared Decision-Making in Mental Health Care: Practice, Research, and Future Directions 2010). They can also provide the technical support providers who have indicated that they need in order to be able to engage in shared decision-making (Shared Decision-Making in Mental Health Care: Practice, Research, and Future Directions 2010).

DAs are distinguished from other patient resources by the "inclusion of exercises designed to promote clarification of the patient's values regarding what is at stake…[and are]… intended to promote 'self-help' in the treatment decision-making process" (Llewellyn-Thomas 1995). Treatment DAs function both as an educational intervention and, by breaking the decision down into a number of specific and sequential steps, as a structure for the decision-making process (Charles et al. 1997).

DAs have become more widely available in recent years and exist in a variety of forms from printed brochures to interactive, web-based electronic tools. Studies on the use of DAs in mental health care have shown them to produce a number positive outcomes including more realistic expectations of treatment outcomes, increased consumer participation in decision making without increased consumer anxiety, and increased agreement between consumers' values and choices. In addition to these outcomes, a systematic review of studies of patient DAs in mental health also found that they reduced decisional conflict by helping patients feel more comfortable with their choices, lowered the number of those unsure what to choose, and stimulated patients to be more active (Schauer et al. 2007).

The Ottawa Hospital Research Institute has developed and compiled a list of various DAs, some of which are designed for use in mental health care decisions that are diagnosis specific as well as others that are more general. They have also designed the *Ottawa Personal Decision Guide for People Facing Tough Health or Social Decisions* (Ottawa Personal Decision Guide for People Facing Tough Health or Social Decisions 2011). This tool guides patients through steps to clarify the decision—explore facets of the decision including support persons, values, knowledge of risks and benefits; identify decision-making needs; and plan next steps based on those needs. Tools such as the *Ottawa Personal Decision Guide for People Facing Tough Health or Social Decisions* can be easily accessed from the web, printed and given to patients to complete during the clinical encounter or prior to the next.

Another program, the CommonGround, is a comprehensive web-based application that supports shared decision-making (CommonGround 2015). Access to the program is provided to individuals receiving services at designated Decision Support Centers prior to their psychiatric visit. The touch-screen application guides them to develop personal goals, "Power Statements," and "Personal Medicine" strategies (2013 APA Gold Award: Amplifying the voices of individuals who use mental health services: a commitment to shared decision making: Decision Support Centers, Community Care Behavioral Health Organization, Pittsburgh, Pennsylvania 2013). The program's other features—including decision support tools as well as inspirational videos on recovery—empower individuals to approach their encounter with the provider in an active and engaged manner.

CommonGround has been implemented in a variety of practice settings and by a variety of organizations. For example, the Community Behavioral Health Care Organization at the University of Pittsburgh Medical Center has implemented CommonGround in its peer-run Decision Support Centers. Other examples include the Two-Way Communication Checklist (Van Os et al. 2004; Van Os et al. 2002), DIALOG (Priebe et al. 2007), and the Right Question Project (Alegria et al. 2008). There is an extensive review of DAs in health care, and standards for health care DAs have been established by the International Patient DAs Standards (IPDAS) (Shared Decision-Making in Mental Health Care: Practice, Research, and Future Directions 2010; Stacey et al. 2014).

The use of DAs should be strongly encouraged in inpatient psychiatric care. It is important to note that the use of DAs and the development of Patient Competencies can be done outside of face-to-face time with the provider and, thus, help to maximize the efficiency and effectiveness of the time the clinician and individual receiving services have with one another. Giving thought to how physician extenders or support staff (e.g., mental health aids, Certified Peer Specialists) can facilitate these processes may be helpful. For individuals who wish to participate, but lack a systematic way of structuring the decision-making process, DAs can provide not only information but also a way of thinking about treatment decision-making that can help them focus on key issues and evaluate relevant options (Charles et al. 1997). As such, the use of these tools not only facilitates the development of patients' decision-making skills, but also communicates the provider's commitment to the shared decision-making endeavor.

## Conclusion

In summary, with regard to clinical decision-making on the inpatient psychiatric unit, shared decision-making provides a viable system of enhancing the engagement of care recipients in treatment and is an essential component of recovery-oriented practice. There is accumulating evidence that the traditional model of decision making is insufficient in psychiatric care and may play a significant role in the reluctance of individuals who need mental health care to seek it and sustain their efforts in it. Inasmuch as it represents a change from the paternalistic model of traditional care, shared decision-making requires a shift in perspective and skill for both the provider and for the individual receiving mental health services. Because behaviors are based on habits, long-held attitudes, beliefs and experiences, it is critical that providers engage in self-examination and ongoing self-reflection and make the effort to learn and employ strategies that facilitate shared decision-making. This involves learning and implementing shared decision-making competencies in oneself and facilitating them in one's patients, as well as using DAs whenever appropriate. These steps can not only greatly enhance the level of shared decision-making in the clinical encounter, but also help to make the most use of limited clinical encounter time. While individual practitioners must adapt these skills and tools to their own practice, it is clear that mental health providers must invest in shared decision-making if it is to take hold in the mental health care system.

## An Illustrative Case of Shared Decision-Making

**Brian Anderson, CPS**

***Do consumers want to participate in shared decision making?***

Yes. As a person that was diagnosed with Clinical Depression and Addictive Disease, I can tell you how important it was for me to have a voice in my recovery. Before shared decision in my treatment, I felt like a robot, following every command to the letter. I remember not trusting myself because I had failed over and over again, and there was an abundance of evidence to support my belief. It was not until I met someone who had been through what I was going through that I realized I had a voice in my own recovery, I had developed GREAT insight on the problem and solution. The power that came from my voice was a life changer; I felt alive again.

***Are consumers able to participate in shared decision-making?***

Yes. I have worked in the field of Mental Health over 25 years, in group homes, mental hospitals, medical centers, etc. I 'have literally seen the "light" come back on when clients started participating in their recovery, advocating for themselves. Given the chance, I have seen clients go back to school and get degrees, become employed, get married, facilitate recovery groups, put on workshops at mental health conferences, and reconnect with their families. All because a clinician, a staff member, a peer, took time to listen to them, their wants, needs, and desires.

***Is it important for mental health professionals to be able to view through the lens of the consumer?***

Absolutely. What a wonderful world it would be if all mental health workers did this one act for every encounter. We want only the best for ourselves—the best treatments, the best relationships, to be treated with respect and dignity—we all need that. That is why I live by this one statement: "I give what I need the most."

***Personal story***

After 28 days in inpatient treatment, I can recall being eager and yet terrified of going back to my hometown. In 28 days, I had been diagnosed, put on medication, gone through withdrawal and intense treatment. I was put on a treatment plan as a part of my release, and one of the "most important" steps I was ordered to take was to attend 90 NA meetings in 90 days. Then, out the doors of safety and back to reality I went. I immediately located the day treatment center and the NA meetings I was ordered to attend. Night after night I went to the NA for about two weeks meetings before something went wrong. (I must stop here and tell you that when I was in treatment for those 28 days on the inpatient unit, I reconnected with the God of my understanding and with the belief that ALL THINGS ARE MADE NEW WHEN YOU RETURN TO HIM). Back to the story, during every NA meeting, there's a statement that is repeated by everyone in attendance. I had to say, "My name is Brian Anderson, and I'm an addict." That statement left me very uncomfortable, feeling like an addict, and remembering all my addict ways, because once again I repeated it over and over and over again. I was in a fight. One of these statements was going to win, either ALL THINGS ARE MADE NEW WHEN YOU RETURN TO HIM or My name is Brian Anderson, and I am an addict. I decided to talk to my father and one of my favorite clinicians at the day treatment center and WE decided (with great input from me) that I would finish my 90 meetings at my Dad's church revival. Now this worked for me—this was my "individual plan of action." NA has worked miracles for many people and I would not dare say that everyone should follow my lead. What I will tell you is that with the help of a GREAT clinician, my dad, and myself, WE worked it out. Shared decision-making at its finest!

## References


2013 APA Gold Award: Amplifying the voices of individuals who use mental health services: A commitment to shared decision making: Decision Support Centers, Community Care Behavioral Health Organization, Pittsburgh, Pennsylvania. (2013). *Psychiatric Services, 64*(10), e7–e9.

Adams, J. R., & Drake, R. E. (2006). Shared decision-making and evidence-based practice. *Community Mental Health Journal, 42*(1), 87–105.

Adams, J. R., Drake, R. E., & Wolford, G. L. (2007). Shared decision-making preferences of people with severe mental illness. *Psychiatric Services, 58*(9), 1219–1221.

Ahmed, A. O., Birgenheir, D., Buckley, P. F., & Mabe, P. A. (2013). A psychometric study of recovery among Certified Peer Specialists. *Psychiatry Research, 209*(3), 721–731.

Ahmed, A. O., Buckley, P. F., & Mabe, P. A. (2012). Latent structure of psychotic experiences in the general population. *Acta Psychiatrica Scandinavica, 125*(1), 54–65.

Alegria, M., Polo, A., Gao, S., Santana, L., Rothstein, D., Jimenez, A., et al. (2008). Evaluation of a patient activation and empowerment intervention in mental health care. *Medical Care, 46*(3), 247–256.

American Psychiatric Association & American Association of Community Psychiatrists. (2011). *Psychiatry and recovery oriented practice: A situational analysis*. Washington, DC: Author.

Angermeyer, M. C., & Matschinger, H. (2003). The stigma of mental illness: Effects of labelling on public attitudes towards people with mental disorder. *Acta Psychiatrica Scandinavica, 108*(4), 304–309.

Barratt, A. (2008). Evidence based medicine and shared decision making: The challenge of getting both evidence and preferences into health care. *Patient Education and Counseling, 73*(3), 407–412.

Bedregal, L. E., O'Connell, M., & Davidson, L. (2006). The recovery knowledge inventory: Assessment of mental health staff knowledge and attitudes about recovery. *Psychiatric Rehabilitation Journal, 30*(2), 96–103.

Benbassat, J., Pilpel, D., & Tidhar, M. (1998). Patients' preferences for participation in clinical decision making: A review of published surveys. *Behavioral Medicine, 24*(2), 81–88.

Bond, G. R., Drake, R. E., & Becker, D. R. (2008). An update on randomized controlled trials of evidence-based supported employment. *Psychiatric Rehabilitation Journal, 31*(4), 280–290.

Boyd, J. E., Katz, E. P., Link, B. G., & Phelan, J. C. (2010). The relationship of multiple aspects of stigma and personal contact with someone hospitalized for mental illness, in a nationally representative sample. *Social Psychiatry and Psychiatric Epidemiology, 45*(11), 1063–1070.

Buckley, P. F., & Ahmed, A. O. (2013). Principles and practices of medication management for people with schizophrenia: Evolution within a recovery-based framework of care. In K. Yeager, D. Cutler, D. Svendsen, & G. Sills (Eds.), *Modern community mental health: An interdisciplinary approach*. New York: Oxford University Press.

Buckley, P. F., Schooler, N. R., Goff, D. C., Hsiao, J., Kopelowicz, A., Lauriello, J., et al. (2015). Comparison of SGA oral medications and a long-acting injectable SGA: The PROACTIVE study. *Schizophrenia Bulletin, 41*(2), 449–459.

Bunn, M. H., O'Connor, A. M., Tansey, M. S., Jones, B. D., & Stinson, L. E. (1997). Characteristics of clients with schizophrenia who express certainty or uncertainty about continuing treatment with depot neuroleptic medication. *Archives of Psychiatric Nursing, 11*(5), 238–248.

Burns, T., & Kendrick, T. (1997). The primary care of patients with schizophrenia: A search for good

practice. *British Journal of General Practice, 47*(421), 515–520.
Charles, C., Gafni, A., & Whelan, T. (1997). Shared decision-making in the medical encounter: What does it mean? (or it takes at least two to tango). *Social Science and Medicine, 44*(5), 681–692.
CommonGround. (2015). Retrieved on 5/25/15 from https://www.patdeegan.com/commonground
Conus, P., Lambert, M., Cotton, S., Bonsack, C., McGorry, P. D., & Schimmelmann, B. G. (2010). Rate and predictors of service disengagement in an epidemiological first-episode psychosis cohort. *Schizophrenia Research, 118*(1–3), 256–263.
Corrigan, P. W., Rafacz, J. D., Hautamaki, J., Walton, J., Rüsch, N., Rao, D., et al. (2010). Changing stigmatizing perceptions and recollections about mental illness: The effects of NAMI's in our own voice. *Community Menalt Health Journal, 46*(5), 517–522.
Corrigan, P. W., River, L. P., Lundin, R. K., Penn, D. L., Uphoff-Wasowski, K., Campion, J., et al. (2001). Three strategies for changing attributions about severe mental illness. *Schizophrenia Bulletin, 27*(2), 187–195.
Corry, P., Hogman, G., & Sandamas, G. (2001). *That's just typical*. London, UK: National Schizophrenia Fellowship.
Cousin, G., Schmid Mast, M., Roter, D. L., & Hall, J. A. (2012). Concordance between physician communication style and patient attitudes predicts patient satisfaction. *Patient Education and Counseling, 87*(2), 193–197.
Deegan, P. E., & Drake, R. E. (2006). Shared decision making and medication management in the recovery process. *Psychiatric Services, 57*(11), 1636–1639.
Deegan, P. E., Rapp, C., Holter, M., & Riefer, M. (2008). Best practices: A program to support shared decision making in an outpatient psychiatric medication clinic. *Psychiatric Services, 59*(6), 603–605.
Diamond, R. J. (2006). Recovery from a psychiatrist's viewpoint. *Postgraduate Medicine,* 54–62.
DiMatteo, M. R., Giordani, P. J., Lepper, H. S., & Croghan, T. W. (2002). Patient adherence and medical treatment outcomes: A meta-analysis. *Medical Care, 40*(9), 794–811.
Doyle, R., Turner, N., Fanning, F., Brennan, D., Renwick, L., Lawlor, E., & Clarke, M. (2014). First-episode psychosis and disengagement from treatment: A systematic review. *Psychiatric Services, 65*(5), 603–611.
Drake, R. E., & Deegan, P. E. (2009). Shared decision making is an ethical imperative. *Psychiatric Services, 60*(8), 1007.
Drapalski, A. L., Medoff, D., Unick, G. J., Velligan, D. I., Dixon, L. B., & Bellack, A. S. (2012). Assessing recovery of people with serious mental illness: Development of a new scale. *Psychiatric Services, 63*(1), 48–53.
Elwyn, G., Edwards, A., Kinnersley, P., & Grol, R. (2000). Shared decision making and the concept of equipoise: The competences of involving patients in healthcare choices. *British Journal of General Practice, 50*(460), 892–899.
Fenton, W. S., Blyler, C. R., & Heinssen, R. K. (1997). Determinants of medication compliance in schizophrenia: Empirical and clinical findings. *Schizophrenia Bulletin, 23*(4), 637–651.
Flynn, K. E., Smith, M. A., & Vanness, D. (2006). A typology of preferences for participation in healthcare decision making. *Social Science and Medicine, 63*(5), 1158–1169.
Godolphin, W. (2009). Shared decision-making. *Healthcare Quarterly, 12 Spec No Patient*, e186–e190.
Gordon, G. H., Joos, S. K., & Byrne, J. (2000). Physician expressions of uncertainty during patient encounters. *Patient Eduucation and Counseling, 40*(1), 59–65.
Hamann, J., Cohen, R., Leucht, S., Busch, R., & Kissling, W. (2007). Shared decision making and long-term outcome in schizophrenia treatment. *Journal of Clinical Psychiatry, 68*(7), 992–997.
Hamann, J., Kruse, J., Schmitz, F. S., Kissling, W., & Pajonk, F. G. (2010). Patient participation in antipsychotic drug choice decisions. *Psychiatry Research, 178*(1), 63–67.
Hamann, J., Langer, B., Winkler, V., Busch, R., Cohen, R., Leucht, S., & Kissling, W. (2006). Shared decision making for in-patients with schizophrenia. *Acta Psychiatrica Scandinavica, 114*(4), 265–273.
Hamann, J., Mendel, R., Cohen, R., Heres, S., Ziegler, M., Bühner, M., & Kissling, W. (2009). Psychiatrists' use of shared decision making in the treatment of schizophrenia: Patient characteristics and decision topics. *Psychiatric Services, 60*(8), 1107–1112.
Hansson, L., Jormfeldt, H., Svedberg, P., & Svensson, B. (2013). Mental health professionals' attitudes towards people with mental illness: Do they differ from attitudes held by people with mental illness? *International Journal of Social Psychiatry, 59*(1), 48–54.
Huhn, M., Tardy, M., Spineli, L. M., Kissling, W., Förstl, H., Pitschel-Walz, G., et al. (2014). Efficacy of pharmacotherapy and psychotherapy for adult psychiatric disorders: A systematic overview of meta-analyses. *JAMA Psychiatry, 71*(6), 706–715.
Improving the Quality of Health Care for Mental and Substance-Use Conditions. (2006). *Improving the quality of health care for mental and substance-use conditions: Quality chasm series*. Washington, DC: National Academic Press.
Kingdon, D., Sharma, T., & Hart, D. (2004). What attitudes do psychiatrists hold towards people with mental illness? *The Psychiatrist, 28*(11), 401–406.
Kreyenbuhl, J., Nossel, I. R., & Dixon, L. B. (2009). Disengagement from mental health treatment among individuals with schizophrenia and strategies for facilitating connections to care: A review of the literature. *Schizophrenia Bulletin, 35*(4), 696–703.
Kriston, L., Scholl, I., Hölzel, L., Simon, D., Loh, A., & Härter, M. (2010). The 9-item shared decision making questionnaire (SDM-Q-9). Development and psychometric properties in a primary care sample. *Patient Education and Counseling, 80*(1), 94–99.

Levinson, W., Kao, A., Kuby, A., & Thisted, R. A. (2005). Not all patients want to participate in decision making. A national study of public preferences. *Journal of General and Internal Medicine, 20*(6), 531–535.

Link, B. G., & Phelan, J. C. (2001). Conceptualizing Stigma. *Annual Review of Sociology, 27*, 363–385.

Llewellyn-Thomas, H. A. (1995). Patients' health-care decision making: A framework for descriptive and experimental investigations. *Medical Decision Making, 15*(2), 101–106.

Loh, A., Simon, D., Hennig, K., Hennig, B., Harter, M., & Elwyn, G. (2006). The assessment of depressive patients' involvement in decision making in audio-taped primary care consultations. *Patient Education and Counseling, 63*(3), 314–318.

Makoul, G., & Clayman, M. L. (2006). An integrative model of shared decision making in medical encounters. *Patient Education and Counseling, 60*(3), 301–312.

Malm, U., Ivarsson, B., Allebeck, P., & Falloon, I. R. (2003). Integrated care in schizophrenia: A 2-year randomized controlled study of two community-based treatment programs. *Acta Psychiatrica Scandinavica, 107*(6), 415–423.

Masand, P. S., Roca, M., Turner, M. S., & Kane, J. M. (2009). Partial adherence to antipsychotic medication impacts the course of illness in patients with schizophrenia: A review. *Prim Care Companion Journal of Clinical Psychiatry, 11*(4), 147–154.

Maslach, C. (1982). *Burnout: The cost of caring*. New York: Prentice Hall.

Mistler, L. A., & Drake, R. E. (2008). Shared decision making in antipsychotic management. *Journal of Psychiatric Practice, 14*(6), 333–344.

Noordsy, D. L., Torrey, W. C., Mead, S., Brunette, M., Potenza, D., & Copeland, M. E. (2000). Recovery-oriented psychopharmacology: Redefining the goals of antipsychotic treatment. *Journal of Clinical Psychiatry, 61*(Suppl 3), 22–29.

Nordt, C., Rössler, W., & Lauber, C. (2006). Attitudes of mental health professionals toward people with schizophrenia and major depression. *Schizophrenia Bulletin, 32*(4), 709–714.

O'Connor, A. M. (2001). Using patient decision aids to promote evidence-based decision making. *EMP Notebook, Vol. 6, July/August*.

O'Brien, A., Fahmy, R., & Singh, S. P. (2009). Disengagement from mental health services. A literature review. *Social Psychiatry and Psychiatric Epidemiology, 44*(7), 558–568.

Ottawa Hospital Research Institute. (2015). Retreived from https://decWoSonaid.ohri.ca/

Ottawa Personal Decision Guide for People Facing Tough Health or Social Decisions. (2011). Retrieved on January 6, 2015 from http://med.dartmouth-hitchcock.org/documents/OPDG_2pg.pdf

Patel, S. R., Bakken, S., & Ruland, C. (2008). Recent advances in shared decision making for mental health. *Current Opinion in Psychiatry, 21*(6), 606–612.

Peebles, S. A., Mabe, P. A., Fenley, G., Buckley, P. F., Bruce, T. O., Narasimhan, M., et al. (2009). Immersing practitioners in the recovery model: An educational program evaluation. *Community Menalt Health Journal, 45*(4), 239–245.

Priebe, S., McCabe, R., Bullenkamp, J., Hansson, L., Lauber, C., Martinez-Leal, R., et al. (2007). Structured patient-clinician communication and 1-year outcome in community mental healthcare: Cluster randomised controlled trial. *British Journal of Psychiatry, 191*, 420–426.

Priebe, S., Watts, J., Chase, M., & Matanov, A. (2005). Processes of disengagement and engagement in assertive outreach patients: Qualitative study. *British Journal of Psychiatry, 187*, 438–443.

Roberts, L. W., & Dyer, A. R. (2003). Caring for "difficult" patients. *FOCUS, 1*(4), 453–458.

Robinson, A., & Thomson, R. (2001). Variability in patient preferences for participating in medical decision making: Implication for the use of decision support tools. *Quality Health Care, 10*(Suppl 1), i34–i38.

Rossi, A., Amaddeo, F., Sandri, M., Marsilio, A., Bianco, M., & Tansella, M. (2008). What happens to patients seen only once by psychiatric services? Findings from a follow-up study. *Psychiatry Research, 157*(1–3), 53–65.

Rüsch, N., Angermeyer, M. C., & Corrigan, P. W. (2005). Mental illness stigma: Concepts, consequences, and initiatives to reduce stigma. *European Psychiatry, 20*(8), 529–539.

Schauer, C., Everett, A., del Vecchio, P., & Anderson, L. (2007). Promoting the value and practice of shared decision-making in mental health care. *Psychiatric Rehabilitation Journal, 31*(1), 54–61.

Schaufeli, W. B., & Enzmann, D. (1998). *The burnout companion to study and practice: A critical analysis*. London, UK: Taylor & Francis.

Schrank, B., Bird, V., Rudnick, A., & Slade, M. (2012). Determinants, self-management strategies and interventions for hope in people with mental disorders: Systematic search and narrative review. *Social Science and Medicine, 74*(4), 554–564.

Schulze, B. (2007). Stigma and mental health professionals: A review of the evidence on an intricate relationship. *International Review of Psychiatry, 19*(2), 137–155.

Shared Decision-Making in Mental Health Care: Practice, Research, and Future Directions. (2010). *HHS Publication No. SMA-09-4371*. Rockville, MD: Center for Mental Health Services, Substance Abuse and Mental Health Services Administration.

Simon, D., Schorr, G., Wirtz, M., Vodermaier, A., Caspari, C., Neuner, B., et al. (2006). Development and first validation of the shared decision-making questionnaire (SDM-Q). *Patient Education and Counseling, 63*(3), 319–327.

Stacey, D., Legare, F., Bennett, C. L., Barry, M. J., Eden, K. B., Homles-Rovner, M., et al. (2014). Decision aids to help people who are facing health treatment or screening decisions. Retreived on September 5, 20115 from http://www.cochrane.org/CD001431/COMMUN_decision-aids-to-help-people-who-are-facing-health-treatment-or-screening-decisions

Stewart, M., Brown, J. B., Weston, W. W., McWhinney, I. R., McWilliam, C. L., & Freeman, T. R. (2003). *Patient-centered medicine: Transforming the clinical method* (2nd ed.). Abingdon, UK: Radcliffe Medical Press.

Stowkowy, J., Addington, D., Liu, L., Hollowell, B., & Addington, J. (2012). Predictors of disengagement from treatment in an early psychosis program. *Schizophrenia Research, 136*(1–3), 7–12.

Street, R. L., Gordon, H. S., Ward, M. M., Krupat, E., & Kravitz, R. L. (2005). Patient participation in medical consultations: Why some patients are more involved than others. *Medical Care, 43*(10), 960–969.

Towle, A., & Godolphin, W. (1999). Framework for teaching and learning informed shared decision making. *British Medical Journal, 319*(7212), 766–771.

Valenstein, M., Blow, F. C., Copeland, L. A., McCarthy, J. F., Zeber, J. E., Gillon, L., et al. (2004). Poor antipsychotic adherence among patients with schizophrenia: Medication and patient factors. *Schizophrenia Bulletin, 30*(2), 255–264.

Van Os, J., Altamura, A. C., Bobes, J., Gerlach, J., Hellewell, J. S., Kasper, S., et al. (2004). Evaluation of the two-way communication checklist as a clinical intervention. Results of a multinational, randomised controlled trial. *British Journal of Psychiatry, 184*, 79–83.

Van Os, J., Altamura, A. C., Bobes, J., Owens, D. C., Gerlach, J., Hellewell, J. S., et al. (2002). 2-COM: An instrument to facilitate patient-professional communication in routine clinical practice. *Acta Psychiatrica Scandinavica, 106*(6), 446–452.

Woolf, S. H., Chan, E. C., Harris, R., Sheridan, S. L., Braddock, C. H., Kaplan, R. M., et al. (2005). Promoting informed choice: Transforming health care to dispense knowledge for decision making. *Annals of Internal Medicine, 143*(4), 293–300.

# Part II
# Practice

# 6 Inpatient Treatment Planning

Nirbhay N. Singh, Giulio E. Lancioni, Evelyn Harris and Alan S.W. Winton

## Introduction

There are probably as many ways of undertaking treatment planning as there are clinicians. But most inpatient psychiatric hospitals have or are inching toward an electronic medical records system that sets in stone how each hospital does its treatment planning. The treatment plans in these hospitals range from purely medical models of inpatient psychiatric care, with problem lists and diagnosis-specific treatments, to those that are heavily recovery based, which emphasize each individual's right to self-determination, preferences, and choices that will enable the individual to lead a fulfilling and meaningful life even in the presence of psychiatric disorders (Barber 2016). The nature of the recovery plans may also depend on whether the length of stay is acute or somewhat longer, or even long term due to civil and forensic commitments.

N.N. Singh (✉)
Department of Psychiatry and Health Behavior, Medical College of Georgia, Augusta University, Augusta, GA, USA
e-mail: nisingh@augusta.edu

G.E. Lancioni
Department of Neuroscience and Sense Organs, University of Bari, Bari, Italy

E. Harris
Division of Behavioral Health and Developmental Disabilities, Atlanta, GA, USA

A.S.W. Winton
Massey University, Palmerston North, New Zealand

Spaulding et al. (2016) have described the history and development of the concept of recovery, and Davidson et al. (2016) have cogently articulated the principles for recovery-oriented inpatient care. In this chapter, we present an example of treatment planning in recovery-oriented inpatient care that has been used successfully in state psychiatric facilities to enhance the quality of life of individuals with serious mental illness, including those with forensic involvement. In broad strokes, the chapter focuses on the mechanics of recovery planning for individuals with a length of stay in an inpatient facility that extends beyond acute care, i.e., psychiatric stabilization before discharge within a few days, typically within two weeks of admission. For those needing acute care, the essence of inpatient hospitalization is to provide immediate care, reduce the risk for further psychiatric and behavioral decompensation, attend to immediate medical needs, and to discharge them back to the community for further engagement in their recovery. For those requiring somewhat longer lengths of stay, staff needs to consider how it can support an individual to move from a sense of being burdened with a disability to a more meaningful life, even with mental illness present.

A basic question emerges when staff collaborates with the individual on what a meaningful or fulfilling life would entail for that individual. Most people have what has been termed *experiential interests* and *critical interests* that together



N.N. Singh et al. (eds.), *Handbook of Recovery in Inpatient Psychiatry*, Evidence-Based Practices in Behavioral Health, DOI 10.1007/978-3-319-40537-7_6

make life meaningful (Dworkin 1993). Experiential interests are those that the individual likes to do, such as listening to music, eating out, watching football, taking a walk in nature or the first monsoon rain, making love, or reading a novel. These are activities that the individual finds pleasurable or satisfying because they add something extra to that individual's life. If an individual did not experience these kinds of activities the value of life would not lessen; they simply provide something extra. Critical interests on the other hand are interests whose absence would produce a deficit in the individual's quality of life; with them, life is genuinely better. They involve judgment calls which an individual makes with regard to aspirations in life—to give and receive unconditional love, assist the less fortunate, have close relationships with one's family members, engage in spiritual practices, and so on. When supporting the development of an individual's recovery plan, the individual and staff should ensure the inclusion of both experiential and critical interests because, if sustained in the long term, these interests will give meaning to the individual's life and increase that individual's motivation to stay on the path of recovery. An individualized recovery plan, by definition, must involve more than mere symptoms to control; it must include one's life goals.

## Individualized Recovery Planning Process

An Individualized Recovery Plan (IRP) is the blueprint or roadmap for recovery that is initiated during an individual's admission to an inpatient hospital and the plan continues to be used when discharged to the next level of care in the community. The development of an IRP proceeds from a synthesis of (a) the reason for admission, (b) anticipated placement, (c) discharge criteria, (d) the individual's life goals and choices, (e) treatment and recovery needs identified by risk and multidisciplinary assessments, and (f) the discharge plan. The discharge process begins at admission, and the reason for admission determines the pathway to discharge. A person-centered planning assumes that the individual will (a) take increasing responsibility for his or her engagement in recovery, as treatment, rehabilitation, and enrichment progress, (b) resolve the reasons for admission, (c) overcome discharge barriers with the assistance of hospital and community agency staff to the greatest extent possible, and (d) be discharged to the next level of care. If admitted on forensic charges, the individual's legal status may determine the next level of care; in their absence, however, discharge should be to the most integrated setting available in the community (e.g., permanent housing with wraparound supports).

The IRP is designed to offer the individual in recovery, family members and significant others, conservators and guardians, and other authorized representatives, an opportunity to participate meaningfully in the recovery and discharge process. The IRP is individualized, person-centered, strength-based, and demonstrates respect for self-determination, personal choices, preferences, hopes, aspirations, and cultural and spiritual values, beliefs and practices. As a general rule, staff should always encourage the individual to engage in recovery planning, fully understand the IRP process, and collaborate with his or her Recovery Planning Team (RPT)—traditionally called the *Treatment Planning Team*—to develop goals, objectives, and interventions that are meaningful for that individual. The individual's signature on the signature page of the IRP is necessary, but not sufficient, to show that these conditions have been met. As recovery proceeds, the RPT should engage, encourage, and facilitate the individual to gradually assume increasing responsibility for reviewing and revising his or her IRP.

## RPT

The membership of a RPT is dictated by the particular needs and strengths of the individual in recovery. In addition to the individual, the core team members include a psychiatrist, clinical psychologist, registered nurse, social worker, rehabilitation therapist, and direct care staff (e.g., health service technician, forensic service technician who best knows the individual). The core RPT membership should be consistent and enduring, as staffing permits. Other staff (e.g., behavior specialist, nutritionist, primary care physician, physical therapist, occupational therapist, speech and language pathologist, peer specialist, activity therapist) and family members, significant others, conservators, guardians, advocates, friends, and community treatment provider (as authorized by the individual), may be invited to attend, depending on the specific needs and by request of the individual. The core RPT members must verifiably be competent in the development and implementation of IRPs as well as in the principles of recovery.

## Role of the RPT

A key role of the RPT is to develop and implement an IRP that optimizes the individual's recovery and sustains the individual in the most integrated and appropriate setting. This setting is based on the individual's legal status, life goals, strengths, and functional abilities, and promotes the individual's self-determination, preferences, choices, and independence. The RPT should ensure that the individual has substantive input into the IRP process including, but not limited to, input with regard to focused interventions, psychosocial treatment mall groups, and individual therapies appropriate to his or her assessed needs. In addition, the RPT should educate the individual regarding his or her roles, rights, and responsibilities with regard to developing the IRP, engaging in treatment and rehabilitation, working on discharge goals, and revising and updating the IRP as recovery proceeds.

## Initial Recovery Plan

The initial recovery plan is the individual's first "treatment plan." The admitting physician and the registered nurse develop this plan at the time of admission (i.e., within 24 h of admission). It is based on admission assessments, and includes immediate treatment goals and interventions that focus on the individual's psychiatric, medical, and behavioral concerns, as well as potential risks (e.g., for aggression or suicide). The individual's RPT meets on the second business day of admission and begins the process of updating this plan as new information and assessment data become available. Revision schedules may differ across hospitals, depending on the average length of stay or hospital-specific policies. Usually, the initial recovery plan is updated by the RPT within 72 h of admission. The 72-h update and subsequent periodic updates provide the basis for care of the individual until the first IRP is developed on the 15th day.

## Assessments

The admitting physician/psychiatrist and nurse complete the admission assessment within the first 24 h of admission. Usually the nursing assessments begin at admission and are completed within the first 8 h of admission. The individual's psychiatrist completes the Psychiatric Evaluation within 60 h of admission and the social worker completes the Initial Psychosocial Assessment within 72 h of admission. The RPT clinical psychologist, social worker, and activity therapist complete the Integrated Psychosocial Assessment by the 12th day of admission. The RPT team leader or facilitator synthesizes the assessment findings and recommendations, and presents a holistic picture of the individual when developing the first IRP. This synthesis incorporates other assessments, including the admission assessment, Psychiatric Evaluation, Initial Psychosocial Assessment, violence risk assessment, suicide risk assessment, clinical risk profile, input from the individual (as much as possible, depending on his or her mental health), his or her family (as appropriate) and community sources, as necessary and appropriate.

## Focused Assessments

Periodically, the RPT may request additional assessments, as clinically indicated. Examples include neuropsychological and behavioral assessments, personality tests, speech, dysphagia, nutrition, physical therapy, occupational therapy, and other assessments that may assist differential diagnosis, assessments related to specific psychiatric disorders and psychological distress, and outcome measures. The results of these assessments are also integrated into the IRP.

## Cognitive Assessments

These are a specific example of focused assessments. Individuals with cognitive impairments (e.g., developmental disabilities, dementia, traumatic brain injury, or other conditions that may lead to cognitive decline) should be assessed at admission and periodically after that, as clinically indicated. The purpose of the cognitive assessment is to provide an individual's RPT with information and recovery recommendations so that it can assist the individual to make appropriate choices with regard to treatment, psychosocial rehabilitation, and enrichment activities. These assessments should be in the form of cognitive screening or a full neuropsychological battery, and should specify particular types of cognitive remediation programs that will best enhance the individual's recovery (Hill et al. 2016).

## Strengths

Knowledge of an individual's strengths or protective factors can enable the RPT and care staff to provide specific social and instrumental supports, and enable group facilitators in the Psychosocial Rehabilitation Malls (for details, see PSR Malls below) to motivate the individual to fully participate in recovery activities. In this context, whatever the individual presents (including personal attributes, characteristics, skills, diseases, disability, or disorders) can be used as strengths to achieve symptom and functional recovery, and to enhance quality of life. The *Strengths-Based Conversation* is a 40-item protocol that clinicians can use as the basis for conversing with the individual (see Table 6.1). The aim of this conversation is to facilitate the mutual exploration of the individual's general strengths and highlight specific strengths that the individual wishes to enhance or use in recovering from mental illness. The *Strengths-Based Conversation* is not used as a tool for a structured interview; strengths will emerge from discussions of an individual's life goals. These strengths should be updated as the individual begins to recover and is increasingly able to use identified strengths in the recovery process.

## Stages of Change

In a recovery model of mental health service delivery system, it is important to consider the concept of stages of change. Psychotic behavior may be so serious in terms of severity, frequency, intensity, and duration that it interferes with an individual's quality of life. The clinician may think that the person needs to be in treatment. Whether the individual agrees with this assessment will depend on that individual's understanding of the disorder and the need for treatment, and a willingness to engage in the treatment. To determine the approximate level that treatment should begin, clinicians often assess the individual's stage of change using a transtheoretical model (DiClemente and Prochaska 1998; Prochaska and DiClemente 1983; Prochaska and Velicer 1997). There are five nonlinear stages in the transtheoretical model—precontemplation, contemplation, preparation, action, and maintenance. Stages of change do not assess the individual's capacity to change because that quality is a given in all individuals.

The University of Rhode Island Change Assessment (URICA) is a widely used tool that can be used to assess an individual's stage of change (McConnaughy et al. 1983). Traditionally, the URICA is completed by a clinician who has the greatest rapport with the individual, or by

**Table 6.1** Strength-based conversation

| | |
|---|---|
| Name of Individual: | Age: |
| Hospital ID#: | Admission Date: |
| Unit/Program: | DOB: |
| Dates of Conversation: | Facilitator: |

Respondents, if other than individual (e.g., parents, advocates, siblings):

---

*You can use this instrument as the basis for a conversation with an individual in recovery. It is usually advisable to hold the conversation in a pleasant area, preferably in a social setting where the individual feels comfortable. Invite the individual to have something to eat or drink (e.g., coffee, soda, water) when you have a conversation, or when you are engaged in some task that does not require focused attention (e.g., a walk on the grounds). Make notes following, but not during, the conversation. The areas you should cover are determined by the type of information you need to assist the individual with his or her recovery. For example, if you want to know something about his or her life goals, you can use the Miracle Question and the Possibility Questions, or if you are interested in knowing how the individual will handle discharge, focus on the Discharge Questions as the basis of the conversation. You can use the conversation like a "focused assessment," by developing a conversation around only those areas that are most pertinent at the time.*

---

**Survival Questions:**

1. How have you managed to survive or thrive, thus far, given all the challenges you have had to contend with?
2. What is going well for you right now?
3. What are you willing to do to make things work well for you?

**Support Questions:**

4. Who are the special people on whom you can depend?
5. Who is important to you in your life?

**Exception Question:**

6. In the past, when you felt that your life was better, more interesting, or more stable, what about your world, your relationships, and your thinking was different or special? [Several issues are embedded in this one]

**Possibility Questions:**

7. What do you want out of life?
8. What is important to you in your life?
9. What makes life worth living for you?
10. What are your hopes, visions, and aspirations?
11. If things were different, what would you wish for?
12. If you had three wishes, what would they be?
13. What are you willing to do to make your wishes come true?

(continued)

**Table 6.1** (continued)

**Esteem Questions:**

14. When people say good things about you, what are they likely to say?
15. What do you think is unique about you that people should know?

**Discharge Questions:**

16. Are you anxious about being discharged?
17. Do you have any fears about being discharged?
18. What can we do to make it easier for you to live in the community?
19. Who can you count on in the community to be there for you?
20. What are you willing to do to make this transition successful?

**Housing Questions:**

21. What sort of housing arrangements have worked for you in the past?
22. Under ideal conditions, where would you like to live?
23. When you lived in the community, what sort of place did you live in?
24. What sort of place would you like to live in when you are discharged? Why?
25. How can we help you to find a place like this?
26. What are you willing to do to live in a place like this?

**Employment Questions:**

27. What jobs have you had in the past?
28. Which one(s) did you like the best? Why?
29. What sort of work would you like to do in future?
30. How can we help you get this kind of work?
31. What are you willing to do to get this kind of work?

**Daily Activities Questions:**

32. What do you do in a regular day?
33. What did you do before you were hospitalized (. . . or before your current hospitalization or in your previous Unit)?
34. What would you like to do in the future?
35. What are you willing to do make this possible?

**General Conversation Questions:**

36. What makes you happy?
37. Is religion or spirituality important in your life?
38. What are your priorities in life?
39. Who are the most important people in your life?

**The Miracle Question:**

40. The miracle question is often a good way to stimulate thinking about life goals and aspirations:

    Suppose that while you are sleeping tonight a miracle happens. The miracle is that the issues that you have (e.g., being incarcerated, having mental illness, homelessness) are somehow solved, but you don't know that because you are asleep.

(continued)

**Table 6.1** (continued)

a. What will you notice different tomorrow morning that will tell you that a miracle has happened?
b. What is the first thing you will notice after the miracle happens?
c. What might your ... (family member, friend) notice about you that would give him or her the idea that things are better for you?
d. When he or she notices that, what might he or she do differently?
e. When he or she does that, what would you do?

the individual. The URICA is used for specific issues, and not as a general or global measure of a person's stage of change. It measures the person's stage of change for a specific area of life functioning (e.g., substance use), and this may vary over time or with treatment. A skilled clinician may clinically determine an individual's stage of change without using a rating scale.

## Individualized Recovery Plan

The IRP—traditionally called the *Master Treatment Plan*—is the individualized recovery plan that provides a roadmap for an individual's recovery while in the hospital. It is developed by the 15th day of admission, reviewed for progress on a preset schedule, incrementally completed as new assessment, consultation, and treatment data, or other information become available, and is fully developed by the 60th day of admission, although the days specified might vary with hospital-specific policies.

### Recovery Planning Schedule

Inpatient hospitals usually have specific schedules for initiating, completing, and updating the IRP. In broad terms, these include an initial IRP, followed by monthly, quarterly, and annual reviews. In addition, hospital policy will also specify the tasks that the RPT will undertake for the initial IRP and for the scheduled IRP reviews. Typically, the initial IRP and monthly and quarterly reviews take between 20 and 30 min, while annual reviews take a little longer because of the interval length. In this context, it is useful to remember that the IRP should not be a long document. Although there may be exceptions, a fully developed IRP is usually no more than 8–12 pages in length, and is written at the reading and comprehension level of the individual.

### IRP for Internal Transfers

When an individual is transferred between units or programs, a RPT conference is scheduled on the day following the transfer, and then the regular cycle from the original admission date is continued. If the transfer is made within five business days of a scheduled conference, the RPT may complete the 15-day, monthly, quarterly, or annual IRP in lieu of the one-day post-transfer IRP review. The receiving RPT is required to review the entire IRP and make revisions based on current information and as clinically indicated.

### IRP for Readmissions

Some individuals may be discharged and readmitted to the hospital for a number of reasons (e.g., court returns, outside medical care, failure to integrate fully in the community). When an individual is readmitted in less than 90 days after discharge, an IRP is completed within the first 24 h. The individual's RPT meets on the second business day of admission and updates the individual's original IRP (from the previous admission). The first RPT conference is scheduled on the 15th day following readmission. If the integrated assessments indicate no major changes in condition, the individual is placed on a monthly

IRP review cycle from the date of the previous admission. If the integrated assessments indicate major changes in the individual's condition, the RPT should follow the new admission sequence for review meetings. In either case, the assessment findings should be documented in the Present Status section of the individual's IRP. For readmissions longer than 90 days, the individual should be treated as a completely new admission.

### IRP for Transfer to Another Hospital

When an individual is transferred to another inpatient hospital, all assessments and the recovery plan follow the individual. Clinicians at the receiving inpatient hospital complete new assessments after meeting with the individual, but the process may be treated like an update, as the receiving hospital should utilize the information from the sending facility. The first IRP is based on the final IRP before discharge of the individual from the prior hospital. The first IRP meeting is an opportunity to update, revise, or add any new goals and objectives to the IRP, and will allow the recovery team to work with the individual to identify the interventions that are available at the receiving hospital to meet the recovery goals and objectives of the individual.

## Sample IRP Template

A sample IRP template is provided in Table 6.2. This can be modified to suit the specific requirements of any inpatient hospital. Typically, the IRP is a part of the hospital's electronic medical records, and the RPT members, together with the individual, collaboratively discuss and complete the form. In addition to inserting the demographics, the RPT team leader assists the members to conceptualize the case and develop goals, objectives, and interventions.

### Case Formulation

A case formulation assists an individual in recovery to understand the likely origins of his or her problems, what triggers them, and what maintains them. It assists the individual's RPT to collaborate with the individual to develop optimal treatment and support options that put the individual on a trajectory to recovery. The case formulation is developed by the RPT, not just by a single team member. Using a team process to develop, review, and revise the case formulation ensures that the team is focusing on the individual as a person opposed to just specific diseases, disorders, or deficits of that individual.

There are numerous ways that cases can be formulated. For example, in this IRP, the case formulation is structured as follows:

#### Pertinent History

History can be within any timeframe, but typically includes historical information that may impact current treatment. The individual's pertinent history is not repeated in other sections of the case formulation. The following sequence can be used to describe pertinent history: (a) *Personal*: Includes a brief sketch of the individual's social history (i.e., age, education, employment, family of origin, course of life, current support system); (b) *Psychiatric, Behavioral, and Medical*: Includes a brief description of the individual's history of mental illness (i.e., psychiatric history, course of illness, past hospitalizations including reasons for admission), maladaptive behaviors, and a medical history; and (c) *Legal*: Includes a brief description of the individual's legal history (i.e., interaction with the legal system) and, if applicable, a very brief statement of the instant alleged offense.

#### Predisposing Factors

A predisposing factor is any condition that predisposes the individual to possible adverse

**Table 6.2** Individualized recovery plan

| | | | |
|---|---|---|---|
| **Individual's Name:** | | **ID Number:** | |
| **Admission Date:** | | **Date Of Continuous Admission** | |
| **Date of IRP:** | ☐ 15-Day ☐ Monthly ☐ Quarterly ☐ Annual | | |
| **Legal Status:** | | | |
| | | | |
| **CASE FORMULATION** | | | |
| **Pertinent History** | | | |
| | | | |
| **Predisposing Factors** | | | |
| | | | |
| **Precipitating Factors** | | | |
| | | | |
| **Perpetuating Factors** | | | |
| | | | |
| **Previous Treatments and Response** | | | |
| | | | |
| **Present Status** | | | |
| | | | |
| **PREFERRED METHOD OF DE-ESCALATION** | | | |
| | | | |
| **DIAGNOSIS** | | | |
| Date of Diagnosis: | | | |
| **Diagnoses** | | | |
| | | | |
| **Medical Conditions** | | | |
| | | | |
| **Psychosocial and Contextual Factors** | | | |
| | | | |
| **Disability** | | | |
| | | | |
| **INDIVIDUAL'S LIFE GOALS** | | | |
| | | | |
| | | | |
| **DISCHARGE PROCESS** | | | |
| **Reason For Admission** | | | |
| | | | |
| **Discharge Criteria For Anticipated Placement** | | | |
| | | | |
| **Discharge Plan** | | | |
| | | | |
| **Discharge Barriers** | | | |

(continued)

**Table 6.2** (continued)

| | | | |
|---|---|---|---|
| | | | |
| | | | |
| **GOAL # 1** | | **DATE INITIATED:** | |
| | | | |
| **OBJECTIVES** | | | |
| **OBJ. #** | **OBJECTIVE DESCRIPTION** | | **NEXT REVIEW DATE** |
| | | | |
| | | | |
| **INTERVENTIONS** | | | |
| **INT. #** | **INTERVENTION DESCRIPTION** | | |
| | | | |
| | | | |
| | | | |
| **GOAL # 2** | | **DATE INITIATED:** | |
| | | | |
| **OBJECTIVES** | | | |
| **OBJ. #** | **OBJECTIVE DESCRIPTION** | | **NEXT REVIEW DATE** |
| | | | |
| | | | |
| **INTERVENTIONS** | | | |
| **INT. #** | **INTERVENTION DESCRIPTION** | | |
| | | | |
| | | | |
| (Delete or add blank rows in each section as needed)<br>(Add more goals, as needed) | | | |
| | | | |
| **DEFERRED ISSUES** | | | |
| | | | |
| | | | |
| **SOCIAL SUPPORT** | | | |
| Relationship to Individual in Recovery | Contact Person | | Telephone |
| | | | |
| | | | |
| | | | |
| | | | |
| | | | |

outcomes. At a minimum, if the individual's clinical risk profile has identified high risks (psychiatric, behavioral, or medical), it includes those that could be predisposing factors for conditions that may occur in the absence of preventative interventions. An example of a statement of a predisposing factor is, "Francis has diagnoses of dyslipidemia and hypertension, and a BMI of 35; thus, he is at risk for developing metabolic syndrome." In addition, other documented risk conditions identified in assessments should be considered as predisposing factors.

### Precipitating Factors

A precipitating factor is any condition that has been found, through assessment or observation, to precipitate the occurrence or exacerbation of an adverse outcome (e.g., maladaptive behavior, medical condition, psychological distress, or psychiatric disorder). These factors are based on the individual's current clinical condition and assessments, and any recorded behavioral challenges (e.g., instances of aggressive or destructive behavior). An example of a precipitating factor due to a medical condition would be: "Judy is very irritable when she is hypoglycemic. If a staff member makes a demand when she is irritable, she is likely to be verbally and, occasionally, physically aggressive. With Judy, low blood sugar level precipitates irritation, which may lead to verbal and physical aggression under demand conditions." If an individual is admitted for pretrial evaluation or competency restoration, the focus is on the psychiatric symptoms or behaviors that may interfere with the individual's ability to proceed and participate in the legal process.

### Perpetuating Factors

A perpetuating factor is any variable that is untreatable or may continue to perpetuate adverse conditions or outcomes for the individual if left untreated. In some cases, identifying a perpetuating factor (e.g., treatment, or medication non-adherence) may enable an effective treatment to be developed and implemented. In other cases (e.g., cancer), while the disease itself may not be fully treatable, the condition that the disease perpetuates may be (e.g., depression). For example, "Bruce is depressed because of the pain and suffering due to cancer. His cancer is a perpetuating factor for his depression." Certain psychosocial factors (e.g., crowded rooms, unsupervised transition times, fear of discharge in long-term inpatients) are also perpetuating factors for some behaviors. In some cases, there may be an overlap between precipitating and perpetuating factors, and occasionally among predisposing, precipitating, and perpetuating factors.

### Previous Treatment and Response

Previous treatment includes treatments utilized throughout the course of the individual's psychiatric and medical illnesses, treatments for maladaptive behavior, including culture-based treatments, and psychosocial interventions (e.g., PSR Mall groups, behavior plans, outpatient programs). The response to these treatments and any adverse effects of psychotropic and other medications should be described. It is useful to include symptoms or target behaviors for which the treatments were provided and not just the psychiatric diagnosis. In addition, it is clinically relevant to include any treatments that were discontinued during the review period. For long-stay individuals, it is acceptable to consider the impact of previous treatments and responses on current treatment for only the preceding 12–24 months. The narrative is a synthesis and not a chronological listing of previous treatments.

### Present Status

This section includes a clear description of the individual's current overall status as it pertains to the time period being reviewed (i.e., monthly, quarterly, or annual). It provides a clinical picture across relevant multiple domains, current efforts to provide treatment, and discharge readiness. Again, it is written as a synthesis rather than a chronological listing. The narrative usually begins with symptom status and includes any current signs and symptoms of psychiatric disorders, maladaptive behaviors, and psychological distress. For each symptom, there should be the current interventions (i.e., appropriate medications, psychosocial interventions, and behavioral interventions) and the responses to them. Then there should be a description of all medical conditions, with an update on their current status and treatment and any medication side effects.

This is followed by the current status of any risk profile—psychiatric, medical, or behavioral (e.g., violence, suicide, assault)—or other vulnerabilities covered under predisposing, precipitating, and perpetuating factors. Examples of medical risks include: bowel obstruction, choking, pneumonia, diabetes, falls, fractures, blood or body fluid diseases, metabolic syndrome, osteoporosis, seizures, refractory seizures, status epilepticus, electrolyte imbalance, impaired skin integrity. Include all incidents and behavioral events such as aggressive acts to self, aggressive acts to others, alleged abuse/neglect/exploitation, illicit substance use, property destruction, elopement, specified observations, restraints, seclusion, suicide, victimization, and unsubstantiated allegations.

Then follows a description of functional status in terms of what the individual is able to do at present (e.g., self-care, adherence to the recovery plan, skills, and strengths). The focus is on skills that may be considered essential at the next level of care (e.g., ADL skills, job skills, independent living skills). It should include a description of the individual's attendance and participation in the PSR Mall groups, level of achievement with current objectives and interventions, and the rationale for changing or maintaining goals, objectives and interventions. It is useful to incorporate any cultural issues that may impact the individual's interventions and wellness and also any general wellness concerns, and areas in need of further intervention. Finally, if applicable include current legal status as related to discharge status.

## Preferred Method of De-escalation

Occasionally individuals get irritated, agitated, or aggressive. Often staff can de-escalate the situation by engaging in methods that the individual has found to be particularly effective in the past. In this section, include any de-escalation methods that the individual, on becoming upset, would prefer the staff to use. For example, key information from the initial Personal Safety Interview (see Table 6.3), and updated information based on staff observations, can be included in this section. The key issue is that the information should be practical—staff should be able to understand and use the information to preempt maladaptive or challenging behavior.

## Diagnosis

Typically, this information is aligned with the most recent psychiatric evaluation or psychiatric progress note. Documentation of diagnosis is included, with separate notations for psychosocial and contextual factors, as well as disability.

## Individual's Life Goals

This is a statement of the individual's vision of recovery, including dreams, hopes, and aspirations. It may include what the individual would like to do while at the hospital, but it is intended to help the individual envision life following discharge. It is best stated as quotations in the individual's own words. If the individual declines to state life goals, document this. The individual's life goals are elicited in strength-based conversations prior to a RPT conference, but never during it. If the RPT feels that the individual's life goals represent delusional thinking, the team records what the individual has stated anyway. However, the team revisits and revises the life goals periodically as the individual's psychiatric condition improves. The main thing to remember is that, notwithstanding any mental illness, it is critical to know what the individual envisions his or her life could be, if given hope and tools for recovery (Shafer et al. 2016). The individual's life goals are updated periodically as they change depending on current recovery status.

## Discharge Process

### Reason for Admission

This includes a brief statement of the reason(s) why the individual was admitted to the hospital. The statement includes the precursor behavior that resulted in the admission. For example, if the individual was admitted for assault, assault or aggression would be the reason listed, but what is more important for informed intervention is what led to the aggression (e.g., medication non-adherence worsened the individual's underlying psychosis, and the assault occurred during a psychotic episode). At admission, it would be important to assess why the individual was medication nonadherent, and the inpatient treatment or training should focus on this reason.

If an individual is admitted for a pretrial forensic evaluation or competency restoration, this should be stated as the reason for admission, as well as the specific current symptoms or

**Table 6.3** Personal safety interview

**INSTRUCTIONS**: Interview the individual to complete this form or give it to the individual to complete (if preferred). Information can be updated through staff observations.

1. What are some of the things or "triggers" that make you irritated, upset, or angry?

| | | |
|---|---|---|
| Being Touched | Bedroom door open | Particular time of day (When?) |
| Loud noise | Being isolated | Time of year (When?) |
| People in uniform | | Being around men or women |
| Not having control (explain): | | |
| Other (Please list): | | |

2. It is helpful for our staff to be aware of how you might behave when you get irritated, upset, or angry. How will our staff know that you are getting upset? What behaviors should they look for? (That is, do you start pacing the floor? Do you begin talking to yourself? Do you clench your fists?)

________________________________________
________________________________________
________________________________________

3. How can staff members help you when they notice that you are getting irritated, upset or angry? (That is, what should they do, not do, say or not say when they notice you are getting irritated, upset or angry?)

________________________________________
________________________________________
________________________________________

4. Do you have preferences or concerns regarding who serves you (such as gender, race, language, culture)? ☐ Yes ☐ No
If yes, describe:

________________________________________
________________________________________

5. Seclusion and Restraint:
Have you ever been placed in a seclusion room? ☐ Yes ☐ No
Have you ever been restrained? ☐ Yes ☐ No
If yes, what led up to the incident(s)? Tell me about the experience(s) for you:

________________________________________
________________________________________

(continued)

**Table 6.3** (continued)

6. Is there anything you find helpful in emergency situations that could prevent seclusion or restraint being used? ☐ Yes ☐ No
If yes, describe:

____________________________________________

____________________________________________

7. Do you have any medical conditions or physical disabilities and limitations that may place you at risk if seclusion or restraint is used? ☐ Yes ☐ No
If yes, describe:

____________________________________________

____________________________________________

8. If you have to be placed in seclusion or restraint to help keep you and others safe, would you want us to notify someone? ☐ Yes ☐ No
If yes, what is that person's name and telephone number and his/her relationship to you?

____________________________________________

____________________________________________

9. Does it bother you if people get close to you and touch you? ☐Yes ☐No
If yes, describe:

____________________________________________

____________________________________________

10. Trauma History:
Have you experienced any incidents of: (a) Physical abuse? ☐ Yes ☐ No
(b) Sexual abuse? ☐ Yes ☐ No
If yes, are there things that remind you of the abuse and are difficult for you or cause you to act differently? ☐ Yes ☐ No
If yes, describe:

____________________________________________

____________________________________________

Would you find it helpful to discuss these issues with staff? ☐Yes ☐ No
Would you like more information on these issues in classes or support groups?
☐Yes ☐ No

11. Is there anything else you would like to tell me or discuss? ☐ Yes ☐ No
If yes, describe:

____________________________________________

____________________________________________

| Date/Time | Individual's Signature | RN's Signature (Print and sign name) |
|---|---|---|

behaviors that prompted the need for the evaluation or restoration. Also to be referenced are any evaluations that bear on the legal status (e.g., if newly admitted as Incompetent to Stand Trial (IST), what information in the pretrial report is relevant to the finding of incompetency). For forensic admissions, it is critical that only the official account (i.e., law enforcement or court documentation) is used, so that potentially discoverable, legally prejudicial information revealed by the individual is not recorded on his or her chart.

If it is a civil commitment, the narrative should explain the clinical condition and behavior that warranted hospitalization. It is best to describe the specific context of the individual's behavior that led to the hospitalization. If it is a readmission, the reason why the individual was not able to maintain community placement should be clearly stated. Being specific in describing the reason (i.e., the precipitating behavior) helps the PRT and the individual to collaboratively develop goals, objectives, and interventions for overcoming barriers to maintaining community placement upon next discharge.

## Discharge Criteria for Anticipated Placement

*Anticipated Placement.* This is where the individual may be discharged to when discharge ready, or with the court's agreement. If known, the name of the placement is provided; if unknown, the generic class of placement is stated (e.g., independent living, supported apartment, group home). In the recovery model, placement consideration begins at the highest independent level (e.g., independent apartment with supportive services) and works its way down to lower levels, if necessary.

*Discharge Criteria.* Typically, the hospital's discharge criteria are the admission criteria specified by the receiving agency, or those determined by the legal system (i.e., the penal code specifies competency requirements). The criteria are individualized and, as much as possible, are stated in behavioral and measurable terms. The criteria should be written in simple and clear language in terms of what the individual must do in order to be discharged to a specific place. If a specific placement is not available, the RPT can work on the basis of what the individual must do to be discharged to the most integrated setting available in the community.

The discharge criteria are written in language that the individual understands at first reading. A good way to do this is by (a) discussing each discharge criterion with the individual, (b) asking the individual to restate each criterion in his or her own words, and (c) if stated correctly, recording the individual's version of each discharge criterion. This will ensure that the individual has understood what he or she needs to do and, when the discharge criteria are read to that individual again, will understand these correctly without further discussion or training. It is useful to remember that the discharge criteria are written in terms of what the *individual* needs to do to be discharged. The criteria should be clinical in nature (with the exception of those individuals with a forensic legal status) and translate into goals, objectives, and interventions in the IRP, based on prioritized needs as determined by the individual's RPT.

## Discharge Plan

The discharge plan is a chronological sequence of all tasks that hospital staff (i.e., Social Worker, Case Manager, RPT) and/or community agencies will initiate and complete that will enable the individual to be discharged when the last item on the discharge plan is completed and all discharge criteria have been met. For accountability, the actual names of hospital and community agency staff responsible for each step, as well as realistic timelines, are listed. The timelines are specified only for the initial steps, with further timelines provided at successive reviews of the discharge plan. The discharge plan includes action steps specific to the individual as opposed to generic plans that may vaguely apply to all hospitalized individuals. The discharge plan does not pertain to the clinical services that staff provides to the individual (e.g., PSR Mall group, individual therapy), as these are addressed in the goals, objectives, and interventions in the IRP. The discharge plan is written in terms of what the *staff* needs to do to enable the individual to be discharged expeditiously. A person-centered discharge planning is accomplished in collaboration with all stakeholders, the individual, hospital staff, family, and friends, as well as the community providers. As the RPT determines appropriate community treatment services, it is important to identify other resource needs that an individual may need to achieve successful community tenure. These resource needs may include assisting the individual to obtain both federal and state-funded programs to assist with housing, medical and prescription insurance, transportation, and so on.

The discharge plan for pretrial evaluations and individuals designated as IST should state that they are discharged to the jail as competent. All notifications and recommendations given to the jail regarding continuity of care (e.g., continued medication, suicide watch, conditions needing monitoring/observation) are included in the discharge packet. If the charges are minor and it is likely that the individual will be discharged from the jail to the community, then the standard discharge plan is followed.

### Discharge Barriers

These include all systems barriers that arise from implementing the action steps in the Discharge Plan such as legal issues, shortage of a specific type of housing, financial resources, citizenship status, and so on. Only those barriers that are actually encountered when implementing the action steps are listed, as opposed to anticipated barriers. Legal status is not a discharge barrier until the court has denied the hospital's recommendation for consideration of release (e.g., waiting on a court date is not a discharge barrier). Until an actual barrier is identified, it is useful to note, "None identified at this time." When a barrier is identified, the RPT ensures follow up in terms of steps that will be taken to overcome it.

Typically, discharge barriers do not include the clinical status of the individual (e.g., psychiatrically unstable, major medical problems, psychiatric or behavioral decompensation) because this is covered in the individual's IRP. An exception is that they may include any behaviors that the individual engages into thwart placement (e.g., when discharge is imminent, the individual engages in aggressive behavior to purposely delay discharge). When such a barrier is identified, it is followed up with an assessment and appropriate treatment, and documentation in the goals, objectives, and interventions.

## Goals

A goal statement documents an assessed treatment, rehabilitation, or recovery need of the individual. In non-recovery terminology, it is the "problem statement" described in behavioral terms. As much as possible, the RPT members collaborate with the individual in determining his goals before developing goal statements. The goal statements are kept realistic and simple by defining the goal as clearly as possible. Forensic goals follow the same basic format, but Forensic RPTs need to be cognizant of the individual's legal status and prioritize goals and objectives based on the reason for the forensic admission.

### Goals for Competency Restoration

For individuals who are admitted for competency restoration, the primary goal is to describe the behavior that is believed to be the underlying cause of the individual's inability to participate in court proceedings. The goal should not be simply "Restore the individual to competency." The goal should explain the factors that are leading to incompetency and then the objectives should specifically target these factors. An individual who, due to cognitive impairments, is not competent to understand the roles of courtroom personnel or the adversarial nature of court proceedings, would have a very different recovery plan from that for an individual who cannot work with an attorney because that individual thinks the attorney works for the CIA.

### Goals for Pretrial Evaluations

For individuals who are admitted for pretrial evaluations, the primary goal focuses on the reason for the evaluation being completed on an inpatient basis. As most pretrial forensic evaluations are completed on an outpatient basis, the rationale for bringing an individual for evaluation as an inpatient is critical and should be clearly delineated in the goal statement. If the reason is an attempt to make the person competent on a pretrial basis (circumventing the long IST process), then everything under Competency Restoration applies. If it is to rule out malingering, then the first goal should be related to clarifying a particular behavior (i.e., the behavior that gives rise to the suspicion of malingering). It is not enough to simply state, "rule out malingering;" the suspected malingering behavior needs to be stated so that all staff members will know what behavior they are to observe. Given that the recovery plan is shared with the individual, the context and explanation for this goal should be carefully crafted. An example of a thoughtfully crafted goal would be, "Mr. Dempsey is being evaluated for his competency to stand trial. His self-reported symptoms of seeing little green men and elephants as well as his use of nonsense words in sentences could potentially interfere with his ability to assist his attorney. The goal for this hospitalization is to determine whether the current symptoms are related to a mental illness and for Mr. Dempsey to be able to participate in his trial without symptom interference."

## Goals for Civilly Committed ISTs or NGRIs

For individuals with civil commitment designations of IST or Not Guilty by Reason of Insanity (NGRI), the recovery plans would look very similar to mental health recovery plans for long-term stay individuals, emphasizing skills needed to live in the community. Due to a focus on the safety of the individual and the community, the plan should also specify factors identified as contributing to the index offense(s) and any significant historical aggression, and how those risk factors have been ameliorated or managed.

## Objectives

Once a goal is clearly defined, the RPT members develop the steps the individual can take to accomplish the goal. When a goal is broken down into small steps then the individual can incrementally engage to achieve it. These small steps form the objectives for the individual. So an objective is written in terms of what the individual is capable of doing to achieve the goal. An objective is always an action statement, e.g., "John will learn (or use) a mindfulness-based strategy to self-manage his rising anger when he cannot get what he wants." In addition, the objective is written in behavioral, observable, and/or measurable terms, and in language that the individual will understand easily and is free of jargon. To make it measurable, it includes performance and termination criteria. The majority of the objectives in a recovery-focused IRP are learning-based, but a few may be service-based. Learning-based objectives are those where the objectives specify what the individual will learn. Service-based objectives are those where the staff, usually the individual's psychiatrist and nursing staff, provides a service to the individual (e.g., prescribe or administer medication, provide specific medical treatments).

Recovery team members use these basic principles when developing or revising learning-based objectives. Each objective is (a) linked to a goal of hospitalization, (b) written in terms of what the individual in recovery is going to learn or do, (c) written in behavioral, observable, and/or measurable terms to provide the individual and staff with specific thresholds for measuring outcomes of interventions, (d) focused on what the individual can do within a specific timeframe, (e) attainable given the individual's current level of cognitive functioning and engagement level, (e) functional and meaningful to the individual, and (f) taught within the context in which the individual will use the skill. In addition, each objective should pass the *dead man's test*, which means that it should focus on not only what the individual should not do (e.g., not engage in aggressive acts for 6 months)—which a dead person can pass—but also alternative positive behaviors (e.g., learning anger management skills). Furthermore, each learning-based objective includes the following four components: (a) what the individual will accomplish (e.g., learn, identify, state, demonstrate, discuss, read, draw, play, make, and so on) in measurable terms, (b) a performance criterion, (c) a termination criterion, and (d) where the individual's performance will be documented.

## Interventions

Interventions are written in terms of what staff will do to assist the individual achieve the relevant objective. There are two types of interventions: (1) those that pertain to PSR Mall groups (i.e., those typically referred to as active treatment and which count towards the 20 h that individuals are typically scheduled to attend per week), and (2) those that are done in the units (i.e., service interventions).

As noted above, in a recovery model of mental health service delivery system, it is important to consider the concept of stages of change. For example, an individual's substance abuse may be serious enough to interfere with the individual's quality of life, and therapists may think that the person needs to be in treatment. Whether the individual agrees with this assumption or recommendation will depend on the individual's understanding of the disorder, the need for treatment, and agreement to engage in appropriate treatment. To determine the approximate level at which treatment should begin, a clinician (usually a clinical psychologist) assesses the individual's stage of change using the *University of Rhode Island Change Assessment* (URICA).

The following are the five stages of change:

1. **Precontemplation** is the stage in which individuals have no intention of changing their behavior in the foreseeable future. Many individuals in this stage are unaware or not fully aware that they are addicted to one or more substances.
2. **Contemplation** is the stage in which individuals are aware that a problem exists and are seriously thinking about overcoming it, but have not yet made a commitment to take action.
3. **Preparation** is a stage that combines intention and behavioral criteria. Individuals in this stage intend to take action or have just started to take action. These individuals may have unsuccessfully taken action in the past.
4. **Action** is the stage in which individuals modify their behavior, experiences, or environment in order to overcome their addiction. Action involves the most overt behavioral changes and requires considerable commitment of time and energy.
5. **Maintenance** is the stage in which individuals work to consolidate the gains attained during action, and to prevent relapse.

An assessment of an individual's stage of change, as well as readiness to engage in treatment or rehabilitation, provide the RPT with a starting point for developing interventions and affording the individual choice in selecting one or more PSR Mall groups or individual therapy that are appropriate for that individual. In general, an individual at the precontemplation level will benefit most from therapies that aim to change cognition, i.e., the individual's thinking about his or her condition or functional status. An individual at the other end of the continuum will benefit most from behavioral or action-oriented therapies (see Table 6.4). Interventions for substance abuse are written in exactly the same manner as for other objectives, but are aligned with the mall group or individual therapy offered at the same stage of change, as stated in the objective.

## Deferred Issues

Occasionally, there will be issues that RPT members know about and wish to include in the individual's IRP, but cannot do so because the individual does not have the prerequisite skills, the needed supports have not been developed, or the individual's anticipated length of stay is too

**Table 6.4** Stages of change continuum and matching of interventions

| Stages of change continuum | Approaches to psychiatric rehabilitation |
|---|---|
| Stage 1: Precontemplation | |
| • Denial<br>• Defensive<br>• Unwillingness to change<br>• Feels coerced into treatment<br>• Pressured by others to seek treatment<br>• Uncommitted or passive in treatment<br>• Unaware of having a disease, disorder, disability, or deficit<br>• Unaware of the causes and consequences of the disease, disorder, disability, or deficit<br>• Unaware of the need for treatment and rehabilitation<br>• Lack of motivation to engage in treatment and rehabilitation<br>• Pros of the behavior outweigh the cons | • Consciousness-raising interventions, e.g., sharing observations, confronting the individual with specific consequences of their behavior<br>• Therapeutic alliance or relationship building with the practitioner; understanding and emotional relationship<br>• Nonpossessive warmth—the practitioner relates to the person as a worthwhile human being; shows unconditional acceptance of the person (as opposed to the behavior, e.g., addiction, offense)<br>• Empathic understanding—extent to which the practitioner understands what the individual is experiencing from the individual's frame of reference<br>• Catharsis—expression of emotion; practitioner engages in active listening skills, empathic observations, and gentle confrontation (reality checks)<br>• *Motivational interviewing*—a person centered, directive method for enhancing intrinsic motivation to change by helping the individual to explore and resolve his or her "issues;" practitioner facilitates the individual to resolve his or her ambivalence with regard to change. Based on four general principles for practitioners: express empathy, develop discrepancy, roll with resistance, and support self-efficacy<br>• *The intervention*—confronting the individual in a nonjudgmental, caring, and loving manner<br>• *Node-link mapping*—a visualization process tool that enables practitioners and individuals to develop and study the relationships between and among nodes (circles or squares) that contain elements of ideas, feelings, actions, or knowledge. Builds alliance between practitioner and individual, focuses the individual's attention on areas of concern, and enhances treatment readiness<br>• Practitioner approaches—authoritarian approaches to behavior change lead to greater resistance to engage in change<br>• Practitioner emotional well-being—poor emotional well-being inhibits an individual's progress, positive well-being facilitates positive intervention outcomes |
| Stage 2: Contemplation | |
| • Aware of their issues ("problems")<br>• Knows the need for change<br>• Not yet committed to change<br>• Wants to know more about their issues<br>• Not yet ready to engage in change process<br>• Thinking about engaging in change process<br>• May have attempted to take action in the past<br>• May be distressed with their situation<br>• May express a desire to take control of the situation<br>• Assessing pros and cons of their behavior and of making changes | • Continue with precontemplative stage consciousness-raising interventions and slowly introduce new interventions<br>• Receptive to bibliotherapy interventions<br>• Receptive to educational interventions<br>• *Presuppositional questions* (from SFT)—used to encourage individuals to examine and evaluate their issues, situation, or predicament. Practitioners can use presuppositional questions to think about change in a non-threatening context. As an example, consider an individual who thinks he does not have a problem and is waiting to be released to CONREP. The practitioner's |

(continued)

**Table 6.4** (continued)

| Stages of change continuum | Approaches to psychiatric rehabilitation |
|---|---|
| | presuppositional question could be, "Let's agree that what you are saying is true… 'How would you know when you are ready to be released to CONREP?'"<br>• *Circular questions*—used in a nonthreatening manner to ask a question about the individual's issues, situation or predicament from the perspective of an outsider. Consider the individual used in the example above. The practitioner may ask: "How would the CONREP representative know when you know that you are ready to be released?"<br>• *Miracle questions* (from SFT)—used as a method to assist an individual in imaging change and with goal setting. Classic example: "Suppose you go to bed tonight, and while you are asleep a miracle happens and all your issues, situations, or predicaments disappear. Everything is resolved to your liking. When you wake up in the morning, how will you know that the miracle happened? What would be the first thing you would notice that is different? |
| Stage 3: Preparation | |
| • Ready to change—behavior and attitude<br>• Needs to set goals and priorities for future change<br>• Receptive to treatment plans that include specific focus of interventions, objectives, and intervention plans<br>• Ready to engage in rehabilitation<br>• Engaged in change process<br>• Cons of not changing outweigh pros | • Continue with contemplative stage awareness enhancing interventions and slowly introduce new interventions<br>• Practitioners encourage the individual's sense of "self-liberation" and foster a sense of personal recovery by taking control of his or her life<br>• Discrimination training and stimulus control interventions can be introduced at this stage. The practitioner enhances the individual's awareness of the conditions that give rise to his issues, situations, or predicaments. Focus is on the presence or absence of antecedents, setting events, and establishing operations<br>• *Scaling question* (from SFT)—used as a tool by the individual to "buy into" the treatment planning process. Practitioners can use it to obtain a quantitative measure of the individual's issues, situation, or predicament, as perceived and rated by the individual and then assist the individual to think about the next step in the change process. Example: "On a scale of 1–10, with 1 being totally not ready and 10 being totally ready, how would you rate your current readiness to be discharged to CONREP?" If the individual self-rates as a 4, the practitioner can follow this up with, "During the next month, what steps can you take or what can you work on to get from 4 to 5?" Scaling questions can be used to (a) obtain a quantitative baseline, (b) assist the individual to take the next step in the process of recovery, and (c) encourage the individual to achieve recovery by successive approximations (i.e., in incremental steps—one point at a time, one month at a time) |
| Stage 4: Action | |
| • Committed to and is engaged in change process<br>• Demonstrates motivation to change<br>• Follows suggested change processes and activities | • Cognitive-behavioral approaches<br>• Explore and correct faulty cognitions—catastrophizing, overgeneralizing, magnification, excessive |

(continued)

**Table 6.4** (continued)

| Stages of change continuum | Approaches to psychiatric rehabilitation |
|---|---|
| • Makes successful efforts to change<br>• Develops and implements strategies to overcome barriers<br>• Requires considerable self-effort<br>• Noticeable behavioral change takes place<br>• Target behaviors are under self-control, ranging from a day to six months | responsibility, dichotomous thinking, selective abstraction<br>• Learning-based approaches<br>• Action-oriented approaches<br>• Skills and support rehabilitation |
| Stage 5: Maintenance | |
| • Meets discharge criteria<br>• Is discharged<br>• Maintains wellness and enhance functional status with minimum professional involvement<br>• Lives in environments of choice<br>• Is empowered and hopeful<br>• Engages in self-determination through appropriate choice-making<br>• Develops and implements strategies to sustain and enhance wellness<br>• Avoids relapse through positive action<br>• Expresses fear or anxiety about relapse<br>• Avoids high risk behaviors or situations that may trigger relapse<br>• Engages in a variety of wellness activities<br>• Seeks social supports for maintaining wellness | • Adapt and adjust to situations to facilitate maintenance<br>• Develop and use personal wellness recovery plans<br>• Utilize coping skills in the rhythm of life, without spiraling down (i.e., if substance use is a problem, cope with distressing or faulty cognitions without using drugs)<br>• Continue with dynamic change process<br>• Accept that change is a spiral rather than a linear process<br>• Strengthen social supports and build alliances in the community<br>• Learn about mindfulness, especially unconditional acceptance, loving kindness, compassion for self and others, and letting go<br>• Practice and use mindfulness strategies in daily life |

NNS 06-27-05

short to even begin working on the particular issue or problem. In addition, when an individual has too many goals and objectives, there is a need to prioritize them in terms of what the individual can focus on immediately, leaving the rest as substitutes after these are achieved. In this section, the RPT lists all issues that have been deferred, including the reason for deferral. If there are absolutely no deferred issues, the RPT may state, "No deferred issues at this time." It will be very rare for an individual not to have at least one deferred issue.

Deferred issues include only those that the RPT plans to address during the current hospital admission, or refer to the community if the individual is discharged before the team is able to address them. Deferred issues cannot be high-risk issues (e.g., aggressive behavior), or medical conditions for which the individual receives or must receive treatment (e.g., pre-diabetes). RPTs review and update the deferred issues at each scheduled review of the individuals' recovery plan.

## Social Support

This is a list of all persons that the individual has approved as members of his or her social support group that can be contacted on behalf of the individual. It is updated periodically because an individual's social supports may change with length of stay at the hospital.

## Psychosocial Rehabilitation Mall (PSR Mall)

A PSR Mall is a centralized approach to delivering services that enables an inpatient hospital to maximize the therapeutic time for the individuals it serves by providing them with an array of mental health services that they can select from and attend (Bopp et al. 1996; Matthews et al. 2015; Webster et al. 2009). As much as possible, mall interventions are provided in the context of real-life functioning and in the rhythm of life of each individual. Thus, a PSR Mall extends beyond the context of a building or place, and its services are based on the needs of the individual, and not the needs of the program, the staff, or the hospital. PSR Malls are designed to ensure that each individual receives intensive and individualized services to promote that individual's increased wellness, enhanced quality of life, and the ability to thrive in the community. All decisions regarding what is offered in a PSR Mall are driven by the needs of the individuals served. Mall services are provided in an environment that is culturally sensitive and strength-based.

## Hours of Attendance

An individual is typically scheduled to attend groups for four hours a day (i.e., two hours in the morning and two hours in the afternoon, each weekday) in a PSR Mall that is usually in an off-residential location. These services are directly linked to an individual's assessed needs and documented in the intervention section of his or her IRP. The interventions include the treatment, rehabilitation, and recovery needs of individuals. Services provided in the PSR Mall include groups, individual therapy, and activities designed to help with symptom management, personal skills development, and life enrichment. The PSR Mall capitalizes on clinical and support staff resources from the entire hospital, to provide a larger diversity of interaction and more realistic experiences for all individuals attending the mall groups.

## Choice of Groups

The choice of a PSR Mall group begins with an assessment of the individual's needs in terms of treatment, rehabilitation, and enrichment. Assessed needs are written as goals for the individual, as described above. Each goal has at least one objective, which is written in terms of what the *individual* needs to do, and for each objective there is at least one intervention—within a PSR Mall group or in individual therapy. In addition, it is expected that what is taught in the PSR Mall group or individual therapy is reinforced in the therapeutic milieu. The individual makes a choice of PSR Mall group based on the relevant mall groups or individual therapies identified by his or her RPT. Typically, an inpatient service will have a PSR Mall catalog of mall groups and individual therapies that the individual can consult before being assigned to a mall group of his or her choice.

As an example, when an individual has an objective to learn a coping strategy, the RPT may:

1. Review the PSR Mall catalog for all groups that teach coping strategies and find likely groups (or individual therapies) that would enable the individual to learn the required coping strategy;
2. Sort out any qualifiers that narrow down the choices (e.g., stage of change, cognitive level, learning style, group size, mode of presentation, time of group);
3. Present to the individual the relevant groups, describing their characteristics;
4. Request the individual to choose one group for this objective; and
5. Assign the individual to the group the individual has chosen.

The choice is not between what the individual would like to do (e.g., play volleyball) and a PSR Mall group (e.g., coping skills group), but between groups (or individual therapy) that the RPT has identified would help the individual fulfill an assessed need for treatment, rehabilitation, or enrichment. However, group selection can include simultaneous consideration of what the individual likes to do and what the individual needs to be able to do; they do not always have to be mutually exclusive. For example, for an individual who likes to play sports, but who has anger problems, a tai chi or a power yoga group might be appropriate choices for learning anger management. For an individual who likes to play music, but who lacks social interaction skills, a rhythm instruments group may benefit the learning of social skills. This can facilitate motivation and promote adherence to and participation in groups that an individual needs to attend in order to meet discharge criteria.

The total number of groups, and frequency of attending groups is linked to the individual's discharge criteria, and mental and cognitive status. For example, if the individual needs to control physical aggression as a condition of discharge, it would help the individual to have a higher dosage of an anger management group. Thus, the individual may be scheduled to attend an anger management group three times a week, but only one volleyball group a week, as an enrichment activity. Similarly, if an individual has been admitted for competency restoration, the dosage could be at least one PSR Mall group per day, depending on mental and cognitive status.

## Levels of Support in PSR Mall Services

The RPT determines the level of support that an individual needs in a particular PSR Mall activity, given the individual's cognitive level, strengths, and weaknesses. The RPT psychologist is responsible for providing the PSR Mall with the individual's level of cognitive functioning. Levels of support can be graded as follows:

1. **Advanced**: Mall activities labeled as "advanced" would be reserved for those individuals who can self-start and direct their own learning with little assistance. These individuals also might be able to teach others.
2. **Independent**: Mall activities labeled as "independent" are aimed at individuals who have the basic skills necessary to continue in a mall activity without any special assistance in learning. These individuals can listen to a facilitator, take basic notes, ask and answer questions without much stress or difficulty. Individuals in an independent mall activity could take a written pre- and post-test.
3. **Assisted**: Mall activities labeled as "assisted" are aimed at individuals who have learning deficits that may require additional support (i.e., reading/writing deficits, poor listening comprehension, short attention spans), but have the basic skills necessary to partake in a mall activity. The content of these courses would not require individuals to do much independent work (i.e., homework) unless a study hall or tutor was available to assist at other times. The in-group content of these classes may include more activities and experiential exercises (i.e., games, role plays) than traditional "chalk and talk" groups.
4. **Supported**: Mall activities labeled as "supported" provide the highest level of support to an individual. Individuals appropriate for these activities mostly struggle to function independently, particularly when it comes to learning. Supported activities might involve individuals who do not possess even the most basic skills to participate effectively in a mall activity (i.e., sitting still for periods of time, turn taking, tolerating others). The staff to individual ratio in these mall activities would probably be no less than 1:3.

## Delivery of Interventions in Groups

The majority of services offered in a PSR Mall are in a group format. Although the group is the context for providing treatment, rehabilitation, or enrichment activities, the majority of the groups do not have a group objective. That is, all groups in core service areas have a theme or focus (e.g., job skills, ADL skills, social skills, coping skills, anger management), but each individual's objective is taught within the group. For example, in a social skills group, Katrina may have an objective to refine turn-taking skills in dyadic interactions while Sandi may have an objective to increase her social conversations. In some cases, the group objective may be the same as the individual's objectives. For example, a group objective may be to teach individuals to play basketball and all individuals enrolled in the group may have an objective in their IRP to learn to play basketball as an enrichment activity.

## Individual Therapy

If the RPT assesses that an individual requires individual therapy, this is provided. As for PSR

Mall groups the requirements for individual therapy are that:

1. There is an objective in the IRP that requires the individual to participate in individual therapy for a specific purpose;
2. The objective states how progress will be measured;
3. The intervention corresponding to the objective specifies who will provide the individual therapy; and
4. Progress is assessed prior to the individual's next scheduled RPT planning meeting.

The individual's progress is quantified as much as possible for both groups and individual therapy. Some hospitals may require that individual therapy can be provided outside of regular PSR Mall hours because of staffing issues. Individual therapy provided as a requirement in the IRP will be counted as a part of the individual's active treatment regardless of when or where the therapy is provided. Individual therapies vary in scope and include, among others, psychopharmacological treatment (Van Sant 2016), psychological services (Phillips 2016), and nursing services (Myers 2016).

## Nonadherence to Therapy

By the second monthly IRP the individual is scheduled to attend 20 h of therapy each weekday, or there should be clinical justification documented in the Present Status section for fewer scheduled hours. While individuals do not have the option of unilaterally dropping out of scheduled group or individual therapy, they often do. If an individual does not attend PSR Mall groups, the RPT should develop alternative strategies for encouraging the individual to re-engage in them. The team may refer the individual for assessment of the reasons for nonadherence and for subsequent treatment, using cognitive behavior therapy, motivational interviewing, node-link mapping, or other evidence-based interventions. Of course, this assumes that at least some of these therapeutic services are offered in the PSR Mall.

## Engagement in the PSR Mall

In the context of recovery, engagement is the process of encouraging an individual to fully participate in not only the process of treatment, but also its content (Jackman 2016). Clinicians often rely on their therapeutic alliance with the individual to involve and motivate the individual to engage in treatment (Jackman 2014). A majority of individuals attend, participate, and learn new skills in their assigned PSR Mall groups. Their engagement is dependent on a number of factors that include personal motivation, the goodness of fit between what the individual needs and what is offered, the nature of the group, the ability of the group facilitator to make the group process and learning interest, boredom, and personal variables (e.g., medication effects, cognitive level, stage of change).

A PSR Mall group facilitator can enhance engagement by using various "tested" techniques that have proven to be effective teaching tools. These include some of the following techniques.

### Cold Call

Group facilitators like to engage all members in their group by asking questions, waiting for a show of hands, and then choosing someone with a raised hand. However, this often leads to only a few individuals actively participating while others drift into inattention and other activities (e.g., sleep, daydreaming). What would be ideal is for all individuals in the group to pay attention and anticipate being called upon to answer questions, regardless of whether they raise their hands or not. Cold Call is a system that encourages all group members to pay attention, to prepare answers to all questions in their minds, but to respond only when called upon.

A prerequisite for Cold Call is that the group facilitator has the names of all group members. The procedure is simple: The facilitator asks a question, and then calls on the group member to answer the question regardless of whether a hand is raised. After a short while, the group members will realize that the facilitator may call on anyone in the class, so everyone must be ready to answer the question. This will: (a) increase engagement by the group members; (b) decrease and eventually eliminate inattention and daydreaming; (c) increase learning time because the group facilitator does not have to ask a question, wait for individuals to raise their hand, ask individuals other than the usual three or four members to raise their hand, ask an individual to respond, and then wait for an answer—the facilitator asks a question, and then immediately asks an individual to respond; and (d) it enables the facilitator to distribute the questions broadly across the group members—it signals to them that not only are they likely to be asked, but also the facilitator is interested in their answers and opinions. They had better be prepared!

Used skillfully, Cold Call is very productive in encouraging engagement by individuals who are shy or reluctant to raise their hands. If used consistently, it is predictable—it builds an expectation that anyone can be asked a question. Thus, it is a positive behavior change technology; group members begin paying more attention and mentally prepare answers in anticipation of being asked a question. Some group facilitators keep a visible chart that tracks who has been called upon, thereby sending a clear message that everyone gets their share of questions, and that engagement is an expectation, not a choice.

### Scaffolding

Most groups have individuals at different cognitive levels, with varying degrees of knowledge of the topic covered by the group. Scaffolding can be paired with Cold Call very effectively, especially if the group facilitator begins with simple questions and progresses to more difficult ones in each session. This enables the group facilitator to engage all group members at their skill level, reinforcing what they already know and challenging them to learn more by listening to others in the group with greater knowledge of the topic.

Typically, a group facilitator begins with a simple question that is at the skill level of a group member to whom the question is directed. Once this individual is engaged, the group facilitator "unbundles" a single larger question into a series of smaller but graduated questions, and directs the questions at the skill level of successive group members, ending with the most difficult question directed at the most accomplished group member. The sequence involves calling on several, though not necessarily all, group members in rapid succession with incrementally more difficult questions. Scaffolding enables the group facilitator to parse a question to multiple group members instead of just one, thus increasing group engagement, learning, and cohesion. One useful strategy is to begin with what the group members learned in prior sessions, and then move the questions systematically into the topic that is to be covered in the present session. This enables the group members to think their way into the next topic.

Cold Call and Scaffolding work best if the group facilitator asks a question, follows it with a pause while the group members formulate their responses, and then asks a specific individual to answer the question—i.e., Question, Pause, Name. This ensures that every group member hears the question and mentally prepares the answer in anticipation of being asked to respond. If the sequence is changed and the individual's name is called first, there is some likelihood that all other group members will sit back with a sigh, knowing that they have been excused from answering at least this question!

### Call and Response

In many cultures, call and response is a form of spontaneous verbal and nonverbal interaction between a speaker and listeners in which the statements (calls) of the speaker are punctuated by responses from the listeners. Group facilitators can utilize this form of engagement in a number of ways. For example, the group facilitator can ask a question and ask all members of the group to respond together. The group facilitator can ask questions in rapid succession, and ask different individuals from the group to respond to each question. Another form of this involves the group facilitator directing a question to a specific person, who responds correctly, and then asking the entire group for a response to the same question. This is akin to high-energy performance where there is a lot of fun because the entire group is involved in calling out the answers to the group leader's questions in rapid succession. It invigorates the entire group, motivates high attendance, and enables learning to occur in the context of positive engagement.

### Everybody Writes

In some groups, the group facilitator describes the topic, and follows it with a question to the group. When there is silence, the group facilitator is either flustered or simply answers it and moves on. This is not atypical in many groups. One way of engaging the group members is to give them some time to respond to the question by asking them to write their responses before discussing the answers verbally. Once the group members have had time to write their responses, the group facilitator can use Cold Call and Scaffolding to elicit the group's responses, e.g., "What did you write, Max?" This will promote engagement, both in terms of writing and responding verbally. Using a Participant Workbook will serve this purpose beautifully!

These are just some ways of engaging individuals in mall groups in the PSR Mall. The methods chosen will depend on contextual factors—nature of the topic, group characteristics, motivational level of the participants, cognitive status, skill level of the group facilitator, and so on. However, regardless of how well we do, a minority of group members will be nonadherent. They may refuse to attend the group, or attend but refuse to participate. These individuals may require different kinds of interventions to get them incrementally or fully engaged.

## Conclusion

A recovery-focused treatment planning system is based on asking what would make the individual's life better from the perspective of the individual. Given that the individual is in an inpatient psychiatric hospital, it does not mean that the right to recovery is sacrificed in the interests of treating the individual's mental illness by way of symptom control. Indeed, the individual may never need to agree with a diagnosis of a mental illness, as long as that individual knows how to engage in self-care activities when feeling unwell, low, or out of touch with reality. If the individual has developed a set of skills to not only manage in the real world, but also thrive in terms of his or her own goals, then that individual is on a successful path to recovery. In a general sense, recovery is a journey and the journey is the goal. On this journey, the individual invests in experiential and critical interests that provide meaning to his or her life. Like life itself, recovery has its ups and downs, highs and lows, sun and rain, but the individual can learn to navigate through these. The role of clinicians is to support individuals on their particular journey of life.

## References


Barber, J. W. (2016). Psychiatric services. In N. N. Singh, J. Barber, & S. Van Sant (Eds.), *Handbook of recovery in inpatient psychiatry*. New York: Springer.

Bopp, J. H., Ribble, D. J., Cassidy, J. J., & Markoff, R. A. (1996). Re-engineering the state hospital to promote rehabilitation and recovery. *Psychiatric Services, 47*, 697–701.

Davidson, L., Carr, E., Bellamy, C., Tondora, J., Fossey, E., Styron, T., et al. (2016). Principles for recovery-oriented inpatient care. In N. N. Singh, J. Barber, & S. Van Sant (Eds.), *Handbook of recovery in inpatient psychiatry*. New York: Springer.

DiClemente, C. C., & Prochaska, J. O. (1998). Toward a comprehensive, transtheoretical model of change: Stages of change and addictive behaviors. In W. R. Miller & N. Heather (Eds.), *Treating addictive behaviors*. New York: Plenum Press.

Dworkin, R. M. (1993). *Life's dominion: An argument about abortion, euthanasia, and individual freedom*. New York: Vintage.

Hill, B. D., Sofko, C., & Boettcher, A. (2016). Cognitive remediation in mental health. In N. N. Singh, J. Barber, & S. Van Sant (Eds.), *Handbook of recovery in inpatient psychiatry*. New York: Springer.

Jackman, M. M. (2014). Mindful occupational engagement. In N. N. Singh (Ed.), *Psychology of meditation* (pp. 241–278). New York: Nova Science Publishers.

Jackman, M. M. (2016). Occupational therapy services. In N. N. Singh, J. Barber, & S. Van Sant (Eds.),

*Handbook of recovery in inpatient psychiatry*. New York: Springer.
Matthews, A. N., Beecher, B., Hofer, P. J., & Short, R. A. (2015). An exploratory evaluation of a treatment mall at a state psychiatric hospital. *American Journal of Health Sciences, 6*, 83–90.
McConnaughy, E. A., Prochaska, J. O., & Velicer, W. F. (1983). Stages of change in psychotherapy: Measurement and sample profiles. *Psychotherapy: Theory, Research and Practice, 20*, 368–375.
Myers, R. E. (2016). Mental health nursing services. In N. N. Singh, J. Barber, & S. Van Sant (Eds.), *Handbook of recovery in inpatient psychiatry*. New York: Springer.
Phillips, J. (2016). Psychological services. In N. N. Singh, J. Barber, & S. Van Sant (Eds.), *Handbook of recovery in inpatient psychiatry*. New York: Springer.
Prochaska, J. O., & DiClemente, C. (1983). Stages and processes of self-change of smoking: Toward an integrative model of change. *Journal of Consulting and Clinical Psychology, 51*, 390–395.
Prochaska, J., & Velicer, W. (1997). The transtheoretical model of health behavior change. *American Journal of Health Promotion, 12*, 38–48.
Shafer, M. S., Staples, V., & George, L. (2016). Self-advocacy and empowerment. In N. N. Singh, J. Barber, & S. Van Sant (Eds.), *Handbook of recovery in inpatient psychiatry*. New York: Springer.
Spaulding, W. D., Montague, E., Avila, A., & Sullivan, M. E. (2016). The idea of recovery. In N. N. Singh, J. Barber, & S. Van Sant (Eds.), *Handbook of recovery in inpatient psychiatry*. New York: Springer.
Van Sant, S. (2016). Psychopharmacological services. In N. N. Singh, J. Barber, & S. Van Sant (Eds.), *Handbook of recovery in inpatient psychiatry*. New York: Springer.
Webster, S. L., Sheitman, B. B., Barboriak, P. N., Harmon, S. H., Paesler, B. T., Gordon, P.A., et al. (2009). Integrating forensically and civilly committed adult inpatients in a treatment mall program at a state hospital. *Psychiatric Services, 60*, 262–265.

# Psychopharmacological Treatment

7

Scott Van Sant

## Introduction

What is the role of pharmacotherapy in the process and attainment of recovery? There is quite a spectrum of opinions on the effect of psychopharmacological agents on individuals ranging from the writings of Patricia Deegan in reference to her own early negative experiences, to multiple reviews and practice algorithms that discuss the virtues of antidepressants, antipsychotics, and mood stabilizers in their role in stabilization and maintenance of psychiatric symptoms in severe mental illness. Deegan (2007) described the abject hopelessness she felt when she was told by her psychiatrist that she had a "chronic lifelong illness" from which there was no recovery. Instead of viewing the antipsychotics prescribed to her as a panacea, she found them "noxious" and "dangerous" and likened the side effects to, "walls as thick and impenetrable as any institution" and leaving her "isolated and alienated." In describing her first hospitalization, Houghton (1982) likened her confinement to an "entombment" and the medications as the "embalmment" as she "walked among the dead."

S. Van Sant (✉)
Department of Psychiatry and Health Behavior, Medical College of Georgia, Augusta University, 997 St., Sebastian Way, Augusta, GA, USA
e-mail: svansant@gru.edu

That is not to say that those involved in the recovery movement think that psychotropic medications are needless. Actually, great strides toward obtaining recovery for many suffering from severe mental illness are due, in fact, to advances in pharmacotherapy over the past few decades. For these people, medications have paved the way for utilizing other treatment modalities in obtaining symptom remission and improvement of functional status. There have been descriptions of the changes in "mind, body, and social experience" that occur with illness, and the subsequent treatment that helps the person take control, reinforcing her ability to "reclaim" her life (Bizub 2013). Alternatively, in the words of Henderson (2004), traveling from being paralyzed by depression, emotional turmoil, poor memory and concentration, and sleeplessness to being gainfully employed and having meaningful relationships where she was "thriving not just surviving" and accepting her diagnosis and need for medication as important elements of her eventual recovery.

Some patients have seen newer psychotropic medications as being the foundation for recovery, along with support, rehabilitation, training, and acceptance (Paquette and Navarro 2005), or simply that medications meant "not being sick" (O'Neal 1984). In a study describing patient's perceptions and experiences while being treated with long-acting depot antipsychotics, Svedberg et al. (2003) described individuals reporting the state of psychosis as having been "lost in an



N.N. Singh et al. (eds.), *Handbook of Recovery in Inpatient Psychiatry*,
Evidence-Based Practices in Behavioral Health, DOI 10.1007/978-3-319-40537-7_7

estranged world" and where they felt "anguish and insecurity." Moreover, these periods of psychosis actually interfered with aspects of life that were key to recovery, such as work, education, family interactions, parenting, and financial independence. They were motivated by distressing memories of episodes where they had been off medication with subsequent relapse and loss of control. They understood the medications as being a prerequisite for maintenance of health and functioning, and attributed regaining "hope" to the medications. Side effects were described as a "necessary evil" to obtain this (Svedberg et al. 2003).

Often hospital settings are the first exposure people have to adjust with the mental health system early in the course of severe mental illness, and this experience can affect their attitudes toward the treatment that are offered for years, if not life. Psychotropic medications are frequently a large part of the armamentarium offered during this stage. In a qualitative study of subjective experiences of illness recovery in persons treated for first episode psychosis several themes were noted, including symptom recovery, reconciliation of the meaning of the illness, regaining control, and finally negotiation and acceptance of treatment including medications (Windell et al. 2012, 2015). Symptom resolution was identified as an important "turning point" in the beginning process of obtaining recovery, and "finding the right medication" was a significant element of this. In this study, it was also found that medications had other meanings that affected a person's outcome, including acceptance they were "ill" which led to initial nonadherence. This illustrated that there is a process that persons go through before they fully accepted their illness, and the idea of the need for external sources of stability may not have been automatic. Specifically, persons spoke of the difficulties involved in the process of accepting the need for medications, especially when the medications were not initially effective in treating symptoms, or when side effects interfered with other "valued states" such as alertness or activities that required cognitive performance. For some, medications were seen as an integral part of recovery because of the associated symptom reduction attributed to medications, but others saw the need to take medications as a barrier because it implied that the illness may return and was a chronic condition.

Deegan and Drake (2006) stipulated that "choice, self-determination, and empowerment" are foundational values for persons with disabilities, and many view recommended treatments as worse than the condition. They also pointed out that the research from which our medication treatment algorithms are derived is usually based on population averages, not individuals and their "unique concerns, values, and life context." Medications can be seen as unnecessary, ineffective, or an interference with the process of recovery. Persons may feel that they lose who they are with the effects of medications. One way to reframe this issue is the "illness" versus "wellness" model. In the first, the person has a diagnosis with associated symptoms, the doctor prescribes medications to treat these symptoms, and either the illness is cured or managed chronically. The second entails the person's aspiration for a meaningful life including hope, empowerment, self-determination, relationships, and employment. These viewpoints are not mutually exclusive. Medications can be an important tool for many in taking the first steps in obtaining eventual recovery. The mistake the clinician can make is to assume that cessation of auditory hallucinations, or depression, or other debilitating symptoms is the desired ultimate result of treatment, thinking that a pill will instill "hope and empowerment." Actually, a pill may cause adverse effects that the person finds worse than the symptoms, or the person may feel like they will be irrevocably changed by the medication, and not be "his self" any longer (Piat et al. 2009).

Medications are just one tool that is available to persons with mental illness to be utilized in a collaborative fashion with a clinician's guidance. With a view of the human continuum as encompassing suffering, loss, and grief as well as joy, accomplishment, and purpose, interventions provided by the medical-model, specifically medications, are not enough in helping people discover their own paths to recovery. Some postulate that physicians are only treating superficial behavioral manifestations of the complicated internal processes that lead to mental illness. An individual can feel that administering medications may actually alter his thought processes and emotions, leaving him with a sense of loss that is greater than the illness itself. The interventions proposed by the recovery model can fill the void left by the "extinction" of these symptoms. As stated by Lunt (2002), "in the views of many people with mental illnesses, the biochemical solution alone will only propel one partially down the road to recovery."

## Emergency Involuntary Care

When discussing recovery-oriented pharmacotherapy in inpatient settings, it is impossible to avoid the issue of forced psychotropic medications. The primary psychiatric diagnoses that prevail in inpatient settings include Schizophrenia, Bipolar Disorders, and Major Depressive Disorders (Watanabe-Galloway and Zhang 2007) and these conditions often affect cognition and thought processes needed to make rational decisions about care during times of crisis and decompensation (Austin et al. 2001; Martinez-Aran et al. 2004; O'Leary et al. 2000). By default, clinicians may resort to paternal medical decision-making when the person is impaired. There can be conflict when a person, or his caregivers, do not agree with the clinician's recommendations, regardless that they originate from current evidence-based treatment algorithms.

Frese et al. (2001) discussed a person's ability to accept or reject evidence-based care, and suggested that more disabled persons may need the more paternalistic medical model until they have progressed to the point where they are capable of making their own decisions. They and other authors have also suggested that regardless of a person's functioning, the instillation of hope, responsibility, and internal control is necessary at all stages of treatment (Bellack 2006; Fisher and Ahern 2002; Frese et al. 2001). Many authors support the notion that when individuals lack decision-making capacity due to the severity of his or her symptoms, other means must be utilized such as processes for involuntary treatment or preferably psychiatric advanced directives (Davidson et al. 2006; Drake et al. 2010), but the question arises on how to ensure that at least a foundation for recovery-oriented principles is developed and respected during this crucial period?

## Informed Consent

With the advent, in the late 1970s, of the legal concept of the right of psychiatric patients to refuse treatment, including psychotropic medications, different jurisdictions have developed varying approaches in adopting the *treatment* versus *rights* model of care. Depending on which side of this argument a particular jurisdiction has adopted, processes for involuntary treatment can be instituted with dominance of clinical versus judicial decision makers (Appelbaum 1988; Menninger 2001). See Table 7.1 for an outline of the requirements for *Informed Consent*.

Other authors have suggested a "sliding scale" for determining capacity as related to the dangerousness of the condition being treated versus

**Table 7.1** Requirements for informed consent

| |
|---|
| According to legal standards for the informed consent process, one must have the ability to: |
| 1. Express a choice |
| 2. Understand information relevant to the decision about treatment |
| 3. Appreciate the significance, for one's own situation, of the information disclosed about the illness and possible treatments |
| 4. Manipulate information rationally (or reason about it) in a manner that allows one to make comparisons and weigh outcomes |

Adapted from Wirshing et al. (1998)

the treatment provided. An example would be initiating low risk intervention known to improve outcomes versus an invasive, high-risk, non-proven procedure for the same condition. The first would only require assent, where the second would require a higher level assessment of decision-making capacity (Drane 1984). The presumption for some is that persons suffering from major mental illness cannot, by definition, participate in the informed consent process. In one retrospective study examining people with schizophrenia who participated in research protocols, it was determined that this was not the case. Taking the selection bias into account, (persons who were too ill to give consent were not included) the authors found that through the implementation of systematic and thorough informed consent procedures, including repetition and education about risks and benefits, that a large portion of study subjects were able to comprehend and retain all the critical components necessary for informed consent. They did find that "conceptual disorganization" was correlated with poor performance on informed consent procedures, but that psychosis per se did not interfere with comprehension and retention (Wirshing et al. 1998).

Many proponents of the recovery process do not see this aspect as an absolute issue. There are times when individuals cannot make decisions for themselves, and safety concerns are predominant. This can be seen as carrying the concepts of recovery further, as it emphasizes not just the rights of an individual to make decisions about his care, but his responsibility to the community he lives into not pose a danger to himself or others (Davidson et al. 2006). Also, taking personal responsibility for health and wellness, and one's own illness management, including acceptance of psychotropic medication when needed, can be seen as important components of obtaining recovery.

During times when involuntary treatment is necessary, recovery-oriented approaches are most critical, otherwise, "the treatment relationship is likely to disintegrate into a policing relationship that discourages the client's growth, development of new skills and acceptance of illness" (Noordsy et al. 2002). Deegan (2007) pointed out that most treatment algorithms do not make allowances for shared-decision making. There is literature that supports the fact that many persons with severe mental illness do have the capacity to understand their illness and treatment choices, and are capable about making rationale decisions. For those with temporary incapacity in emergency situations, Psychiatric Advanced Directives are a viable option consistent with recovery-oriented principles (Deegan and Drake 2006; Drake et al. 2010; Sowers and Quality Management Committee of the American Association of Community Psychiatrists 2005).

## Psychiatric Advanced Directives

This intervention was inspired by initiatives around patients' rights of self-determination at end-of-life that began in the early 1990s, and subsequently laws have been enacted in large percentage of jurisdictions in the United States and several western countries. There is as well a great deal of advocacy support for this concept with the hope of respecting individual's wishes during times of incapacitation due to decompensation. There are several alternative terms that are in use that refer to documenting these wishes including: advanced crisis planning, anticipatory psychiatric planning, joint crisis planning, and "Ulysses directive."

The two primary forms of psychiatric advanced directives focus on treatment decisions where the person outlines what treatments are preferred and what is not acceptable, versus identification of who will be a proxy decision maker during times of incapacitation. Proposed advantages of this approach encompass enhanced autonomy, reduced familial conflict over treatment decisions, clinician acceptance of patient self-determination, and decreased service use, e.g., hospital admissions, length of stay, involuntary commitment, and interaction with law enforcement.

Despite the widespread support and enactment of these types of directives, the penetrance into common use has fallen short. There are of course some real barriers to appropriate implementation, such as concerns over the person's capacity to enact this type of legal document (the same issues that would occur with end-of-life advanced directives, health-care powers-of-attorney, wills, and other binding contracts); clinician willingness to follow directives; the liability associated with following or not following directives; directives that contradict actual current treatment guidelines; and availability of the documents during times of crisis, i.e., midnight in the emergency room. This of course is not an all-inclusive list, but does illustrate there are valid barriers that have to be addressed (Campbell and Kisely 2009; Nicaise et al. 2013). One very important issue is the reality that most people will not have the foresight to create this type of document before they have their first episode of severe psychiatric illness.

Several groups have examined outcomes related to implementation of these types of directives, since their advent. In the strict methods of the Cochrane Review, no improvement was found in general outcomes such as voluntary and involuntary admissions, hospital length of stay, interaction with law enforcement, or outpatient contact. In their review, they did not find data on social functioning, imprisonment, quality of life, self-esteem, accommodation status, or career/family satisfaction, all purportedly important factors in recovery. They did mention one non-randomized study that demonstrated improvement in working relationships with clinicians and satisfaction with mental health treatment on short-term follow up. They also suggested that more intense methods such as joint crisis planning might have some positive effect on reducing involuntary admissions (Campbell and Kisely 2009). In another systematic review of research related to this topic, Nicaise et al. (2013) identified three frameworks for expected benefits of psychiatric advanced directives: (1) enhancement of the user's autonomy, (2) improvement of the therapeutic alliance, and (3) integration of care through health providers working in partnership. They also demonstrated that these benefits have not been adequately assessed, but rather the focus has been on organizational outcomes.

The *American Association of Community Psychiatrists Guidelines for Recovery-Oriented Services* stipulated that there will be crisis management and hospital diversion plans with "participatory" psychiatric medication management. Providing information for informed decisions when persons are capable of participating is seen as critical. In these recommendations, coercive treatment is not considered compatible with recovery-oriented care. Though it is acknowledged that at times this is necessary, the time should be kept to a minimum, and voluntary care instituted as soon as possible. Moreover, even during times of involuntary care, compassion and respect are tantamount (Sowers and Quality Management Committee of the American Association of Community Psychiatrists 2005).

## Stabilization Versus Recovery: Phased-Linked Treatment

There is a body of literature that reports the occurrence of recovery in people with schizophrenia who were not maintained on antipsychotics, though most research does indicate better outcomes with early aggressive identification and treatment of psychosis, and subsequent maintenance on antipsychotic medication (Bellack 2006). Psychotropic medications have been shown to reduce debilitating symptoms and risk of relapse in both bipolar disorder and severe recurrent and major depressive illness as well (Geddes et al. 2003; Kaymaz et al. 2008; Moller and Nasrallah 2003; Sachs and Rush 2003). Some authors see the installation of hope in periods of greatest instability as crucial to eventual recovery. In keeping with this viewpoint, the *how* is as important as the *what* with regard to treatment delivered. Even during instability is the individual encouraged to participate and take personal responsibility? Does the clinician instill hope instead of paternalistic blame? Evidence-based practices are not incompatible with recovery, but ideally implemented in partnership (Bellack 2006).

From the perspective of a psychopharmacologist, the clinician establishes symptom clusters that indicate diagnosis, and therefore suspected etiology of illness. Current methods of research focus on reduction or elimination of these symptoms, while ideally avoiding unbearable and/or dangerous side effects. The focus of rehabilitation is strengths driven toward the goal of improving functioning in aspects of the illness that are not amenable to chemical interventions. Psychopharmacology can be conceptualized as a stepping-stone that supports re-attainment of healthy functioning. Specific examples given are the improvement in functioning that occurs with treatment of positive symptoms (delusions, hallucinations, paranoia, disorganized thinking), while not worsening debilitating side effects such as extrapyramidal symptoms or cognitive dysfunction.

With direct reference to schizophrenia, several symptom clusters are countered to obtaining recovery. Positive symptoms are inversely correlated with "life-satisfaction," and are associated with dangerous behaviors that can lead to hospitalization. Negative symptoms are thought to be strongly associated with functional disability and poor self-care, and interfere with independent living skills, vocational status, and quality of life. The practice of psychopharmacology can enhance, or at least not impede promotion of hopefulness, personal responsibility, self-control, and life "beyond illness" (Noordsy et al. 2000; Tandon et al. 2006).

In his book, *Recovery From Disability: Manual of Psychiatric Rehabilitation,* Liberman (2008, pp. 101–103) presented the concept of phase-linked treatment, which involves periods of prodromal illness, periods of acute symptoms and potential associated crisis, the period of stabilization, and then subsequent stability where the person hopefully progresses to full recovery. These are not seen as static phases that occur in linear fashion, but individual paths where people may fluctuate between various aspects of illness and recovery. When traversing these phases, movement is not a regimented and lock step, but rather a dynamic, individual process.

By definition, persons newly admitted to the hospital would qualify as being in the acute or stabilization phase which precludes taking the next steps to full recovery until resolved (an exception may be long-term forensic units where the individual is still hospitalized for legal reasons, not psychiatric instability). As the person moves from the acute phase through the different stages, symptoms will become less prominent and debilitating, and the person will regain psychosocial functioning. During the acute and stabilization phases, symptoms are at their peak or starting to resolve. Cognitive abilities and resilience are limited. Interventions must be adjusted to avoid over taxation of the person's capacities and possible exacerbation of symptoms. The treatment team will have to take a more direct responsibility in interventions to encourage adherence, though this does not preclude collaborative approaches. During the stable phase, the individual can tolerate more intensive, evidence-based rehabilitation that can be personalized to improve vocational and social functioning.

From a pharmacological viewpoint, the highest priority during the acute and stabilization phases is to control and alleviate symptoms and associated problematic behaviors. This requires appropriate diagnosis of the condition with identification of predominant symptoms (i.e. psychosis, mania, depression) and provision of optimal diagnostic-specific psychopharmacological interventions, if indicated. Throughout all of these phases, collaboration between the care recipient and clinicians is necessary and marked by mutual respect, shared decision-making principles, and engagement in treatment adherence for pharmacological and non-pharmacological interventions. The focus during the acute and stabilization phases is on reducing symptoms and minimizing side effects, to move the person past dangerous behavior, and begin reintegration into the community so that the process of full recovery can begin (Liberman 2008; Tandon et al. 2006).

## Recommendations for Initial Medication Choices

Tandon et al. (2006) focused on the management of schizophrenia, but their approach in maximizing effectiveness of treatment is generalizable to other conditions. This involves ongoing monitoring and management of four outcome domains: symptom of disease, disease burden, treatment burden, and overall health and wellness. Symptoms of disease involve positive and negative symptoms, aggressiveness, hostility, mood dysfunction, and cognitive dysfunction. This could include manic and depressive symptoms associated with other serious mental conditions as well. Treatment burden includes side effects such as extrapyramidal symptoms, metabolic issues, sexual dysfunction, and other adverse effects resulting from psychotropic medications. Disease burden encompasses the impact on family, caregivers, social supports, healthcare cost, as well as vocational, interpersonal, and educational functioning. Last, overall health and wellness include social reintegration, independence, vocational/educational functioning, and physical health. In this model, psychopharmacology is seen as a component of the multiple psychosocial interventions that promote recovery (Tandon et al. 2006).

The first issue to address is "evidence-based care" being provided? Part of the impetus for quality improvement initiatives in mental health systems was the widespread evidence that many mental health systems were not following the prescribing guidelines, providing newer possibly more effective and less-toxic pharmacological agents, nor access to appropriate care, both in crisis and community settings. Part of this push came from regulatory and professional bodies, but several consumer advocacy groups have asked for access to newer treatments and adherence from their providers to prescribing guidelines (Drake et al. 2001; Kingsbury et al. 2001; Lehman and Steinwachs 1998; Torrey et al. 2001).

The second is to remember that though there is good research to support current recommendations for the pharmacological treatment of the major diagnostic categories of mental illness, these are based on statistical averages in large population groups, not individuals. Third, research directly linking pharmacotherapy to recovery is scant. At present, we examine domains which can be tied to elements that are associated with recovery, e.g., time to relapse, decrease in hospitalization rates, decrease in symptom clusters that cause distress and disability, improvement in elements of cognition (Liberman and Kopelowicz 2005). All important issues, but again are they directly linked to a person's ability to recover, with its subjective elements of hope, empowerment, self-direction, self-sufficiency? Another consideration is that laypersons may have different concepts of what "evidence-based" means, or may not even be aware of the methods behind formulation of treatment recommendations (Tanenbaum 2008; see Table 7.2).

In the *Roadmap* developed by Weiden et al. (2007), they discussed expansion of the maintenance model where the emphasis is placed on stabilization, maintenance of stability, and relapse prevention to include the next steps in the recovery model, where the individual obtains further gains in physical and emotional health. These two models, maintenance and recovery

**Table 7.2** Consumer perspectives on evidence-based care in public mental health

| |
|---|
| 1. Consumers want information, including but not limited to scientific information, about recommended treatments |
| 2. Though consumers take this information seriously they are focused on their individual experience as opposed to aggregate data collected in research protocols |
| 3. They are experts in their own illnesses |
| 4. Communication and discussion about treatment options with their psychiatrist is key, even if they do not agree |
| 5. Medications are only a small part of what they need and only give the person a "chance to learn and see." |

Adapted from Tanenbaum (2008)

oriented, are not seen as contradictory or in opposition, but rather logical extensions of each other. In times past, it was thought to be too risky to alter medication treatment regimens once stability was obtained. With inclusion of recovery concepts into the medical model, continued improvement in functional outcomes is expected.

Pharmacological management is one tool that actively facilitates continued recovery beyond initial stabilization and associated medication side effects. With the maintenance model, the goals would be achievement of stability, prevention of relapse, and worsening of symptoms (especially those associated with potential harm) and avoidance of adverse effects of treatment. These all are important objectives, but with recovery-oriented care continued efforts to improve health and wellbeing would also involve the reduction of overall burden of side effects, continued improvement from that obtained at initial stabilization, reduction in other functional impairments, and ultimately the lack of psychiatric symptoms and disease. Though addressing one of these can threaten or worsen another aspect, e.g., dose reduction to minimize side effects leading to recurrence of psychotic symptoms (and possibly destabilization). With these objectives in mind, detailed knowledge of psychopharmacology is needed to address efficacy for specific conditions, possible side effects in the context of treating an individual, general physical health issues that can be influenced by psychopharmacological agents, and interactions related to polypharmacy both for somatic and psychiatric medications.

There are multiple respected algorithms/guidelines from different organizations that cover recommended psychopharmacological treatment for the primary diagnoses of persons with severe mental illness. Examples of these guidelines include but are not limited to those for schizophrenia (Hasan et al. 2012; Moore et al. 2007), bipolar disorders (Sachs et al. 2000; Yatham et al. 2013), and severe major depressive disorders (American Psychiatric Association 2010; Bauer et al. 2013). These were developed by clinical and research experts in the field and are valuable in that they reduce the overwhelming, and sometimes conflicting, body of published research into digestible documents for clinicians (Mellman et al. 2001). They are based on a synthesis of drug trial data, which, for the most part, are based on large groups of people though, not individuals. Often these protocols severely limit variation in their subject matter (diagnosis, age, health status, co-morbidities, substance use, adherence), and hence may not be completely applicable to both the psychological and physical health needs of individuals. Therefore, both pharmacodynamic (what drugs do to the body, e.g. receptor binding) and pharmacokinetic (what the body does to the drug, e.g. half-life, metabolism, drug clearance) must be an integral part in making collaborative decisions with individuals regarding their care (Weiden et al. 2007).

## Individualization of Pharmacological Interventions: Efficacy Versus Side Effects

### Pharmacokinetic and Pharmacodynamic Interactions

There are several determinants of drug response/efficacy and the potential for adverse effects. The drug binds has an intrinsic effect on the site of action, e.g., a neuron receptor, ion channel, chemical transporters, or cell-associated enzymes (Stahl 2013, Chap. 2). In order for the drug to have an effect, it must reach the site of action in sufficient concentration. This is determined by how efficiently the body absorbs the drug, where the drug is distributed (i.e., determined by relative blood flow in different areas of the body, storage in fat cells, and protein binding), by what mechanism and rate the body metabolizes the substance (e.g. liver; and eventually how it is eliminated, e.g. urine, feces). There is biological variation, which can shift the usual dose response curve making the individual more or less sensitive to both clinical effectiveness and incidence of adverse reactions to a drug. These include, but are not limited to genetics, age, co-occurring health problems, and the individual's internal environment (Weiden et al. 2007).

Several mechanisms are involved, including metabolic interactions that raise or lower plasma drug levels, clearance and excretion, distribution of the drug in the body, and either potentiation or competition at the primary site of action (e.g. neurotransmitter receptor). Pharmacokinetic interactions involve the effect the body has on the drug, which increases or decreases the concentration of drug available in the body. There are four primary phases involved in this, including absorption, distribution, metabolism, and excretion. With few exceptions, psychotropic drugs are lipophilic agents that are extensively metabolized in the liver. Most pharmacokinetic interactions occur at a metabolic level and usually involve changes in the activity of the liver cytochrome P450 system. The activity of this system is genetically determined and may be profoundly influenced by environmental factors such as concomitant administration of other drugs, primarily through enzyme inhibition or induction. Enzyme inhibition usually involves competition with another drug at the enzyme-binding site, while induction occurs when a drug stimulates the synthesis of more enzyme proteins. There are also pharmacodynamic interactions that alter the effect the drug has at its site of action. Two drugs can interact at the same or interrelated receptor sites, resulting in additive, synergistic, or antagonistic effects (Besag and Berry 2006; Spina et al. 2003).

Polypharmacy has become very common and often antipsychotics, antidepressants, and mood stabilizers are prescribed together, in addition to many medications prescribed for co-occurring somatic conditions. There are several reasons for polypharmacy, and some are justified such as combinations of different classes of agents for treatment of acute mania, treatment of persistent residual symptoms of depression, and refractory psychosis. Additional agents can be utilized to treat known side effects such as anticholinergics for antipsychotic-induced extrapyramidal symptoms. Sometimes there are co-occurring conditions, e.g., a person with schizophrenia and posttraumatic stress disorder, or bipolar disorder and HIV. A person may have multiple symptom clusters warranting different agents, such as a person with schizoaffective disorder needing a mood stabilizer and antipsychotic. There are several possible interactions between these medications plus any other prescribed, over-the-counter, or herbal agents people may be taking for other conditions. These interactions can have both positive and negative actions on efficacy.

Though not all of these interactions are clinically relevant, there is the chance of an increased risk for adverse effects that can affect quality of life, and even safety. Factors that have to be taken into account when evaluating clinical relevance of interactions are drug, patient, and epidemiological-related factors. Drug-related factors include concentration, therapeutic effect of substrate, extent of metabolism of substrate through affected enzyme, and presence of active or toxic metabolites. Patient-related factors include phenotype and genotype of the person involved, and special populations that are at increased risk, e.g., the elderly. Epidemiological factors basically involve whether there is a chance the drugs will be used concurrently, meaning are they both available to the population involved (Spina et al. 2003).

Almost all medications have dose response curves where efficacy increases with dosage to a certain point, then side effects, and eventually toxicity predominates (occurs at different rates and concentrations for different drugs). There are variations in these curves between individuals, and the factors described above can all influence them as well, so the dose for efficacy, side effects, and toxicity can change during treatment for an individual. These issues must also be taken into account when discontinuing or changing doses/types of psychotropic medication. If a drug has a narrow therapeutic index, it is more likely to be at subtherapeutic or toxic levels. For example, serotonin-specific-reuptake-inhibitors (SSRIs) have a wide therapeutic index. They have many reactions through either induction or inhibition of their metabolism, but these interactions are less likely to have clinical relevance related to their levels. They can cause adverse effects through the interference of metabolism of other agents though. For example, fluoxetine inhibits the metabolism of haloperidol and fluphenazine, and therefore potentially raises the blood concentrations of these drugs, thereby increasing the risk for extrapyramidal symptoms. Second-generation antipsychotics are only weak inhibitors of CYP isoenzymes at therapeutic concentrations, and thus are less likely to interfere with the elimination of co-administered drugs. The administration of inhibitors or inducers of their metabolism can raise or lower their levels though, e.g., fluvoxamine can double olanzapine levels, ketoconazole can quadruple quetiapine levels, whereas phenytoin can reduce the quetiapine by 80 % (Spina et al. 2003).

Psychotropic drugs also make persistent changes in the neurotransmitter receptor profiles in the nervous system, which can become important when changing doses or medication regimens. An example is the withdrawal dyskinesia that can occur with antipsychotic induced upregulation of dopamine receptors and subsequent full or partial withdrawal of the blockade (Cerovecki et al. 2013), or anxiety induced by withdrawal of serotonergic antidepressants (Fava et al. 2015). If not explained to the person, this can have long-term effect on the person's willingness to adhere to future recommendations or other agents (as the new agent may be blamed). When medication changes do occur, the dosing and speed of a switch depends on possible withdrawal and rebound effects (Weiden et al. 2007). Discussed below are some of the variables that have to be taken into account when establishing psychiatric drug treatment regimens with care recipients.

**Gender**. Though there are gender-based metabolic differences regarding psychotherapeutic drugs, there are physiological differences that are more clinically relevant. There are differences in how men and women absorb, metabolize, and excrete a drug due to gastric motility, expression and activity of intestinal and liver enzymes, sex hormones (specifically estrogen), and protein binding. The main differences in how medications are absorbed and distributed are due primarily to factors such as differences in body mass index, body composition, plasma volume, organ blood flow, and the extent of tissue and plasma protein binding. Women generally have a higher body-fat percentage, decreased body weight, decreased plasma volume, and decreased organ blood flow as compared to men, leading to disparities in the rate and extent of drug distribution. Due to these factors, there is a potential for increased clinical effect or side effects with psychotropic medications (e.g. the potential for reduction in psychotic symptoms, but also increased extrapyramidal side effects with antipsychotics). Women generally need lower doses of antipsychotics than men, and there is some evidence that women are more prone to both the neurological (i.e. EPS and tardive dyskinesia) and metabolic effects of antipsychotics (Gandhi et al. 2004).

**Pregnancy**. Many women under the care of inpatient facilities are of reproductive age, or even sometimes pregnant during their psychiatric hospitalization. Even if a woman is not expectant, the potential for future childbirth is an important issue for many. There are several non-medication-related issues involved in pregnancy, including the potential adverse outcomes associated with untreated psychiatric illness due to possible direct physiological derangements, poor physical health of the mother, interference with child care in the postnatal period, and unfortunately sometimes harm committed by mother to the infant due to depression or psychosis. When counseling women on these issues, the potential effect of psychiatric medications on the fetus is unavoidable and must be taken into account when making treatment recommendations to such persons, including the possible congenital malformations associated with psychotropic medications when administered during the pregnancy. There are definite malformations associated with drugs such as valproate or carbamazepine. There are possibly serious issues with commonly prescribed antidepressants such as an elevated risk of miscarriage, preterm birth, decreased birth weight, and postnatal pulmonary hypertension. There are also outcomes associated with antidepressants such as increased incidence of low birth weight infants, preterm birth, or delivery complications (e.g. post-natal adaption syndrome). Medications may have strong effect on the mother such as increasing the risk of gestational diabetes, obesity, metabolic syndrome, and hypertension all of which can increase the risk to the fetus. Finally, many psychotropic medications are excreted in the breast milk. These are all valid concerns, but none absolutely preclude administration of psychotropic medications in pregnancy and the postnatal period, if indicated. Many women will have concerns over ingesting psychiatric medications, and these concerns have to be respected and addressed with her and her partner, if present (De Hert et al. 2011a, b; Pearlstein 2013).

**Children and Adolescents**. It is beyond the scope of this chapter to cover treatment recommendations for children and adolescents. In addition, the question of choice and self-determination is less relevant because legally the parents are the ultimate decision makers in deciding what care their children will receive. Though parents can certainly be exposed to and educated about recovery-oriented concepts, and clinicians should utilize the same approaches, there is a different context for these discussions.

**The Elderly**. The primary concerns with the elderly are etiology of psychiatric symptoms and their increased susceptibility to medication adverse effects. As a general rule, the later the onset of symptoms (mood and psychosis) the more likely there is an underlying medical reason such as cerebral vascular disease, cancer, Parkinson's, Alzheimer's, and even arthritis, which must be ruled out first and much more aggressively than would be the case for a younger population (Krishnan et al. 2002). Furthermore, many psychiatric symptoms such as depression, anxiety, mild cognitive issues, and impulse control issues can be the hallmark of various types of dementia, and precede the full onset by months to even years. Aggressive identification and treatment of these conditions are crucial as often the conditions can be reversed or at least mitigated, providing the person with years more of fruitful and fulfilling life (Alexopoulos et al. 2002; Charney et al. 2003). Ideally, this should occur before the person starts losing decisional capacity.

Regarding medication side effects, the elderly heightened sensitivity is due to several factors. The elderly react differently to medications, exhibiting a different response to drugs as compared to younger persons and to adverse effects of these same medications. The elderly have less functional reserve, both mental and physical, which is a natural occurrence with the aging process. There are physiological changes that occur, which affect both metabolism and clearance of medications and also add to drug–drug interactions (Campanelli 2012). Particular side effects of concern are sedation, anticholinergic side effects, and postural instability caused by hypotension. Regarding the gastrointestinal system, they have decreased stomach acid, smaller absorptive surface, decreased intestinal motility, and possible delayed absorption due to more common use of antacids. The elderly have increased total body fat so fat-soluble medications are distributed and stored more extensively. They have lower serum albumin levels, affecting protein binding and hence increasing plasma concentration of the drug. Their livers do not function as well so they have decreased ability to metabolize drugs. Finally, their kidneys have decreased functional capacity so many drugs and their metabolites are not excreted as efficiently. Other issues that have to be considered with the elderly are their greater propensity for poor nutrition, co-morbid medical conditions, and concomitant medications that may interfere with the metabolism or therapeutic effect of a psychiatric medication (David 2010; Mangoni and Jackson 2004; Pollock et al. 2009).

**Co-morbid Medical Issues**. There is evidence of increased medical co-morbidity among people with mental illness, which can affect the person's sensitivity to psychopharmacological agents, the risk of side effects, and severe adverse events. Persons in this class have also been found to have a higher incidence of multiple co-morbidities, e.g., a person with schizophrenia, respiratory disease, hypertension, and diabetes (Dickey et al. 2002). People with severe mental illness (i.e., schizophrenia, bipolar disorder, and major depressive disorders) have 2–3 times the mortality and 13–30-year shorter life spans than the general population, largely attributed to medical co-morbidities. This increased risk is multifactorial, including genetics, diet, smoking, level of exercise and physical activity, illness associated issues, and disparities in health care access and utilization. Specific diseases associated with increased risk in the context of severe mental illness include tuberculosis, HIV, Hepatitis B and C, obesity-related cancer, osteoporosis/decreased bone mineral density, poor dental status, impaired lung function, sexual dysfunction, and obstetric complications. There are also pre-existing issues with cardiovascular disease (CV) including myocardial infarction, cerebral vascular disease including stroke, and obesity-related metabolic disturbances of diabetes, dyslipidemia, and metabolic syndrome (De Hert et al. 2011a, b).

**Genetic Variation**. There has been a great deal of research and interest in genetic polymorphisms, or natural variations in genes, DNA sequences, or chromosomes that do not have adverse effects on an individual and occur with high frequency in populations. These variations are not necessarily an advantage or disadvantage (like blood types), but do increase overall variability of the species (U.S. National Library of Medicine 2015). Areas that are being studied include genes encoding metabolic enzymes, blood-brain barrier transport mechanisms, neurotransmitter receptor expression, and neurotransmitter storage and degradation. Of particular interest is relative responsiveness to medications and risk of adverse effects. There is evidence of these variations with regard to antipsychotics, antidepressants, and mood stabilizers (Brandl et al. 2014; Fabbri et al. 2014; Kato and Serretti 2010).

One example to elucidate this topic is the differences in the liver cytochrome system, where variability in genes that encode for this system affect enzyme activity, and subsequent metabolism of medications, including many psychotropics. Genes encoding for the CYP system are highly polymorphic with 80 variations known for one element the CYP2D6 alone, which is involved in the metabolism of many antipsychotics. There are differences in incidence of these genes within ethnic groups and between different cultural groups. Based on the combinations of these variations, people can be ultra-high, intermediate, or poor metabolizers, e.g., carriers of the allele that is defective for CYP2D6 function can have up to 80 % higher plasma levels of risperidone (a commonly used second generation antipsychotic). Though there are no strong data that supports differential treatment responses to antipsychotics based on this particular variation, there is good evidence of its effect on the incidence of adverse events, particularly antipsychotic-induced weight gain, tardive dyskinesia, and extrapyramidal symptoms (Brandl et al. 2014). Though testing for these differences has not reached mainstream clinical utility yet, the science behind this will definitely affect how psychiatric drugs are developed, and consequently prescribed in the future (Malhotra et al. 2004).

## Medication Side Effects

As described above, there are many variables that affect both effectiveness and the incidence of adverse medication effects. When looking at several measures associated with domains of recovery, fewer medication side effects (among other measures) were associated with general life satisfaction, hope, and empowerment (Resnick et al. 2004). The person's internal experience with medications needs to be addressed, as some adverse effects may not be well elucidated in tables derived from safety and tolerability trials. Just as with efficacy measures, information gathered on medication side effects is based on large population groups included in research. Often inclusion criteria for safety and efficacy protocols are severely restricted and do not reflect the diversity of co-morbidities, age, and health status of the general population.

Safety and tolerability profiles differ across individuals, and psychopharmacological plans should be customized to reflect the needs of an individual. Individuals have described the effects of medications as "strange and threatening," especially because the people involved did not know that the medications were causing these experiences. Other complaints included feelings

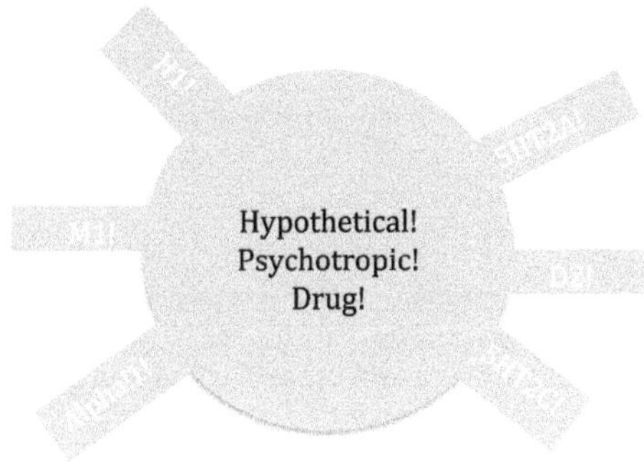


**Fig. 7.1** Hypothetical psychotropic drug illustrating receptor site of action associated with potential clinical efficiency and or side effects

of tiredness, dullness, feeling like a "zombie," and being cut off from life and creativity. Some felt this was worse than psychosis (Svedberg et al. 2003). Absence of side effects is not realistic, but there is a balance of symptom reduction versus medication side effects that should be taken into account in a collaborative fashion with an individual when making treatment decisions. This also applies to the emergence of adverse outcomes later in the course of treatment (Tandon et al. 2006). See Fig. 7.1 and Table 7.3 for an example of the complex interplay between psychotropic drug interaction with neurotransmitter receptors and subsequent efficacy and/or side effects.

The recent update of the World Federation of Societies of Biological Psychiatry (WFSBP) guidelines for treatment of schizophrenia (Hasan et al. 2013) stated that the main goals of the stabilization phase in the treatment of schizophrenia are to facilitate continued symptom reduction, consolidate remission, and promote the process of recovery. They continued with the following stipulations for the first few months post hospitalization: ongoing symptom remission must be ensured; there should be maintenance or improvement in the person's level of functioning and quality of life; that there is continued monitoring for adverse treatment effects; and steps are taken to ensure relapse prevention. In these guidelines, they stated that psychopharmacologic management must be individually tailored to the needs and preferences of the person, focusing on relapse prevention, symptom suppression, and improvement in subjective wellbeing and quality of life. Based on their review of the literature, they stated that continued treatment with adequate dosing of antipsychotic medication would reduce the risk of relapse after a psychotic episode. They also stated that medications that were effective in eliminating or reducing psychotic symptoms in the acute phase should be continued for at least six months post discharge (Hasan et al. 2013).

The purpose in outlining these recommendations is to emphasize the importance of medication adherence after a person has been hospitalized, to help ensure ongoing stability so the individual can continue on his or her path to full recovery. Relapse of symptoms, decompensation, and rehospitalization all are barriers to this goal. One of the most often cited reasons for medication discontinuation, or expression of choice, in persons with serious mental illness is side effects. No matter the stage of stabilization versus recovery a person is in, the clinician needs to take this into account when developing a pharmacotherapy plan. Side effects have several realms, including the initial discomfort (sometimes actually expected with many psychotropic medications), long-term health concerns (metabolic issues, tardive dyskinesia), and stigma associated with being on psychotropic medications (Tandon et al. 2006).

In one recent large study based on interviews of 876 persons identified as having schizophrenia that were prescribed antipsychotic medication, it was determined that side effects were prevalent at about 86.19 % (Dibonaventura et al. 2012). In addition, 42.5 % of this group acknowledged at least partial nonadherence with psychotropic medications. The categories of side effects that were found to be significantly associated with nonadherence were extrapyramidal symptoms, sedation, prolactin/endocrine derangements, and metabolic disturbances. They also found that this nonadherence was associated with an increased frequency of emergency room visits, hospitalizations, and healthcare resource utilization.

It is necessary to assess side effects that have been present in the acute phase and to adjust pharmacotherapy accordingly in order to

**Table 7.3** Examples of neurotransmitter-associated potential positive clinical effect versus adverse side effects (not all-inclusive)

| Neurotransmitter receptors affected by psychotropics | Potential positive clinical effect | Potential adverse side effect |
|---|---|---|
| *Dopamine* | | |
| D2 | Antagonism reduces psychotic symptoms | Antagonism leads to: Prolactin elevation-amenorrhea, galactorrhea in women; gynecomastia in men; sexual dysfunction in both sexes<br>Parkinsonian symptoms (EPS)-dystonias, tremors, bradykinesia<br>Long-term blockade thought to lead to Tardive Dyskinesia<br>Antagonism can possibly aggravate cognitive issues in Schizophrenia<br>Blockade can possibly aggravate apathy, anhedonia, decreased motivation, loss of interest, and joy from social interactions |
| *Serotonin* | | |
| 5HT2A | Antagonism reduces EPS, prolactin elevation<br>Antagonism possibly reduces depressive symptoms<br>Antagonism may result in an increase in cortical dopamine improving cognition | Sexual dysfunction<br>Antagonism can lead to over activation with increased agitation, anxiety, and insomnia<br>Agonism can cause EPS symptoms |
| 5HT2C | Antagonism increases dopamine and norepinephrine in certain areas of the brain and possibly reduces depressive symptoms and improves cognition | Antagonism thought to lead to weight gain<br>Antagonism can lead to over activation with increased agitation, anxiety, and insomnia |
| *Acetylcholine* | | |
| M1 | Antagonism can ameliorate parkinsonian symptoms | Antagonism leads to: Sedation and deficits in memory and cognition<br>Anticholinergic effects:<br>Dry mouth, Constipation,<br>Tachycardia, Blurred vision<br>Urinary retention |
| *Histamine* | | |
| H1 | | Antagonism leads to:<br>Sedation<br>Increased hunger<br>Weight gain<br>Postural dizziness |
| *Alpha-adrenergic* | | |
| Alpha 1 | | Antagonism leads to: Orthostatic Hypotension<br>Dizziness<br>Tachycardia<br>Sedation<br>Priapism |

Derived from Ferguson (2001), Newcomer et al. (2013), Stahl (2013), Stahl et al. (2013)

minimize adverse outcomes. The relative benefits of the drugs versus their associated risk profiles, in conjunction with the person's personal experience, have to be taken into account when discussing treatment options with an individual. Quality of life is rarely a primary outcome measure in clinical trials. Therefore, it is usually not powered to detect differences between drugs (i.e. drug A has been shown to significantly increase quality of life over drug B). Citing the CATIE and Cutlass trials, Hasan et al. (2013) stated there was no difference between individual antipsychotics and between first- and second-generation antipsychotics in improving employment outcomes, participation in psychosocial rehab, quality of life, and quality adjusted life years, although there was a hint that there may be an increased subjective wellbeing with second-generation antipsychotics. However, they found that antipsychotic-induced side effects negatively influenced quality of life.

The primary groupings of antipsychotic-induced side effects, or as Nasrallah et al. (2005) termed "treatment burden," include extrapyramidal symptoms involving parkinsonian-like symptoms, such as muscle rigidity or tremors; metabolic issues including weight gain, diabetes, lipid abnormalities; anticholinergic side effects including blurry vision, dry mouth, constipation; elevation of prolactin which can lead to amenorrhea, galactorrhea, gynecomastia, decreased libido, and erectile dysfunction. All of these issues can possibly lead to secondary sequelae that can be as debilitating as the primary side effect, e.g., antipsychotic-induced obesity leading to sleep apnea, insomnia, and hypertension. Antipsychotic associated side effects of EPS, sexual dysfunction, and psychological experiences as described above are associated with a decreased sense of wellbeing with related negative influence on medication adherence (Fenton et al. 1997; Karow et al. 2007).

**Extrapyramidal Symptoms (EPS) and Tardive Dyskinesia (TD)**. In registration trials and other studies, EPS is one of the largest offenders cited for drug discontinuation. First-Generation Antipsychotics (FGAs) are known in general to have a higher incidence of extrapyramidal symptoms and tardive dyskinesia thought to be due to their differential effect on certain dopaminergic pathways in the brain involved in movement. There are also differential effects between the newer agents with some having a greater propensity for these conditions than others, again mostly due to relative differences in dopamine blockade. The primary treatments for EPS are anticholinergics, which are known to worsen cognition, one of the most debilitating symptoms of schizophrenia and other conditions, plus other side effects associated with anticholinergics themselves, such as dry mouth, constipation, blurred vision. Avoidance of these conditions is at least possible and certainly should be part of the discussion with people receiving these types of medications (Minzenberg et al. 2004; Nasrallah et al. 2005; Weiden et al. 2007).

**Weight and Cardiometabolic risk**. Persons with schizophrenia and other major mental illness have been shown to die younger primarily from CV and are more prone to risk factors associated with CV disease, including obesity, diabetes, smoking, dyslipidemias, and hypertension. Psychotropic medications, with particular concern over newer antipsychotic agents but mood stabilizers and antidepressants as well, are known to be associated with several of these risk factors and can possibly exacerbate them (Weiden et al. 2007).

**Obesity**. Obesity increases the risk for diabetes, hypertension, cardiovascular disease, dyslipidemias, respiratory difficulty, reproductive hormone difficulties, and certain cancers that have an association with obesity, e.g., colon. Persons with severe mental illness are at increased risk for obesity, and this increased risk occurs before progression of their illness and initiation of psychotropic drug use. There are disease-specific risk levels, with schizophrenia (2.8–3.5× risk) > bipolar disorders > major depression. As mentioned previously, this is multifactorial, including lifestyle, illness specific, and medication side effect-related issues. Lifestyle refers to the association of these conditions with decreased physical activity and poor diet in general. Illness-specific issues include negative symptoms, disorganization of thought and behavior, and depression itself all leading to reduced physical activity and poor self-care.

Antipsychotics, antidepressants, and mood stabilizers are all associated with sedation and its associated sequelae, but also they may directly cause or worsen obesity. Antipsychotics have been identified as the worst culprit, associated with weight gain in 15–72 % of persons receiving them. There is a differential effect among antipsychotics with some posing a greater risk than others, clozapine and olanzapine having the greatest risk, quetiapine and risperidone intermediate risk, and aripiprazole, asenapine, amisulpride, and ziprasidone having little effect. For the most part, FGAs have less risk, but have a stronger association with motor adverse effects. No antipsychotic should be considered to be totally weight neutral though.

**Metabolic Syndrome**. A grouping of conditions, including central obesity, hypertension, hypercholesterolemia, elevated triglycerides, and glucose intolerance or insulin resistance (incudes diabetes). Persons with metabolic syndrome have a five to sixfold elevated risk of developing diabetes, and three to sixfold increased mortality from coronary artery disease. Despite this well-known risk, and position statements from the American Diabetes Association, American Psychiatric Association, American Association of Clinical Endocrinologists, and North American Association for the Study of Obesity, screening by primary care physicians and psychiatrists is inadequate for these conditions (Clark 2004).

**Diabetes**. There are several modifiable risk factors for the development of diabetes, including obesity, lack of physical activity, diets low in whole grains and vegetables, and smoking. People with schizophrenia, schizoaffective disorder, and bipolar disorder have 2–3 times increased risk for the development of diabetes. The risk for persons with severe depression is lower, but still increased as compared to the general population. Antipsychotics are associated with this increased risk with the same pattern as seen for weight gain.

**Cardiovascular disease**. Cardiovascular disease is one of the leading causes of death for people with major depressive disorder, schizophrenia, and bipolar disorder. The risk for bipolar disorder and schizophrenia is 2–3 times higher. Depression is an independent risk factor associated with morbidity and mortality from cardiovascular disease. The main factor linking depression and poor outcomes from cardiovascular disease is lack of physical activity. Depression also increases the risk of myocardial infarction 2.5 times in persons who have coronary artery disease. Here is an illustrative case example.

> Mr. B. was a 38-year-old male with a history of Schizophrenia who already had several of these risk factors, which if not dealt with would lead to long-term physical disability and possibly mortality at a relatively early age. He started suffering from a severe mental illness during his college years and had only obtained stability, and subsequent recovery, on olanzapine, an agent strongly associated with weight gain. His weight had increased by 30 lb since the start of treatment, but when discussing this issue he said that under no circumstances did he want to go back to the time when he suffered from distressing psychotic episodes and frequent hospitalizations. He was concerned about his weight and diabetes though because his dad died at 55 from a myocardial infarction. He has a wife, a job, and two young children and did not want to put them through this. Would it be recovery oriented to tell this man he has to come off this medication because of his other health problems, or to tell him he can't because of the possible decompensation that may occur?

**Cerebral vascular attacks**. Again associated with all the issues mentioned above, but there is an increased risk ranging from 1.3–3.3 times in persons with severe mental illness. Besides the association of antipsychotics with weight gain and obesity, there is a direct association with increased risk of cerebral vascular attacks.

**Elevated prolactin**. Due to the dopamine D2 receptor blockade caused by many antipsychotic medications, there is a risk of elevated prolactin levels (a hormone involved in regulation of the reproductive endocrine system), which can have serious and uncomfortable side effects in both men and women. In women, this can lead to menstrual disturbances, cessation of menses, and abnormal lactation. In men, this can result in gynecomastia or development of breast tissue, decreased libido, impotence, and ejaculatory dysfunction. There is a differential risk for this side effect as follows:

haldol > risperidone > ziprasidone > olanzapine > aripiprazole > clozapine > quetiapine.

Though not part of normal screening, prolactin levels can certainly be drawn in persons complaining of symptoms consistent with elevated levels, and other medication options that are not associated with this issue can be discussed (Weiden et al. 2007). Here is an illustrative case example.

Ms. M. was a 35-year-old African American lady with a diagnosis of schizoaffective disorder who had been a long-term resident of a state operated psychiatric facility. When decompensated, she exhibited symptoms of paranoia regarding people stealing her possessions and trying to poison her, which had resulted in violence directed toward family, neighbors, and care givers in residential settings. In addition, she would have periods of "mania" where she would become sexually promiscuous and proposition strangers in her neighborhood. Other periodic problem behaviors included walking out in traffic and not attending to her physical conditions, which included obesity, diabetes, and hypertension. One persisting symptom was her delusional belief that she was pregnant, despite being provided with repeated laboratory results that showed she was in fact, not pregnant.

For these conditions, she was prescribed divalproex sodium, oral haloperidol, and long-acting injectable risperidone. As long as she adhered to her medications most of these symptoms were controlled, but she often refused her medications, which had repeatedly led to residential placement failures and periods of instability in the hospital. This was the main barrier to her reintegration into the community. Her treatment team was frustrated by this, and during many discussions, she reported her reason for her medication refusal was her concern she may harm her baby as she was pregnant. Her psychiatrist at the time did have a good relationship with her, but was often stretched due to census, staffing, and acuity issues at the hospital. One day, things were calm, and two standing administrative meetings were canceled, so he decided to sit down with Ms. M and convince her that she was indeed not pregnant and therefore should be happy to take the medications he had prescribed. She was shown multiple recent pregnancy tests and a recent Ob-Gyn checkup that proved she was not carrying a fetus. She responded that the information provided was not accurate because she knew she was pregnant since her breasts were engorged and she occasionally lactated. The proverbial light bulb went off for the psychiatrist and he ordered a prolactin level, which came back at 165 ng/ml (normal for non-pregnant females < 25 ng/ml). He explained these results to Ms. M., which she accepted, and together they came up with a new pharmacological treatment regimen involving medications that were less likely to cause this adverse effect. With this change, her side effects subsided, her adherence improved dramatically, and she was successfully transitioned to the community three months later.

**Osteoporosis**. The three diagnostic groupings associated with severe mental illness are all associated with decreased bone mineral density. Again, this is multifactorial with smoking, reduced physical activity, alcohol abuse, vitamin D and calcium deficiency, and polydipsia. Antidepressants, particularly SSRIs are associated with worsening this condition and consequently an increased risk of fractures in the elderly (De Hert et al. 2011a, b).

**Oral health**. In general, people with severe mental illness have poor dental health. Besides many of the multifactorial issues mentioned above, including poor self-care, antipsychotics, antidepressants, and mood stabilizers are associated with xerostomia, or decreased salivary flow. This adversely affects the oral environment aggravating caries, gingivitis, and periodontal disease (De Hert et al. 2011a, b).

**Constipation**. Medication-induced constipation is common, but often under recognized and has not been a focus of research. In addition to the discomfort this can cause, there are severe sequelae associated with this condition, including paralytic ileus, bowel occlusion, and death. Active screening, monitoring, and treatment are recommended (De Hert et al. 2011a, b; Ozbilen and Adams 2009).

## Medication Adherence and Transition to the Community

Inpatient settings are an artificial environment that will not be sustained upon a person's discharge. Environmental stressors that may have contributed to the need for hospitalization have been temporarily suspended, but may return in full force. Schedules are controlled with definite "pill calls" and staff who diligently remind the person to take their prescribed treatments. Medication side effects can be addressed immediately, and for the most part illicit substances and alcohols are not available. Upon discharge, the person typically has more control over management of the medications and individual barriers to ongoing adherence need to be identified and addressed as part of the discharge process.

Issues around medication adherence are complex. It would be nice if we simply could institute psychoeducational groups during the hospital stay and say that we have positively affected care recipient's adherence rates, but the research support for these assertions are equivocal (Barkhof et al. 2012; Zygmunt et al. 2002). In addition, there are many types of people who require psychiatric hospitalization, all of whom have different risk factors and who may require individualized approaches to improving medication adherence. Some issues that may arise, which adversely affect adherence, are the care recipient's insight into the illness and symptoms, active symptoms that may interfere with the cognitive aspects of health behavior, medication side effects, therapeutic alliance, environmental supports, and ongoing substance abuse.

Concerning people with schizophrenia receiving antipsychotic treatment, methodological factors cause large variation in adherence rates, ranging from estimates of 10–80 %, though this averages out to about a 50 % nonadherence rate. There are individual, medication, and environment-related reasons for this nonadherence and modifiable factors which should be targeted. In one study, Dolder et al. (2003) found that education alone was not adequate in changing adherence rates. They found that more intense interventions using behavioral and "affective" techniques in addition to education were effective in improving adherence. Education can be in verbal or written formats with a knowledge-based emphasis designed to convey information, e.g., one-on-one or group teaching with educational materials providing information about the purpose and potential side effects of medications. Behavioral interventions involve targeting or reinforcing specific behavioral patterns, e.g., skill-building practice activities, behavioral modeling, contracting, medication packaging, and dosage modification. This includes interventions such as simplifying regimens, teaching skills, and external cues such as medication reminder devices. "Affective" interventions influence medication adherence through appeals to feelings, emotions, social relationships, and social supports and involve psychotherapeutic modalities such as family support, counseling, and home visits. The last two modalities can help individuals cognitively reframe negative attitudes and learn to become more effective collaborators in their treatment (Dolder et al. 2003; Lacro et al. 2002).

Lacro et al. (2002) also discussed the *health belief model* which involved a summation of a person's susceptibility to illness, his perceived severity of illness, what he would see as benefits of taking health action, and perceived barriers (or costs) and cues to taking action. Improving an individual's assessment of the costs and benefits requires addressing diverse risk factors such as poor insight, negative attitudes toward medications, substance abuse, and the alliance with the therapist. What is the patient's motivation to adhere? In their review medication, side effects were not directly tied to non-adherence but were connected to the cost analysis of medication benefits, "…tipping the cost-benefit ratio against adherence."

All that said, psychoeducational groups are still considered an important part of the treatment armamentarium utilized in hospital settings. Examples of specific psychoeducational topics that can be addressed include the establishment of medication routines, identification of side effects, use of PRN medications if prescribed, negotiating medication changes with physicians, and development of crisis plans centered around medication choices in times of crisis (Noordsy et al. 2000). In addition, educational activities for family members and other care givers have been found to be effective in improving outcomes for both individuals being treated and their significant others (Resnick et al. 2004). With post discharge follow up rates of approximately 50 %,

**Table 7.4** Strategies for ensuring continuity of treatment at discharge

| |
|---|
| 1. Provide enough medication at discharge to last several days to allow for time to have a prescription filled |
| 2. Ask how the patient will obtain the medication on an outpatient basis |
| 3. Find out if the patient has insurance coverage and if it will cover the medication being considered |
| 4. If insurance will not cover the medication, ask about patient's/family's ability to pay out of pocket |
| 5. Choose a medication that the patient will be able to afford or obtain free of charge |
| 6. If patient cannot pay for the medication you believe is indicated, and then contact the pharmaceutical company to see if they will supply medication free of charge or at a reduced cost |

Adapted from Weiden et al. (2007)

steps need to be taken to encourage connection with appropriate outpatient services. One tool that is available is the "Community Reentry Module" that has been shown to be effective in both private and public hospitals (Rossotto et al. 2004). Of course an important step in obtaining and maintaining recovery is cessation of conditions that led to hospitalization (Weiden et al. 2007). See Table 7.4 with regard to medication adherence management.

## Conclusion

This chapter has elucidated the role of pharmacotherapy which can play in assisting individuals on their path to recovery. There is a great deal of research on the "efficacy" of psychotropics, and also potential safety issues that are required in registration trials. Most of our current research, by necessity, looks at large populations with relatively strict inclusion criteria that often do not reflect the reality of people in the community receiving the treatments. There are some efficacy measures that can be indirectly tied to recovery (e.g. time to relapse, symptom reduction), but often the current research falls short of demonstrating our pharmacological armamentarium actually contributes to a person's personal process of obtaining hope, destigmatization, empowerment, self-acceptance, meaningful relationships, gainful employment, independence, and health.

As we continue to develop the operational definitions of "recovery" there needs to be a focus on outcomes that can be utilized in pharmacological research. Measurement of intensity, frequency, and duration of symptoms is of course important in determining efficacy of pharmacotherapeutic agents, but this frequently does not take into account the fluctuating nature of many psychiatric illnesses whose presentations change over time. Moreover, symptom remission alone is an inadequate measure, as often a return to premorbid functioning which is not obtained with mere removal of symptoms. There has to be an assessment of psychosocial functioning, with attention on matters such as work, school, family life, friends, recreation, and independent living.

In putting forward this research agenda, there needs to be a consensus of stakeholders including practitioners, researchers, patients, and family members in determining areas of psychosocial functioning that will be used to establish efficacy in relation to recovery. As with other diseases, when rates of recovery are reported in replicable, reliable, and valid terms, stigma is decreased (Liberman and Kopelowicz 2005). Until such research goals are met, we should fulfill our role in partnering with care recipients to develop evidence-based treatment strategies that minimize adverse effects, are truly individualized, and address amenable aspects of the person's illness he or she finds to be a barrier to his or her recovery.

## References

Alexopoulos, G. S., Borson, S., Cuthbert, B. N., Devanand, D. P., Mulsant, B. H., Olin, J. T., & Oslin, D. W. (2002). Assessment of late life depression. *Biological Psychiatry, 52*(3), 164–174.

American Psychiatric Association. (2010). *Practice guideline for the treatment of patients with major depressive disorder* (3rd ed.). Washington, DC: American Psychiatric Publishing Inc.

Appelbaum, P. S. (1988). The right to refuse treatment with antipsychotic medications: Retrospect and prospect. *American Journal of Psychiatry, 145*(4), 413–419.

Austin, M. P., Mitchell, P., & Goodwin, G. M. (2001). Cognitive deficits in depression: Possible implications for functional neuropathology. *British Journal of Psychiatry, 178*, 200–206.

Barkhof, E., Meijer, C. J., de Sonneville, L. M., Linszen, D. H., & de Haan, L. (2012). Interventions to improve adherence to antipsychotic medication in patients with schizophrenia—A review of the past decade. *European Psychiatry, 27*(1), 9–18.

Bauer, M., Pfennig, A., Severus, E., Whybrow, P. C., Angst, J., & Moller, H. J. (2013). World Federation of Societies of Biological Psychiatry (WFSBP) guidelines for biological treatment of unipolar depressive disorders, part 1: Update 2013 on the acute and continuation treatment of unipolar depressive disorders. *World Journal of Biological Psychiatry, 14*(5), 334–385.

Bellack, A. S. (2006). Scientific and consumer models of recovery in schizophrenia: Concordance, contrasts, and implications. *Schizophrenia Bulletin, 32*(3), 432–442.

Besag, F. M., & Berry, D. (2006). Interactions between antiepileptic and antipsychotic drugs. *Drug Safety, 29* (2), 95–118.

Bizub, A. L. (2013). A hard pill to swallow: Medication, empathy, and the value of collaborative recovery. *Community Mental Health Journal, 49*(3), 338–343.

Brandl, E. J., Kennedy, J. L., & Muller, D. J. (2014). Pharmacogenetics of antipsychotics. *Canadian Journal of Psychiatry. Revue Canadienne de Psychiatrie, 59*(2), 76–88.

Campanelli, C. M. (2012). American geriatrics society updated Beers criteria for potentially inappropriate medication use in older adults. *Journal of the American Geriatrics Society, 60*(4), 616–631.

Campbell, L. A., & Kisely, S. R. (2009). Advance treatment directives for people with severe mental illness. *Cochrane Database Systematic Reviews,* (1), CD005963.

Cerovecki, A., Musil, R., Klimke, A., Seemuller, F., Haen, E., Schennach, R., & Riedel, M. (2013). Withdrawal symptoms and rebound syndromes associated with switching and discontinuing atypical antipsychotics: Theoretical background and practical recommendations. *CNS Drugs, 27*(7), 545–572.

Charney, D. S., Reynolds, C. F., 3rd, Lewis, L., Lebowitz, B. D., Sunderland, T., & Alexopoulos, G. S. (2003). Depression and Bipolar Support Alliance consensus statement on the unmet needs in diagnosis and treatment of mood disorders in late life. *Archives of General Psychiatry, 60*(7), 664–672.

Clark, N. (2004). Consensus development conference on antipsychotic drugs and obesity and diabetes. *Diabetes Care, 27*(2), 596–601.

David, G. (2010). The pharmacology of aging. In H. Fillit, K. Rockwood, K. W. Woodhouse, & J. C. Brocklehurst (Eds.), *Brocklehurst's textbook of geriatric medicine and gerontology* (7th ed., pp. 138–144). Philadelphia, PA: Saunders/Elsevier.

Davidson, L., O'Connell, M., Tondora, J., Styron, T., & Kangas, K. (2006). The top ten concerns about recovery encountered in mental health system transformation. *Psychiatric Services, 57*(5), 640–645.

De Hert, M., Correll, C. U., Bobes, J., Cetkovich-Bakmas, M., Cohen, D., Asai, I., & Leucht, S. (2011a). Physical illness in patients with severe mental disorders. I. Prevalence, impact of medications and disparities in health care. *World Psychiatry, 10*(1), 52–77.

De Hert, M., Hudyana, H., Dockx, L., Bernagie, C., Sweers, K., Tack, J., & Peuskens, J. (2011b). Second-generation antipsychotics and constipation: A review of the literature. *European Psychiatry, 26* (1), 34–44.

Deegan, P. E. (2007). The lived experience of using psychiatric medication in the recovery process and a shared decision-making program to support it. *Psychiatric Rehabilitation Journal, 31*(1), 62–69.

Deegan, P. E., & Drake, R. E. (2006). Shared decision making and medication management in the recovery process. *Psychiatric Services, 57*(11), 1636–1639. doi:10.1176/appi.ps.57.11.1636

Dibonaventura, M., Gabriel, S., Dupclay, L., Gupta, S., & Kim, E. (2012). A patient perspective of the impact of medication side effects on adherence: Results of a cross-sectional nationwide survey of patients with schizophrenia. *BMC Psychiatry, 12*, 20.

Dickey, B., Normand, S. L., Weiss, R. D., Drake, R. E., & Azeni, H. (2002). Medical morbidity, mental illness, and substance use disorders. *Psychiatric Services, 53* (7), 861–867.

Dolder, C. R., Lacro, J. P., Leckband, S., & Jeste, D. V. (2003). Interventions to improve antipsychotic medication adherence: Review of recent literature. *Journal of Clinical Psychopharmacology, 23*(4), 389–399.

Drake, R. E., Deegan, P. E., & Rapp, C. (2010). The promise of shared decision making in mental health. *Psychiatric Rehabilitation Journal, 34*(1), 7–13.

Drake, R. E., Goldman, H. H., Leff, H. S., Lehman, A. F., Dixon, L., Mueser, K. T., et al. (2001). Implementing evidence-based practices in routine mental health service settings. *Psychiatric Services, 52*(2), 179–182.

Drane, J. F. (1984). Competency to give an informed consent. A model for making clinical assessments. *Journal of the American Medical Association, 252*(7), 925–927.

Fabbri, C., Porcelli, S., & Serretti, A. (2014). From pharmacogenetics to pharmacogenomics: The way toward the personalization of antidepressant treatment. *Canadian Journal of Psychiatry. Revue Canadienne de Psychiatrie, 59*(2), 62–75.

Fava, G., Gatti, A., Belaise, C., Guidi, J., & Offidani, E. (2015). Withdrawal symptoms after selective serotonin reuptake inhibitor discontinuation: A systematic review. *Psychotherapy and Psychosomatics, 84*, 72–81.

Fenton, W. S., Blyler, C. R., & Heinssen, R. K. (1997). Determinants of medication compliance in schizophrenia: Empirical and clinical findings. *Schizophrenia Bulletin, 23*(4), 637–651.

Ferguson, J. M. (2001). SSRI antidepressant medications: Adverse effects and tolerability. *Primary Care Companion to the Journal of Clinical Psychiatry, 3*(1), 22–27.

Fisher, D. B., & Ahern, L. (2002). Evidence-based practices and recovery. *Psychiatric Services, 53*(5), 632–634.

Frese, F. J, 3rd, Stanley, J., Kress, K., & Vogel-Scibilia, S. (2001). Integrating evidence-based practices and the recovery model. *Psychiatric Services, 52*(11), 1462–1468.

Gandhi, M., Aweeka, F., Greenblatt, R. M., & Blaschke, T. F. (2004). Sex differences in pharmacokinetics and pharmacodynamics. *Annual Review of Pharmacology and Toxicology, 44*, 499–523.

Geddes, J. R., Carney, S. M., Davies, C., Furukawa, T. A., Kupfer, D. J., Frank, E., et al. (2003). Relapse prevention with antidepressant drug treatment in depressive disorders: A systematic review. *Lancet, 361*(9358), 653–661.

Hasan, A., Falkai, P., Wobrock, T., Lieberman, J., Glenthoj, B., Gattaz, W. F., et al. (2012). World Federation of Societies of Biological Psychiatry (WFSBP) Guidelines for Biological Treatment of Schizophrenia, part 1: Update 2012 on the acute treatment of schizophrenia and the management of treatment resistance. *World Journal of Biological Psychiatry, 13*(5), 318-378.

Hasan, A., Falkai, P., Wobrock, T., Lieberman, J., Glenthoj, B., Gattaz, W. F., et al. (2013). World Federation of Societies of Biological Psychiatry (WFSBP) guidelines for biological treatment of schizophrenia, part 2: update 2012 on the long-term treatment of schizophrenia and management of antipsychotic-induced side effects. *World Journal of Biological Psychiatry, 14*(1), 2–44.

Henderson, H. (2004). From depths of despair to heights of recovery. *Psychiatric Rehabilitation Journal, 28*(1), 83–87.

Houghton, J. F. (1982). First person account: Maintaining mental health in a turbulent world. *Schizophrenia Bulletin, 8*(3), 548–553.

Karow, A., Czekalla, J., Dittmann, R. W., Schacht, A., Wagner, T., Lambert, M., et al. (2007). Association of subjective well-being, symptoms, and side effects with compliance after 12 months of treatment in schizophrenia. *Journal of Clinical Psychiatry, 68*(1), 75–80.

Kato, M., & Serretti, A. (2010). Review and meta-analysis of antidepressant pharmacogenetic findings in major depressive disorder. *Molecular Psychiatry, 15*(5), 473–500.

Kaymaz, N., van Os, J., Loonen, A. J., & Nolen, W. A. (2008). Evidence that patients with single versus recurrent depressive episodes are differentially sensitive to treatment discontinuation: A meta-analysis of placebo-controlled randomized trials. *Journal of Clinical Psychiatry, 69*(9), 1423–1436.

Kingsbury, S. J., Yi, D., & Simpson, G. M. (2001). Psychopharmacology: Rational and irrational polypharmacy. *Psychiatric Services, 52*(8), 1033–1036.

Krishnan, K. R., Delong, M., Kraemer, H., Carney, R., Spiegel, D., Gordon, C., et al. (2002). Comorbidity of depression with other medical diseases in the elderly. *Biological Psychiatry, 52*(6), 559–588.

Lacro, J. P., Dunn, L. B., Dolder, C. R., Leckband, S. G., & Jeste, D. V. (2002). Prevalence of and risk factors for medication nonadherence in patients with schizophrenia: A comprehensive review of recent literature. *Journal of Clinical Psychiatry, 63*(10), 892–909.

Lehman, A. F., & Steinwachs, D. M. (1998). Patterns of usual care for schizophrenia: Initial results from the Schizophrenia Patient Outcomes Research Team (PORT) Client Survey. *Schizophrenia Bulletin, 24* (1), 11–32.

Liberman, R. P. (2008). Illness managment. In R. P. Liberman (Ed.), *Recovery from disability* (pp. 100–119). Washington, DC: American Psychiatric Publishing, Inc.

Liberman, R. P., & Kopelowicz, A. (2005). Recovery from schizophrenia: A concept in search of research. *Psychiatric Services, 56*(6), 735–742.

Lunt, A. (2002). A theory of recovery. *Journal of Psychosocial Nursing and Mental Health Services, 40*(12), 32–39.

Malhotra, A. K., Murphy, G. M, Jr., & Kennedy, J. L. (2004). Pharmacogenetics of psychotropic drug response. *American Journal of Psychiatry, 161*(5), 780–796.

Mangoni, A. A., & Jackson, S. H. (2004). Age-related changes in pharmacokinetics and pharmacodynamics: Basic principles and practical applications. *British Journal of Clinical Pharmacology, 57*(1), 6–14.

Martinez-Aran, A., Vieta, E., Reinares, M., Colom, F., Torrent, C., Sanchez-Moreno, J., et al. (2004). Cognitive function across manic or hypomanic, depressed, and euthymic states in bipolar disorder. *American Journal of Psychiatry, 161*(2), 262–270.

Mellman, T. A., Miller, A. L., Weissman, E. M., Crismon, M. L., Essock, S. M., & Marder, S. R. (2001). Evidence-based pharmacologic treatment for people with severe mental illness: A focus on guidelines and algorithms. *Psychiatric Services, 52*(5), 619–625.

Menninger, J. A. (2001). Involuntary treatment: Hospitalization and medications. In J. L. Jacobson & M. Alan (Eds.), *Psychiatric secrets* (2nd ed., pp. 477–484). Philadelphia, PA: Harley and Belfus Inc.

Minzenberg, M. J., Poole, J. H., Benton, C., & Vinogradov, S. (2004). Association of anticholinergic load with impairment of complex attention and memory in schizophrenia. *American Journal of Psychiatry, 161* (1), 116–124.

Moller, H. J., & Nasrallah, H. A. (2003). Treatment of bipolar disorder. *Journal of Clinical Psychiatry, 64* (Suppl 6), 9–17.

Moore, T. A., Buchanan, R. W., Buckley, P. F., Chiles, J. A., Conley, R. R., Crismon, M. L., et al. (2007). The Texas medication algorithm project antipsychotic algorithm for schizophrenia: 2006 update. *Journal of Clinical Psychiatry, 68*(11), 1751–1762.

Nasrallah, H. A., Targum, S. D., Tandon, R., McCombs, J. S., & Ross, R. (2005). Defining and measuring clinical effectiveness in the treatment of schizophrenia. *Psychiatric Services, 56*(3), 273–282.

Newcomer, J. W., Weiden, P. J., & Buchanan, R. W. (2013). Switching antipsychotic medications to reduce adverse event burden in schizophrenia: establishing evidence-based practice. *Journal of Clinical Psychiatry, 74*(11), 1108–1120.

Nicaise, P., Lorant, V., & Dubois, V. (2013). Psychiatric Advance Directives as a complex and multistage intervention: A realist systematic review. *Health Social Care Community, 21*(1), 1–14.

Noordsy, D. L., Torrey, W. C., Mead, S., Brunette, M., Potenza, D., & Copeland, M. E. (2000). Recovery-oriented psychopharmacology: Redefining the goals of antipsychotic treatment. *Journal of Clinical Psychiatry, 61*(Suppl 3), 22–29.

Noordsy, D. L., Torrey, W., Mueser, K., Mead, S., O'Keefe, C., & Fox, L. (2002). Recovery from severe mental illness: An interpersonal and functional outcome definition. *International Review of Psychiatry, 14*, 318–326.

O'Leary, D. S., Flaum, M., Kesler, M. L., Flashman, L. A., Arndt, S., & Andreasen, N. C. (2000). Cognitive correlates of the negative, disorganized, and psychotic symptom dimensions of schizophrenia. *Journal of Neuropsychiatry and Clinical Neurosciences, 12*(1), 4–15.

O'Neal, J. M. (1984). First person account: Finding myself and loving it. *Schizophrenia Bulletin, 10*(1), 109–110.

Ozbilen, M., & Adams, C. E. (2009). Systematic overview of Cochrane reviews for anticholinergic effects of antipsychotic drugs. *Journal of Clinical Psychopharmacology, 29*(2), 141–146.

Paquette, M., & Navarro, T. (2005). Lives recovered. *Perspectives in Psychiatric Care, 41*(3), 95–96.

Pearlstein, T. (2013). Use of psychotropic medication during pregnancy and the postpartum period. *Womens Health (Lond Engl), 9*(6), 605–615.

Piat, M., Sabetti, J., Couture, A., Sylvestre, J., Provencher, H., Botschner, J., et al. (2009). What does recovery mean for me? Perspectives of Canadian mental health consumers. *Psychiatric Rehabilitation Journal, 32*(3), 199–207.

Pollock, B., Forsyth, C., & Bies, R. (2009). The critical role of clinical pharmacology in geriatric psychopharmacology. *Clinical Pharmacology and Therapeutics, 85*(1), 89–93.

Resnick, S. G., Rosenheck, R. A., & Lehman, A. F. (2004). An exploratory analysis of correlates of recovery. *Psychiatric Services, 55*(5), 540–547.

Rossotto, E., Wirshing, D. A., & Liberman, R. P. (2004). Rehab rounds: Enhancing treatment adherence among persons with schizophrenia by teaching community reintegration skills. *Psychiatric Services, 55*(1), 26–27.

Sachs, G. S., Printz, D. J., Kahn, D. A., Carpenter, D., & Docherty, J. P. (2000). The expert consensus guideline series: Medication treatment of bipolar disorder 2000. *Postgraduate Medicine, Spec No*, 1–104.

Sachs, G. S., & Rush, A. J. (2003). Response, remission, and recovery in bipolar disorders: What are the realistic treatment goals? *Journal of Clinical Psychiatry, 64*(Suppl 6), 18–22.

Sowers, W., & Quality Management Committee of the American Association of Community Psychiatrists (2005). Transforming systems of care: The American Association of Community Psychiatrists Guidelines for Recovery Oriented Services. *Community Mental Health Journal, 41*(6), 757–774.

Spina, E., Scordo, M. G., & D'Arrigo, C. (2003). Metabolic drug interactions with new psychotropic agents. *Fundamental & Clinical Pharmacology, 17*(5), 517–538.

Stahl, S. M. (2013). *Stahl's essential psychopharmacology: Neuroscientific basis and practical applications. Chapter 2: Transporters, receptors, and enzymes as targets of psychopharmacological drug action*. Cambridge: Cambridge University Press.

Stahl, S. M., Lee-Zimmerman, C., Cartwright, S., & Morrissette, D. A. (2013). Serotonergic drugs for depression and beyond. *Current Drug Targets, 14*(5), 578–585.

Svedberg, B., Backenroth-Ohsako, G., & Lutzen, K. (2003). On the path to recovery: patients' experiences of treatment with long-acting injections of antipsychotic medication. *International Journal of Mental Health Nursing, 12*(2), 110–118.

Tandon, R., Targum, S. D., Nasrallah, H. A., Ross, R., & Treatment Effectiveness in Schizophrenia Consortium. (2006). Strategies for maximizing clinical effectiveness in the treatment of schizophrenia. *Journal of Psychiatric Practice, 12*(6), 348–363.

Tanenbaum, S. J. (2008). Perspectives on evidence-based practice from consumers in the US public mental health system. *Journal of Evaluation in Clinical Practice, 14*(5), 699–706.

Torrey, W. C., Drake, R. E., Dixon, L., Burns, B. J., Flynn, L., Rush, A. J., et al. (2001). Implementing evidence-based practices for persons with severe mental illnesses. *Psychiatric Services, 52*(1), 45–50.

U.S. National Library of Medicine. (2015). Polymorphism. *National Institute of Health Retrieved from* http://ghr.nlm.nih.gov/glossary=polymorphism

Watanabe-Galloway, S., & Zhang, W. (2007). Analysis of U.S. trends in discharges from general hospitals for episodes of serious mental illness, 1995–2002. *Psychiatric Services, 58*(4), 496–502.

Weiden, P. J., Preskorn, S. H., Fahnestock, P. A., Carpenter, D., Ross, R., Docherty, J. P., et al. (2007). Translating the psychopharmacology of antipsychotics to individualized treatment for severe mental illness: A Roadmap. *Journal of Clinical Psychiatry, 68 Suppl 7*, 1–48.

Windell, D. L., Norman, R., Lal, S., & Malla, A. (2015). Subjective experiences of illness recovery in individuals treated for first-episode psychosis. *Social Psychiatry and Psychiatric Epidemiology, 50*(7), 1069–1077.

Windell, D., Norman, R., & Malla, A. K. (2012). The personal meaning of recovery among individuals treated for a first episode of psychosis. *Psychiatric Services, 63*(6), 548–553.

Wirshing, D. A., Wirshing, W. C., Marder, S. R., Liberman, R. P., & Mintz, J. (1998). Informed consent: Assessment of comprehension. *American Journal of Psychiatry, 155*(11), 1508–1511.

Yatham, L. N., Kennedy, S. H., Parikh, S. V., Schaffer, A., Beaulieu, S., Alda, M., et al. (2013). Canadian Network for Mood and Anxiety Treatments (CANMAT) and International Society for Bipolar Disorders (ISBD) collaborative update of CANMAT guidelines for the management of patients with bipolar disorder: Update 2013. *Bipolar Disord, 15*(1), 1–44.

Zygmunt, A., Olfson, M., Boyer, C. A., & Mechanic, D. (2002). Interventions to improve medication adherence in schizophrenia. *American Journal of Psychiatry, 159*(10), 1653–1664.

# Cognitive Remediation in Mental Health

8

Benjamin D. Hill, Channing Sofko and Anneliese C. Boettcher

## Introduction

Cognitive deficits are common in psychiatric conditions and they are often core features of the disorders. Cognitive impairments in severe psychiatric disorders can be quite dramatic and can significantly interfere with quality of life and treatment outcomes. As such, techniques for improving cognitive functioning in psychiatric populations are garnering attention and becoming a focus of intervention research. These techniques are typically categorized as cognitive rehabilitation or cognitive remediation. We will generally use the term cognitive remediation throughout this chapter. However, some experts contend that cognitive rehabilitation refers to interventions that are general in nature and cognitive remediation is more concerned with techniques developed for specific etiologies. The distinction between these two intervention categories will be discussed in more detail, but we will use the term cognitive remediation to categorize a range of behavioral interventions using targeted training exercises designed to improve cognitive functioning (Eack 2012).

Cognitive remediation was designated a "best practice" treatment for severe mental disorders by the APA/CAAP Task Force on serious mental illness and severe emotional disturbance (2007) and these interventions typically focus on improving cognitive processes, such as attention, memory, and higher level executive functions, including social cognition. The goal is to train and strengthen specific cognitive processes that will then generalize and result in long-term improvement (Medalia 2010). Remediation interventions are often used in conjunction with compensation approaches that attempt to circumvent deficits, but these are conceptually distinct rehabilitation techniques (Pella et al. 2008).

## Neuroplasticity

The field of cognitive remediation capitalizes on neuroplasticity (Bruel-Jungerman et al. 2007). Neuroplasticity is the neurobiological process by which learning and environmental factors alter cognitive processing. An example of neuroplasticity is when individuals who lose motor skills following brain injury are able to improve motor functioning through practiced approximations of the lost skills resulting in neurobiological changes in the affected cortex (Robertson and Murre 1999). Many of the guiding principles of cognitive remediation that are currently used in practice were initially developed in the realm of brain injury rehabilitation. (e.g., Ben-Yishay et al. 1985; Hogarty and Flesher 1999). The guiding principle in brain injury rehabilitation is to

B.D. Hill (✉) · C. Sofko · Anneliese C.Boettcher
Department of Psychology, UCOMM 1500,
University of South Alabama, Mobile, AL 36688,
USA
e-mail: bdhill@southalabama.edu



N.N. Singh et al. (eds.), *Handbook of Recovery in Inpatient Psychiatry*,
Evidence-Based Practices in Behavioral Health, DOI 10.1007/978-3-319-40537-7_8

acutely intervene to reduce damage to the brain damage and stabilize the initial pathology then shift to recovery and rehabilitation as the primary clinical focus (Pella et al. 2008). This is a different paradigm than what is typically done in mental health as severe psychopathology often has a more chronic course requiring ongoing treatment leading cognitive remediation to frequently occur concurrently with treatment of the underlying psychopathology.

## Common Elements in Programs

Cognitive remediation programs vary widely in complexity, domains addressed, and methods of implementation. For instance, some programs are administered individually while others involve group administration. Most programs have traditionally focused on basic cognitive abilities such as attention and memory (Pella et al. 2008) but newer approaches are emphasizing higher level executive functions such as social cognition. Despite these nuances, some common elements span across most cognitive remediation programs. The following were proposed by Eack (2012) as the principle components of cognitive remediation therapy for individuals with schizophrenia: (1) *strategic*: the purpose of the intervention is to assist individuals in developing cognitive strategies to complete tasks; (2) *drill and practice*: repetition of the cognitive strategies continues over multiple sessions until performance improvement is noted; (3) *hierarchical*: the approach to cognitive abilities proceeds from simple activities to those that are more complex; (4) *cueing*: using external auditory or visual aids to support cognitive abilities; (5) *fading*: slowly removing cues and external aids as progress is made to increase difficulty; (6) *adaptive*: adjustment of the difficult of cognitive tasks so they continue to be challenging and interesting; (7) *anchoring*: linking those skills learned in remediation training to real-word behaviors; and (8) *integration with other treatments*: using other treatments for schizophrenia in conjunction with remediation to increase the potential benefits. Eack's nomenclature provides a useful tool for comparing elements across different programs and evaluating the literature in this area.

Some experts contrast cognitive remediation with cognitive rehabilitation by defining the latter as a broad range of behavioral therapy approaches that target cognitive deficits, regardless of the etiology of the deficits (Medalia 2010). Cognitive rehabilitation can be thought of as a therapeutic service individualized to address deficits in cognition and behavior as measured through neuropsychological assessment procedures (Cicerone et al. 2000). This therapeutic service is systematic, although the particular intervention approach can vary. For example, one intervention includes relearning and reestablishing previously learned patterns of behavior while a second form includes establishing new patterns of behavior.

## Evaluating Efficacy and Effectiveness

As with any clinical intervention, it is important to examine the efficacy of cognitive remediation. A typical approach to examining the effectiveness of the approaches has been through the use of single-subject designs. Although randomized clinical trials (RCTs) are the ideal method for conducting this type of research, they are often extremely difficult if not impossible to conduct as a result of limited financial funding resources for such trials. Furthermore, application of the RCT methodology is difficult due to the lack of consensus as to the type of treatments, methodology of the intervention, and assessment of outcomes (Cappa et al. 2005). Single-subject designs are beneficial for the fields of cognitive remediation because they allow researchers to see if a treatment intervention is working for a specific individual. However, many argue that this approach is difficult to apply broadly because what may work for one individual may not work in exactly the same way for another.

Cognitive remediation research has been systematically reviewed and studies have been divided into a typical class structure to help explain the various quality indicators with respect to methodology. Class I studies are defined as prospective, randomized controlled trials. Class II studies are defined as prospective cohort studies, retrospective case-control studies, or clinical series with well-designed controls. Finally, Class III studies are defined as clinical series without concurrent controls, or studies with appropriate single-subject methodology. Cicerone et al. (2000) advised researchers to conduct psychometrically sound, single-subject (Class III) research designs or controlled multiple-baseline designs across subjects or interventions in order to minimize potentially problematic methodology.

Although there are some benefits to single-subject designs they also have the previously mentioned limitations. One major criticism of using small sample sizes is the difficulty in extrapolating the findings of one study with a particular sample (e.g., outpatient adults with regular pharmacological management of schizophrenia) and generalizing to a larger population (individuals in inpatient settings with comorbid conditions). In other words, researchers are challenged with the question of efficacy versus effectiveness. Current studies suggest that cognitive remediation may be beneficial for inpatient psychiatric patients with specific conditions such as schizophrenia and eating disorders. Further, individuals experiencing psychosis following traumatic brain injury (TBI) and stroke have often remained in inpatient psychiatric units for longer durations than those without concurrent psychotic features. Individuals suffering from TBI and/or stroke and psychotic features share many of the same symptoms of behavioral and cognitive dysfunction seen in other psychotic disorders. There is evidence to suggest that general cognitive remediation has been very beneficial for psychosis following TBI and stroke, with implications for specific cognitive remediation documented (Batty et al. 2013; Fujii and Ahmed 2014; Molloy et al. 2011). These diagnoses with demonstrated efficacy for cognitive remediation will be the focus of this chapter.

## Practice Effects in Cognitive Remediation

Before reviewing the literature on the effectiveness of cognitive remediation, it is imperative to make note of an important caveat in this field that we believe is commonly misunderstood by researchers in this area. Specifically, we want to address practice effects on neuropsychological measures and consider the effect sizes of practice effects. Practice effects are defined as learning that results from repeated exposure to testing materials (e.g., Beglinger et al. 2005). They can be thought of as improved test scores that occur regardless of an individual's ability on a particular construct; accordingly, these effects can compromise the validity of findings (Calamia et al. 2012). Inaccurate findings as a result of neglecting to account for practice effects have been found to mask cognitive decline in longitudinal studies and limit the ability to determine whether or not an intervention was beneficial. In particular, simply taking a measure at pretest and posttest led to gains in the control group of nearly one-half of a standard deviation (Brown et al. 2007).

Practice effects associated with cognitive remediation may be especially prominent in individuals with severe mental illness, such as schizophrenia, as illustrated by high variability among reported effect sizes in this population. Practice effect sizes in individuals with schizophrenia have been reported as $d = 0.36$ (Goldberg et al. 2007), $d = 0.45$ (Keefe et al. 2008), $d = 0.22$ (Mishara and Goldberg 2004), $d = -0.02$ to 0.53 (Szoke et al. 2008), and $d = 0.17$–0.46 (Woodward et al. 2007). These results support that cognitive remediation studies in severe mental illness need to be interpreted in the context of possible practice effects that may contribute substantially to intervention outcomes.

One approach to reducing practice effects has been the use of alternative forms. However, Benedict and Zgaljardi (1998) found that the use of alternate forms may not be as helpful in reducing practice effects if both versions of the form are assessing a novel concept or if they assess visuospatial learning or graphomotor responses. In particular, Beglinger et al. (2005) found that the Paced Auditory Serial Addition Test and the Stroop interference test had the largest practice effects because they involve novel concepts and strategies. Practice effects across alternate forms have also been found on tests of numerous cognitive domains and specific tests in which these effects were found include Digit Span, Digit Symbol Coding, Letter Number Sequencing, Trail Making Test, and Paced Auditory Serial Addition Test (Fastenau et al. 2002). Perhaps the best approach to controlling for practice effects is to give the baseline assessment more than once prior to any intervention in order to account for improvement due to practice effects leading to erroneous findings of improvement due to treatment.

## Cognitive Remediation in Clinical Groups

We will now move on to examining cognitive remediation in specific clinical samples. The main focus will be on a review of the extant literature on the use of cognitive remediation in individuals with schizophrenia and anorexia nervosa. Cognitive rehabilitation in TBI and cerebrovascular accident/stroke will also be discussed, as these individuals are likely to be seen in inpatient settings and commonly have a neuropsychiatric presentation (Batty et al. 2013; Fujii and Ahmed 2014; Molloy et al. 2011). Currently available intervention strategies will be discussed in the context of each study. The use of cognitive remediation and associated mindfulness techniques will be reviewed in the context of available outpatient remediation options and preventative measures. Finally, factors that could affect clinical implementation of the interventions, such as medication interference effects and patient/therapist variables will be discussed.

## Cognitive Remediation and Schizophrenia

Schizophrenia can be seen as a heterogeneous diagnostic category associated with impaired occupational and social functioning. Diagnostic symptoms include a range of cognitive, behavioral, and emotional dysfunction with no single symptom being pathognomonic of the disorder (American Psychiatric Association 2013), but center on delusions, hallucinations, or disorganized speech. Grossly disorganized or catatonic behavior and/or negative symptoms, such as diminished emotional expression or avolition, may also be present. Individuals with schizophrenia may also display inappropriate affect, a dysphoric mood, a disturbed sleep pattern, a lack of interest in eating, as well as develop anxiety and specific phobias. While it is important to identify mood symptoms, it is vital to identify cognitive symptoms in order to accurately diagnosis schizophrenia. Individuals may lack insight into their condition, leading to non-adherence to treatment, and lack of awareness is predictive of higher relapse rates, an increased number of involuntary treatments, poorer social functioning, aggression, and an overall poorer course of illness.

### Cognitive Effects of Schizophrenia

Individuals with schizophrenia may experience cognitive changes that result from disrupted neurotransmitter systems, changes in structure, connectivity and other physiological changes in addition to possible affective and psychotic symptoms (Schaefer et al. 2013). Meta-analyses have indicated moderate to large raw effect sizes ($d > 0.60$) across 22 measures that assessed seven major cognitive domains further demonstrate the presence of widespread cognitive effects (Heinrichs and Zakzanis 1998). On average, individuals with schizophrenia perform one to two standard deviations below the general population in the cognitive domains of attention, memory, and problem solving (Reichenberg and Harvey 2007). Specific decrements can include impairments in declarative memory, working memory, language functioning, processing speed, and various aspects of executive functioning (American Psychiatric Association 2013). These findings highlight the need for intervention to attempt to remedy these cognitive disparities.

## Theories of Schizophrenia

Currently, there are no radiological or laboratory tests that determine whether or not schizophrenia is present. However, differences in multiple brain regions exist between healthy controls and individuals with schizophrenia, with evidence from neuroimaging, neuropathology, and neurophysiological studies supporting these differences (American Psychiatric Association 2013). Several theories exist in an attempt to explain the presence of schizophrenia. Theories relating to the pathological process and etiology of schizophrenia consider specific neurotransmitters, neural systems, and developmental factors (Tamminga and Medoff 2000). Although the etiology of the condition is unclear, these insights allow guidance of intervention approaches.

***The role of dopamine***. A reduction in psychotic symptoms following the administration of antipsychotic medications that block dopamine receptors have led early researchers to hypothesize that dopamine dysregulation may be a cardinal biological feature leading to the observed symptoms characteristic of schizophrenia (Carlsson and Lindquist 1963). More recently, this theory has been adapted and termed the "revised dopamine hypothesis," which proposes hyperactive dopamine transmission in the mesolimbic areas of the brain and hypoactive dopamine transmission in the prefrontal cortex (Brisch et al. 2014). Current research has supported the role of dopamine antagonists in reducing the psychotic symptoms associated with the condition (Laurelle et al. 1999). Despite this, there is little evidence that dopamine alone could be responsible for the global changes.

***Neural pathways***. DeLong (1990) proposed that neural pathways between the frontal cortex and subcortical areas which affect the basal ganglia, thalamus, and caudate nucleus may play a part in observed symptoms. This theory centers on the dysfunction seen in the frontal cortex and proposes that disruption in the dynamic dopamine system, combined with changes in the balance of neurotransmitters and modulators released by the basal ganglia, and the thalamic relay system lead to these frontal changes (Andreasen et al. 1994; Carlsson and Carlsson 1990; Laurelle et al. 1999). In addition, connections associated with the cerebellum have been found to differentiate persons with schizophrenia from those without, suggesting the inclusion of pathways to the cerebellum (Yu et al. 2013).

***Developmental factors***. Walker and Diforio (1997) proposed a neural diathesis-stress model to describe the onset of schizophrenia. This model incorporates aspects of environmental stress with the biological view of heightened dopamine receptor sensitivity in the striatum. Specifically, the researchers posit that environmental insults that occur during the prenatal or perinatal periods and psychosocial stressors are environmental factors that can place individuals at a biological risk. This risk may include altered function or structure of the hippocampus due to early life insults or changes in the hypothalamus-pituitary-adrenal axis (HPA), a major axis involved in stress modulation. Further, the HPA axis and the hippocampus function are mutually influential and the effects on the HPA axis can lead to increased cortisol release. This increase in cortisol activates the subcortical dopamine system which in turn feeds into the HPA axis and further cortisol release. When this process occurs the outcome is symptom onset or exacerbation.

## Cognitive Remediation Approaches for Inpatients with Schizophrenia

One well-studied cognitive remediation program is the Neuropsychology Educational Approach to Cognitive Remediation ([NEAR]; Medalia and Freilich 2008; Medalia and Choi 2009) intervention. The NEAR approach was developed based on information from educational psychology, cognitive psychology, learning theory, and neuropsychology and it was designed for use with psychiatric patients. The NEAR program consisted of twice weekly computer-based training sessions and a 30–60 min group meeting once per week. The NEAR approach has been implemented in research settings, acute and chronic inpatient psychiatric units, outpatient programs, intensive psychiatric rehabilitation units, and in forensic settings (Medalia and Richardson 2005). Attention, memory, verbal fluency, motor speed, information processing, executive function, and verbal and working memory abilities are domains targeted by the computer-based intervention. The weekly group sessions serve to help patients generalize the skills they learned via computer training to their daily activities.

In an attempt to remedy the concern of practice effects, researchers have investigated structural changes concurrent with cognitive remediation. Evidence suggests cognitive remediation is associated with changes in critical expressive language areas, the prefrontal cortex, and the process of information transfer across brain hemispheres (Penadés et al. 2013; Pu et al. 2014; Vianin et al. 2014). Pu et al. (2014) examined the effectiveness of the NEAR cognitive remediation approach by measuring the resulting effect on prefrontal and temporal perfusion during working memory tasks. Perfusion was measured using near-infrared spectroscopy imaging of the brain to assess hemodynamic changes. Both inpatient residents and outpatients with mild to moderate schizophrenia or schizoaffective disorder were included. Unfortunately, there was no random assignment to the treatment or control groups and medication dosage levels were not controlled. Additionally, differences between the groups at study onset included more chronicity of illness in the control group and lower daily dosages of antipsychotic medications but no significant differences were noted for level of cognitive function. Cognitive outcomes were measured using a brief measure employed both pre and posttreatment for the treatment and control groups. The treatment group showed significant improvement in processing speed and executive functioning and increased activation in the right frontal area when scores were compared to the control group. NEAR was also implemented and assessed in a Japanese sample and significant improvements in cognitive function were observed (Ikezawa et al. 2012). Interesting, improvement was noted despite limitations in software access. These results are not surprising as past research demonstrated that using NEAR educational software alone, without an instructional component, did not results in significant changes in neuropsychological functioning (Dickinson et al. 2010).

In addition to NEAR, the effectiveness of integrated psychological therapy (IPT) has been meta-analytically reviewed in both inpatient and outpatient settings and results suggest it is related to improvements in cognitive functions including social cognition, psychosocial functioning, and negative symptoms when compared to placebo and usual care conditions (Roder et al. 2011). IPT is a manualized group-based treatment available in 13 different languages (Roder et al. 2010). The premise is that cognitive dysfunction affects social skills and social functioning. Thus, treatment aims to target cognitive functioning, communication, social skills, and problem-solving abilities within relationships. The review of IPT included 36 studies spanning 12 countries including North and South America, Asia, and Europe. Articles reviewed in this meta-analysis used a variety of control groups, differing numbers of modules, and various environments. They found that programs using all five modules of the intervention did not significantly differ from those who used one module or a combination of modules though they found therapy including all five modules resulted in more pronounced effects at follow-up approximately 8 months after the intervention. Importantly, they found that combining the cognitive module with social cognition and/or social perception modules led to larger effects on cognitive variables versus the cognitive module alone. They also found that the dropout rate for cognitive programs alone was higher than in interventions using more than one of the modules.

Other researchers have assessed for global structural and functional changes attributable to cognitive remediation using both diffusion tensor imaging (DTI) and functional magnetic resonance imaging (fMRI). Penadés et al. (2013) conducted a RCT using a treatment group, an active control group receiving a cognitive social skills intervention, and a healthy control group. The treatment group received an individualized and scaffolded cognitive remediation therapy based on a manualized intervention by Wykes and Reeder (2005) and completed tasks from a Spanish translation of an executive functioning program for schizophrenia (Delahunty and Morice 1993). The program entailed 40 1-hour sessions occurring two to three times per month for 4 months. The researchers highlighted three modules related to executive functions, such as set shifting, working memory, and planning. The active control group received an adapted social skills intervention (Liberman and Kopelowicz 1995), which was expected to assist in symptom control without having any effects on cognitive abilities. Results suggested improvement in the cognitive remediation treatment group for both the executive functioning network and the default network (or the functioning of the brain in an unfocused state) as well as greater white matter integrity in the anterior corpus callosum.

Another supported program is the Cognitive Remediation Program for Schizophrenia and other related disorders or RECOS (Vianin 2013), which incorporates modalities, such as problem-solving training (D'Zurilla and Nezu 2007) and verbal mediation (Franck et al. 2013). Cognitive training domains included selective attention, working memory, reasoning, memory, and visuospatial skills. This program combines computer-based training with paper and pencil activities. The intervention was administered individually to 16 diagnosed with schizophrenia. Increased activation of Broca's area, a cortical region associated with fluent expressive speech, was found using fMRI after cognitive remediation training using RECOS. This was thought to reflect remediation of the decrease in language lateralization that is typical of schizophrenia. The intervention was part of a 14-week randomized, single blind trial of cognitive remediation versus treatment as usual without cognitive training.

## Interventions for Outpatients with Schizophrenia

***Cognitive enhancement therapy***. Cognitive enhancement therapy was developed as an intervention to enhance neurocognitive and social thinking abilities designed for use with individuals with schizophrenia whose symptoms have been stabilized (Hogarty et al. 2004). It incorporates aspects of programs developed for those with TBI (Ben-Yishay et al. 1985), integrative cognitive strategies (Brenner et al. 1992) and human development theory (Brainerd and Reyna 1990). The program encourages movement away from concrete thought to more abstract reasoning through the use of in vivo social interactions. Participants engaged in 75 h of computer-based training relating to problem-solving, attention, and memory and engaged in over 50 group sessions focusing on social cognition. Individuals worked on computer programs in pairs and were instructed to support and encourage one another. Aspects of the cognitive training component were taken from Ben-Yishay et al. (1985). Remediation Module and the PSSCogReHab computer-based program (Bracy 1995) were used for memory and problem solving. Group activities involved solving real-life social dilemmas, abstraction of themes from newspaper editorials, and categorization exercises among others. Results of this 2-year RCT revealed significant effects between groups on all behavioral and cognitive domains except for residual symptoms.

***Neurocognitive Enhancement Therapy***. Neurocognitive enhancement therapy is another technique that has been employed as a cognitive remediation approach for individuals with schizophrenia (Bell et al. 2005). This therapy involves three specific parts: (1) feedback from the vocational cognitive rating scale (Greig et al. 2004), (2) approximately 5 hours per week of cognitive exercises for a duration of 26 weeks, and (3) participation in a weekly social processing group. Rewards were also used as patients were paid a small amount per hour for time spent doing cognitive exercises and they received a bonus payment for reaching the maximum five hours of cognitive training. The cognitive exercises were implemented on a computer and targeted the domains of attention, memory, and executive functioning. The computer program (PSSCogRehab; Bracy 1995) was tailored to meet the request of the researchers. The social processing group was based on Ben-Yishay et al. (1985) cognitive remediation program for TBI. Neurocognitive enhancement therapy was used as one component within a larger intervention that included work therapy (employment at a Veteran's Administration Medical Center) and a job coach. The primary focus of the intervention was to determine whether adding a cognitive remediation component to a work involvement program would improve functional outcomes in individuals with schizophrenia or schizoaffective disorder. Differences between the neurocognitive enhancement therapy group and the neurocognitive enhancement therapy group plus work training did not emerge until a 6 month follow-up was completed and were maintained at 1 year follow-up. Specifically, at the time of follow-up those in the cognitive remediation program combined with work therapy had significantly more employment hours than those in work therapy group alone.

***Mindfulness Interventions for Schizophrenia and Psychosis***. There has been recent interest in the use of mindfulness interventions with psychosis and schizophrenia. Mindfulness-based programs can be conceptualized as a type of cognitive remediation due to their intense focus on attentional exercises. Meta-analyses to date have found such interventions to be moderately effective in treating negative symptoms of schizophrenia and more research is warranted (Khoury et al. 2013). Mindfulness interventions generally focus on embracing present-moment experiences instead of using avoidance or suppression to cope with unwanted experiences. Qualities encouraged by mindful practice include nonjudgment, nonreactivity, detachment, acceptance, and compassion among others. Accordingly, interest has been placed on applying these principles to controlling psychotic symptoms (e.g. Chadwick et al. 1996). The goal in mindful approaches to psychotic disorders is to delineate the difference between the self and psychotic sensations that are transient experiences and not part of the self (Chadwick et al. 2005). In other words, the unpleasant sensations associated with psychosis are experienced but the individual refrains from reacting and experiencing additional distress.

In their meta-analysis of 13 studies that included both inpatient and outpatient sample, Khoury et al. (2013) found moderate effect sizes (Hedge's $g = 0.52$) for mindfulness interventions in pre-post analyses. However, the effect sizes were small to moderate when intervention groups were compared with control conditions (Hedge's $g = 0.41$). In studies in which follow-up data was available, the results were still significant for pre-post test designs (Hedge's $g = 0.62$), but were only approaching significance for controlled studies.

***Cognitive remediation as a preventative approach***. The success of cognitive remediation therapies for schizophrenia has led researchers to consider using this approach to prevent progression from prodromal features to first-episode psychosis or to attenuate subsequent cognitive decline in individuals who experience first-episode psychosis. Essentially, cognitive remediation is used as a maintenance strategy in either approach. The efficacy of this idea was demonstrated in a multicenter RCT of an integrated psychological intervention (cognitive-behavioral therapy, group skills training, cognitive remediation, and multifamily psychoeducation) versus supportive counseling (Bechdolf et al. 2012). While the focus of the integrated psychological intervention was to improve coping and provide participants with stress management techniques consistent with the stress-vulnerability paradigm of schizophrenia (Nuechterlein and Dawson 1984), cognitive remediation was a component of the intervention. The researchers found that the intervention significantly reduced conversion to psychosis at both 1 year and 2-year follow-up.

Another recent study suggests cognitive remediation may influence long-term course and outcomes in individuals with schizophrenia though an indirect effect on cognition (Trapp et al. 2013). Inpatients diagnosed with schizophrenia were assigned to either an experimental group that received cognitive remediation or control group that received occupational therapy. The cognitive remediation group participated in four 60-min sessions per week for 3 weeks of the computerized X-Cog® program. Promising long-term effects were found for cognitive remediation but the generalizability of this intervention may be hindered by the number of diverse treatments individuals in both groups were receiving concurrently with the study, such as antipsychotic medication, sports therapy, and music therapy. Still, the average time spent in periods of psychosis was significantly shorter for those in the cognitive remediation group ($M = 75$, $SD = 51$) versus the control group ($M = 140$, $SD = 124$) with a Cohen's $d$ effect size of 0.58. Cognitive remediation was associated with improved problem solving, memory, and attention. Overall, they found an indirect effect for cognitive remediation therapy influencing variables that affected days until relapse and time in psychosis. Specifically, memory at baseline and participation in cognitive remediation were significant predictors of post-intervention memory performance and cognitive training indirectly affected time spent in psychosis. Taken together, these findings suggest cognitive remediation training may have some influence on the long-term course of schizophrenia and that cognitive functions improved by training in addition to employment status predicted time to first relapse and time spent in psychosis.

## Patient and Clinician Factors Affecting Outcomes

Medalia and Richardson (2005) examined patient and therapist factors that mediate cognitive remediation outcomes in schizophrenia. For patient factors, they found motivation and the manner in which individuals approach work tasks to be significant predictors while age, education, socioeconomic status, gender, and ethnicity were not significantly related to outcome. Cognitive ability was deemed as possibly affecting outcome. Many illness variables analyzed were surprisingly not related to outcome. Symptom acuity, diagnosis, and symptom profile were unrelated to outcome while years spent hospitalized was possibly related to outcome. Treatment factors appeared to have the largest impact on outcome with clinician experience, intensity of the program, and type of training significantly affecting outcome measures. Information regarding the effects of type of medication on outcome was unclear.

More recent research, though limited by a small sample size, disputes these findings by suggesting that patient factors may have more measurable effects on cognitive remediation outcome in schizophrenia (Vita et al. 2013). Results of cognitive improvement in this sample were similar to the nearly 50 % improvement reported in other studies (Medalia and Richardson 2005). Vita et al. (2013) suggest cognitive remediation may be more effective in younger patients with schizophrenia, those who are less cognitively disorganized, and patients that are less cognitively impaired overall. Further, these results suggest it may be more effective in those who took lower doses of antipsychotic medications. It was unclear if this was due to the fact that lower dosing may reflect less severe psychopathology or those antipsychotic medications interfered with the effectiveness of cognitive remediation programs in a dose-response manner.

## Computer-Assisted Cognitive Remediation

Computer-assisted cognitive remediation therapy has been supported in the literature and improvements have been noted in neuropsychological performance, self-esteem, and quality of life. Recently, there has been an interest in discerning the active agents of change within these programs. Garrido et al. (2013) examined the effectiveness of a 48-session, 6-month, computer-assisted cognitive remediation program with a RCT in outpatients with schizophrenia and an active control group. Outcomes assessed included quality of life, self-esteem, verbal intelligence, attention, psychomotor speed, phonemic fluency, working memory, verbal learning, and executive functioning. The remediation therapy consisted of individualized 1-hour sessions. The program involved over 1500 computer exercises that were available to participants and were classified by domain and difficulty level so the program could be tailored to each participant's level of neuropsychological performance. The program encouraged errorless learning and a scaffolding approach was used where tasks were made less difficult if performance fell below an 85 % correct response rate. Participants assigned to the active control condition watched hour-long videos on a computer, answered multiple-choice questions, and wrote down feedback regarding the documentaries they viewed. Results indicated improvement in the remediation therapy group in the domains of processing speed, working memory, reasoning, problem solving, quality of life, and self-esteem when compared with the control group.

Lee (2013) also assessed a computerized cognitive remediation program for individuals with schizophrenia in an inpatient setting. Individuals were randomly assigned to the computerized intervention group where they received cognitive remediation in addition to their standard rehabilitation or a control group who received only standard rehabilitative care. The intervention group received training using Cog-trainer software (Lee et al. 2008), which was based on the Yongin cognitive-behavioral rehabilitation training (Y-CBRT; Lee et al. 2004) manual. This program targeted many of the same neuropsychological domains addressed by other interventions but also included tasks that transcended-specific domains and targeted cultural knowledge and language. Scaffolding was employed and an errorless learning environment was encouraged. The cognitive remediation group demonstrated significant improvement in attention and working memory in addition to evidence of improved job skills. There was no evidence of a positive effect on pathological symptoms.

Kurtz et al. (2007) sought to examine the active agents of change among computerized cognitive remediation interventions with a sample of outpatients diagnosed with either schizophrenia or schizoaffective disorder. These researchers improved upon other studies by utilizing multiple neuropsychological measures within each broad domain. Further, they exposed the control group to many of the same elements as the treatment group (e.g., same duration exposure to a computer, interaction with a clinician) to better deconstruct the critical elements of the intervention. The intervention was 12 months in duration with approximately 100 h total of training for each participant. Cognitive remediation involved computerized training across cognitive domains and, more specifically, drill and practice techniques described in PSSCogRehab Version 95 (e.g., Bell et al. 2001; Bracy 1995; Seltzer et al. 1997). The active control group was designed to create a similar overall environment while eliminating the domain-specific cognitive training aspects of the intervention. The control group received equivalent interaction with a clinician as was available in the treatment group. The active control group received a computer skills-based course for 12 months with a target goal of 100 h of intervention. The skills course involved tutorials on the use of Microsoft Office and individuals received training in word processing, internet usage, and spreadsheet management skills. Overall, analyses indicated that exposure to computers, interactions with clinicians and non-specific forms of cognitive challenge experiences led to nonspecific improvements on neuropsychological measures. However, those in the cognitive remediation group experienced incremental benefits for more specific aspects of neuropsychological functioning. The authors argued that the nonspecific cognitive changes are not likely explained by practice effects, familiarity with tasks, or long-term pharmacological management as past research has suggested neuropsychological functioning in adults with schizophrenia is relatively stable without intervention (e.g., Censits et al. 1997).

Improved neuropsychological functioning is the global target of cognitive remediation interventions. However, screenings for symptomology are included in many programs and small changes in symptom severity have been noted following cognitive remediation (Wykes et al. 2011). Cella et al. (2014) argued that past research has neglected an important area in the assessment of symptom changes as a result of cognitive intervention. Specifically, they argued for assessing symptomology beyond the traditional positive and negative symptoms and instead propose adding the assessment of mood, excitement, and disorganization. They had outpatients with schizophrenia engage in 40 session of individual therapy that targeted neuropsychological domains. The sessions were held 3 times per week and based on a flexible application of Wykes and Reeder (2005) manualized intervention. Compared to a treatment as usual group, those in the intervention group showed a significant reduction in disorganized symptoms as well as a reduction in negative symptoms associated with schizophrenia.

## Comparison of Treatment Delivery Approaches in Schizophrenia

***Cognitive remediation versus Integrated Psychological Therapy***. Two approaches to cognitive remediation dominate the literature: computer-assisted cognitive remediation and IPT. Computer-assisted programs have been discussed in-detail thus far. However, reviews addressing IPT (Brenner et al. 1994) have found positive effects on symptom severity, psychosocial functioning, and neurocognitive performance over treatment as usual groups (Roder et al. 2006). IPT is a group-based program for individuals with schizophrenia and includes the following components: Cognitive differentiation (attention and conceptual processes are targeted), social perception (stimulus discrimination and interpretation/assessment of social interactions), verbal communication (basic conversation skills and semantic processes), Social Skills (interpersonal skills, and self-instructions), and interpersonal problem solving (overcoming obstacles to meet social goals). Vita et al. (2011) sought to compare the efficacy of computer-assisted programs versus IPT versus a noncognitive control psychosocial intervention program in a prospective study. The study included these interventions within the normal standard of care of inpatient psychiatric rehabilitation. Those in the cognitive remediation condition used Cogpack (Marker Software) computerized neurocognitive training.

***Individualized Neurocognitive Training versus Social Skills Individualized Training***. A comparison study of outpatients with schizophrenia randomly assigned individuals to either a cognitive remediation individualized training group or a social skills individualized training group (Bucci et al. 2013). Outcome measures included symptomology, cognitive functioning, and quality of life. Neurocognitive individualized training involved a computerized training program, RehaCom, (HASOMED GmbH) which allowed the leaders of the training to alter the level of difficulty for each module. The attention and concentration module required individuals to compare several pictures to find an exact match. The verbal memory module involved the presentation of a short story followed by multiple-choice questions asking the individual to recall specific content. Another module, memory for faces, presented unfamiliar faces, and individuals were later asked to remember them; individuals were required to recall these faces as well as related jobs, names, and telephone numbers at a more difficult level of the module. The logical thinking module required individuals to identify a rule from a series of pictures and select the next relevant picture from a matrix. In the shopping module, the individual performed as if he or she were carrying out the steps involved in planning, shopping, and paying for groceries. The day planning module involved viewing a list of appointments and a map with nine buildings and individuals must choose the shortest routes, make efficient choices, and complete the appointments in a limited amount of time (Galderisi et al. 2010). The computer program offered immediate feedback on performance after each task and at the end of each training session. The participants received corrective feedback or praise on their skills training process and each individual attended two individual 1-hour sessions per week for 6 months to remediate any necessary skills. The social skills individualized training was developed to target social and emotional skills by increasing perception and understanding of emotions while encouraging appropriate emotional expression. Training was conducted within a group setting and role-play enabled participants to assist one another by providing corrective feedback. Tasks involved included recognizing unpleasant emotions, expressing these emotions, apologizing for inappropriate behaviors, sharing fears, sustaining conversations, and actively listening to others. To practice social skills outside of sessions, individuals were given homework assignments and a tracking log.

The researcher found that cognitive remediation training led to significant improvements in attention, verbal memory, and a decrease in perseveration errors on executive functioning measures up to 6 months after the intervention. Importantly, they found that the social skills training program did not improve cognitive functioning and, in some cases, a decline actually occurred. Finally, they found the two programs affected quality of life differently such that cognitive training was related to an improvement in interpersonal relationships while social skills training was related to improvements on a measure of occupational role functioning. Results of this study suggest cognitive remediation is more effective than social skills training on several cognitive domains and on measures of real-world social functioning. The authors indicate that the cognitive remediation program inherently involved many social skills training aspects and they suggested a balance between the two programs so that the synergistic aspects are maintained.

## Cognitive Remediation Therapy in Anorexia Nervosa

Outside of schizophrenia, the effectiveness of cognitive remediation has been most studied in eating disorders, such as anorexia nervosa. Anorexia nervosa has been characterized by three essential features: persistent energy intake restriction; intense fear of gaining weight or persistent behavior that interferes with weight gain; and a disturbance in self-perceived weight or shape (American Psychiatric Association 2013). To meet the DSM-5 criteria for anorexia nervosa, an individual must meet criteria for maintaining a body weight that is below a minimally normal level for age, sex, developmental trajectory, and physical health (American Psychiatric Association 2013). In addition, the intense fear experienced by the individuals meeting diagnostic criteria is not typically alleviated by weight loss, but rather worsens even as they lose weight. A lack of insight or denial that there is a problem is also common to this diagnosis suggesting metacognitive impairment.

The use of cognitive remediation therapies has recently been investigated to target what are believed to be important maintaining factors of anorexia nervosa: cognitive inflexibility and extreme attention to detail. These traits are thought to interfere with daily functioning as well as engagement in psychotherapy (Tchanturia et al. 2013) and are thus a leading target for intervention. The intervention is applied to those with anorexia nervosa by promoting a more flexible cognitive style by teaching individuals to prioritize information and employ estimation strategies to combat perfectionist tendencies. Metacognition is encouraged through engagement in nonthreatening behavioral tasks, such as changing one's hairstyle or clothing style) before targeting symptoms and rules related to the illness. Tchanturia et al. (2013) reviewed the current research in the field and found medium to large effect sizes in cognitive flexibility and tasks aimed to decrease attention to detail. Overall, they found low dropout rates (around 10–15 %) and concluded that this approach is highly tolerable for patients and therapists (Easter and Tchanturia 2011).

An initial investigation and pilot study for the effectiveness of cognitive remediation therapy for anorexia nervosa included four adult inpatients whose duration of illness ranged from 7 to 24 years (Tchanturia et al. 2007). This pilot study revealed improvements in set-shifting with medium to large effect sizes. These encouraging findings led to further investigation into the use of this therapy with individuals with anorexia nervosa.

Tchanturia et al. (2008) studied 23 consecutively referred inpatients engaged in a bi-weekly individual cognitive remediation program that included 10 total sessions. Importantly, the same cognitive measures were administered at baseline and after the intervention and results should be interpreted with caution due to the possibility of practice effects. Improvements were noted in cognitive performance and, more specifically, improvements included a reduction in time and errors on cognitive-set shifting measures and improvements in style and organization in a figure-copy task.

Genders and Tchanturia (2010) also conducted a brief, four session pilot study to assess the effectiveness of cognitive remediation therapy on self-reported cognitive flexibility, self-esteem, and motivation to change in a group of inpatients with anorexia nervosa. Beyond a focus of translating skills to daily life, sessions included elements of psychoeducation, practical exercises, reflection, and planning of homework assignments. The first session involved psychoeducation regarding cognitive remediation therapy, cognitive styles, and cognitive processing in the brain. An exercise in more broad levels of thinking was used. The focus of the second session was on increasing cognitive flexibility using visual illusions posters that were available online. Card games and discussions were used to again target cognitive switching during the third session. The final session consisted of a review of the main content and an emphasis was placed on reviewing the benefits of flexible thinking through different activities. The brief pilot program concluded with a discussion of motivational quotes that were intended to promote future behavioral change practice and to highlight the positives of flexible cognitive styles. Patients in this group provided feedback regarding the program and many mentioned the benefits of talking and sharing experiences. Others found the hands-on practical tasks used to encourage flexible thinking as helpful. A small number of participants endorsed the homework as helpful. Despite the promising evidence to support the use of cognitive remediation therapy on cognitive outcomes, there is currently no evidence that these intervention techniques lead to improved overall treatment outcomes. Future research should investigate effects of treatment beyond the cognitive measures and should include symptom reduction as a measure.

## Cognitive Rehabilitation Therapy in Traumatic Brain Injury and Stroke

It has been estimated that up to 10 % of individuals who have suffered a TBI also experience symptoms of psychosis (Batty et al. 2013). This results in a large number of individuals with a history of TBI requiring psychiatric services. Individuals with neuropsychiatric symptoms related to the TBI share many of the same symptoms of behavioral and cognitive dysfunction seen in other psychotic disorders. For instance, behavioral changes can include reduced behavioral control, disinhibition, and a motivation. Cognitive deficits are also seen and are prominent in domains of language, memory, processing speed, attention, and executive functioning (Batty et al. 2013). Additionally, individuals with a dual diagnosis of TBI and a psychiatric disorder have significant impairments in occupational and social functioning, creating increasing dependency on family members, caregivers, and social isolation (Molloy et al. 2011). There is evidence to suggest that general cognitive rehabilitation has been very beneficial for psychosis following TBI and stroke, with implications for specific cognitive remediation documented (Batty et al. 2013; Fujii and Ahmed 2014; Molloy et al. 2011).

For individuals who have suffered a TBI or cerebrovascular accident/stroke, treatment has typically been provided as cognitive rehabilitation, since behavioral therapy approaches that target cognitive deficits tend to be broad-based and generally designed to improve overall cognitive functioning (Pella et al. 2008). Cicerone et al. (2000, 2005, 2011) have conducted three systematic reviews on the effectiveness of evidence-based cognitive rehabilitation for individuals who have suffered a TBI and/or stroke. The first review was published in 2000 and covered 171 published research articles. Results from this early review revealed strong evidence for using treatment interventions for language and visuospatial perception after stroke (Cicerone et al. 2000). Cicerone et al. (2000) also indicated effectiveness of treatment intervention for attention, memory, functional communication, and executive functioning after TBI. Recommendations for future research included examining outcome measures tailored to the level of disability as well as the duration of intervention post injury.

A second evidence-based review was published in by Cicerone et al. (2005) and spanned the years from 1998 to 2002. The analysis compared 47 different treatment interventions from class I studies. Within this review, they found evidence supporting that TBI and stroke patients benefit from cognitive rehabilitation. They found continued evidence supporting the efficacy of visuospatial and language rehabilitation following strokes leading to aphasia and neglect syndromes and efficacy of memory, attention, and language rehabilitation for individuals with TBI. They found cognitive rehabilitation interventions useful for increasing specific behaviors rather than improving actual overall memory. Cicerone et al. (2005) stressed the need to replicate interventions that have been shown to be effective as well as to compare the techniques that have been shown to be effective. Furthermore, they recommend examination of treatment effect sizes in order to obtain greater clarity of treatment impact.

Shortly thereafter, a third review conducted by Cicerone et al. (2011) was published. This review examined the cognitive rehabilitation literature published from 2003 to 2008. Results of this review revealed significant evidence for the use of direct attention training and metacognitive training after TBI. Cicerone et al. (2011) stated that direct attention training will promote development and help individuals to strategize to real world tasks and activities. They further recommend comprehensive-holistic neuropsychological rehabilitation after moderate to severe TBI, visuospatial rehabilitation for stroke, cognitive-linguistic interventions for aphasia and gestural strategy training for apraxia.

In contrast to cognitive remediation, both occupational and speech-language therapies have been found to be effective rehabilitation techniques for individuals who have suffered from language and visuospatial skill deficits (Cicerone et al. 2000; MacDonald and Wiseman-Hakes 2010; Schoenberg et al. 2008; Wolf 2011). Occupational therapy interventions focus on adapting the environment, modifying the task, teaching the skill, and educating the client in order to increase participation in and performance of daily activities. Wolf (2011) reviewed articles published from 2009 to 2010 in the American Journal of Occupational Therapy to summarize and evaluate occupational therapy for practice in a neurological population. He indicated that the field of occupational therapy is still somewhat novel, with research focused on basic science and efficiency studies and therefore the effectiveness of the field has not fully been addressed. Despite this, Wolf was still able to find that treatments targeting problem-solving strategies, improvement of learning or memory, community reintegration, and improvement of self-care abilities to be effective for those suffering from a TBI. Wolf also found evidence for the effectiveness of treatments targeting upper-extremity dysfunction, motor impairment, self-care, and activities of daily living for individuals suffering from stroke.

Speech-language pathologists provide a wide range of services, mainly on an individual basis, but also as support for individuals, families, support groups, and providing information for the general public. Speech services begin with initial screening for communication and swallowing disorders and continue with assessment and diagnosis, consultation for the provision of advice regarding management, intervention and treatment, and provision counseling and additional follow-up services (MacDonald and Wiseman-Hakes 2010). Both occupational and speech-language therapies focus on tasks to promote overall activities of daily living. They both focus on tailoring treatments to the individual's level of need. Both occupational therapy and speech-language therapy have been found to be efficacious treatments for individuals who have suffered from stroke and TBI (MacDonald and Wiseman-Hakes 2010; Schoenberg et al. 2008). However, the researchers in support for these treatments have also expressed concerns regarding the lack of RCTs and large sample sizes necessary to generalize these findings (Smith et al. 2003; Wolf 2011). Despite the novelty of these two fields and their research findings, it is important to recognize that these two fields are in existence to treat deficits in speech and language or visuospatial skills.

Cicerone et al. (2000, 2005, 2011) consistently found support for cognitive rehabilitation for stroke patients in the areas of speech and language and visuospatial skills. Results for other injuries across the different cognitive domains remain more inconclusive and it appears there may be other factors moderating the treatment effect. Based on these main findings and the current status of this area of research, there are several recommendations for future research to consider including leveling out the high percentage of single-subject designs and to develop more homogeneous control conditions. These are two of the largest voids within the literature examining cognitive rehabilitation. Furthermore, the literature is varied in terms of defining a control group with some outpatient studies utilized true notreatment groups and others utilized placebo comparison groups or inpatient comparison groups that were administered standard treatments. Other problematic findings of the cognitive rehabilitation literature include the confounding variables of treatments by etiology, age, and recovery level, making a goal of future research to be to employ methodology that may control for such confounds (Pella et al. 2008). Summing up the current literature, cognitive rehabilitation appears to work best with stroke patients who have circumscribed deficits in speech and language or visuospatial skills. Clinicians can best improve client outcomes by working in collaborative multidisciplinary teams with neuropsychologists, occupational therapists and speech pathologists to provide specific cognitive remediation for these inpatients.

## The Effects of Medications and Treatment on Cognitive Functioning

It is important to consider the potential effects of medications and treatments frequently used within inpatient settings on memory and other cognitive processes. Although no studies examining the effects of these medications in the context of cognitive remediation are currently available, literature indicated certain classes of medications can negatively affect cognitive processes, thus individuals taking these medications may not achieve the same benefit from cognitive remediation groups. Further, some treatments that are used with severe, chronic mental illness may be encountered in an inpatient setting and these may have negative effects on cognition.

### Benzodiazepines

Benzodiazepines are known to have acute effects across domains and may produce drowsiness, lead to psychomotor slowing and anterograde amnesia, and lead to difficulties learning new information (Barbee 1993; Buffett-Jerrott et al. 1998). It has been hypothesized that these difficulties learning new information are related to the sedative properties of the medication that affect memory indirectly through an effect on memory (Barbee 1993). The effects of benzodiazepines on individuals who have taken the medication on a long-term basis have historically been contested with some researchers reporting no long-term effects and others reporting significant changes; however, a recent meta-analytic review revealed changes associated with long-term use. Specifically, the results of the meta-analysis noted impairment in visuospatial and visuomotor abilities have been reported and impairments in visuospatial abilities are believed to be the most frequently reported cognitive effect associated with long-term use (Barker et al. 2004; Golombok et al. 1998; Tata et al. 1994).

Further, reports of decreased IQ, psychomotor speed, processing speed, motor abilities, verbal learning, response time, and concentration have been reported in the literature (Barker et al. 2004; Buffett-Jerrott et al. 1998; Golombok et al. 1998, Gorenstein et al. 1995). Importantly, cognitive changes are likely to be more pronounced in certain groups of patients. For instance, the risk of cognitive change is higher for males, individuals who require higher doses, older adults, and those who take medications with anticholinergic effects (Barker et al. 2004; Barbee 1993). The results of this meta-analysis challenge past research that claimed long-term benzodiazepine use to be association with cognitive changes. Luki et al. (1986) asserted that long-term use did not differentially affect psychomotor function, motor speed, sustained attention, or verbal memory in patients who took benzodiazepines long-term versus those who did not. While controversy remains, withdrawal of benzodiazepines has led to recovery in many cognitive domains but impairment exists when compared to controls suggesting long-term effects providing further support for the notion that long-term changes may result from prolonged medication use (Barker et al. 2004).

Others have suggested that benzodiazepine use may specifically affect individuals' abilities to recall psychoeducational information presented during group therapy sessions (Westra et al. 2004). Specifically, in the context of group therapy for individuals with panic disorder, those who used benzodiazepines performed more poorly than controls on an immediate recall task of psychoeducational information that was presented via videotape. More important clinically may be the finding that while non-medication individuals recalled roughly three-fourths of the information presented, those using benzodiazepines recalled, on average, only half of the presented information.

Recent research has begun to assess the effects of benzodiazepines on cognition in healthy older adults in a double-blind, placebo-controlled, randomized cross-over study (Pietrzak et al. 2012). The researchers examined acute effects of a single 1 mg dose of alprazolam in seventeen healthy older adults. They examined the effects on two specific domains: visual paired associate learning, and memory. Visual paired associate learning involved pairing visual stimuli so that later exposure to one of the stimuli will support recall of the other (Stark and Squire 2001). Overall, they found decrease in visual paired associate learning and memory. They suggested this may be related to an interruption in the process of memory consolidation.

## Anticholinergics

An individual working in an inpatient psychiatric facility is likely to encounter individuals taking anticholinergic medication as this class of medications were the first to be used in the treatment of Parkinson's disease symptoms and their use for this purpose has continue (Katzenschlager et al. 2002). Further, extrapyramidal symptoms are often treated with this class of medications (Pringsheim et al. 2011). Further, many medications are known to have anticholinergic side effects; antipsychotics, antidepressants, and over-the-counter medications such as antihistamines are some of the medications known to elicit these side effects (Mintzer and Burns 2000).

In a systematic review of the literature Katzenschlager et al. (2002) found, in six of eight reviewed studies with the necessary information, evidence of adverse neuropsychiatric or cognitive effects. The most frequently reported adverse effect was confusion. One study involved objective assessment of cognitive functioning and a 10 % decrease in performance on an immediate memory recall measure was observed. Others have investigated the impact of anticholinergic medications on responsiveness to cognitive training in individuals with schizophrenia and have found a relationship between serum levels and cognitive performance (Vinogradov et al. 2009). Participants were 55 clinically stable adults with schizophrenia whose baseline cognitive abilities and serum anticholinergic activity levels were assessed. They were randomly assigned to either a computerized auditory training condition or a control condition in which they engaged in computer games for one hour per day, 5 days per week for approximately 10 weeks. No changes in dose of medication greater than 10 % occurred during the course of the investigation but medication use varied widely by participant. At baseline, higher serum anticholinergic activity levels were related to lower scores on measures of auditory working memory and auditory learning and memory. Statistically, significant improvements in global cognition and auditory learning and memory were observed when the computerized cognitive training group was compared to the computer-based controls. However, those with higher levels of serum anticholinergic activity showed lower levels of response to the computerized cognitive training program.

Fortin et al. (2011) retrospectively examined the effects of multiple medications believed to have anticholinergic properties in older adults; the most frequently prescribed medication in their sample were as follows: furosemide, hydrochlorothiazide, digoxin (cardiovascular), paroxtine, sertraline, fluoxetine (antidepressant), and oxybutynin chloride (antispasmodic). Overall, they found using medications with anticholinergic properties had a significant negative effect on verbal episodic memory though other cognitive functions measured remained intact.

## Antipsychotics

The effects of benzodiazepines on cognition have been well addressed in the literature but the available literature on the effects of antipsychotics on these cognitive domains is significantly less well developed. A meta-analysis of randomized controlled trials found that antipsychotic medications generally led to enhanced cognitive function; they found the most positive effects for Quetiapine and olanzapine, followed by risperidone, ziprasidone, amisulpride, and haloperidol respectively (Désaméricq et al. 2014). One controlled study that examined the relationship between antipsychotics and cognitive changes found significant associations only in the domain of verbal fluency; verbal memory abilities in individuals with schizophrenia are believed to be one of the most impaired cognitive domains (Tuulio-Henriksson et al. 2011) and antipsychotics were found to have a deleterious effect (Albus et al. 2006).

Imaging studies have led to the contention that an association exists between higher doses of antipsychotic medications and greater reduction in brain volume in individuals during their first episode of schizophrenia (Andreasen et al. 2013). This reduction in brain volume has been associated with decreased cognitive functioning in individuals with schizophrenia (Gur et al. 1998). A recent observational 9-year study elucidated the effects on learning and memory (Husa et al. 2014) and specifically addressed the effects of dose and the domain of verbal memory. They examined changes in this domain over nine-years in a cohort of 40 individuals with schizophrenia (or a schizophrenia spectrum disorder) and 73 controls with no history of psychosis. Verbal learning and memory was assessed at both time points using the California Verbal Learning Test

(CVLT; Delis et al. 1987). Record reviews provided information on lifetime antipsychotic medication use and all antipsychotic medications were converted to a common metric of dose-years of 100 mg of chlorpromazine per day (see Kroken et al. 2009, for more information on conversion procedures). They found higher dose-years were associated with a decline in some facets of learning and memory at the time of 9-year follow-up when individuals were in mid-life. Interestingly, they found that higher dose-years before the baseline testing were especially association with decline and poorer baseline functioning. They found no significant differences in decline between low-dose cases and those in the control group. The researchers were unable to differentiate differences in effects based on typical versus atypical antipsychotic status because many individuals had used a variety of antipsychotics during their lives. Still, they found that both typical and atypical agents had significant effects on cognitive functioning. As such, these medications present a potential confound for studies examining cognitive remediation in groups with psychotic symptoms and may hamper potentially positive benefits of cognitive remediation when used therapeutically.

## Electroconvulsive Therapy

Estimates indicate approximately 100,000 individuals in the United States receive electroconvulsive therapy (ECT) every year to treat persistent and severe psychiatric conditions such as treatment resistant major depressive episodes (Abrams 2002). Semkovska and McLoughlin (2010) asserted that literature on electroconvulsive therapy lacked specificity in terms of memory impairments following the procedure. They aimed to address this lack of specificity in their review of 24 cognitive variables from 84 studies of electroconvulsive therapy. The meta-analysis addressed the following cognitive domains: cognitive status screening, processing speed, attention/working memory, verbal episodic memory, visual episodic memory, spatial problem solving, executive functioning, and intellectual ability. No standardized measures of retrograde amnesia were available for analysis but more recent research suggests that electroconvulsive therapy is not related to significant lasting retrograde amnesia (Meeter et al. 2011).

The review found evidence that ECT is associated with significant cognitive impairment in the first 2 weeks following the procedure; they described the first 3 days post-treatment as the time of the most severe impairment. When compared to individuals' baseline performance, deficits generally resolved within 2 weeks and most cognitive functions improved in subsequent weeks. When individual domains are analyzed, the meta-analysis provides more specific information regarding changes in cognitive functioning. Medium to large deficits in episodic memory and executive functioning were noted up to 3 days after the procedure. Executive functioning measures showed medium to large levels of impairment and were the most consistently affected domain in this acute period following the procedure. In addition, delayed recall abilities were affected to a greater extent than immediate recall and verbal episodic memory was more impaired that visual episodic memory. Unstructured information that was presented verbally showed greater impairment than when information was already organized in the form of a story and this form of immediate recall appeared to be spared by the latent effects of electroconvulsive therapy. In the acute 3 day period, attention and working memory abilities appeared to have been spared while processing speed, spatial problem solving abilities, and global cognition showed only small deficits. While most domains of cognitive functioning improved, verbal paired associates delayed recall remained below baseline levels during the short-term follow-up period which extended to 15 days in most studies; however, it is important to note that all but one study analyzing this variable involved sine-wave electroconvulsive therapy which may not generalize to contemporary brief-impulse electroconvulsive therapy. Based on these findings, cognitive remediation within a month of ECT is not recommended as the individual is still in a possible recovery phase for cognitive functioning.

## Conclusion

Overall, cognitive remediation appears to have some positive benefit for ameliorating cognitive deficits associated with schizophrenia and anorexia nervosa. There is significant evidence that it leads to improvements in cognitive functioning in TBI and stroke and has a beneficial effect on psychotic aspects of brain injury sequelae. Based on these results, we believe it also has possible therapeutic utility in other conditions where psychotic symptoms are present. While the literature in this field is improving, there is still a need for high-quality studies demonstrating treatment efficacy for cognitive remediation in specific clinical populations.

Much of the recent research that has supported cognitive remediation as an effective intervention has been done using proprietary computerized programs and this introduces the possibility of researchers having a financial stake in demonstrating the effectiveness of the program. While this possibility does not invalidate the obtained results, it would be helpful for the clinical community to see these results validated by researchers with no potentially vested interest in the product being evaluated.

Overall, the field of cognitive remediation is being hindered by heterogeneous patient groups, particularly in TBI samples, making it difficult to state any conclusions broadly. The field also has a large number of one-time treatment studies, an overreliance on small sample sizes and single-subject designs, and very few replications (Proto et al. 2009). Furthermore, cognitive remediation research is often criticized for its lack of effect size calculations as this hampers the ability to know to what degree findings are meaningful. Lastly, the field of cognitive rehabilitation rarely uses performance validity tests measuring suboptimal effort. Due to these limitations, much of the existing scientific record contains weak and conflicting evidence that makes a definitive judgment regarding the effectiveness of candidate treatments difficult. What is truly needed are dismantling studies where researchers systematically evaluate a large number of components from cognitive remediation approaches and determine which are necessary for positive treatment outcomes. We believe that cognitive remediation approaches have significant potential to help patients with severe mental illness improve cognitive functioning, return to work, and have fuller and happier lives. However, this potential has to be standardized, empirically demonstrated, and tailored for efficient service delivery before cognitive remediation can be fully implemented in mental health care settings.

## References

Abrams, R. (2002). *Electroconvulsive therapy* (4th ed.). New York: Oxford University Press.

Albus, M., Hubmann,W., Mohr, F., Hecht, S., Hinterberger-Weber, P., Seitz, N., et al. (2006). Neurocognitive functioning in patients with first-episode schizophrenia: Results of a prospective 5-year follow-up study. *European Archives of Psychiatry and Clinical Neuroscience, 256*, 442–451.

American Psychiatric Association. (2013). *Diagnostic and statistical manual of mental disorders* (5th ed.). Arlington, VA: American Psychiatric Publishing.

Andreasen, N. C., Arndt, S., Swayze, V., Cizadlo, T., Flaum, M., O'Leary, D., et al. (1994). Thalamic abnormalities in schizophrenia visualized through magnetic resonance image averaging. *Science, 266*, 294–298.

Andreasen, N. C., Liu, D., Ziebell, S., Vora, A., & Ho, B. C. (2013). Relapse duration, treatment intensity, and brain tissue loss in schizophrenia: A prospective longitudinal MRI study. *American Journal of Psychiatry, 170*, 609–615.

APA/CAAP Task Force on Serious Mental Illness and Severe Emotional Disturbance. (2007). *Catalog of clinical training opportunities: Best practices for recovery and improved outcomes for people with serious mental illness*. http://www.apa.org/practice/resources/grid/catalog.pdf

Barbee, J. G. (1993). Memory, benzodiazepines, and anxiety: Integration of theoretical and clinical perspectives. *Journal of Clinical Psychiatry, 54*(Suppl.), 86–97.

Barker, M. J., Greenwood, K. M., Jackson, M., & Crowe, S. F. (2004). Persistence of cognitive effects after withdrawal from long-term benzodiazepine use: A meta-analysis. *Archives of Clinical Neuropsychology, 19*(3), 437–454.

Batty, R. A., Rossell, S. L., Francis, A. J. P., & Ponsford, J. (2013). Psychosis following traumatic brain injury. *Brain Impairment, 14*(1), 21–41.

Bechdolf, A., Wagner, M., Ruhrmann, S., Harrigan, S., Putzfeld, V., Pukrop, R., et al. (2012). Preventing progression to first-episode psychosis in early initial prodromal states. *The British Journal of Psychiatry: The Journal of Mental Science, 200*(1), 22–29.

Beglinger, L. J., Gaydos, B., Tangphao-Daniels, O., Duff, K., Kareken, D. A., Crawford, J., et al. (2005). Practice effects and the use of alternate forms in serial neuropsychological testing. *Archives of Clinical Neuropsychology, 20*, 517–529.

Bell, M., Bryson, G., Greig, T., Corcoran, C., & Wexler, B. E. (2001). Neurocognitive enhancement therapy with work therapy: Effects on neurocognitive test performance. *Archives of General Psychiatry, 58*(8), 763–768.

Bell, M., Bryson, G., Greig, T., Fiszdon, J., & Wexler, B. (2005). Neurocognitive enhancement therapy with work therapy: Productivity outcomes at 6- and 12-month follow-ups. *Journal of Rehabilitation Research and Development, 42*(6), 829–838.

Benedict, R., & Zgaljardic, D. (1998). Practice effects during repeated administrations of memory tests with and without alternate forms. *Journal of Clinical and Experimental Neuropsychology, 20*, 339–352.

Ben-Yishay, Y., Piasetsky, E. B., & Rattok, J. (1985). A systematic method for ameliorating disorders in basic attention. In M. J. Meir, A. L. Benton, & L. Diller (Eds.), *Neuropsychological rehabilitation* (pp. 165–181). New York: Guilford Press.

Bracy, O. (1995). *PSS CogRehab version 95*. Indianapolis, IN: Psychological Software Services Inc.

Brainerd, C. J., & Reyna, V. F. (1990). Gist is the grist: Fuzzy trace theory and the new intuitionism. *Developmental Review, 10*, 3–47.

Brenner, H. D., Hodel, B., Roder, V., & Corrigan, P. (1992). Treatment of cognitive dysfunctions and behavior deficits in schizophrenia. *Schizophrenia Bulletin, 18*, 21–26.

Brenner, H., Roder, V., Hodel, B., Kienzie, N., Reed, D., & Liberman, R. (1994). *Integrated psychological therapy for schizophrenic patients*. Seattle, Washington: Hogrefe & Huber.

Brisch, R., Saniotis, A., Wolf, R., Bielau, H., Bernstein, H., Steiner, J., et al. (2014). The role of dopamine in schizophrenia from a neurobiological and evolutionary perspective: Old fashioned, but still in vogue. *Frontiers in Psychiatry, 5*, 1–11.

Brown, E. S., Frol, A. B., Khan, D. A., Larkin, G. L., & Bret, M. E. (2007). Impact of levetiracetam on mood and cognition during prednisone therapy. *European Psychiatry, 22*, 448–452.

Bruel-Jungerman, E., Davis, S., & Laroche, S. (2007). Brain plasticity mechanisms and memory: A party of four. *Neuroscientist, 13*, 492–505.

Bucci, P., Piegari, G., Mucci, A., Merlotti, E., Chieffi, M., De Riso, F., et al. (2013). Neurocognitive individualized training versus social skills individualized training: A randomized trial in patients with schizophrenia. *Schizophrenia Research, 150*, 69–75.

Buffett-Jerrott, S. E., Stewart, S. H., Bird, S., & Teehan, M. D. (1998). An examination of differences in the time course of oxazepam's effects on implicit vs explicit memory. *Journal of Psychopharmacology, 12* (4), 338–347.

Calamia, M., Markon, K., & Tranel, D. (2012). Scoring higher the second time around: Meta-analyses of practice effects in neuropsychological assessment. *The Clinical Neuropsychologist, 26*(4), 543–570.

Cappa, S. F., Benke, T., Clarke, S., Rossi, B., Stemmer, B., & van Heugten, C. (2005). EFNS guidelines on cognitive rehabilitation: Report of an EFNS taskforce. *European Journal of Neurology, 12*, 665–680.

Carlsson, M., & Carlsson, A. (1990). Interactions between glutamatergic and monoaminergic systems within the basal ganglia: Implications for schizophrenia and Parkinson's disease. *Trends in Neurosciences, 13*(7), 272–276.

Carlsson, A., & Lindquist, L. (1963). Effect of chlorpromazine or haloperidol on formation of 3-methoxytyramine and normetanephrine in mouse brain. *Acta Pharmacologica et Toxicologica, 20*, 140–145.

Cella, M., Reeder, C., & Wykes, T. (2014). It is all in the factors: Effects of cognitive remediation on symptom dimensions. *Schizophrenia Research, 156*, 60–62.

Censits, D. M., Ragland, J. D., Gur, R. C., & Gur, E. (1997). Neuropsychological evidence supporting a neurodevelopmental model of schizophrenia: A longitudinal study. *Schizophrenia Research, 24*, 289–298.

Chadwick, P. D. J., Birchwood, M. J., & Trower, P. (1996). *Cognitive therapy for delusions, voices and paranoia*. Chichester, UK: Wiley.

Chadwick, P., Taylor, K. N., & Abba, N. (2005). Mindfulness groups for people with psychosis. *Behavioral and Cognitive Psychotherapy, 33*(3), 351–359.

Cicerone, K. D., Dahlberg, C., Kalmar, K., Langenbahn, D. M., Malec, J. F., Bergquist, T. F., et al. (2000). Evidence-based cognitive rehabilitation: Recommendations for clinical practice. *Archives of Physical Medicine and Rehabilitation, 81*, 1596–1615.

Cicerone, K. D., Dahlberg, C., Malec, J. F., Langenbahn, D. M., Felicetti, T., Kneipp, S., et al. (2005). Evidence-based cognitive rehabilitation: Updated review of the literature from 1998 through 2002. *Archives of Physical Medicine and Rehabilitation, 86*, 1681–1692.

Cicerone, K. D., Langenbahn, D. M., Braden, C., Malec, J., Kalmar, K., Fraas, M., et al. (2011). Evidence-based cognitive rehabilitation: Updated review of the literature from 2003 through 2008. *Archives of Physical Medicine and Rehabilitation, 92*, 519–530.

D'Zurilla, T. J., & Nezu, A. M. (2007). *Problem solving therapy: A positive approach to clinical intervention* (3rd ed.). New York, NY: Springer.

Delahunty, A., & Morice, R. (1993). *The frontal executive program, a neurocognitive rehabilitation program for schizophrenia* (2nd ed.). Albury, Australia: Department of Health.

Delis, D. C., Kramer, J. H., Kaplan, E., & Ober, B. A. (1987). *California verbal learning test*. New York: Psychological Corporation.

DeLong, M. R. (1990). Primate models of movement disorders of basal ganglia origin. *Trends in Neuroscience, 13*(7), 281–285.

Désaméricq, G., Schurhoff, F., Meary, A., Szoke, A., Macquin-Mavier, I., Bachoud-Levi, A. C., et al. (2014). Long-term neurocognitive effects of antipsychotics in schizophrenia: A network meta-analysis. *European Journal of Clinical Pharmacology, 70*(2), 127–134.

Dickinson, D., Tenhula, W., Morris, S., Brown, C., Peer, J., Spencer, K., et al. (2010). A randomized, controlled trial of computer-assisted cognitive remediation for schizophrenia. *American Journal of Psychiatry, 167*, 170–180.

Eack, S. M. (2012). Cognitive remediation: A new generation of psychosocial interventions for people with schizophrenia. *Social Work, 57*(3), 235–246.

Easter, A., & Tchanturia, K. (2011). Therapists' experiences of cognitive remediation therapy for anorexia nervosa: Implications for working with adolescents. *Clinical Child Psychology and Psychiatry, 16*, 233–246.

Fastenau, P. S., Hankins, W. T., McGinnis, C. M., Moy, T., & Richard, M. (2002). Effects of alternate forms on retest effects in clinical testing. *Journal of International Neuropsychological Society, 7*(2), 151.

Fortin, M., Rouch, I., Dauphinot, V., Gédéon, C., Genthon, S., Bonnefoy, M., et al. (2011). Effects of anticholinergic drugs on verbal episodic memory function in the elderly. *Drugs and Aging, 28*(3), 195–204.

Franck, N., Duboc, C., Sundby, C., Amado, I., Wykes, T., Demily, C., & Members of the Cognitive Remediation Network. (2013). Specific vs. general cognitive remediation for executive functioning in schizophrenia: A multicenter randomized trial. *Schizophrenia Research, 47*, 68–74.

Fujii, D. E., & Ahmed, I. (2014). Psychotic disorder caused by traumatic brain injury. *Psychiatric Clinics of North America, 37*, 113–124.

Galderisi, S., Piegari, G., Mucci, A., Acerra, A., Luciano, L., Rabasca, A. F., et al. (2010). Social skills and neurocognitive individualized training in schizophrenia: Comparison with structured leisure activities. *European Archives of Psychiatry and Clinical Neuroscience, 260*, 305–315.

Garrido, G., Barrios, M., Penadés, R., Enríquez, G. M., Aragay, N., & Vendrell, J. (2013). Computer-assisted cognitive remediation therapy: Cognition, self-esteem and quality of life in schizophrenia. *Schizophrenia Research, 150*, 563–569.

Genders, R., & Tchanturia, K. (2010). Cognitive remediation therapy for anorexia in group format: A pilot study. *Eating and Weight Disorders, 15*, 234–239.

Goldberg, T. E., Goldman, R. S., Burdick, K. E., Malhotra, A. K., Lencz, T., Patel, R. C., et al. (2007). Cognitive improvement after treatment with second-generation antipsychotic medications in first-episode schizophrenia: Is it a practice effect? *Archives of General Psychiatry, 64*, 1115–1122.

Golombok, S., Moodley, P., & Lader, M. (1988). Cognitive impairment in long-term benzodiazepine users. *Psychological Medicine, 18*, 365–374.

Gorenstein, C., Bernik, M. A., Pompéia, S., & Marcourakis, T. (1995). Impairment of performance associated with long-term use of benzodiazepines. *Journal of Pharmacology, 9*(4), 313–318.

Greig, T. C., Bryson, G. J., & Bell, M. D. (2004). Development of a scale for the assessment of cognitive impairments in vocational rehabilitation: Reliability and predictive validity. *Journal of Vocational Rehabilitation, 21*, 71–81.

Gur, R. E., Cowell, P., Turetsky, B. I., Gallacher, F., Cannon, T., Bilker, W., et al. (1998). A follow-up magnetic resonance imaging study of schizophrenia. Relationship of neuroanatomical changes to clinical and neurobehavioral measures. *Archives of General Psychiatry, 55*, 145–152.

Heinrichs, R. W., & Zakzanis, K. K. (1998). Neurocognitive deficit in schizophrenia: A quantitative review of the evidence. *Neuropsychology, 12*(3), 426–445.

Hogarty, G. E., & Flesher, S. (1999). Practice principles of cognitive enhancement therapy for schizophrenia. *Schizophrenia Bulletin, 25*, 693–708.

Hogarty, G. E., Flesher, S., Ulrich, R., Carter, M., Greenwald, D., Pogue-Geile, M., et al. (2004). Cognitive enhancement therapy for schizophrenia. *Archives of General Psychiatry, 61*, 866–876.

Husa, A. P., Rannikko, I., Moilanen, J., Haapea, M., Murray, G. K., Barnett, J., Jones, P.B., Isohanni, M., Koponen, H., Miettunen, J., & Jääskeläinen, E. (2014). Lifetime use of antipsychotic medication and its relation to change of verbal learning and memory in midlife schizophrenia — An observational 9-year follow-up study. *Schizophrenia Research*, 158(1–3), 134–41.

Ikezawa, S., Mogami, T., Hayami, Y., Sato, I., Kato, T., Kimura, I., et al. (2012). The pilot study of a neuropsychological educational approach to cognitive remediation for patients with schizophrenia in Japan. *Psychiatry Research, 195*, 107–110.

Katzenschlager, R., Sampaio, C., Costa, J., & Lees, A. (2002). Anticholinergics for symptomatic management of Parkinson's disease. *Cochrane Database of Systematic Reviews, 3*. Art. No.: CD003735.

Keefe, R. S., Malhotra, A. K., Meltzer, H. Y., Kane, J. M., Buchanan, R. W., Murthy, A., et al. (2008). Efficacy and safety of donepezil in patients with schizophrenia or schizoaffective disorder: Significant placebo/practice effects in a 12-week, randomized, double-blind, placebo-controlled trial. *Neuropsychopharmacology, 33*, 1217–1228.

Khoury, B., Lecomte, T., Gaudiano, B. A., & Paquin, K. (2013). Mindfulness interventions for psychosis: A meta-analysis. *Schizophrenia Review, 150*, 176–184.

Kroken, R. A., Johnsen, E., Ruud, T., Wentzel-Larsen, T., & Jørgensen, H. A. (2009). Treatment of schizophrenia with antipsychotics in Norwegian emergency wards, a cross-sectional national study. *BMC Psychiatry, 9*, 24.

Kurtz, M. M., Seltzer, J. C., Shagan, D. S., Thime, W. R., & Wexler, B. E. (2007). Computer-assisted cognitive remediation in schizophrenia: What is the active ingredient? *Schizophrenia Research, 89*, 251–260.

Laurelle, M., Abi-Dargham, A., Gil, R., Kegeles, L., & Innis, R. (1999). Increased dopamine transmission in schizophrenia: Relationship to illness phases. *Biological Psychiatry, 46*, 56–72.

Lee, W. K. (2013). Effectiveness of computerized cognitive rehabilitation training on symptomatological, neuropsychological and work function in patients with schizophrenia. *Asia-Pacific Psychiatry, 5*, 90–100.

Lee, W. K., Lee, W. H., & Hwang, T. Y. (2004). *Yongin-cognitive behavioral rehabilitation therapy (Y-CBRT)*. Seoul, Korea: Hakjisa.

Lee, W. K., Lee, W. H., & Hwang, T. Y. (2008). *Cog-trainer*. Seoul, Korea: Maxmedica.

Liberman, R. P., & Kopelowicz, A. (1995). Basic elements in biobehavioral treatment and rehabilitation of schizophrenia. *International Clinical Psychopharmacology, 9*, 51–58.

Luki, I., Rickels, K., & Geller, A. M. (1986). Chronic use of benzodiazepines and psychomotor and cognitive test performance. *Psychopharmacology, 88*, 426–433.

MacDonald, S., & Wiseman-Hakes, C. (2010). Knowledge translation in ABI rehabilitation: A model for consolidating and applying the evidence for cognitive-communication interventions. *Brain Injury, 24*(3), 486–508.

Medalia, A. (2010). *Ask the experts*. [Web log post]. Retrieved from http://asp.cumc.columbia.edu/psych/asktheexperts/ask_the_experts_inquiry.asp?SI=300

Medalia, A., & Choi, J. (2009). Cognitive remediation in schizophrenia. *Neuropsychology Review, 19*(3), 353–364.

Medalia, A., & Freilich, B. (2008). The neuropsychological educational approach to cognitive remediation (NEAR) model: Practice principles and outcome studies. *Journal of Psychiatric Rehabilitation, 11*(2), 123–143.

Medalia, A., & Richardson, R. (2005). What predicts a good response to cognitive remediation interventions? *Schizophrenia Bulletin, 31*(4), 942–953.

Meeter, M., Murre, J. M. J., Janssen, S. M. J., Birkenhager, T., & van den Broek, W. W. (2011). Retrograde amnesia after electroconvulsive therapy: A temporary effect? *Journal of Affective Disorders, 132*, 216–222.

Mintzer, J., & Burns, A. (2000). Anticholinergic side-effects of drugs in elderly people. *Journal of the Royal Society of Medicine, 93*(9), 457–462.

Mishara, A. L., & Goldberg, T. E. (2004). A meta-analysis and critical review of the effects of conventional neuroleptic treatment on cognition in schizophrenia: Opening a closed book. *Biological Psychiatry, 55*, 1013–1022.

Molloy, C., Conroy, R. M., Cotter, D. R., & Cannon, M. (2011). Is traumatic brain injury a risk factor for schizophrenia? A meta-analysis of case-controlled population-based studies. *Schizophrenia Bulletin, 37* (6), 1104–1110.

Nuechterlein, K. H., & Dawson, M. E. (1984). A heuristic vulnerability/stress model of schizophrenic episodes. *Schizophrenia Bulletin, 10*(2), 300–312.

Pella, R., Hill, B. D., Kendra, K., & Gouvier, W. D. (2008). Cognitive rehabilitation. In A. Horton & D. Wedding (Eds.), *Neuropsychology handbook* (3rd ed.). New York, NY: Springer.

Penadés, R., Pujol, N., Catalán, R., Massana, G., Rametti, G., Garcia-Rizo, C., et al. (2013). Brain effects of cognitive remediation therapy in schizophrenia: A structural and functional neuroimaging study. *Biological Psychiatry, 73*, 1015–1023.

Pietrzak, R. H., Scott, J. C., Harel, B. T., Lim, Y. Y., Snyder, P. J., & Maruff, P. (2012). A process-based approach to characterizing the effect of acute alprazolam challenge on visual paired associate learning and memory in healthy older adults. *Human Psychopharmacology, 27*(6), 549–558.

Pringsheim, T., Doja, A., Belanger, S., & Patten, S. (2011). Treatment recommendations for extrapyramidal side effects associated with second-generation antipsychotic use in children and youth. *Pediatrics and Child Health, 16*(9), 590.

Proto, D., Pella, R. D., Hill, B. D., & Gouvier, W. D. (2009). Assessment and rehabilitation of acquired visuospatial and proprioceptive deficits associated with visuospatial neglect. *NeuroRehabilitation, 24* (2), 145–157.

Pu, S., Nakagome, K., Yamada, T., Ikezawa, S., Itakura, M., Satake, T., et al. (2014). A pilot study on the effects of cognitive remediation on hemodynamic responses in the prefrontal cortices of patients with schizophrenia: A multi-channel near-infrared spectroscopy study. *Schizophrenia Research, 153*, 87–95.

Reichenberg, A., & Harvey, P. D. (2007). Neuropsychological impairment in schizophrenia: Integration of performance-based and brain imaging findings. *Psychological Bulletin, 133*(5), 833–858.

Robertson, I. H., & Murre, J. M. J. (1999). Rehabilitation of brain damage: Brain plasticity and principles of guided recovery. *Psychological Bulletin, 125*, 544–575.

Roder, V., Mueller, D.R., Brenner, H.D., & Spaulding, W. (2010). *Psychological Therapy (IPT) for the Treatment of Neurocognition, Social Cognition and Social Competency in Schizophrenia Patients*. Seattle, WA: Hogrefe & Huber.

Roder, V., Mueller, D. R., Mueser, K. T., & Brenner, H. D. (2006). Integrated psychological therapy (IPT) for schizophrenia: Is it effective? *Schizophrenia Bulletin*, (Suppl. 1), 81–93.

Roder, V., Mueller, D. R., & Schmidt, S. J. (2011). Effectiveness of integrated psychological therapy (IPT) for schizophrenia patients: A research update. *Schizophrenia Bulletin, 37*(Suppl. 2), 71–79.

Schaefer, J., Giangrande, E., Weinberger, D. R., & Dickinson, D. (2013). The global cognitive impairment in schizophrenia: Consistent over decades and around the world. *Schizophrenia Research, 150*, 42–50.

Schoenberg, M. R., Ruwe, W. D., Dawson, K., McDonald, N. B., & Forducey, P. G. (2008). Comparison of functional outcomes and treatment cost between a computer-based cognitive rehabilitation teletherapy program and a face-to-face rehabilitation program. *Professional Psychology: Research & Practice, 39*(2), 169–175.

Seltzer, J., Cassens, G., Ciocca, C., & O'Sullivan, L. (1997). Neuropsychological rehabilitation in the treatment of schizophrenia. *Connecticut Medicine, 61*(9), 597–608.

Semkovska, M., & McLoughlin, D. M. (2010). Objective cognitive performance associated with electroconvulsive therapy for depression: A systematic review and meta-analysis. *Biological Psychiatry, 68*(6), 568–577.

Smith, H. A., Phil, M., & Connolly, M. J. (2003). Evaluation and treatment of dysphagia following stroke. *Topics in Geriatric Rehabilitation, 19*, 43–59. Retrieved from http://web.ebscohost.com.libproxy2.usouthal.edu

Stark, C. E. L., & Squire, L. R. (2001). Simple and associative recognition in the hippocampal region. *Learning and Memory, 8*, 190–197.

Szoke, A., Trandafir, A., Dupont, M. E., Meary, A., Schurhoff, F., & Leboyer, M. (2008). Longitudinal studies of cognition in schizophrenia: Meta-analysis. *British Journal of Psychiatry, 192*, 248–257.

Tamminga, C. A., & Medoff, D. R. (2000). The biology of schizophrenia. *Dialogues in Clinical Neuroscience, 2*(4), 339–348.

Tata, P. R., Rollings, J., Collins, M., Pickering, A., & Jacobson, R. R. (1994). Lack of cognitive recovery following withdrawal from long-term benzodiazepine use. *Psychological Medicine, 24*(1), 203–213.

Tchanturia, K., Davies, H., & Campbell, I. C. (2007). Cognitive remediation therapy for patients with anorexia nervosa: Preliminary findings. *Annals of General Psychiatry, 14*, 6–14.

Tchanturia, K., Davies, H., Lopez, C., Schmidt, U., Treasure, J., & Wykes, T. (2008). Neuropsychological task performance before and after cognitive remediation in anorexia nervosa: A pilot case-series. *Psychological Medicine, 38*, 1371–1373.

Tchanturia, K., Lloyd, S., & Lang, K. (2013). Cognitive remediation therapy for anorexia nervosa: Current evidence and future research directions. *International Journal of Eating Disorders, 46*, 492–495.

Trapp, W., Landgrebe, M., Hoesl, K., Lautenbacher, S., Gallhofer, B., Günther, W., et al. (2013). Cognitive remediation improves cognition and good cognitive performance increases time to relapse—results of a 5-year catamnestic study in schizophrenia patients. *BMC Psychiatry, 13*(184).

Tuulio-Henriksson, A., Perälä, J., Saarni, S. I., Isometsä, E., Koskinen, S., Lönnqvist, J., et al. (2011). Cognitive functioning in severe psychiatric disorders: A general population study. *European Archives of Psychiatry and Clinical Neuroscience, 261*, 447–456.

Vianin, P. (2013). *LaRemédiation cognitive dans la schizophrénie. LeProgramme RECOS.* Bruxelles: Mardaga.

Vianin, P., Urben, S., Magistretti, P., Marquet, P., Fornari, E., & Jaugey, L. (2014). Increased activation in Broca's area after cognitive remediation in schizophrenia. *Psychiatry Research: Neuroimaging, 221*, 204–209.

Vinogradov, S., Fisher, M., Warm, H., Holland, C., Kirshner, M. A., & Pollock, B. G. (2009). The cognitive cost of anticholinergic burden: decreased response to cognitive training in schizophrenia. *American Journal of Psychiatry, 166*, 1055–1062.

Vita, A., De Peri, L., Barlati, S., Cacciana, P., Deste, G., Poli, R., et al. (2011). Effectiveness of different modalities of cognitive remediation on symptomatological, neuropsychological, and functional outcome domains in schizophrenia: A prospective study in a real-world setting. *Schizophrenia Research, 133*, 223–231.

Vita, A., Deste, G., De Peri, L., Barlati, S., Poli, R., Cesana, B. M., et al. (2013). Predictors of cognitive and functional improvement and normalization after cognitive remediation in patients with schizophrenia. *Schizophrenia Research, 150*, 51–57.

Walker, E. F., & Diforio, D. (1997). Schizophrenia: A neural diathesis-stress model. *Psychological Review, 104*(4), 667–685.

Westra, H. A., Stewars, S. H., Teehan, M., Johl, K., Dozois, D. J. A., & Hill, T. (2004). Benzodiazepine use associated with decreased memory for psychoeducation material in cognitive behavioral therapy for panic disorder. *Cognitive Therapy and Research, 28* (2), 193–208.

Wolf, T. J. (2011). Centennial vision-rehabilitation, disability, and participation research: Are occupational therapy researchers addressing cognitive rehabilitation after stroke? *American Journal of Occupational Therapy, 65*, e46–e59. doi:10.5014/ajot.2011.002089

Woodward, N. D., Purdon, S. E., Meltzer, H. Y., & Zald, D. H. (2007). A meta-analysis of cognitive change with haloperidol in clinical trials of atypical antipsychotics: Dose effects and comparison to practice effects. *Schizophrenia Research, 89*, 211–224.

Wykes, T., Huddy, V., Cellard, C., McGurk, S. R., & Czobor, P. A. (2011). Meta-analysis of cognitive remediation for schizophrenia: Methodology and effect sizes. *American Journal of Psychiatry, 168*, 472–485.

Wykes, T., & Reeder, C. (2005). *Cognitive remediation therapy for schizophrenia: Theory and practice*. London: Routledge.

Cogpack. *Marker software*. Retrieved from http://www.markersoftware.com/

HASOMED Gmbh. *RehaCom-cognitive therapy*. Retrieved from http://www.hasomed.de/en/products/rehacom-cognitive-therapy.html

RehaCom. *HASOMED GmbH*. Retrieved from www.hasomed.de

X-Cog®. Retrieved from www.x-cog.de/xcogen.html

Yu, Y., Shen, H., Zeng, L., Ma, Q., & Hu, D. (2013). Convergent and divergent functional connectivity patterns in schizophrenia and depression. *PLoS ONE, 8*(7), 1–11.

# Psychiatric Services

# 9

Jack W. Barber

## Introduction

The current, though still maturing, conception of recovery-oriented services is the derivative of decades of braiding a number of sometimes conflicting developments impacting the mental health system and the individuals needing services from it (Anthony and Farkas 2012; Liberman 2008; SAMHSA 2006). These include the "myth of mental illness" (Szasz 1974), deinstitutionalization, civil rights, consumerism, the general neglect of state hospitals and individual abuses, and professional evidence relative to treatment adherence (Brown and Bussell 2011; Zygmunt et al. 2002). Today, the factors of mental health parity, the Olmstead decision, United States Department of Justice actions relative to the Civil Rights of Institutionalized Persons Act and the United States Supreme Court's Olmstead Decision, highly publicized violent incidents, Center for Medicare and Medicaid Services regulations, peer provided services, inconsistent funding of public mental health systems and, for psychiatrists, the ever present reality of medical liability are among the factors impacting the integration of recovery principles into inpatient psychiatric treatment. The not uncommon dialectic of the "recovery model" versus the "medical model" (e.g., Roberts and Wolfson 2004), in which neither has a clear and consistent definition for individuals, may have facilitated conflict rather than thoughtful integration. Further, the necessity of managing clinical risks responsible for involuntary hospitalizations while maintaining a recovery-oriented focus can produce complexities not easily addressed by "one size fits all" policies or practices.

Given the complexity of development, the continuing evolution of recovery-oriented services, and the potential delicacy of integrating recovery principles into high risk clinical/legal situations, it is not surprising that its translation and consequent challenges lack consistency generally, but also in the specific situation of providing treatment to involuntary or otherwise forensic individuals in inpatient settings. This may be especially so in public state and community hospitals treating individuals who commonly manifest multidimensional challenges related to aggression, self-injury, severe or refractory symptoms, losses relative to employment, family, housing, or medical health, legal charges, and the denial of the need for treatment. It is not the purpose of this chapter to explore any of these factors or developments, just as it will not describe the particulars of diagnosis or psychopharmacology, which are essential functions of psychiatric practice. First, it will focus on how key recovery principles should manifest in the assessment, planning, and treatment activities conducted by

J.W. Barber (✉)
Department of Behavioral Health and Developmental Services, Richmond, VA 23219, USA
e-mail: Jack.barber@dbhds.virginia.gov



N.N. Singh et al. (eds.), *Handbook of Recovery in Inpatient Psychiatry*,
Evidence-Based Practices in Behavioral Health, DOI 10.1007/978-3-319-40537-7_9

psychiatrists and other professionals in their roles as treatment team members. Second, it will address how recovery principles should be integrated into tasks primarily conducted by psychiatrists in public inpatient settings.

A psychiatrist in an inpatient setting is typically charged with a number of essential responsibilities. These include admission/discharge, diagnosis, prescribing medication, and making decisions and/or recommendations relative to capacity to consent, involuntary or emergency administration of medications, privilege determinations, and the use of restrictive interventions ranging from special observation to the use of seclusion or restraints. Beyond this, however, many psychiatrists are the designated leaders for treatment teams or are responsible for the individual's overall treatment within the hospital. At the very least, they will be essential members of the individual's treatment team. In this capacity, the necessity of developing an holistic understanding of the individual, the roles the treatment providers need to play in the individual's path of recovery, the interventions necessary to help the individual move forward on that path, and the actions to establish a recovery-oriented environment become essential for all members of the treatment team. For recovery principles to have meaning and effect, they must be integrated into the assessment, treatment planning, treatment interventions, and discharge planning that constitute the essential work of psychiatrists, other treatment team professionals, and direct care staff.

It is a hallmark of inpatient care that safety is the essential "bottom line". Safety has a number of dimensions relative to the physical environment, having an adequate number of staff, completing assessments, implementing plans based on those assessments, anticipating and preventing risk situations, attending effectively to medical conditions and medication risks, examining incidents and medication errors, conducting fire and medical emergency drills, and so forth. What has become clear over the past two decades is that effective attention to the implementation of recovery principles such as hope, respect, choice, connection to others, purpose, and sensitivity to trauma reduce risk in the aggregate. Individuals who feel connected, respected, and included in decisions related to the treatment are less likely to be aggressive or self-injurious. There are obviously exceptions and individuals with serious mental disorders who are unable to absorb or metabolize such approaches are more likely to find their way into state hospitals. However, one of the advantages to such settings is that they typically have the option of more lengthy stays during which there are opportunities for developing more effective treatment strategies, mitigating past traumatic experiences, and establishing more complete connections with individuals consequent to more shared experiences in the treatment setting. Establishing and carefully nourishing a treatment environment in which behavioral events can be treated as exceptions and examined as such is an essential component of a well functioning service. Facilities that default to treating exceptional events as the norm will typically regress to the "us and them", anxiety and fear-driven efforts to over-control individuals that lead to more incidents and compromise the fundamental necessity of a safe environment in which to begin or renew the recovery process.

The most critical source of real and perceived conflict relative to implanting recovery principles centers on individual "choice" and "safety" (Davidson et al. 2006; Hillbrand et al. 2010; Parks et al. 2014). Despite policy statements from SAMHSA (2011, pp. 25–26), such as, "Honoring self-determination, however, does not require, and is not equal to, doing whatever the person wants.... Mental health professionals are bound both by their professional ethics and by their societal obligation to act in the person's and community's best interests, even if that may be in conflict with the person's wishes at the time", these dilemmas do not play out consistently or thoughtfully. Questions, at times offered quite pointedly, such as, "So you want me to let her kill herself if she chooses", "He is going to kill someone if he refuses treatment", or "He will not survive three days if I let him leave like he wants to" reflect the hard, if hyperbolized, edges of the dilemma between self-determination and clinical risk management or between "choice" and required treatment. Less dramatic or more subtle variants face individuals and clinicians daily in state hospitals:

> George is an individual with congenital deafness committed involuntarily after being found Not Guilty by Reason of Insanity (NGRI) for a rape-murder of an elderly woman who was unable, despite many years of attempted treatment to accept his role in the crime or that the potential risks relative to re-offending had any relationship to him personally. Periodic allegations of unwanted advances persisted. As the population of individuals with deafness declined to the point that operating a special program was no longer feasible (or perhaps legal), he strongly advocated for being placed in a co-ed environment versus in an all-male unit.
>
> Alice has been found Not Guilty by Reason of Insanity, has persistent grandiose and paranoid delusions despite taking fluphenazine, and refuses to consider any other antipsychotic agent to the point of threatening to attack anyone who tries to give her a different medication. The content of the delusions precludes her from considering potential discharge placements or other requirements necessary for her to be released.
>
> Susan is a young woman with a history of multiple self-injurious events, a substantial trauma history, intermittent substance use, and predilection for entering abusive sexual relationships who demands, after involuntary commitment for the fourth time in two months, to be discharged to live her life the way she wants to live it with her new boyfriend who has multiple psychological and substance use issues.

Two important principles related to choice will be discussed below. These are: (1) that life is a limited menu (for everyone) and (2) that an inability to make one or more choices does not mean that many other choices cannot be made. However, it is important to note in the beginning that self-determination and choice, like the other essential recovery principles of hope, meaning, respect, connection, and sensitivity to trauma does not exist in a vacuum. It is an important aspect to a recovery orientation that has other important aspects. Knitting the various threads together with safety and treatment into a cohesive and consistently applied tapestry is the essential work of creating and sustaining a recovery-oriented service. The specific details to be applied will be determined by the condition, circumstances, strengths and protective factors, predilections, and input of each individual committed for treatment.

In order to provide a foundation for this discussion, it is essential to delineate the essential principles of recovery-oriented treatment that are best applied to and integrated in the processes of inpatient treatment. These are hope, self-determination/choice, purpose or meaning, respect, and a connection to helpful others as well as an assessment of and sensitivity to trauma. As a practical matter, however, the application of three other broad principles provides the framework within which these principles are applied and integrated. First, it is essential to understand the purpose of inpatient treatment relative to an individual's personal recovery journey, even when the individual has not yet conceptualized or initiated such a path. In general, this is to provide the treatment, support, and discharge planning necessary to return the individual to the community with an opportunity to succeed in establishing or reestablishing a more integrated life in that community. The particulars will vary based on individual strengths, symptoms, and circumstances. An individual involuntarily committed consequent to severe, but treatment responsive manic symptoms may require little more than expeditious symptom resolution, support during the crisis, education, and establishing an aftercare plan. A person with serious chronic psychotic symptoms that have responded in limited fashion to medications, lacks effective coping or problem-solving skills, has become estranged from family and other supports, and lacks a place to live will require the implementation of a much more holistic plan of care and discharge planning. An individual ordered into inpatient treatment to restore their capacity to stand trial will require treatment as well as preparation for court proceedings and a plan for "what comes after."

The essential point is that the inpatient treatment should help the person advance their recovery journey with the clear recognition and demonstration that recovery does not end with discharge. Its focus is not to become a successful inpatient. The length of stay or time available for this phase of treatment will obviously hinge on the interface between the individual's legal status and the resolution or mitigation of the risks responsible for the hospitalization. Nonetheless, the general principle that an inpatient treatment episode is part of a recovery path as opposed to a circumscribed, essentially isolated, episode that concludes with discharge represents a critical change in the framework of inpatient treatment.

> Eli is a young man with Aspergers Syndrome admitted involuntarily after his plan (and preparations) for conducting a mass shooting at a local shopping mall was discovered. Consultations with experts concluded that the risk of his following through with his plan were extremely high, having been foiled only by his father's aggressive efforts to prevent his obtaining weapons. His viscous preoccupation with "all things mass shooting", lack of symptoms of psychosis or affective illness, developmental immaturity, lack of anxiety or distress relative to his plans, inability to manifest anger in any form, and lack of any future orientation with respect to work or relationships presented no obvious options for him or his treatment team.
>
> Ultimately, it was determined that a potential path lay in the advantage of his relative youth and immaturity as well as his intelligence, i.e., that if treatment was designed to help him mature emotionally and socially while providing options to exercise his intelligence then he would develop more capacity to discuss and address the issues driving his plans. If so, then there would be an opportunity to mitigate the risks posed by his ideas while having him more prepared to resume college, find employment or other purpose, and improve his opportunities for relationships. Over time, other avenues may present themselves and, hopefully, he will develop more capacity for self-determination toward non-dangerous ends.

In this case, the treatment team had to develop a pathway based on their assessments as a means of getting the recovery process started.

Second, it must be demonstrably understood that each person is an individual as dimensional as "anyone else". A person is not an illness. While the illness may be overwhelming at times, it does not define "who they are" any more than having hypertension, diabetes, arthritis, or hypothyroidism defines a person with any of those conditions. It is common for parents, spouses, and other family members to state, "I have my son back" or "We have our mother back" and in so doing reflect the recovery of an individual from the storms of a psychotic or affective illness. In the end, we are to help the person recover to the point they can begin living their lives and managing their illness. To do so, requires an approach recognizing the person at every stage of treatment.

Third, we must treat each individual as we would wish to be treated or as we would wish a family member to be treated. It may read as a platitude that virtually all clinicians would agree to, but the ultimate test is whether the individual (and family or friends) feel that they were treated in this manner as they prepare to leave. The tyranny of caseloads, behavioral crises, difficult or complicated problems, paperwork, scheduling, and all of the other pressures of inpatient care can and do impede clinicians' capacity for the kind of demonstrable respect, kindness, and clarity of communication we all aspire to.

Finally, as described in the case of Eli above, psychiatrists and inpatient treatment teams must be prepared to take up more of this joint venture when the individual is less able to do so. As Bellack (2006) noted in discussing the management of risks presented by individuals, "... the balance of power may need to shift towards the professional when the consumer is highly impaired and has diminished decisional capacity" (p. 441). This is true for all aspects of recovery-oriented treatment. In simple terms, when an individual is without hope, it is the obligation of the treatment providers to help the individual restore it; when an individual has lost control of their behavior, relationships, purpose, or life in general, it is for the providers to develop a path for him to regain it; when an individual has become isolated, it is the staff's task to help them find connections to others; and when an individual cannot see a life in the community or a life beyond incarceration, it is our job to try to construct one to "see if it fits", recognizing that it will be adapted as the individual becomes more able to engage in the process.

## Forensic Patients

Prior to discussing the central recovery concepts it is worth considering those individuals transferred to state psychiatric hospitals from jails for the restoration of competency, emergency treatment, or other categories of treatment or evaluation. Many of these individual have a major mental illness and considerable overlap symptomatically with individuals who have been involuntarily detained or committed. The context within which they are to be treated differs, however, in terms of the increased oversight, accountability, security provisions, and stigma commonly related to forensic processes (Simpson and Penney 2011).

The specific parameters placed upon an individual under forensic status must be part of the recovery-oriented thinking that is applied in such cases. First, the legal charges may or may not limit their choices in terms of discharge. Some may be able to return to Court and leave from the next applicable hearing in which case discharge planning is similar to that for civil individuals. Others may face a period of time in jail, the length and eventual outcome of which may not be known. Second, these individuals will typically need to be educated regarding the functioning of the Court, the potential pleas that may be available, and the procedures applicable as they reenter the criminal justice system. Third, the criteria by which discharge or internal privilege decisions are made may be different, the provisions for security on and off the primary residential unit may be different, and there may be different rules governing phone calls, visitation, contraband, patient rights, and so on. At the same time, these differences are relative to the details of an individual's case rather than the general premises of recovery-oriented treatment. All individuals need to adapt to or cope with the external reality which is applicable to them and that does not change. For example, an individual with a recurrent psychotic disorder who will likely be found guilty once restored to competency may be facing some period of jail time. This reality frames what will be necessary to provide him the best opportunity to be successful after discharge differently than someone leaving to go into the community, but the principle of treatment is the same. Another example would be an individual admitted from jail to a unit that requires all of the individuals to wear the same outfit. However, the fact that each individual has no choice in terms of their wardrobe does not convey that they have no choice in what they select for their diet, what groups they may attend outside of those required to restore their competency, what they prefer to be called, or who they choose to spend their time with. Ultimately, they may have a choice relative to their plea or respond to a plea bargain or whether they serve time in jail or state prison, all of which may become an important component in charting their recovery journey. The hope for immediate release may be unrealistic, but the need for hope is present, nonetheless, and may require attention.

For individuals admitted to the hospital after an NGRI decision, the requirements necessary to achieve Conditional Release are very likely to be different than the discharge criteria that would be applied for an individual on civil status. Satisfying the applicable criteria, probably in stepwise fashion, becomes a reality for treatment and an additional component of the eventual discharge plan. It does not change the goal of success in the community, the need for hope, the making of choices, being treated with respect, making connections with people who are perceived to be of help, and receiving treatment sensitive to their applicable trauma history.

## Hope

Hope and optimism is of essential significance in many people's accounts of recovery (Roberts and Wolfson 2004). It is often sufficient to understand hope as it typically is: "I can get better", "I can feel better", "I can be discharged", "I can get a job", "I can be with my family", "I can find a girlfriend", and so forth. Encouragement, statements of confidence, references to the resolution of prior episodes, recognition of strengths, and validating feedback on clinical progress may be sufficient. For some individuals, a clear statement of the plan, its basis, and the clinical steps toward and through discharge are required to give hope some tangible markers to restore the individual's confidence. For each, treatment teams have to determine the language or currency with which hope can be transmitted to and received by the individual.

There are two circumstances, however, in which the foundation for hope has to be reestablished, if not demonstrated, before the individual can connect meaningfully with the therapeutic optimism vital to eventual success. In the first group are individuals for whom their experiences have oppressed any real sense that life can get better. This may be due to persistent psychotic symptoms, psychosocial losses, and limited or evaporative responses to treatment. In certain individuals afflicted with severe borderline personality disorder and the associated trauma history the psychological preparation for, and tolerance of, optimism is lacking. In such cases, a series of successful steps will be required as well a demonstrable commitment from providers to persist in the "hard work" until success is achieved.

Beth is a young woman treated several decades ago with severe Borderline Personality Disorder who had progressed from short admissions to longer and longer hospitalizations featuring repeated self-inflicted lacerations, occasional overdoses, emotional discord, and gains and losses relative to special observations and privileges. Part of the repeated message given to her was that the time would come when she was not so afflicted by her "emotional storms" (her words), would not feel so compelled to harm herself, and would feel that she was emotionally strong enough to leave the hospital, but that no one could possibly know how long that would take. Well before state hospitals became attendant to recovery principles, she noted as she was leaving that this was an essential part of the treatment.

For a second group, it is necessary to keep in mind that embedded in "hope" is the want or desire for something of meaning or value to the individual. Very few people wish to engage in treatment for the sake of being in treatment. Virtually no one takes medication because they merely want to take their medication. People engage in activities and behaviors that serve a purpose for them. Thus, the treatment must connect to helping the individual achieve or maintain something they value and they must have some hope that they can be successful. Few clinicians who have worked any length of time in a state hospital have not encountered an individual who wants or hopes for no more than they have in the hospital. Such an individual will typically perform whatever tasks are required to maintain the status quo of their current situation, but have no interest in participating in anything that would advance them toward a return to community life. Treatment teams often describe such a person as "hospital dependent", a concept that unfortunately offers no basis for planning interventions tailored to the individual. The individual lacks hope for anything more or different, without which further clinical progress is unlikely. Among the tasks of the treatment is to envision a path that the individual is unable to visualize, attempt its construction, and see if it proves attractive to the individual.

Dave is a middle aged man with a long history of Schizophrenia who had, for a number of years, been reasonably well compensated from the standpoint of symptoms and was hopeful and contented with the prospect of remaining in the hospital "forever". Repeated attempts to involve him in community activities or show him possible places he could live left him entirely nonplussed and uninterested. He finally connected with one of the Clinical Department Heads who spent many hours with Dave over almost two years, eventually talking about what he might be able to do if he left the hospital. A part of the eventual discharge plan was for him to serve on the local Human Rights Committee as well as to participate in the governance of the local clubhouse program.

Kent was a similar gentleman with much more substantial ongoing psychotic symptoms who had refused for a number of years to entertain any thought of leaving the hospital. Over the years, he had acquired a significant amount of musical equipment and his own storage room on the unit. In reviewing the case it was determined, rather obviously, that the hospital was encouraging his remaining rather than helping him realize a more integrated life in the community. An administrative decision was made to eliminate his storage room. From the consequent angst there derived a plan to find an apartment that could hold his equipment and, leveraging that interest, part-time work with Goodwill Industries. A lengthy transition was required, but Kent lived in the community for a number of years pleased with his work and apartment.

## Self-determination and Choice

Operationalizing choice in an inpatient setting for individuals who have been involuntarily detained and also lack the capacity to make certain decisions related to their treatment can be a source of uncertainty, confusion, and conflict (Mountain and Shah 2008). The ability to make choices over one's life is an essential element of liberty and personal control. Furthermore, the reality is that once a person is discharged most, if not all, more and less important decisions will be theirs to make. To the extent an individual has developed an ownership for managing their illness and recovery and practiced making decisions, the opportunity to achieve success is improved. While legitimately framed as a "right", the practical, clinical importance of improved decision-making is substantial. Developing the skills necessary for decision-making requires the experience of making them. Nonetheless, legal and medical-legal realities as well as institutional limits and efficiency may challenge the best implementation of this principle.

Two important concepts to facilitate navigating these potential ambiguities are that (1) "life is a limited menu" (Barber 2007) and (2) the fact that an individual may lack the capacity or authority to make one type of decision does not mean there are not a number of other decisions that they can make. The first represents a reality based premise that facilitates decision-making and problem-solving while mitigating extreme choice positions that are not supported by law, regulation, clinical judgment, or pragmatism. In truth, no one has a freedom of choice unconstrained by limits related to financial resources, work and family obligations, geography, personal limitations, health, and opportunity. The normal human condition is that "wanting something does not make it so". Everyone has to, for example, wait in line to get a driver's license, vote, or eat in a cafeteria. Each of us can only afford to buy what we can afford, marry someone who agrees to marry us, or work in a job that someone has been willing to hire us to do. Recognizing this, staff may work with an individual regarding the choices that they do have, the choices that can be restored or achieved, and how to work to create better choices in the future. It is also true, and sometimes of motivational importance, that residing in an institution provides fewer choices than living in an apartment or personal home. For example, mealtimes are typically set as are medication times, when groups are offered, and when outdoor and recreational spaces are accessible. Such things may be limited outside the hospital, but typically less so than within an institution.

It is common in state hospital settings for an individual to have been assessed as lacking the capacity to make particular treatment decisions, especially the decision regarding taking antipsychotic medication or when they are ready for discharge. However, such an individual may well be able to determine whether they will take a traditional or atypical antipsychotic agent or take, for example, olanzapine versus risperidone or quetiapine, even if they lack the capacity to refuse medication altogether. A variety of less essential decisions related to food choices, what to wear, when to shower, who to sit with during meals, some group or activity selections, who they will allow to visit them, what they listen to or watch on television, and what information they choose to access from the Internet (within limits as necessary) are generally possible. Encouraging such choices and overtly recognizing them as choices can increase the individual's feeling of control and awareness of making choices as well as serve as building blocks toward more important decisions.

It is worth noting that people make many choices without being aware of doing so. Increasing the awareness of choices made can be of value as it recognizes the individual exerting personal control over their actions and thoughts, whether they are participating in a Cognitive Behavioral Therapy program or not. The institutional rigidity of prior eras was both disempowering and devaluing of the individual, but also poor preparation for the reality of personal decision-making after discharge. Wasting an individual's ability to make or recognize choices by overregulating all aspects of their inpatient experience, "telling them what to do", or denying choices that are neither unsafe nor beyond the hospital's capacity for flexibility have similar effects today. From the standpoint of achieving success after discharge, making choices as a tangible aspect to self-determination is a more narrowly defined treatment issue as well as a key recovery principle.

At the same time, psychiatrists and other clinicians must provide for an individual's safety and treatment while they are in the hospital. A presently suicidal individual may not be left unsupervised, an actively aggressive individual may require restrictions on where they can be, who they can be with, and how closely they must be supervised, a forensic patient may require a Security presence when outside a locked unit, and an individual with active psychotic symptoms causing or facilitating a risk to themselves or others may require medication whether they choose to accept that or not. Serious injuries, death, prolonging a hospital stay due to elopement, and legal charges, future guilt, or placement limitations consequent to aggression are all impediments to recovery and require declarative action. When such risks are derived from acute symptoms or crisis states, the clinical decision-making is relatively straightforward. However, when the risks are chronic or impulsively episodic, the interface between the empowering personal control of choice and the risks of a "bad outcome" with all the attendant consequences for the individual, clinician, and hospital the matter becomes more complicated and imperfect.

Perhaps the clearest examples are found in the cases of individuals with severe borderline personality disorder, a history of repeated self-injurious behaviors, occasional suicide attempts, and virtually complete external locus of control whose ultimate recovery hinges on the development of improved internal regulation of emotions, making conscious decisions, and developing greater trust in themselves and others. Continuous supervision and restriction of activities promotes the regression that is directly related to risk while the exercise of autonomy, sometimes at a relatively basic level, may produce the anxiety and perceived abandonment that produces an acute, "impulsive" risk. In such cases, clinicians must engage the individual in the dilemma, establish parameters for making decisions based on the individual's history and assessment of the current clinical state, develop plans that can be consistently implemented such that the consequences of safe and unsafe behaviors are known in advance, and document the rationale for decisions made when risks are present with any decision. In such cases, as in others perhaps less dramatically, one cannot divorce choice from the other important dimensions of hope, respect, connection, meaning, and sensitivity to trauma without ill effect.

## Respect

Respect is embedded in the central tenets of recovery practices of self-determination, being treated as an individual rather than an illness, participating in both care decisions and policy development, and recognizing the importance of peer services (Anthony and Farkas 2012). Beyond the well-articulated means of demonstrating respect and treating individuals with dignity there are three further dimensions of respect essential for treatment providers and psychiatrists. The first is the respect for the gravity of an individual's condition and experience. The development of a language applying terms such as "client" or "consumer" to involuntarily hospitalized individuals combined with the necessity of being overtly hopeful and optimistic can result in a devaluing of the person's lived experience. The vitally necessary therapeutic optimism must recognize and validate the seriousness of an individual's condition and experiences which have greatly eroded, if not crushed, their personal hope or optimism that things can improve. Furthermore, clinicians must be sensitive to the individual for whom empowerment and personal autonomy do not (yet) match their feeling of personal competence, which must be met with equal respect.

The second dimension of respect involves practicing at the standard of care. This is discussed in a manner more specific to prescribers below, but it is a measure of respect that all disciplines practice to their standard of care. Doing so encompasses everything from professional boundaries and ethics to conducting psychological testing, to nursing standards of care with respect to assessment and medication administration, and to conducting therapies by any of the professional disciplines. Practicing safe and effective medicine, and discussing both positive and negative treatment developments, are tangible demonstrations of respect by physicians, but they are no less so for the other professional disciplines.

The third point regarding respect is applicable to only a small number of cases and relates to a treatment colluding with an individual's unrealistic ideas about their treatment or circumstance when doing so precludes the individual from making clinical progress toward discharge and returning to community life.

Jackie is a woman in her late thirties with a diagnosis of Schizoaffective Disorder who was found Not Guilty by Reason of Insanity for a felony assault with a pair of scissors and had been in the hospital for almost five years. Intelligent, sometimes charming, and creative she disagreed with the NGRI finding and demonstrated an unwillingness to accept the parameters required for advancing through the privilege system to Conditional Release. These parameters basically require an individual to take the medications as prescribed, control any risk behaviors, and demonstrate that they are able to follow the rules in order to demonstrate that they will comply with the parameters of their Conditional Release plan. Jackie's position was that she had been in the hospital many times and had always been able to be discharged without "going through all of this". Thus, her progress was impeded by repeated violations of the hospital's no smoking policy, inconsistent attendance at groups, engaging in sexual activities, failing to return to her unit on time, and engaging in verbal skirmishes with the staff regarding meal quantities, snacks, showers, washing her clothes, and so forth. It came to our attention that her treatment team was overtly agreeing with her that she would have been discharged long ago if she had been a civil patient, making repeated pleas to the privileging committee making a similar argument, and implicitly encouraging her efforts to have her attorney get the NGRI ruling overturned (which was unrealistic even if it were legally possible). The treatment team's stance was clinically inappropriate (because it impeded her making any progress toward release), but was also disrespectful in facilitating her pursuing a false path and essentially wasting her time. After being transferred to another unit with a team that repeatedly held the position that she would have to meet the requirements under the NGRI system in order to gain the release she did badly want. It was a difficult course for much of the next year, but eventually she began demonstrating the required behaviors and was able to achieve her Conditional Release.

A variant of this type of situational impasse created at the interface between the individual and treatment team is demonstrated by the case of Albert.

Albert is a man in his mid-forties with a longstanding diagnosis of schizophrenia who demonstrated some vague paranoid thoughts and secretiveness, but who presented no behavioral risks. However, after almost two years in the hospital he refused to discuss any discharge plans, instead making references to plans he was making in this regard which he would not share with the team, the unit Social Worker, or his Community Liaison. He refused to take more than a very small dose of medication and had been successful almost a year before in persuading a Special Justice that he could make his own decisions. His case was presented due to his "hospital dependency" and lack of progress. The summary of the consultation was that it was most likely that his refusal to discuss discharge actually reflected persistent delusional ideation about threats he felt would be present in the community and that it was essential for him to have an adequate trial of treatment. The psychiatrist, rather than passively accepting as permanent a judicial decision made a year before that essentially consigned Albert to permanent hospitalization, needed to petition the Special Justice for substitute consent and make it clear that Albert had no future other than living in the institution unless a more effective medication regimen could be implemented. This was done, a more effective medication regimen was prescribed, the psychotic symptoms further attenuated, and a successful discharge was implemented.

In this case, a clinical legal process that appeared to be respecting of the individual's autonomy was, in fact, placing the individual's life at the mercy of psychotic symptoms that could be treated. It is not respectful to waste a year of an individual's life when it can be avoided.

## Connection to Helpful Others

Psychiatrists and other professionals invest significant time and training in learning how to establish and maintain a therapeutic relationship. Doing so is vital to understanding an individual and collaborating with them in their treatment and highly valued by the receivers of care (Lakeman 2010). However, the connection of importance to the recovery process is the individual's perceived connectedness to another person who is of help or support to them. This may, of course, be a psychiatrist or other professional but is more likely to be a peer, a family member, a friend, a Pastor, or a direct care or support staff member. Feeling connected to others combats the isolation that may afflict individuals with a mental disorder, severe or not, as well as provides a source of tangible support necessary for the recovery process. In addition, such perceived connections decrease the risk of suicide which may be highly correlated with the sense of isolation (Van Orden et al. 2010). The essential point is that it is the connection as perceived by the individual receiving help that is of value in recovery. Professional as well as direct care staff interactions need to keep this important dimension in mind in order to maximize the chance that the individual will feel that others are interested in his well-being and are steadfast in their attempts to understand him and try to help him "get better". In an inpatient setting, it is not possible to anticipate who the individual will most keenly feel a valid and supportive connection with, thus all staff are required to be mindful of this key recovery principle in order to maximize its chances of development.

To achieve recovery-oriented treatment, such treatment must be delivered in a culturally competent manner to convey respect, assist self-determination, and best assure an opportunity for therapeutic connection (The President's New Freedom Commission 2003; SAMHSA 2006). For an individual to experience a confidence that they are being understood, supported, validated, or helped psychologically some understanding on the part of staff regarding their cultural background and traditions will be necessary. This can be a substantial challenge for state hospitals in less diverse areas treating individuals from urban centers and other geographic areas that feature many primary languages and cultures. In addition to training and education programs to enhance staff recognition of and sensitivity to the importance of culture and its impact on individuals, state hospitals have to recognize that the isolation derived from a lack of common language or culture produces additional risk. Such risks may range from suicide when a person feels alone in their suffering to aggression derived from misunderstanding.

In addition to mitigating strategies, such as the use of translation, additional efforts to assure the individual can remain connected to family or friends, direct acknowledgement of not understanding adequately (while continuing to attempt to do so using the individual, family, and other sources of information) state hospital staff must be mindful of communications that are nonverbal. This relates to individual demeanor and expression, but also to how clear hospital routines are within and off the units. The sooner an individual's environment is more predictable to them as far as when things happen, who does what, and where things are the less anxiety provoking, threatening, and isolating it is. Attention to making such routines as obvious as possible "without words" may not just be useful for individuals who do not speak the language, but also for individuals with ongoing psychotic symptoms who may have more difficulty processing verbal information.

## Meaning or Purpose

This aspect of recovery is well discussed by others (Anthony et al. 2002; Anthony and Farkas 2012; Liberman 2008) and requires only a few points to elaborate on in regard to the treatment of severely ill inpatients. First, treatment staff need to demonstrate their understanding that the purpose of treatment is to help an individual live a more satisfying life in the community. Thus, within legal and temporal constraints as applicable for each case, the objectives for the individual and the interventions by the staff are aligned with the goal of discharging the individual with an opportunity to be successful upon return to the community. This is the purpose of the work that the individual is participating in with the treatment staff. Basic hygiene, proper clothing, safety, attention to physical health, resolving psychiatric symptoms, developing social or problem-solving skills, collaborating with discharge planners, learning Court procedures, and everything else has a purpose with respect to the ultimate goal of successfully living in the community. While this demonstration is not what is intended by this recovery concept it supports and reinforces the individual's sense of purpose.

Second, for an individual in the midst of an acute or ongoing psychotic illness complicated by behavioral, medical, and psychosocial problems the prospect of meaningful engagement, employment or other purpose post-discharge can be easily lost as a consideration. As noted above, the burden may fall more to the treatment providers to recognize its long term importance and bring the matter to attention even if in a preliminary way. As will be discussed later in regard to medications there must be an answer to the question, "Why would this individual accept or engage in the treatment planned or provided?" It may be possible to gain assent and cooperation in an inpatient setting, but this can obscure the larger need for the individual to have meaning or purpose for their life if they are to be motivated to pursue treatment and recovery in the community. If there is no answer to this question, it must become a task for the treatment process, as individuals who lack purpose are likely to require help in order to find it.

Third, one of the substantial, nonspecific improvements in state hospital services has been the implementation of off-unit psychosocial rehabilitation (PSR) groups and activities. In addition to the opportunities to tailor education, practice, problem solving, creative, and recreational activities to the individual, such programs provide a reason for individuals to get up, dress, and eat breakfast if they wish before the work and socialization that accompanies such a PSR program begins. At the least, there is a point to engaging the day, but much more typically the change in location, classroom-type settings, interactions with peers in purposeful conversation or activity, and learning that takes place reinforces the purpose of getting better and preparing for life in the community.

The fourth point relates to the particular challenge of working with that subset of inpatients that have no sense of purpose or meaning in their lives, lack aspiration, and have no genuine hope for living a life any different from what they have in the hospital or have had in the past. Absent a sense of purpose or aspiration, there can be little genuine motivation to engage in treatment or pursue a path to recovery. Two case examples may help illustrate this situation.

Gus is a man in his mid-forties whose prospects for becoming a lawyer had been devastated by the development of severe psychotic symptoms during his early twenties, extended periods of treatment non-adherence and insufficient responses to medications, and multiple hospitalizations. Once his more acute psychotic symptoms and erratic behavior stabilized, he entered a long period in which he cooperated with treatment, presented no behavior problems, and refused all efforts to engage him in any discussion of discharge. He stated he was "perfectly content" to remain in the hospital. Through patient and painstaking efforts over the course of more than a year his treatment team was finally able to identify that he seemed to enjoy the idea of being of help to others and attract him (very cautiously) to the idea of working with Goodwill Industries and living in his own apartment decorated with his possessions. Still, he refused to sign papers necessary to place his financial affairs in order (which was necessary to allow him to rent an apartment). Months of patiently building his commitment to his work via passes, work with him and his father on their expectations, and, ultimately, the development of a situation in which he had no choice but to "sign or lose access" to his funds accompanied the steady nourishment of the idea of his own apartment, what furniture he might have, in what general location, and what size. After almost two years and a number of trial passes during which he developed a sense of pride in the work he was doing, he was discharged. Two years later, he is living successfully in the community, managing his own affairs, and working part-time with Goodwill.

Earl is an individual of similar psychiatric history, but who was found Not Guilty by Reason of Insanity. While his psychiatric symptoms were relatively stable and he no longer demonstrated the kinds of aggressive behavior that he had in the past, he appeared to have no interest in further progress or discharge. In consulting with the treatment team, who knew him well, they were unable to identify anything that he wanted in the community and were at an impasse as to how to help him. In a lengthy discussion with them, we were able to establish that it had been many years since he lived outside of an institution, his life had not gone well during prior periods out of the hospital or jail, he was content with his family visiting him at the hospital and had no interest in going to live with them. He appeared to have no real interests other than he did seem to enjoy small mechanical devices or discussing small motors and car engines, about which he had some knowledge and experience. It was determined that the clearest path to living in the community would have to begin with the quiet nourishment of his interest in small engines by finding him some to work on while in the hospital. If that work could be established as a gratifying endeavor then it might be possible to build from that toward a discharge plan that featured working in small engine repair or some similar activity. The task for the treatment team was to take advantage of knowing him well, envision a future that it appeared that he might relate to, and begin taking steps to nourish that vision to see if it would become his own.

## Trauma Informed Care

It is reported that the rates of trauma exposure in individuals with a serious mental illness range from 49 to 100 % (Grubaugh et al. 2011). The principles and growing penetration of Trauma Informed Care in care delivery (SAMSHA 2014) feature significant operational overlap with those of recovery-oriented services. The assessment for historical trauma and sensitivity to minimizing a triggering or reenactment of such trauma constitute important advances for inpatient treatment. It is essential to be mindful of the fact that the circumstances and process of involuntary hospitalization or arrest and subsequent hospitalization may frequently involve further trauma or an emotional activation derivative of prior trauma. At the same time, a small percentage of such individuals will manifest agitated, aggressive behavior or repeated self-injurious acts that, at times, may require the use of seclusion, restraint, or forced medication when the situation is emergent and the safety of the individual or others can be accomplished in no other way. Staff can be uncertain or confused as to how they are to respond when faced with the potential to re-traumatize an individual versus allowing someone to get hurt in the context of their indecision. When there is peer-to-peer aggression, the matter can be more complicated. Obviously, there is no simple answer to such situations, but there are several things that may mitigate the potential consequences.

First, hospitals must acknowledge that such circumstances arise and provide guidance to staff. If the trauma informed care champions and trainers are unfamiliar with inpatient work or are isolated from clinical and risk management staff practices will be inconsistent, organization splitting will occur, and staff will be left "to their own devices". Staff must be trained in recovery and trauma informed principles and act in a manner consistent with those principles. Seclusion or restraint must be the interventions of last resort when nothing else will achieve safety for the individual or others. They must be competent in utilizing less restrictive interventions to prevent and respond to situations presented the risk of aggression or self-harm as well as in physical techniques to be used when necessary. Treatment teams and psychiatrists must be attentive to the factors that produce risk in an individual and implement treatment strategies and interventions to mitigate such risks. Allowing an individual with an aggressive history, current evidence of ongoing tension and irritability, and paranoia to go without medications in order "not to upset him" is a too common antecedent to an aggressive incident in which the individual and others end up at risk, if not injured. Failing to incorporate known triggers and calming interventions into the treatment plan or failing to educate direct care staff about them is another too common error. If staff demonstrate hope, choice, respect, and sensitivity to trauma consistently, are taught to observe for and intervene early to prevent dangerous escalations, and are competent to handle such emergencies as they occur there will be fewer such escalations and, when they do occur, there will be some mitigation of the potential trauma.

After such an incident it is important for staff to reestablish their demonstration of recovery-oriented interactions, process the incident with the individual, review the current treatment plan, and attempt to learn, with the individual, what could be done should there be a subsequent recurrence. It must be kept in mind that acts of aggression toward the individual or others delay or impede progress toward discharge and may limit the individual's choices. The fact is that it is also traumatic for other patients as well as staff when one of their peers is threatening, tense and irritable, or behaving aggressively as it may activate fears from their own trauma histories. To add to the complexity, it may also be traumatic to see one of their peers secluded or restrained. For all of these reasons, as well as the fact that being a direct care staff member is among the highest risk occupations, the importance of preventing aggression to avoid the need for restrictive interventions and fear in the milieu cannot be overstated. It is redundant, but important to reiterate that the prevention of aggression does not begin once an individual is agitated or threatening. It begins with establishing the proper treatment environment, thinking ahead about the potential risks an individual may present, and implementing strategies to prevent the development of states and circumstances in which aggression is more likely followed by responding appropriately to acute situations that do develop. It is worth noting that teaching mindfulness to direct care staff has been shown to mitigate aggressive incidents in individuals with intellectual disabilities and may hold promise for behavioral health settings as well (Singh et al. 2009, 2015).

## Peer Provided Services

The penetration, acceptance, and effectiveness of peer provided services have increased steadily during the past two decades (Nelson et al. 2006, 2007; Repper and Carter 2011). The roles available for peers within state hospitals are varied and include conducting group therapies, developing Wellness Action Recovery Plans, operating peer resource centers, providing support to individuals at both admission and discharge, and participating on hospital committees. The effectiveness of peers in reducing hospitalizations, increasing confidence and self-determination, and promoting hope are all reasons that treatment teams need to make use of these resources to help individuals move forward in recovery. In addition, for some individuals, becoming a provider of peer services becomes central to their own recovery, providing a way to derive meaning and purpose from their lived experience. The increasing recognition of the value of including people with lived experience on governmental task forces and policy committees provide further avenues for those individuals who wish to utilize their experiences in contributing to system change and effectiveness.

## Direct Psychiatric Services

To this point, our attention has been how key recovery principles apply in the overall care of psychiatric inpatients, with particular attention to those who have been admitted involuntarily or on forensic status. The psychiatrist is an essential member of the treatment team, if not the assigned leader of the team with responsibility for the overall treatment plan. For inpatient treatment to be effective a consistent, shared commitment to and understanding of how the recovery principles will be implemented and how they intersect with the clinical risk management required for individuals admitted on the basis of behavior deemed dangerous to themselves or others. However, psychiatrists have tasks and responsibilities that are not shared with other professionals. These typically include admission, diagnosis, prescribing medications, monitoring for side effects and medication risks, ordering emergency interventions, and discharge. In addition, the psychiatrist will make decisions, render opinions, or make recommendations to the Court regarding an individual's capacity to make informed decisions related to their treatment.

### Admission

In the case of involuntarily admitted individuals, the actual decision to admit the person is typically made by others, particularly for state hospitals. Thus, the psychiatrist is receiving the individual for treatment rather than making a decision to admit the person. The admission process varies across facilities, sometimes encompassing several physician assessments so the discussion will relate to the overall process rather than specific details. There are a number of points to be made as to the integration of the basic admission assessment process with key recovery-oriented principles. Some, like other points made above, may seem so commonplace or part of standard practice that their mention is unnecessary. However, their conscious inclusion mitigates taking them for granted or assuming that they are necessarily incorporated on a consistent basis. Depending upon the individual's clinical condition and the circumstances with which they arrive more or less information may be reliably obtained proximate to the time of admission. Nonetheless, it is important to create an opportunity for the interaction and information to be productive, if not satisfying, for the individual to the greatest extent possible. Our job, while collecting the required information as completely as circumstances permit, is to convey, as well as possible, that the hospital is a safe place where individuals are respected, helped, and involved in their treatment. Finally, it is a place from which everyone is expected to be discharged with the goal of living successfully in the community.

The physician assessment will be one of the first interactions for the individual once they arrive. As such, attention is necessary to convey respect and hope as well as creating an opportunity for interpersonal connection and providing choices when possible. Examples of choice might include asking for their preferred name, offering a choice of two chairs to sit in, asking whether they would like a drink of water or to use the restroom prior to beginning, and so forth. It may be helpful to explain that this is a treatment facility and what the next several steps in the admission process will be. Individual capacity for hearing or exchanging information will obviously vary based on the individual, their clinical status at the time of admission, the immediate circumstances of the admission, and a number of other factors. Clinical judgment will dictate the specific means by which to attempt to establish the recovery principles so long as the physician understands this is an important part of the admission process.

The physician must identify any immediate risks to the individual or others. While attention will be paid to behavioral risks, this assessment must include medical risks as well. It is a simple notion, but in the same way that there can be no recovery after suicide, there can be no recovery after a death from a medical complication either. Again, the care with which this is done conveys value and respect in addition to addressing the task at hand with due medical diligence.

In the recovery literature value is placed on the telling of one's personal narrative. Recognition of this fact may allow the physician to combine the taking of the psychiatric and medical history with some opportunity for the individual to tell their story. As a practical matter, time will not permit more than a portion of the narrative, but the impression made by a professional listening with interest and attention can be significant and contribute to restarting (or starting) the recovery process.

The final point would be, in addition to beginning the process of identifying an individual's personal strengths, to try to solicit where the person wishes to go after discharge and whatever details may emerge efficiently from that discussion. This not only begins building the information required for a full, holistic assessment, but also conveys that the individual will get better and leave the hospital. This latter message may get conveyed even if the responses are infected with delusions or other psychotic symptoms.

## Diagnosis

From a clinical standpoint in a recovery-oriented service, the essential importance of making the proper diagnosis is that medications are approved by the Federal Drug Administration primarily for diagnostic indications. It may also serve as a starting point for educational activities for the individual or family related to the individual's condition. As with medication practices and the monitoring of risks, it is a measure of respect as well as the standard of practice to collect the requisite information and integrate that information into the assignment of the proper diagnosis. Furthermore, when the diagnosis is unclear, it is required to take steps to clarify the diagnosis through further observation, the collection of more history from other sources, the review of prior records, or the utilization of psychological or laboratory testing.

As already noted in different fashion, a diagnosis describes an illness or condition, not a person. The diagnosis is not the person any more than another individual is simply a "hypertensive", "diabetic", or "arthritic". Our task is to attempt to align with the individual to treat or manage the symptoms that they are experiencing, which have resulted in their suffering or impeded their ability to live a satisfying life in the community. This essential point was made at a recent presentation regarding multi-dimensional efforts to prevent psychosis in young people. The presenter noted that, "in the end, it was not so important whether psychosis was prevented so long as the adolescent's life stayed on its expected trajectory" (Sale 2015). Our purpose is to help the individual get their life on track with treatment of the symptoms of a particular diagnosis subsumed in service of that overarching goal.

## Capacity for Treatment Decisions

With the priority given to empower individuals to take control of their treatment, it is perhaps understandable to find psychiatrists relying on assent for willing patients, despite a lack of true capacity, believing that doing so satisfies this priority. Unfortunately, this practice constitutes a medical-legal risk should complications develop and provides the individual "control" only so long as they go along with the psychiatrist's plan to "control their behavior". Too often, should the individual decide to refuse treatment, another assessment is made concluding that they now lack the capacity for such decisions. The clinical-legal process of assuring that a person able to weigh the risks and benefits of treatment is making decisions for the individual is intended as a protection of an individual who is unable to do so. In the situation of using assent as a replacement for consent, the intended protection may be subverted into a coercive process. Furthermore, it does not constitute the kind of active, bilateral engagement in treatment planning or treatment that promotes genuine partnership and, ultimately, ownership. At worst, it can be the equivalent of treatment teams that make sure the individual signs the treatment plan at the end of each review, whether there has been any evidence of the individual participating in the process or not. Failing to clearly address a lack of capacity when it exists will typically delay treatment, cause medication treatment to be sub-therapeutic and, at times, increase the chances that the individual will engage in dangerous behavior, prolonging their hospitalization and reducing their placement options in the community.

Recovery-oriented treatment does not require clinical or legal standards to be attenuated. It does require that treatment efforts be made to help an individual who lacks capacity regain such capacity so that they can make decisions regarding their care. Such efforts may include medications, education related to medications, other treatments, and side effects as well as rehabilitative activities to improve problem-solving or cognitive skills. At the same time it is important for the individual to participate in the processes designing their care, to have the opportunity to make other choices, for staff to highlight those choices as discussed above, and to participate in activities that facilitate decision-making skills. Allowing the individual to express their preference, engaging them in discussions related to their treatment, and providing information about their treatment are all actions that continue despite a formal lack of capacity and treatment decisions being made by others. Recovery is not a matter of pretending, but of a relentless lack of acceptance that the inpatient status quo is "all there is" and persistence in trying to help the individual develop the skills and symptom stability to live in the community.

Once an individual regains capacity for some or all of the relevant treatment decisions such decision-making must be restored to them in a timely fashion. In addition, such achievement should be recognized and used to facilitate other clinical gains necessary for returning successfully to the community.

## Medications

Virtually all of the individuals who are admitted involuntarily will need medication in order to treat their illness or otherwise mitigate symptoms of distress that are impeding their ability to live in a community setting. This reality makes the prescription of medications and ongoing attention to medication risks and side effects a critical function for psychiatrists, physicians, and other prescribers. Medication nonadherence is a substantial problem in all fields of medicine, including psychiatry (Brown and Bussell 2011; Nockowitz 1998).

Practitioners are well aware of this reality, but the focus is often on the reasons individuals do not adhere to the prescribed regimens (Peselow 2007; Zygmunt et al. 2002). In such discussions, attention is consistently given to the complexity of the regimen, side effects, and lack of apparent ill effect when medications are not taken. While interventions have included education, family support, simplifying medication regimens, and managing stress, an important question from a recovery orientation standpoint is, "why would the individual want to take the medication as prescribed?" The medication benefits and risks must help the individual achieve or maintain important aspects of their lives such as work, relationships, feeling better, or relief of distress.

For some problems and medications, the consequences of not taking the medicine are more consistently immediate, e.g., pain medications and hypnotics. In such situations, adherence is likely to be more reliable so long as the medication is needed. However, with many medications, for many people, not taking a prescribed agent makes no readily discernable difference on a day-to-day, week-to-week basis. Most individuals do not notice an increase in their cholesterol level or blood pressure from a symptomatic standpoint. Individuals with bipolar disorder or a recurrent depression are likely to be able to go extended periods of time off of medication without notice.

Given that individuals outside of hospital settings are largely free to choose whether and when to take their prescribed medications, it is important that medications help the individual achieve or maintain things that are important to them, and for them to understand and maintain awareness of how the medication relates to those dimensions of their lives. Being able to work, maintain good relationships with friends and family, and enjoy pleasurable activities as well as avoid losses or disruptions in these areas, future hospitalizations, debts, or legal charges relate more directly to why an individual would choose to adhere to a medication (and any other) treatment regimen. While most people will take medications in a hospital setting in order to "get out", relieve their immediate distress, or because "everyone else does," these motivations will be of little value after discharge. Thus, aside from that group of people who will faithfully do "whatever the Doctor says", if there is no clear reason that would motivate a person to take the medication, it is unlikely that they will consistently do so over time. Telling a person to take their medications because "I said so" or "the Doctor said so" will be insufficient for many people. Likewise, the idea that the medication should be taken to treat "the illness" may be similarly limited in effect. The essential point is that medication is more likely to be taken when doing so helps an individual meet their personal recovery goals and the linkage between the medication and achieving or maintaining those goals must be at the center of medication treatment.

In this context, there are four particular aspects to prescribing medication in a recovery-oriented manner, not including decisions related to emergency treatment that will be discussed below. First, he prescriber is charged with addressing two, often congruent, objectives with medication treatment. Medications are generally approved by the FDA for diagnostic indications. Thus, in addition to diagnostic fidelity, the medication must be prescribed for an approved indication or deployed "off label" by providing a documented justification based on the literature, specific pharmacological effects, or experience consistent with the standard of professional practice. At the same time, medications need to be prescribed with the goal of success in the community as operationalized for each person. In most cases, relieving the symptoms of an illness resulting in an involuntary admission or legal charges will provide a foundation for making use of other treatments and a path to returning to the community. The two cases below contrast situations in which the successful treatment of the illness per se produced problems for the individual in "real life" in relation to a recovery model of care.

Sarah is a woman in her late thirties who experienced moderately severe anxiety, depression, and poor sleep leading to suicidal thoughts. She was successfully treated with a combination of an antidepressant and benzodiazepine, but complained of ongoing mild sedation and cognitive slowing that prevented her from completing her work tasks as a newspaper editor and engaging in her previous exercise program resulting in some weight gain. Her treatment was changed to feature a gradual discontinuation of the benzodiapine, with an expedited engagement in mindfulness activities and Cognitive Behavioral Therapy as well as changing jobs to go to work as a magazine editor with less rigorous day-to-day deadlines. With these changes she re-engaged her exercise routines and felt that she had achieved the recovery she desired.

In contrast to Sarah, 30 years ago, Sergio was a young man attempting to develop a career as a pianist when he developed severe symptoms of Schizophrenia accompanied by agitated and aggressive behavior leading to an involuntary hospitalization. He adamantly opposed any treatment with antipsychotic medications due to their effect on his fine motor coordination as this was essential to his being able to play at the level required. He was eventually treated, his symptoms were substantially attenuated, and he was discharged. Unfortunately, no discussion was held regarding the impact of the successful treatment of his illness on his occupational goals.

Each clinical situation is different, but when presented with the problem of being unable to meet both diagnostic and recovery goals at the same time the psychiatrist should: (1) attend to the individual's immediate safety first, (2) treat the illness so as to restore the individual to full decision-making capacity, and then (3) collaborate with the individual on the potential strategies to both treat the illness and achieve the individual's recovery goals. Ultimately, the issue is treatment for a life rather than simply treating an illness recognizing that this process will often require effort after the individual leaves the inpatient setting.

The second intersection between recovery-oriented treatment and medications relates to medication risks and side effects. It is a demonstrable measure of respect to practice at the standard of care in terms of medication risks, and to manifest interest and commitment to working with individuals on side effects that may develop during treatment. This is straightforward with some medications and risks. It is required that white blood cell counts be regularly monitored with clozapine, thus leukopenia can hardly be missed. Likewise, an acute dystonic reaction presents with an urgency that cannot be ignored. However, other monitors require the practitioner to order, conduct, or review at the appropriate frequency, typically defined in the hospital's medication guidelines. Still others, such as weight, BMI, mild cognitive effects, constipation, or restlessness, require unit staff to observe and communicate in order to be effective. This requires the prescriber to communicate with staff and attend to their reports in a timely way to reinforce the integrity of the monitoring system. Attention must be paid to side effects, such as weight gain without laboratory evidence of metabolic consequence or the sometimes subtle cognitive slowing that occurs with a number of psychotropic agents, that may compromise an individual's confidence or feeling about themselves without yet posing a health risk to the individual. The psychiatrist must demonstrate a willingness to discuss these less critical side effects with the individual and make adjustments as necessary. Practicing safe medicine and discussing both positive and negative treatment developments are tangible demonstrations of respect, in addition to being the standard of care.

The third intersection involving medications and recovery relates to the necessity of assuring the integration of medications with behavioral treatment and/or other interventions. This intersection may be more subtle than the others as it relates primarily to making sure that treatment is efficient and that it facilitates the individual achieving treatment objectives to improve confidence and reinforce personal control. For example, with an individual with psychotic symptoms who has a behavior plan for recurrent aggression, it is necessary to assure that the medication treatment is optimized to prevent psychotically driven aggression from impeding the effectiveness of the reinforcement strategy. In another example,

> Sam was an individual with a number of positive and negative symptoms of Schizophrenia hospitalized for the restoration of competency who was identified for case review due to a pattern of staying in bed all morning and missing all of the groups designed to aid in the restoration. Upon review it was clear that his meeting treatment objectives related to group attendance and identifying the roles of various Court officials were being impeded by large bedtime doses of olanzapine initiated consequent to agitation and poor sleep at the time of admission a number of weeks ago. Having made significant clinical improvement with respect to his psychotic symptoms and agitation he had become more sedated, particularly in the mornings when the seminal groups were being held. By making medication adjustments it became possible for him to more consistently (and alertly) attend his groups and make progress toward his restoration goals.

The fourth intersection applies when the inpatient formulary does not match the formulary within the jail or community service in which the individual will receive services after discharge. It also relates to individuals who have Medicare Part D coverage and may have limitations related to their specific Prescription Drug Plan. Unless there are clinical contraindications or other clear reasons to do otherwise the prescriber should utilize medication(s) that will be available after discharge because success after discharge is the preferred purpose of inpatient treatment. To use a medication that will not be available sets up a risk after discharge that the new medication will be ineffective and result in a relapse. Alternatively, the need to change medications prior to discharge to assure that symptom control can be maintained results in a longer length of stay, delaying the individual's return to the community. Neither is consistent with recovery-oriented treatment unless there are strong, competing reasons to do so. That said, when an individual is severely ill and suffering, and does not appear to have responded to medications that would be available after discharge, the priority becomes helping the individual improve symptomatically so that they can fully participate in their treatment decisions. At that point the prescriber can collaborate with the individual on the best course to take. It can also be that the individual, having capacity or not, expresses a strong preference for a particular agent or is unwilling to take any of the to be available agents. Each situation is different, but in such circumstances it can be helpful to reinforce the individual's choice, avoid the potential conflicts related to a different agent that may compromise the therapeutic connection, and expedite the individual improving. Doing so has the potential to provide a much better foundation for the subsequent discussion regarding what medication may be available after discharge and how to address that issue.

A final point related to medications, particularly for individuals with more severe conditions whose symptoms have responded inadequately to standard medication trials and doses, is the need to keep trying to achieve adequate symptom relief until all safe means have been attempted. It is not acceptable to allow a person to remain an inpatient for extended periods of time without making available medication changes to try to help them achieve discharge. The difficulty lies in maintaining appropriate attention to medication risks while continuing to try new agents and combinations to achieve symptom reduction. Central to practicing in this tertiary fashion is identifying target symptoms and measures of success. Too often, in such situations, one medication is added to another, and then another, absent clear evidence of effectiveness or eliminating medications that lack such evidence. The ultimate result is a complicated medication regimen of inadequate effectiveness, thereby exposing the individual to all applicable risks in return for limited benefit. Thus, it is essential to identify the target symptoms for the medication trial in advance so that the effect can be measured against the desired benefit. If a medication trial does not address the target symptoms effectively then the medicine can be discontinued and another trial instituted. When a new agent is added to a combination of agents successfully, then attention needs to be paid to whether agents in the prior regimen can be withdrawn. The task is that of providing aggressive medication treatment when such is necessary, as well as providing a reasonable opportunity for success after discharge without lapsing into unnecessary polypharmacy that exposes the individual to untoward risks without discernable benefit.

Rachel is an individual in her early sixties who has been hospitalized for more than a decade under an NGRI order. She has persistent symptoms of paranoia and thought disorganization as well as chronic delusions that impede her ability to make any progress toward Conditional Release or rationally discuss discharge in any fashion. In consultation with the treatment team it became apparent that she has been on fluphenazine decanoate for more than seven years because she "refuses" to take anything else. Even though she is not her own decision-maker, the team did not want to "put her through" the possibility of receiving a different medication over objection.

Unfortunately, this thinking had the effect of sentencing Rachel to life in the hospital, as she clearly could not progress through the NGRI system in the clinical condition she had at present. What the psychiatrist needed to do was identify some of the agents not yet tried (examining the risks in the context of Rachel's current medication conditions), engage the treatment team in how to best work with Rachel to take it, secure consent from her decision maker, and proceed to try to achieve better symptom control.

## Medications in an Emergency

The final intersection between medications and recovery-oriented treatment features the most potential conflict. This is the relatively infrequent need to "force" medication. The circumstances in which medications can be given against an individual's will are the subject of regulations and law, which govern the specific details and vary by setting and state. Given that one of the original strands leading to the modern recovery principles derived from the anti-medication, anti-psychiatry movement, and the much broader importance of choice as a patient right and precursor of the kind of ownership for managing one's illness, the objections to forced medication are readily apparent. Indeed, there are but two exceptions in clinical practice to the general preclusion of medicating a person against their will aside from the Sell decision relating to legal provisions regarding the administration of medication to restore an individual's competency to participate in criminal justice proceeding of compelling interest to the state.

The first, and clearest exception, involves emergency situations in which the safety of the individual or others is in immediate jeopardy and, in the judgment of the physician, medication is required to mitigate that danger. Recovery is not served by an individual harming themselves and it is also not served by them harming others. If a serious injury should occur, there is the additional trauma, the likelihood of remorse, and the reality that future choices regarding placement, work, access to programs, and relationships can be compromised by aggressive actions. Depending on the individual's capacity and motivation legal charges may ensue, further limiting future choices while burdening the recovery process. Any of these developments can complicate the dimensions of hope, connection, and purpose as the individual goes forward. If the hospital has established a recovery-oriented treatment environment, then the potential harm to the recovery process can be mitigated. If the environment is demonstrated to be unsafe, then the maintenance of a recovery orientation is deeply compromised.

The second exception is less clear, may depend on whether the objection is verbal or physical, obviously requires that the individual lack capacity and, in some locations, may be precluded by regulations. However, in the circumstance in which an individual who lacks capacity presents with such symptoms that discharge is impossible, alternative strategies to persuade or reinforce taking indicated medications have been attempted and failed, and there is a reasonable likelihood that medication treatment will produce sufficient symptom relief to allow progress toward discharge and/or mitigate the risk of future aggression or self-injury, it is reasonable to pursue treatment over objection. When the lack of medication treatment is essentially the equivalent of a permanent sentence to inpatient commitment, likely at some risk to the individual or others, for an individual deemed incapable of making a choice based upon the rational assessment of risks and benefits, such a course is inconsistent with the concept of recovery. It is also inconsistent with the broader purpose of inpatient care to provide the individual an opportunity to live more successfully in the community after discharge.

## Discharge

Psychiatrists or other physicians are responsible for writing the discharge order so that an individual may officially leave the hospital. As a practical matter, with exceptions for discharges driven by Court decisions, the discharging physician will bear the liability that goes with a discharge and, thus, must be satisfied that the discharge is a safe and appropriate one. However, the discharge will typically be the result of the efforts of a number of individuals, will reflect an improvement in symptoms as manifested in a reduction in behavior of risk to the individual or others, will be based in an aftercare plan and placement assessed to be sufficient for the individual's immediate and, perhaps, ongoing needs for treatment, supervision, and support.

When an individual who has been civilly committed can or must be discharged derive from local and state laws and regulations, the available community resources, and work processes as developed for the system in which the individual is being discharged to and from. Despite the variations this involves from one place to another there are some common provisions within discharge planning and discharge that should be present in a recovery-oriented service.

As a matter of respect, self-determination, and hope, it should be made clear to the individual, in language that he can understand what he must do or avoid doing in order to be discharged. This "discharge criteria" should serve to focus the individual and the treatment providers as to what needs to be accomplished during the hospitalization. It should be examined in the context of what is necessary for the individual to be able to do or avoid in order to have an opportunity to live successfully in the community.

Discharge criteria should not describe what the staff will do in order to accomplish the discharge. The criteria should be shaped by the anticipated discharge placement and aftercare services to be provided. For example, an individual whose anticipated placement is a group home with 24/7 supervision and medication administration services does not need to learn to self-administer his medications as a criteria for discharge. An individual returning to live alone in his own apartment may not need to demonstrate an ability to socialize with others. The criteria are likely to be different for an individual leaving to go to an apartment versus one leaving to go to a group home or adult home as these destinations are likely to require different capabilities in order to be successful. It is beyond the scope of this chapter to review discharge planning, but it is essential that the individual know what is expected in order to be discharged, that the discharge criteria be individualized to the person, that they reflect what the individual needs to be able to do or avoid in order to be successful in the community after discharge and that the discharge takes place in a timely fashion upon the individual meeting the discharge criteria. Such a process provides respect, an opportunity to exert and be reinforced for exerting personal choice and control, and establishes a pathway that can help establish and reinforce hope.

## Treatment Team Work Processes and Recovery

Psychiatrists are commonly designated to provide leadership to the treatment team, typically without any real supervisory authority for any of the team members. Many books have been written about leadership, reflecting an inherent elusiveness in our ability to describe and teach what appears to come very naturally to a few (e.g., Collins 2001; Kouzes and Posner 2007). Our focus with this chapter is, fortunately, much more narrow and limited to constructing and maintaining a recovery-oriented treatment environment. To this end, the psychiatrist, as well as other professionals, needs to manifest active attention on the recovery principles of hope, purpose, respect, interpersonal connection, choice, sensitivity to trauma while providing the assessments and treatment necessary to provide the individual an opportunity to be successful in the community after discharge. This attention to recovery principles should also manifest in the working relationships among team members and direct care staff, and in the various meetings necessary to conduct the team's work. It is difficult, if not impossible to produce a recovery-oriented treatment environment absent a recovery-oriented culture that extends into the work environment. It is beyond the scope of this chapter to address the many dimensions of the work environment or the working relationships among various staff members, however, "meeting behavior" is so essential that a paragraph on meetings in relationship to recovery is necessary.

Treatment team meetings are an essential aspect of work in a psychiatric hospital. The manner and spirit with which they are conducted should reflect the same recovery orientation with which treatment is to be conducted. The demonstrable mindset is that the team can help the individual get better and that hope for symptom improvement and success after discharge is possible for each individual. For any particular individual, "getting better" will have its own unique characteristics shaped by the relevant clinical symptoms, behaviors, stresses, strengths, goals, and legal requirements of the hospitalization. Likewise, how the individual would assess or define success after discharge will vary for each case. It is then logically consistent that how a given treatment team will demonstrate their ongoing commitment to recovery principles will be unique as well in order for the commitment to manifest its genuineness or authenticity for any individual. However, within such singularity there are some commonalities. These would include, but not be limited to: an opportunity to participate and contribute to the assessment and treatment of the individuals on their unit, to have an opportunity to provide input to decisions related to individual treatment and the operation of the treatment unit, to have their time respected and not wasted in the conduct of meetings, rounds, or required work duties, and to not be subject to or traumatized by unreasonable job stresses, fear, exposure, or humiliation. As with individuals, there must be the hope that problems, however difficult, can be mitigated if not solved. Ideally, the larger organization allows for the career advancement and encourages such improvement to provide additional dimensions of hope and choice for staff. Creating an environment that seeks to learn from incidents and misfortune rather than blame is the parallel to creating a path for recovery in individual treatment.

Psychiatrists, other professionals and physicians have a substantial influence on the day-to-day, week-to-week environment in which individuals are treated and staff members work. For this environment to support a recovery orientation for treatment, it must support the equivalent orientation in the work processes and working relationships.

## Psychiatrist Administrators

For some psychiatrists, there are administrative or supervisory responsibilities that impact upon the hospital at large, e.g., Medical Directors, Unit Medical Directors, Chiefs of Staff, and Medical Staff Presidents. The nature of the specific position will determine the extent to which the administrative psychiatrist has direct authority over the clinical operation of the hospital or is simply in a position of influence within the hospital's over all administration. Through the avenues available to them, their efforts and/or influence need to be aligned toward several particular objectives to facilitate a recovery-oriented environment and culture.

First, the vision for a recovery-oriented service needs to drive the development and implementation of policies and procedures so that the policies and practices support recovery principles. This begins with the hospital having a goal of success in the community after discharge for each individual admitted and carries through all of the work processes necessary to accomplish that. Second, they need to help establish a professional and work environment that provides the parallel recovery principles for staff members at each level. Third, they must help hospital administration face directly the difficulties possible when recovery principles intersect with clinical risks so that the necessary clinical practices are consistently and coherently applied. Fourth, the general and specific training to all staff members must reflect the integration of recovery principles into the safety and operational responsibilities of the hospital. Efforts must be made to assure that staff demonstrate on a consistent basis the lessons of such training. Fifth, the psychiatrist must help the hospital have an operational paradigm of learning first and blaming only when thorough examination requires it. Incidents, deaths, and trends in quality or risk measures all provide opportunities to learn and improve. While the multiple regulatory requirements can risk making such exercises bureaucratic, if not perfunctory, the principle of learning and improving applies as well to organizations as to individuals in recovery. Finally, the requisite budget processes within a hospital need to reflect the priorities that are driving the clinical operation in a recovery based direction. The overall objective is that, despite the stresses that accompany the operation of a state or publically funded community hospital, the hospital's mission, recovery orientation, work environment, and budget processes are cohesive and aligned with producing success in the community for those individuals admitted to the facility.

## References


Anthony, W., Cohen, M., Farkas, M., & Gagne, C. (2002). *Psychiatric rehabilitation* (2nd ed.). Boston, MA: Center for Psychiatric Rehabilitation, Boston University.

Anthony, W., & Farkas, M. (2012). *The essential guide to psychiatric rehabilitation practice*. Boston, MA: Boston University Press.

Barber, J. (2007). *Recovery plan in response to Inspector General*. Staunton, VA: Western State Hospital.

Bellack, A. S. (2006). Scientific and consumer models of recovery in schizophrenia: Concordance, contrasts, and implications. *Schizophrenia Bulletin, 32*, 432–442.

Brown, M., & Bussell, J. (2011). Medication adherence: WHO cares! *Mayo Clinic Proceedings, 86*(4), 304–314.

Collins, J. (2001). *Good to great*. New York, NY: HarperBusiness.

Davidson, L., O'Connell, M. O., Tondora, J., Styron, T., & Kangas, K. (2006). The top ten concerns about recovery encountered in mental health system transformation. *Psychiatric Services, 57*, 640–645.

Grubaugh, A. L., Zinzow, H. M., Paul, L., Egede, L. E., & Frueh, B. C. (2011). Trauma exposure and posttraumatic stress disorder in adults with severe mental illness: A critical review. *Clinical Psychology Review, 31*, 883–899.

Hillbrand, M., Young, J. L., & Griffith, E. E. (2010). Managing risk and recovery: Redefining miscibility of oil and water. *Journal of the American Academy of Psychiatry and the Law, 38*, 452–456.

Kouzes, J. M., & Posner, B. Z. (2007). *The leadership challenge*. New York, NY: Wiley.

Lakeman, R. (2010). Mental health recovery competencies for mental health workers: A Delphi study. *Journal of Mental Health, 19*(1), 62–74.

Liberman, R. (2008). *Recovery from disability: Manual of psychiatric rehabilitation*. Washington, DC: American Psychiatric Publishing.

Mountain, D., & Shah, P. J. (2008). Recovery and the medical model. *Advances in Psychiatric Treatment, 14* (4), 241–244.

Nelson, G., Ochocka, J., Janzen, R., & Trainor, J. (2006). A longitudinal study of mental health consumer/survivor initiatives: Part 1—Literature review and overview of the study. *Journal of Community Psychology, 34*(3), 247–260.

Nelson, G., Ochocka, J., Janzen, R., Trainor, J., Goering, P., & Lomorey, J. (2007). A longitudinal study of mental health consumer/survivor initiatives: Part V—Outcomes at 3-year follow-up. *Journal of Community Psychology, 35*(5), 655–665.

Nockowitz, R. (1998). Enhancing patient adherence with treatment recommendations. In J. B. Herman, P. L. Slavin, & T. A. Stern (Eds.), *The MGH guide to psychiatry in primary care* (pp. 565–574). New York, NY: McGraw Hill.

Parks, J., Radke, A. Q., & Haupt, M. B. (2014). *The vital role of state psychiatric hospitals*. Alexandria, VA: National Association of State Mental Health Program Directors.

Peselow, E. D. (2007). Adherence with respect to medication management. *Primary Psychiatry, 14*(7), 83–89.

Repper, J., & Carter, T. (2011). A review of the literature on peer support in mental health services. *Journal of Mental Health, 20*(4), 392–411.

Roberts, G., & Wolfson, P. (2004). The rediscovery of recovery: Open to all. *Advances in Psychiatric Treatment, 10*, 37–48.

Sale, T. (2015). *Preventing psychosis in young people*. National Council for Behavioral Health Conference, April, 2015.

Simpson, A. I. F., & Penney, S. R. (2011). The recovery paradigm in forensic mental health services. *Criminal Behavior and Mental Health, 21*, 299–306.

Singh, N. N., Lancioni, G. E., Karazsia, B. T., Myers, R. E., Winton, A. S. W., Latham, L. L., & Nugent, K. (2015). Effects of training staff in MBPBS on the use of physical restraints, staff stress and turnover, staff and peer injuries, and cost effectiveness in developmental disabilities. *Mindfulness, 6*, 926–937.

Singh, N. N., Lancioni, G. E., Winton, A. S. W., Singh, A. N., & Adkins, A. D. (2009). Mindful staff can reduce the use of physical restraints when providing care to individuals with intellectual disabilities. *Journal of Applied Research in Intellectual Disabilities, 22*, 194–202.

Substance Abuse and Mental Health Services Administration. (2006). *National consensus statement on mental health and recovery*. Rockville, MD: Author.

Substance Abuse and Mental Health Services Administration. (2011). *Recovery to practice: Most frequently asked questions* (July, 2011).

Substance Abuse and Mental Health Services Administration. (2014). *Trauma-informed care in behavioral health services*. Rockville, MD: Author.

Szasz, Thomas S. (1974). The Myth of Mental Illness: Foundations of a Theory of Personal Conduct. New York: Harper & Row.

The Presidents New Freedom Commission. (2003). *Achieving the promise, transforming mental health care in America*. Rockville, MD: Author.

Van Orden, K. A., White, T. K., Cukrowicz, K. C., Braithwaite, S., Selby, E. A., & Joiner, T. E. (2010). The interpersonal theory of suicide. *Psychology Review, 117*(2), 575–600.

Zygmunt, A., Olfson, M., Boyer, C., & Mechanic, D. (2002). Intervention to improve medication adherence in schizophrenia. *American Journal of Psychiatry, 159* (10), 653–664.

# 10 Psychological Services

Jeff Phillips

## Introduction

The practice of psychology in an inpatient psychiatric hospital is well suited to the recovery model. The recovery model's emphasis on viewing the person holistically, not as defined by his/her diagnoses, person-centered treatment, hope, wellness, respect, and striving to live a satisfying and meaningful life, are all consistent with the training and practice of psychology. Nevertheless, the inpatient psychiatric hospital presents challenges not so often found in the outpatient setting where psychologists have received much of their training and commonly practice. This chapter describes how the recovery model can be incorporated into the delivery of psychological services in inpatient psychiatric hospitals and some of the dilemmas psychologists encounter.

My reference for the inpatient setting is a state behavioral health hospital in which individuals are typically committed involuntarily on a civil or forensic status with lengths of stay ranging from weeks to months to years. This contrasts with psychiatric units in general hospitals where individuals are hospitalized for a relatively short time and often on a voluntary status. Not only is this the setting I am most familiar with, but it likely presents distinctive challenges and opportunities for psychologists to provide recovery-oriented treatment. There is a dearth of empirical studies on psychological services in inpatient psychiatric hospitals. Nevertheless, I hope that this chapter conveys some of the recovery-oriented services psychologists can offer to individuals with serious mental disorders in public behavioral health facilities.

To provide context for subsequent sections, this chapter begins with a brief description of the patient population and the public mental health hospital. This is not a common site for psychologists in their training or practice (Duffy et al. 2002; Michalski et al. 2011; Norcross et al. 2005). To those with limited experience in public inpatient psychiatric facilities, this description will provide an overview of the patient population and the hospital in which such individuals receive services. To those who already work in such facilities, this description should sound familiar. Following this overview, this chapter describes some of the services psychologists provide. Many of these are traditional services provided by psychologists in other clinical settings, but often need adaptation to the public mental health hospital. Finally, I discuss some of the challenges posed by the recovery model for psychologists working in inpatient psychiatric facilities.

J. Phillips (✉)
Department of Psychology, Western State Hospital,
103 Valley Center Drive, Staunton, VA 24401, USA
e-mail: Jeffrey.Phillips@dbhds.virginia.gov



N.N. Singh et al. (eds.), *Handbook of Recovery in Inpatient Psychiatry*,
Evidence-Based Practices in Behavioral Health, DOI 10.1007/978-3-319-40537-7_10

## Individuals Served and Clinical Setting

The state mental health hospital serves individuals with serious mental illnesses, often with co-occurring conditions, complex psychosocial needs, and limited resources. "Serious mental illness (SMI) is a diagnosable mental, behavioral, or emotional disorder … that results in serious functional impairment. These difficulties substantially interfere with a person's ability to carry out major life activities at home, at work, or in the community" (SAMHSA 2012, p. 10). Although a number of diagnoses fit this definition, common ones include schizophrenia spectrum disorders (notably Schizophrenia and Schizoaffective Disorder), severe mood disorders (such as Bipolar Disorder and Major Depressive Disorder, often with psychotic features), and personality disorders (in particular Borderline Personality Disorder and Antisocial Personality Disorder) (SAMHSA 2012). Substance use disorders commonly co-occur with these severe mental disorders (Bahorik et al. 2013; Fowler et al. 1998; Swartz et al. 2006) and an individual may experience more than one mental disorder. Intellectual Disabilities and Borderline Intellectual Functioning may be present along with a history of traumatic brain injury, all of which compromise cognitive abilities. Individuals with SMI commonly have a history of trauma (Grubaugh et al. 2011) and a high incidence of medical conditions (Parks et al. 2006; Saha et al. 2007). A large percentage of patients are hospitalized on a forensic status, and must concurrently address legal issues. Because many of these disorders have an onset in late adolescence or early adulthood, education, employment, social relationships, and family life are often disrupted. Thus, this population has serious mental disorders, often co-occurring mental or substance use disorders, medical conditions, legal problems, and limited resources, presenting many challenges to care.

Most individuals with SMI reside in the community, not inpatient facilities. For example, in 2009 just under 5% of U.S. adults aged 18 or older had a SMI in the past year representing approximately 11.0 million adults, and of these, 6.8 % received inpatient mental health services in the prior year (SAMSHA 2012). Thus, the individuals served in the public inpatient facility represent a small fraction of individuals with SMI, but they are often those with the most debilitating, treatment refractory, and complex issues.

Individuals admitted to an inpatient facility on a civil status (whether voluntary or involuntary), may have been treated first at a community hospital for several days or weeks, and then transferred because they were not sufficiently well to return to the community. Thus, the state hospital is often the last treatment alternative in the continuum of care. While commitment criteria vary from state to state, they commonly include dangerousness to self or others or an inability to care for oneself or protect oneself from harm. Individuals on a forensic status may be admitted directly to the state facility from a correctional center after having been charged with a criminal offense. They may be admitted for emergency treatment due to dangerousness to self or others, an evaluation of their competency to stand trial, restoration of their trial competency, or an evaluation of their mental state at the time of the alleged offense. Still others may be hospitalized after being adjudicated not guilty by reason of insanity.

Targets of treatment during hospitalization include symptoms associated with these serious mental disorders such as delusions, hallucinations, thought disorganization, negative symptoms, depression, mania, and anxiety; and the reasons leading to hospitalization such as dangerousness to self and others or an inability to care for oneself. While these are traditional areas to address during a hospitalization, and continue to be important, the recovery model considerably broadens the focus of care to include helping individuals assess their own recovery goals and to progress toward building or rebuilding personally satisfying and meaningful lives.

Length of stay in the hospital may range from weeks to years. Even with lengthy hospitalizations the goal is to help individuals return to the community in as independent a setting as is safely possible. Because of the long standing nature of many of these disorders, relapse and rehospitalization are common. Thus, with readmissions and sometimes lengthy hospitalizations, a psychologist may work with an individual over a significant portion of the person's lifetime.

The complexity facing individuals with SMI in an inpatient setting necessitates a multidisciplinary approach including staff members from psychology, psychiatry, nursing, social work, occupational therapy, primary care, and other disciplines. As such, psychologists work as members of a treatment team which may differ from their training and previous experience (Geczy and Cote 2002; Reddy et al. 2010). Psychologists need to be aware of the services provided by other disciplines, the perspectives those disciplines hold, and the responsibilities and authorities of each, all within a system of care with many interested parties within and outside the hospital (Wood et al. 1994).

## The Role of Psychologists in the Treatment of Individuals with Severe Mental Illness in Public Psychiatric Inpatient Hospitals

Despite important contributions by psychologists over the years, and a history of training and employment in settings serving individuals with SMI, currently psychologists are underrepresented in public psychiatry hospitals. In a survey of members of the American Psychological Association (Norcross et al. 2005), in 1960 45 % worked in settings that would likely treat individuals with SMI (psychiatric hospitals, general hospitals, and outpatient clinics). By 2003 the percentage had decreased to 13 %. The percentage working in psychiatric hospitals declined from 15 % in 1960 to 4 % in 2003. Some of this decline in employment in psychiatric hospitals may be attributable to the large reduction in psychiatric beds over this time; nevertheless, this low percentage contrasts considerably with other disciplines. For example, according to data from Duffy et al. (2002), 41.9 % of psychiatrists, 30.9 % of social workers, and 50.8 % of psychiatric nurses were primarily employed in hospitals and clinics compared to 15 % of psychologists. Comparable figures for mental health hospitals were 21 % for psychiatrists, 3.9 % for social workers, 9.9 % for psychiatric nurses, and 3.0 % for psychologists. As Levant et al. (2001) lamented, "Psychology does not currently play a major role in the treatment of persons with serious mental illnesses such as schizophrenia and other psychotic disorders, and is not an important presence in the public sector systems that provide most of their care. Although clinical psychology once specifically defined its purview as serious psychopathology, this area has largely been abandoned to psychiatrists and sub-doctoral personnel. This has been shortsighted for the profession and has not been in the best interest of persons with serious mental illnesses" (p. 81).

A number of reasons may account for this underrepresentation by psychologists in inpatient psychiatric hospitals. In their graduate training, students may have limited coursework and practica relevant to SMI or exposure to faculty for whom this is a primary interest (Hoge et al. 2000; Mueser et al. 2013; Reddy et al. 2010). Psychologists may adhere to outdated models of SMI, especially ones that overly emphasize a medical model, leading to the belief that psychological services are of little value (Roe et al. 2006; Smith et al. 1993). They may be unaware of the many contributions psychologists have made to the field, other models of SMI (including the recovery model), and evidence-based and best practices for SMI (e.g., American Psychological Association and Jansen 2014; APA/CAPP Task Force on Serious Mental Illness and Severe Emotional Disturbance 2007; Dixon et al. 2009; Mueser et al. 2003b; Silverstein et al. 2006b). Finally, psychologists may have a preference for working with individuals who have good insight, motivation, cognitive abilities, and verbal skills, and thus steer away from those with SMI (Roe et al. 2006).

With specific reference to public inpatient psychiatric facilities, psychologists may be discouraged by the problems they encounter (Geczy et al. 1990; Wood et al. 1994). Other disciplines, and even psychologists themselves, may question their level of clinical authority and effectiveness, and whether they have the requisite knowledge, skills, and abilities to practice independently, especially if the facility relies heavily on a medical or disease model. Limited resources, competition for scarce resources, and scrutiny and mandates by outside agencies (e.g., the Centers for Medicare and Medicaid Services, the Joint Commission, and the U.S. Department of Justice) can put considerable pressure on psychologists (and even more so on members of other disciplines) to justify their work and follow certain procedures. Psychologists may then find themselves doing a considerable amount of documentation rather than more satisfying tasks. For example, in one survey, psychologists working in state hospitals in the Midwest reported spending over 27 % of their time doing paperwork (Corrigan et al. 1998). The contributions of psychologists may be undervalued leading to difficulties effecting change within a facility such as implementing or maintaining innovative programs. For example, in Nebraska a long standing state of the art psychosocial rehabilitation program in a state hospital was closed despite good outcomes (e.g., reductions in aggression, discharge of individuals with long stays in the hospital) and being cost-effective (Spaulding et al. 2010; Tarasenko et al. 2013). In light of these trends and obstacles, some have called for revisions to the training of psychologists so that they are well prepared to work with persons with SMI (e.g., Mueser et al. 2013; Wood et al. 1994).

Despite these challenges, psychologists practicing in the public inpatient setting reap many rewards (Geczy and Sultenfuss 1994; Geczy et al. 1990). Psychologists can make significant contributions to the recovery of individuals with severe and debilitating disorders. Psychologists work with individuals from other disciplines who bring their own perspectives and expertise to a common mission. This provides camaraderie and support while dealing with the difficulties faced in this setting. The inpatient setting offers opportunities to supervise and train students and interns which is intellectually stimulating. Finally, public psychiatric hospitals offer flexibility and freedom for psychologists to pursue a variety of tasks such as clinical care, supervision, research, program and policy development, and leadership. With this background, I now turn to specific areas of psychological services provided in public inpatient psychiatric hospitals, how they relate to recovery-oriented principles, and some of the challenges psychologists encounter.

## Assessment

A good assessment is the foundation for treatment and clinical decision-making. Psychologists are well trained to perform assessments, and in a public psychiatric hospital psychologists assess many areas using a variety of methods. Many of these assessments predate the recovery movement; nonetheless, they can be performed in a recovery-oriented manner. For example, in order to provide good care, it is helpful to clarify diagnoses, symptoms, and personality characteristics that impact treatment. These are traditional areas of assessment for psychologists that might be accomplished using objective personality instruments such as the Personality Assessment Inventory (PAI; Morey 1997), the Minnesota Multiphasic Personality Inventory-2 (MMPI-2; Butcher et al. 2001), and the Millon Clinical Multiaxial Inventory-IV (MCMI-IV; Millon et al. 2015). For the most part, these instruments assess symptoms and problem areas, and hence focus on deficits rather than strengths. While the assessment of symptoms and personality characteristics can be very useful, psychologists using such instruments need to bear in mind this narrow focus and that the results do not provide a full assessment of an individual. In contrast, neuropsychological assessments have long been used to identify both strengths and weakness, and to help individuals use their strengths to compensate for their weaknesses (Medalia and Belucci 2012).

### Areas and Functions of Assessment

Psychological assessments help make differential diagnoses, describe current functioning, identify specific symptoms of mental disorders, assess personality characteristics, identify risk factors for harm to self and others, discern factors which mitigate risk, assess cognitive strengths and weaknesses, select therapeutic interventions, monitor change over time, and provide feedback as a therapeutic intervention (Meyer et al. 2001).

Psychological assessments help detect subtle thought disturbances, differentiate major mental disorders from personality disorders, and assess the manner in which personality characteristics impact treatment.

Given these long standing functions of psychological assessments, one may question the ways in which they are consistent with recovery-oriented principles. As noted by a number of writers, the concept of recovery includes the amelioration, if not elimination, of distressing symptoms that interfere with life goals, and having a meaningful life despite ongoing symptoms (e.g., Anthony 1993, Law and Morrison 2014). As such, accurate diagnoses and careful assessment of symptoms inform treatment. Furthermore, since recovery is expected to be nonlinear (Anthony 1993; Substance Abuse and Mental Health Services Administration 2006) and change is often slow, for a number of individuals in public psychiatric hospitals, psychological assessments can track subtle changes over time. Serial assessments document progress, and in doing so instill hope in individuals and their treatment teams. Finally, such assessments may be used therapeutically (Finn and Tonsager 1997; Poston and Hanson 2010). For example, while objective personality tests use fixed choices (e.g., true/false) for standardization, such a format does not allow individuals to qualify their answers. Discussing the overall test results and answers to specific questions can form the basis for therapeutic sessions. With self-report measures, this gives individuals the opportunity to disclose and learn more about themselves. Being better informed helps individuals be more involved in their treatment. For example, I worked with an adolescent woman who had been hospitalized for some time with Borderline Personality Disorder and frequently engaged in self-harm and aggression. In discussing Borderline Personality Disorder, not only did she find many of the characteristics descriptive of her, but she reported some reassurance in knowing that others have had similar experiences and were able to recover (Gunderson et al. 2011, Zanarini et al. 2012).

Because many traditional assessment instruments focus on symptoms and deficits, personal strengths can be overlooked when relying solely on these measures. Strengths should be incorporated into treatment plans and help the individual and treatment providers focus on behaviors to enhance, not just behaviors to suppress. A strengths based approach is especially well suited for positive behavior support plans which reinforce replacement behaviors. Identifying strengths can be done in an interview or with questionnaires, for example, by asking about goals that provide motivation for treatment, sources of support, interests, reasons for living, skills, religious beliefs, and so on.

Assessing the risk of self-harm and violence is especially germane in the public psychiatric facility because these risks are often the basis for persons being committed to the hospital. In terms of recovery, risk assessment is especially important as there can be tension between recovery-oriented principles such as autonomy, on the one hand, and the prevention of serious harm to self or others, on the other (Hillbrand et al. 2010; Pouncey and Lukens 2010). Many risk assessment instruments exist (e.g., the Broset Violence Checklist, Almvik and Woods 1998; the Classification of Violence Risk based on the MacArthur Violence Risk Assessment Study, Monahan et al. 2001; Fazel et al. 2012; the Historical, Clinical, Risk Management-20 version 3, Douglas et al. 2013; the Columbia-Suicide Severity Rating Scale, Posner et al. 2008). These instruments help determine a person's level of risk, factors that increase risk, protective or mitigating factors, and dynamic risk factors to focus on in treatment. Thus, these assessments aid in making decisions about precautions needed to protect the person or others from harm (e.g., one to one, constant, or direct observation), the selection of treatments to reduce risk (e.g., anger management or substance abuse treatment), and reassessing risk over time.

## Assessment Methods

As in outpatient settings, psychologists in public inpatient psychiatric facilities have a wide array of methods available to assess the above areas. Objective personality tests, projective measures (e.g., Rorschach Inkblot Test), intelligence tests, and neuropsychological tests are well known to psychologists in both inpatient and outpatient settings, and it is beyond the purview of this chapter to review these. However, I briefly comment below on a few assessment methods that are especially relevant to the inpatient psychiatric facility even though they are not unique to this setting.

Clinician administered rating scales and behavioral observations are especially helpful as supplements to or substitutes for self-report measures. They may be useful when working with individuals who have limited insight or who may have reasons for not being forthright, such as individuals with legal charges who wish to remain in a hospital rather than return to jail, or individuals with a high level of suspiciousness. Even though such individuals may decline most forms of assessment, clinicians still have an obligation to conduct assessments and provide treatment. Rating scales and observations can be useful in these situations. Examples of clinician administered rating scales include the Brief Psychiatric Rating Scale (BPRS; Lukoff et al. 1986) and the Positive and Negative Syndrome Scale (PANSS; Kay et al. 1987) for multidimensional symptoms, the PSYRATS (Haddock et al. 1999) for hallucinations and delusions, and the Young Mania Rating Scale (Young et al. 1978) for symptoms of mania.

Behavioral assessments, functional analyses, and functional assessments assist in describing challenging behaviors, specifying treatment goals, identifying hypothesized casual variables, selecting interventions, and monitoring treatment outcomes (Haynes et al. 1997; Iwata and Dozier 2008). Although functional analyses, in which hypothesized causal variables are experimentally manipulated, may be difficult to implement in inpatient psychiatric facilities, functional assessment methods can be useful. Interview based instruments, such as the Questions About Behavioral Function in Mental Illness (QABF-MI; Singh et al. 2006) and the Functional Assessment Interview (FAI; O'Neill et al. 1997), identify antecedents to and consequences of challenging behaviors and guide treatment. Similarly, using reinforcer checklists with patients or staff members who know the patient well can identify items or activities to use as reinforcers for replacement behaviors.

Because direct care staff members spend much time with patients in different settings within the hospital, they are important sources of behavioral observations. Behavioral observations can be complex as when an extensive array of behaviors are targeted (e.g., in some token economy systems; Paul and Lentz 1977; Silverstein et al. 2006a), or simple as when just a few behaviors are selected for observation (e.g., performance of activities of daily living, social skills, self-harm, and aggression). While some facilities have developed complex observational systems with good inter-rater reliability, often behavioral observations must be simplified due to minimal staffing, time pressures, and limited training opportunities. Behaviors need to be defined as clearly as possible and sampling intervals should fit the hospital routine. These observations often have high ecological validity in that behaviors that are the focus of treatment are directly observed (e.g., self-harm and aggression), and are especially useful for tracking change over time.

Self-monitoring is another assessment method that can be used in a public inpatient psychiatric facility. Examples include daily mood ratings (e.g., Miklowitz 2011), engagement in pleasant events (e.g., Addis and Martell 2004), and the use of skills learned in dialectical behavior therapy (DBT) via diary cards (Linehan 1993). Self-monitoring forms need to be simple given that many individuals with serious mental disorders in the hospital may be limited by cognitive impairments or the severity of their symptoms. The psychologist or other staff members should check self-monitoring forms frequently to promote completion of the forms. By its very nature self-monitoring provides immediate feedback to individuals, and allows them to see the progress they are making toward their goals. For this reason, as well as to be consistent with a strength-based approach to treatment, the valence of at least some of the target behaviors should be positive. Doing so capitalizes on the reactive effects and treatment functions of self-monitoring (Korotitsch and Nelson-Gray 1999).

Although not always thought of as an assessment method, per se, interviews are perhaps the most commonly used method of assessment in inpatient psychiatric facilities. Interviews may be structured (e.g., various diagnostic interview schedules) or unstructured, which is more common. Interviews are very flexible and serve many of the functions of other forms of assessment (e.g., diagnosis, identification of goals and strengths, development of a therapeutic alliance, assessment of change, formulation of factors contributing to problems impeding progress). Thought of in this way, interviews are subject to the same concerns about psychometrics (e.g., reliability, validity, positive and negative predictive power) as other forms of assessment. Structured interviews can be studied for their psychometric properties, but unstructured interviews cannot because of their lack of standardization. As such, psychologists need to be aware of the limitations of unstructured interviews. For example, individuals often provide different information, have different affective presentations, and may exhibit differences in thought organization and content during an interview with a treatment team than in an individual interview. Finally, collateral information from family members or previous treatment providers can be particularly helpful in corroborating interview and self-report information. In practice, assessments in public inpatient psychiatric hospitals rely on multiple methods rather than a single source, and are ongoing rather than static.

## Interventions

This section describes a number of therapies and interventions psychologists can deliver in public inpatient behavioral health facilities including individual and group psychotherapy (e.g., supportive, brief, and extended therapies from various theoretical traditions), psychoeducation about mental disorders and treatment, and psychosocial or psychiatric rehabilitation (PSR). (The terms psychosocial rehabilitation and psychiatric rehabilitation are used interchangeably.) PSR refers to a set of interventions that focus "… on the reduction of disability and the promotion of more effective adaptation in the individual's environment by using specific interventions to improve coping and behavioral abilities" (Silverstein et al. 2006b, p. 3). Psychologists developed many of these interventions, but they are not used solely by psychologists. Many are evidence-based practices while some are promising or emerging practices (APA/CAPP Task Force 2007; Dixon et al. 2010). The evidence for some of these interventions comes from studies conducted in outpatient settings or with study participants who differ in important respects from individuals in the public inpatient setting (e.g., symptom severity, cognitive impairment, length of stay, etc.). As such, it is often necessary to make adaptations to these interventions, knowing that this impacts the fidelity of their implementation. Many of these therapies can be delivered individually, in groups, or both.

The need for these therapies is well beyond the resources of hospital staff giving psychologists many opportunities to provide them. However, implementation depends on factors such as hospital resources and the willingness and readiness of individuals to avail themselves of these services. Despite its limitations, one advantage of the inpatient facility is that therapeutic interventions can be provided for differing lengths of time and frequencies. For example, for many individuals therapy works well when done in short informal sessions, e.g., 15 min in a consultation room or quiet area of the dayroom. At the other end of the spectrum, while unusual, sessions lasting an hour or longer several times a week can be conducted.

A comprehensive review of specific therapies is beyond the scope of this chapter, nor is this survey exhaustive. Furthermore, public psychiatric hospitals do not provide all the interventions describe here. Instead this section illustrates a range of interventions that psychologists can provide in inpatient facilities with comments on their relevance to recovery principles. For details about specific therapies, refer to the many available resources, especially those that describe interventions that have emerged over the past

20 years (e.g., APA and Jansen 2014; Dickerson and Lehman 2011; Dixon et al. 2010; Silverstein et al. 2006b; Wright et al. 2008).

## Individual Psychotherapy

Lysaker et al. (2010) noted that individual psychotherapy, "an activity wherein a client and therapist develop an alliance and mutual goals, while using client's guided self-exploration in the service of improving functioning and reducing distress, is at present, notably absent from most discussions of recovery focused treatment…" (pp. 76–77). They speculate that the lack of individual psychotherapy may be due to limited resources or the perception that individuals with SMI do not benefit from therapy. For much of the twentieth century psychotherapy for schizophrenia used a psychodynamic paradigm. With the advent of psychotropic medication and studies in the 1980s showing a lack of efficacy for psychodynamic therapy, the study of psychotherapy for schizophrenia declined until the 1990s when cognitive behavior therapies began to appear (Dickerson and Lehman 2011). There are now a number of therapies for individuals with SMI with many outcome studies documenting their efficacy as described below.

Individual psychotherapy serves many functions: emotional support, skill building, illness education, symptom reduction, goal setting, improved self-control over impulses and behavior, and working toward a more meaningful life (Geczy and Cote 2002; Grant et al. 2014; Lysaker et al. 2010). In a study by Coursey et al. (1995), 72 % of individuals with SMI receiving services in psychiatric rehabilitation centers perceived individual psychotherapy as effective. The interventions rated as most useful were getting in touch with one's feelings and practical advice. On average, participants identified 28.5 therapeutic issues that were important to them, including illness-intensified life issues (e.g., independence, self-esteem, interpersonal relationships, feelings), adverse consequences of the illness (e.g., lack of work, stigma), self-management of the disorder, coming to terms with the disability, managing specific symptoms, and normal developmental issues (e.g., dealing with sexual issues and family). Individuals with schizophrenia preferred shorter infrequent sessions while those with bipolar disorder and depression were evenly split between shorter infrequent sessions and longer frequent sessions.

In the inpatient setting, the mode and type of therapy depends on many factors such as the person's course of illness, progress in the hospital, severity of symptoms, past history with mental health services, and cultural issues. When individuals are first admitted to a public psychiatric hospital they may have many reactions. Some may be upset or angry at what they view as an illegal and unnecessary detention, frightened or confused not knowing what to expect, or discouraged by ending up in the hospital. Such reactions may be affected by prior experiences, fears of being harmed in the hospital fueled by paranoia or hallucinations, disorganized thinking making it difficult to understand events, communication difficulties (e.g., those with limited English proficiency, deaf), and cultural factors (e.g., the stigma of mental illness that exists in some cultures, men from some cultures being expected to follow directions from female staff members). On the other hand, some individuals may have positive reactions such as those with paranoia who see the hospital as a haven from those they think want to harm them, and people with suicidal ideation who feel relieved knowing that they will not likely hurt themselves in the hospital.

Given these reactions, in the early days of hospitalization the recovery principles of hope, safety, respect, and individualized person-centered care inform the therapeutic relationship. Developing a good therapeutic relationship has long been recognized as an important component in psychotherapy, in general, and specifically with individuals with SMI (Dickerson and Lehman 2011; Howgego et al. 2003; Kingdon and Turkington 2008; Taylor et al. 2009). For example, in an international Delphi study of service users, mental health professionals, caregivers, and advocates about what promotes recovery in people with long-term mental health problems in institutional settings, "staff attitudes," (e.g., the therapeutic alliance), were ranked second in importance among 11 domains (Turton et al. 2010). Therapeutic interventions, which included psychotropic medications and "talking therapies," were ranked the highest.

Developing a good therapeutic relationship early in the course of hospitalization can be challenging due to the factors noted above. Additionally, tension may exist with patients whose paramount goal is immediate release, but who have been committed involuntarily. In such instances, the psychologist can listen attentively to the person's account, provide information about what led to the admission, identify discharge criteria, and discuss what will help the person return to the community. At times, such discussions may provide some reassurance and shared understanding, but at other times the person may still not feel heard because the explanation did not result in release from the hospital.

In contrast to someone recently admitted to the hospital, for those whose hospitalization has been extended for a long period of time, discouragement, hopelessness, frustration, and resentment may set in, especially if they have limited insight into their illness. In such instances it may be beneficial to provide information about the reasons for continued hospitalization, discharge plans, and what they can do to facilitate discharge so as to instill a sense of agency. The psychologist may help the person identify goals to work on while in the hospital, and convey hope that discharge and other goals will indeed be reached.

Psychotherapy may be especially useful helping people put their illnesses and lives in a larger framework. Citing the literature indicating that many people with schizophrenia recover, Lysaker et al. (2010) speculated that psychotherapy might aid recovery by developing a personal narrative, i.e., a context for individuals' illnesses such that they have a richer understanding of themselves and the world. Such narratives might allow individuals to see themselves as resilient in the face of adversity, understand the illness as a biological disorder for which they are not to blame, reduce the stigma of having an illness, and instill a sense of personal agency.

While applicable throughout life, personal narratives become especially poignant at a couple of points in time. One point is early in the course of the illness. Since many serious mental disorders begin in late adolescence or early adulthood, they often disrupt critical developmental tasks such as completing an education, establishing a career, forming close interpersonal relationships, or creating families. Symptoms and behaviors associated with the illness may lead to withdraw from school, job loss, disrupted relationships, strain within the family of origin, lost social supports, hospitalizations, and legal charges. At such times, individuals may struggle with understanding their illness, the impact the illness is having on their lives, what the future holds for them, and how that future differs from what they had envisioned. The stigma associated with mental disorders adds to the burden. Psychotherapy may help individuals understand their illness and provide hope that by managing it there is much reason to expect that they will have meaningful and satisfying lives. The research on the long-term outcome for individuals with schizophrenia (Jaaskelainen et al. 2013; Lang et al. 2013; Warner 2010) and borderline personality disorder (Gunderson et al. 2011, Zanarini et al. 2012) can be illuminating, as can meeting with peers in recovery or reading books and articles by people with lived experiences (e.g., Jamison 1995; first person accounts in *Schizophrenia Bulletin*).

The other point where personal narratives can be especially poignant is much later in life when individuals look back on lives that had not turned out as they had hoped; lives that may have included many hospitalizations, little time spent in meaningful employment, limited social supports and satisfying relationships, few financial resources, and inadequate housing. Awareness of the illness, hopelessness, and feelings of inadequacy are risk factors for suicide in individuals with schizophrenia (Caldwell and Gottesman 1990; Drake et al. 1984; Siris 2001). At such times, psychotherapy can help individuals develop new goals for themselves and ways they can find meaning in their lives despite the effects the illness has had on them.

## Group Psychotherapy

Group therapies have a number of advantages in public inpatient hospitals in much the same way as in outpatient settings. In public psychiatric facilities resources are limited, especially human resources, and psychologists find themselves spending a considerable amount of time in activities other than the direct delivery of patient care. For example, in a survey of psychologists in state hospitals, 40 % of their time was spent on paperwork and supervision (Corrigan et al. 1998). Thus, group therapies offer an economical and efficient way of delivering services. Beyond this practical advantage, group therapies have many other benefits especially relevant to recovery-oriented principles. Groups allow members to gain support from their peers, learn from the experience of others, and have models of individuals who are further along in their recovery. Other advantages are reality testing for psychotic symptoms, emotional support, and the opportunity to provide feedback and guidance in a nonthreatening setting (Geczy and Cote 2002).

Groups can range from process-oriented groups with relatively little structure to highly structured groups with a clear curriculum and active direction from group leaders. Some structure is often beneficial for individuals with psychotic symptoms, cognitive disorganization, and/or negative symptoms. The effectiveness of inpatient group psychotherapy has empirical support. In one meta-analysis of group therapy, researchers found effect sizes of 0.31 in controlled studies and 0.59 in pre- post-studies, and 0.50 for individuals diagnosed with schizophrenia (Kösters et al. 2006). Many of the interventions described below can be delivered in group as well as individual formats.

## Cognitive Behavior Therapy (CBT) for Psychosis and Mood Disorders

Many readers will be familiar with cognitive behavior therapy (CBT) (Beck et al. 1979) and behavior activation for depression (Addis and Martell 2004; Jacobson et al. 1996). Perhaps less well known are CBT for psychosis (CBTp) (Beck et al. 2008; Kingdon and Turkington 2008) and CBT for bipolar disorder (Basco and Rush 2005; Miklowitz 2011). All of these therapies are useful in inpatient psychiatric hospitals.

Because of the frequency of psychosis in public behavioral health facilities, this section focuses on CBTp, which, like CBT for depression, links thoughts, emotions, and behaviors; and posits a central role for cognition (e.g., schemas, dysfunctional beliefs) and cognitive processes (e.g., overgeneralization, jumping to conclusions) in the presentation of symptoms and functioning. Therapy is individualized and multifaceted. It entails developing a shared understanding of symptoms and treatment goals; identifying the links between thoughts, emotions, and behaviors; collaboratively exploring the evidence for specific beliefs; devising means by which to test core beliefs; and problem solving. In published studies, CBTp has usually been provided in combination with pharmacotherapy.

CBTp has been subjected to much empirical testing and has been recommended in guidelines from the American Psychiatric Association (Dixon et al. 2009), the United Kingdom's National Institute for Health and Care Excellence (2014), and the Patient Outcome Research Team (PORT, Dixon et al. 2010). In a frequently cited meta-analysis of 34 studies, the overall effect sizes for CBTp were 0.37 for positive symptoms, 0.44 for negative symptoms, 0.38 for functioning, 0.36 for mood, −0.19 for hopelessness, and 0.35 for social anxiety (Wykes et al. 2008). In a more recent meta-analysis of 22 studies, smaller effect sizes were found. The effect size for positive symptoms was 0.16, which was still significant, but the effect size for negative symptoms was not significant (Turner et al. 2014). Differences in findings between the two meta-analyses may be due to insufficient power, heterogeneity of patients, differences in specific CBTp models, and the intensity of the therapy (Thase et al. 2014; Turner et al. 2014). In a recent effectiveness study of CBTp, moderate effect sizes were found for positive symptoms, general psychopathology, depression, and functional improvement in work and social relationships (Lincoln et al. 2012). Dropout rates were low, and participants' perceptions of treatment were highly positive (e.g., 98 % rated the therapy as helpful or very helpful, 95 % would recommend it to a friend).

I offer two examples of CBTp from my hospital practice. One was with a middle-aged man with a college degree who had been married for many years and previously held professional jobs. For several years, he believed that there was a vast conspiracy against him such that people were watching him wherever he went. He believed that his family was behind this conspiracy and wanted him to kill himself. He was hospitalized after making threats to harm his family and kill himself. In the hospital he believed that his family continued to have him under surveillance by planting "fake patients" to watch him. As a result of his beliefs, his wife divorced him; he became estranged from his family of origin; and he had not been employed for several years. Early in his hospital stay he was convinced that if he told others his account of events, they too would conclude that he was the subject of a conspiracy. He rated the strength of his belief in the conspiracy at 99 %.

CBTp sessions were held two to three times a week for approximately 3 months. Therapy began by listening carefully and nonjudgmentally to his account of the conspiracy and learning about his life. He was then invited to consider the evidence for his beliefs, the plausibility of his conclusions, and alternative explanations for the events he had experienced. One by one he concluded that the evidence for his beliefs was weak, and by the end of therapy he no longer believed in the conspiracy. With this improvement the focus of therapy shifted to building a satisfying life for himself given what he had gone through over the past several years. As a result he restored relationships with his family of origin and planned to look for work again.

In another example of CBTp, a woman with a long history of psychiatric hospitalizations and several past suicide attempts had been hospitalized three times in just over a year. She was very upset by the thought that she could kill members of her family with her mind and had taken an overdose of her medication to avoid harming them. Therapy sessions took place almost daily for approximately 6 weeks. Treatment included several interventions: exposure to her repetitive thoughts that she could kill her family with her mind; coping skills training to manage stressors which exacerbated her delusions; and engagement in pleasant activities to improve her mood, social relationships, and quality of life. An important part of the CBTp treatment included behavioral experiments. We devised ways to test her belief that she could kill her family with her mind. For example, she thought that she could set her family on fire with her thoughts. She agreed that if she had this power she could easily light a match or raise the temperature of a thermometer using her mind. She also believed that her thoughts could cause her family to die in a car accident. Thus, in other experiments she tried to flatten car tires and burst street lamps at the hospital with the power of her thoughts. When she could not cause these things to happen, she questioned her mental powers such that by the end of therapy she no longer believed that she could kill her family with her mind. Greatly relieved by this new realization, she returned to the community.

As these two examples illustrate, CBTp is a highly collaborative partnership between the individual and the psychologist. Although not always highlighted in studies of CBTp, developing and maintaining a good working relationship is a significant component of therapy. Both individuals in the above examples had been upset that no one believed them, not treatment providers, not even family members; and they appreciated having someone listen to their accounts. CBTp brought relief from distressing and debilitating symptoms, taught coping skills, provided education, and promoted self-efficacy, all of which are consistent with recovery principles.

### Dialectical Behavior Therapy (DBT)

Linehan (1993) developed DBT for the treatment of individuals with Borderline Personality Disorder (BPD). She designed it for outpatient treatment, but a high percentage of individuals with BPD are hospitalized at some time in their lives, and they occupy a high percentage of psychiatric beds (Bohus et al. 2000). Staff members often have strong negative reactions to the volatile emotions and self-injurious and violent behaviors sometimes exhibited by individuals with BPD. Furthermore, some staff members believe that the course of BPD is chronic and unremitting with little likelihood of recovery. However, recent studies have shown high rates of symptom remission and functional improvement (Gunderson et al. 2011, Zanarini et al. 2012). For example, one 10-year follow-up study, found that 85 % of individuals with BPD met the definition of remission (two or fewer diagnostic criteria for BPD) for a 12-month period with a relapse rate of 12 % (Gunderson et al. 2011) although social functioning (e.g., full-time employment, marital or cohabitating relationships, Global Assessment of Functioning ratings) remained at low levels despite statistically significant improvements.

DBT is an evidence-based practice. In a 2-year follow-up study, compared to individuals who received therapy from community experts, those in the DBT group had half the rate of suicide attempts, fewer emergency department visits, and fewer hospitalizations (Linehan et al. 2006). In a more recent 2-year, naturalistic, outcome study, individuals in DBT showed improvement in self-injurious behaviors, symptom severity, utilization of health services, and quality of life at follow-up, but there were no significant differences from those receiving manualized general psychiatric management developed specifically for the study (McMain et al. 2012).

DBT has been adapted to inpatient settings. Swenson et al. (2001) described a program whose components included coming to agreement on treatment goals and plans, skill building, contingency management, behavioral analysis of self-injurious behaviors, staff support, and connections with outpatient therapists. Bohus et al. (2000) developed a 3-month DBT program with three stages: analysis of target behaviors, (especially those that led to hospitalization), education and skill building, and discharge planning. In a small pilot study, many symptoms and the frequency of self-harm improved significantly (Bohus et al. 2000). In another uncontrolled study, after 3 months of inpatient DBT, significant reductions in symptoms were found at post-treatment and 15-month follow-up (Kroger et al. 2006). In a controlled trial in an inpatient facility, compared to a naturalistic wait list control group, those getting DBT showed a reduction in self-injurious behaviors and many symptoms (Bohus et al. 2004). DBT was introduced into the Pennsylvania state hospital system in 2003 in an effort to reduce seclusion and restraint (Smtih et al. 2015).

When DBT is implemented in a public inpatient facility, it may be necessary to make some modifications. Didactic information and skill building often need to be presented at a slower pace than in the outpatient setting. Similarly, abstract DBT concepts are difficult for some patients to comprehend (e.g., wise mind, emotional mind, and reasonable mind; some mindfulness strategies; radical acceptance). Such adjustments to teaching materials and strategies may be necessary because of the cognitive impairments, limited educational attainment, and/or symptom severity of individuals with BPD in public inpatient facilities. Nevertheless, many individuals enjoy learning about BPD and developing skills. For patients and staff alike, it is helpful to realize that they are "doing the best they can," which is quite a challenge during periods of extreme emotional and behavioral dyscontrol that can occur in the inpatient setting. To this end, the DBT core strategy of validation can be very useful. For example, "In cheerleading, the therapist is validating the inherent ability of the patient to overcome her difficulties and to build a life worth living … A key therapist attitude [that says] 'I believe in you'" (Linehan 1993, p. 243). Cheerleading can counter some of the person's self-loathing and negative reactions by staff. Coaching skills is another component of DBT which psychologists working in public psychiatric hospitals can employ frequently, often in vivo and at the time when the skills are needed. For example, an individual may get upset about a conflict with a peer on the unit. The psychologist may be on the unit when this occurs or shortly thereafter to coach DBT skills for that specific situation, and provide praise and encouragement. In these ways, DBT teaches individuals control over their lives and engenders autonomy consistent with a recovery orientation.

## Token Economy and Contingency Management

Token economies and contingency management are based on operant and social learning principles. Their flexibility makes them particularly well suited for long-term inpatient care (Dixon et al. 2010). These programs can address a wide array of behaviors common to many individuals on a treatment unit and/or tailored to a small number of behaviors individualized for a particular person. Examples of target behaviors include activities of daily living, social skills, participation in treatment activities, and improved self-control of aggressive behaviors. Selection of reinforcers is also flexible, ranging from highly individualized ones to generalized reinforcers such as points or tokens that can be exchanged for back-up reinforcers. Reinforcers can be social (e.g., praise), tangible (e.g., snacks), or activity-based (e.g., extra time on a computer). Specific examples include playing basketball or football for half an hour with the unit psychiatrist or psychologist for controlling aggression, going to a restaurant with staff members for attending groups, and earning money for wearing a continuous positive airway pressure (CPAP) machine for sleep apnea.

Token economies have been used for many decades and are supported by research, but they have not been widely implemented in hospitals (Dickerson et al. 2005; Dixon et al. 2010; Paul and Lentz 1977; Silverstein et al. 2006a). Dickerson et al. (2005) pointed out that much of the research on token economies is more than 20-years old and was conducted before the adoption of more objective diagnostic criteria and the introduction of atypical antipsychotic medications. Some of the institutions in which the research was conducted would not have met the basic needs of individuals according to today's standards, and therefore some of the reinforcers used in the studies would not be appropriate today. Finally, by current standards for admission, some of the individuals would probably not have been hospitalized, limiting the external validity of the research (Dickerson et al. 2005).

While seemingly simple, the development, implementation, maintenance, and evaluation of token economies and contingency management programs require considerable care and expertise which psychologists can provide. It is important to insure that deprivation of basic needs is not a part of the program and that patients' rights are upheld. Preferably, the program is overwhelmingly positive; that is, positive reinforcement is provided for adaptive behaviors. Much care must be exercised in the use of restrictive measures such as response cost. Not only are positive programs more likely to be effective, but they encourage patients and staff to work toward desired goals and utilize persons' strengths to build new skills.

Token economies have been criticized for the degree of control exerted by staff. However, as pointed out by Dickerson et al. (2005), hospital staff already exercises a high level of control without the use of token economies, and contingencies are ubiquitous for all individuals whether mentally ill or not. The issue then is how best to structure these contingencies. One way to address this criticism is to make participation in the program voluntary as in the Second Chance program described by Silverstein et al. (2006a). During the first 5 years of the program only one person requested to return to the referring state hospital from which he/she had come, reflecting the participants' favorable impressions of the program.

## Social Skills Training

Social skills training utilizes behavioral principles to teach a broad array of skills necessary for effective functioning in interpersonal situations (Bellack et al. 2004; Kopelowicz et al. 2006; Liberman 2007). Topics include basic communication skills, assertiveness, conflict resolution, problem solving, developing supportive relationships, job interviewing, refusing illicit drugs, and collaborating with mental health care providers. Training is often done in groups and includes goal setting, didactic instruction, modeling, behavioral rehearsal, coaching, feedback, positive reinforcement, and homework assignments. The content is flexible enough so that group members can raise specific situations to address in training.

Social skills training is an evidence-based practice recommended in the PORT guidelines for individuals who have skills deficits in everyday activities (Dixon et al. 2010). A meta-analysis of 22 randomly controlled trials found moderate effect sizes on performance-based measure of social and daily living skills, community functioning, and negative symptoms; a small and significant effect size for relapse; and a small and nonsignificant effect sizes for other symptoms (Kurtz and Mueser 2008). Training needs to incorporate maintenance of skills over time and generalization to everyday settings (American Psychological Association and Jansen 2014; Dixon et al. 2010; Kern et al. 2009).

## Integrated Treatment for Co-occurring Disorders

Individuals with SMI have high rates of alcohol and drug use. Estimates of the co-occurrence of SMI and substance use vary depending on the study sample and methods. In the National Institute of Mental Health Clinical Antipsychotic Trials of Intervention Effectiveness (CATIE) project, 60.3 % of individuals with schizophrenia had at least some substance use including 37 % classified as having a current substance use disorder (Swartz et al. 2006). Rates of current substance use disorders for men and unmarried individuals were over 80 %. In an outpatient sample, almost 60 % of individuals with a diagnosis of schizophrenia currently used alcohol or drugs (Fowler et al. 1998). Over 26 % had a current diagnosis of substance abuse or dependence, and almost 60 % had a lifetime diagnosis of substance abuse or dependence. In the McArthur Violence Risk Assessment Study, 67 % of those with SMI used alcohol within 30 days of hospital admission, and 30 % used marijuana (Bahorik et al. 2013). Substance use in individuals with SMI has been associated with symptoms, recent exacerbations of illness, violence, suicide, hospitalization, poor functioning, criminal charges, and a persistent and severe course (Bahorik et al. 2013; Fowler et al. 1998; Kessler 2004; Roncero et al. 2011; Swartz et al. 2006).

With these rates of substance use and associated risks in individuals with SMI, the PORT guidelines recommend substance abuse treatment for individuals with co-occurring conditions (Dixon et al. 2010). There are three treatment models for individuals with co-occurring disorders (Roncero et al. 2011). In sequential or serial treatment individuals are first provided treatment for either their mental illness or substance use. Once treatment is completed for one disorder, treatment is provided for the other. In parallel treatment both disorders are treated concurrently, but by different treatment teams. In integrated treatment the same team treats both disorders concurrently. The PORT guidelines recommend the integrated treatment model.

Mueser et al. (2003a) and SAMSHA's Center for Substance Abuse Treatment (2005) developed models for integrated treatment for co-occurring disorders. These and other such programs are multifaceted and individualized. Motivational interviewing (Miller and Rollnick 2013) and the transtheoretical model of stages of change (Prochaska et al. 1992) are used to increase motivation and tailor interventions to the individual. Treatment strategies include psychoeducation; training in social skills, coping skills, and relaxation skills; contingency management; family involvement; and relapse prevention.

The inpatient setting lends itself well to integrated treatment because one treatment team is responsible for all aspects of a person's care. However, for hospitalized individuals, especially those involuntarily committed, it is their serious mental illness that led to their hospitalization and commitment, and is often seen as the primary focus of treatment. Nevertheless, inpatient psychiatric facilities provide substance abuse programming, and many of the skills taught to help individuals with their mental disorder can be adapted to problems with substance use (e.g., social skills).

## Cognitive Remediation (CR)/Cognitive Enhancement

Interest in cognitive remediation (also referred to as cognitive enhancement) stems from the finding that individuals with schizophrenia often have impairments in attention, working memory, processing speed, executive functioning, and social cognition (e.g., processing facial expressions, interpreting and responding to social cues, theory of mind, and attributional styles) (Kurtz and Marcopulos 2012). Cognitive skills predict everyday functioning and the ability to benefit from psychosocial rehabilitation (Kurtz 2012).

Cognitive remediation can take the form of restoration or compensation (Medalia and Belucci 2012). Restorative approaches aim to directly improve basic cognitive abilities, such as attention and working memory, without emphasizing how such remediation generalizes to everyday functioning. This approach assumes that generalization will occur. Restorative procedures often use massed drill and practice exercises of specific skills. Many of these systems use computer-based programs, but paper and pencil versions are also available. The frequency of sessions ranges from as little as once a week to daily with the duration of training ranging from several weeks to over a year. McGurk et al. (2013) recommended at least 20 h of training over the course of 10 weeks with multiple sessions per week. Task difficulty can vary, depending on the skills of the individual, so as to be challenging but not too difficult.

Compensatory strategies strive to compensate for deficits by improving functioning without directly targeting basic underlying cognitive skills although change in these skills may be an indirect benefit. They include environmental modifications and training that enlists a person's strengths to overcome or compensate for cognitive deficits. Examples include the use of daily calendars to keep track of appointments, checklists of tasks that need to be completed, alarms as reminders for appointments, and hygiene items placed in convenient locations. As with restorative approaches, compensatory strategies can be highly individualized to meet a person's needs while taking into account cognitive strengths and weaknesses.

Two recent meta-analyses of CR, one including 26 randomized controlled trials and the other covering 40 trials, found moderate effect sizes for global cognitive functioning (mean effects sizes of 0.41 and 0.45) and psychosocial functioning (mean effect sizes of 0.35 and 0.42), with small effect sizes for symptoms (mean effect sizes of 0.28 and 0.17) (McGurk et al. 2007; Wykes et al. 2011). Gains were durable: at follow-up the mean effect size was 0.43 for global cognition, 0.37 for functioning, and 0.17 for symptoms (Wykes et al. 2011). Adding CR to PSR, or integrating the two approaches, results in greater improvements in psychosocial functioning when compared to PSR without CR or CR combined with treatment as usual (McGurk et al. 2013). Especially noteworthy is that almost half of the more than 2000 study participants in the Wykes et al. (2011) meta-analysis were inpatients.

### Illness Management and Recovery (IMR)

Illness Management and Recovery (IMR) was developed as an evidence-based practice "... to help clients with schizophrenia or major mood disorders learn how to manage their illnesses more effectively in the context of pursuing their personal goal" (Mueser et al. 2006, p. S33). The goals of the program are to "learn about mental illnesses and strategies for treatment; decrease symptoms; reduce relapses and rehospitalizations; and make progress toward goals and toward recovery" (SAMSHA 2009, p. 6). IMR incorporates empirically supported strategies identified in a review of the literature: psychoeducation about mental disorders and their treatment, cognitive behavioral strategies for improving adherence to medication, relapse prevention, social skills training, and coping skills training (Mueser et al. 2002a, 2006). Theoretically, IMR is based on the stress-vulnerability model of illness, the transtheoretical model of change, and motivational interviewing (Mueser et al. 2006). It consists of 10 modules beginning with a discussion of the meaning of recovery, identifying personal recovery goals, and developing a plan for achieving those goals. Practical facts about mental illnesses are then discussed followed by modules on the stress-vulnerability model, building social supports, using medications effectively, limiting alcohol and drug use, reducing relapse (e.g., identifying triggers and warning signs), coping with stress and persistent symptoms, and utilizing the mental health system (SAMSHA 2009).

In a review of the literature, individuals in IMR programs, compared to treatment as usual, showed improvement in their knowledge about mental illness, progress toward recovery goals, relapse prevention plans, substance use, and ratings of symptoms by observers (but not by consumers) (McGuire et al. 2014). Evidence was lacking or mixed for long-term effects, such as quality of life, role functioning, community integration, social support, hospitalizations, emergency room visits, medication dosages, incarcerations, or hopelessness, although conclusions about some of these outcomes were limited by the number and quality of studies. In a recent randomized control trial comparing IMR with an active control group, no significant differences were found on any outcome measures, but the participation rates in both groups were low (Salyers et al. 2014).

Most studies of IMR have been in community settings, but IMR has been implemented in state hospital units with diverse populations (e.g., acute admissions, long stay patients with persistent symptoms, individuals with co-occurring substance use disorders, and individuals with cognitive impairment) as a means of operationalizing a recovery philosophy (Bartholomew and Kensler 2010; Bartholomew and Zechner 2014). According to these authors, recovery is enhanced when individuals learn to collaborate with treatment providers, manage their illness, and prevent relapse and rehospitalization. In one study in a New Jersey state psychiatric hospital, for each hour an individual participated in IMR the risk of returning to the hospital over the 5-year study period decreased by 1.1 % (Bartholomew and Zechner 2014).

## Trauma Informed Care and Trauma Specific Treatment

Rates of trauma exposure in individuals with SMI are higher than in the general population, ranging from 49 to 100 % in study samples (Grubaugh et al. 2011). Traumatic events include childhood and adult sexual and physical assault, crime victimization, etc. Similarly, rates for Posttraumatic Stress Disorder (PTSD) in individuals with SMI are higher than in the general population with prevalence rates ranging from 13 to 53 % in the former compared to 7–12 % in the latter (Grubaugh et al. 2011). Despite these rates of trauma exposure, in the public sector individuals with SMI are under-diagnosed with PTSD and trauma related problems (Mueser et al. 1998; Salyers et al. 2004). In addition to their direct effects, the experience of traumatic events and PTSD contribute to the symptoms and course of SMI (Gracie et al. 2007; Mueser et al. 2002b; Scott et al. 2007).

The prevalence of trauma in persons with SMI has led recently to the development of trauma related services. Trauma informed care is a broad-based approach that recognizes the impact of trauma and incorporates that understanding across many aspects of service delivery. It includes support from an organization's leadership, policies and procedures, staff training, attention to the physical environment, assessment of trauma, specific trauma services, providing safety, minimizing retraumatization, and so on (SAMSHA 2014a). In trauma informed care screening for trauma is universal. Strengths are incorporated into treatment, and recovery and resilience are expected (SAMSHA 2014b). Examples of trauma informed care include being aware of triggers based on a person's trauma history (e.g., loud noises, isolation, people arguing, physical characteristics of staff members), and asking individuals what may be helpful if they are distressed (e.g., talking with staff, having a safe and quiet place in which to be alone, listening to music).

While trauma informed care is a broad-based approach, trauma specific treatment directly addresses trauma and its sequelae. Few such treatments for individuals with SMI who also have PTSD have been studied or implemented in the public sector (Frueh et al. 2009a). One such therapy is cognitive restructuring which borrows from cognitive behavior therapy for PTSD (Mueser et al. 2009). The core modules include developing a crisis plan, psychoeducation, breathing retraining, and cognitive restructuring. Most sessions focus on cognitive restructuring, a "… strategy for identifying, evaluating, and changing inaccurate thoughts and beliefs that lead to negative feelings" (Mueser et al. 2009,

p. 57). Similar to cognitive therapy for depression, cognitive restructuring for PTSD makes a connection between thoughts, feelings, and behaviors. Individuals are taught the five steps of cognitive restructuring: describe the situation, identify the strongest negative feeling, identify the thought most closely related to that feeling, evaluate the evidence for and against that thought, and take action either by changing the thought to a more accurate one if it is not supported by the evidence or changing the situation. Unlike some treatments for PTSD in the general population, prolonged exposure to the traumatic stimuli, either in vivo or imaginal, is not done. The developers of the therapy reasoned that exposure procedures might be too stressful for individuals with SMI and might lead to a high dropout rate.

Research studies on cognitive restructuring for PTSD in persons with SMI have found some promising results. In a preliminary study, 59 % of the participants completed the treatment (Mueser et al. 2007). Those who completed treatment had significant reductions in PTSD symptoms and depression from baseline to post-treatment, while those who dropped out did not. In a randomized controlled trial comparing cognitive restructuring to treatment as usual, 81 % assigned to cognitive restructuring completed the program (Mueser et al. 2008). Compared to treatment as usual, those in the cognitive restructuring group improved significantly on PTSD symptoms, depression, anxiety, other symptoms, physical health concerns, and working alliance with their case managers. There was no significant difference in whether individuals retained a PTSD diagnosis.

Unlike the above studies, a small pilot study included exposure therapy along with education, anxiety management, trauma illness management, social skills training, and anger management training for individuals with PTSD and schizophrenia or schizoaffective disorder (Frueh et al. 2009b). Significant improvements were noted in PTSD symptoms and anger, but not depression, anxiety, social activities, or physical health. Many of the gains were maintained at 3-month follow-up. Ten of the 13 individuals who completed treatment no longer met criteria for PTSD. These studies of trauma specific treatment for individuals with SMI are promising, but additional research is needed.

## Positive Psychology Interventions (PPI)

Positive psychology has grown rapidly over the past two decades. Seligman and Csikszentmihalyi (2000) noted, "Psychology has, since World War II, become a science largely about healing. It concentrates on repairing damage within a disease model of human functioning. This almost exclusive attention to pathology neglects the fulfilled individual and the thriving community" (p. 5). Seligman (2011) has called positive psychology a "tectonic upheaval" in psychology with the goal of "… exploring what makes life worth living and building the enabling conditions of a life worth living… [which] is by no means identical with the goal of understanding misery and undoing the disabling conditions of life" (p. 1–2). Although there have been few empirical studies of Positive Psychology Interventions (PPI) with individuals with SMI, PPI is included here because of its congruence with the principles of the recovery model (Resnick and Rosenheck 2006; Schrank et al. 2014a).

Interventions derived from positive psychology are "… primarily aimed at increasing positive feelings, positive behaviors, or positive cognitions, as opposed to ameliorating pathology or fixing negative thoughts or maladaptive behavior patterns" (Sin and Lyubomirsky 2009, p. 469). Most studies using PPI have been conducted with the general public, but a few have included people with specific psychological problems. In one meta-analysis of studies with depressed individuals, the mean effect sizes for PPI on well-being and depression were 0.33 and 0.32, respectively (Sin and Lyubomirsky 2009). In another meta-analysis of 39 studies, the 7 studies that targeted individuals with anxiety or depression found effect sizes of 0.31, 0.59, and 0.78 on measures of subjective well-being, psychological well-being, and depression, respectively (Bolier et al. 2013).

Positive psychotherapy (PPT; Seligman et al. 2006) is a PPI designed specifically for depression.

A group of researchers in the United Kingdom adapted it for individuals with psychosis (Schrank et al. 2014b). Called WELLFOCUS PPT, the primary goal of this intervention is to improve subjective well-being with secondary goals of increasing positive feelings, hope, connectedness, self-worth, empowerment, and meaning; and reducing symptoms. Over the course of 11 group sessions, 10 exercises adapted from PPT target positive experiences, strengths, relationships, and development of a meaningful life narrative. Examples include savoring good things, forgiveness, identifying personal strengths, gratitude, and positive responding. Results from a pilot study with individuals with primary diagnoses of psychosis using specialized mental health services found significant improvement in the WELLFOCUS PPT group, compared to a treatment as usual group, on measures of well-being, symptoms, and depression (Schrank et al. 2015). Clearly more research is needed on the use of PPI with individuals with SMI, but "positive psychology provides a useful framework for professionals seeking to provide services that support the recovery orientation" (Resnick and Rosenheck 2006, p. 120).

### Common Factors

Common factors found in most psychotherapies, such as the therapeutic alliance, empathy, instilling hope, acceptance, understanding, and education (Davidson and Chan 2014), cut across many of the psychological services provided in public inpatient psychiatric facilities. Common factors are consistent with recovery-oriented practice and can form the foundation for many psychological services. Individuals with SMI have identified many of these factors as important to their recovery. In one study, of the top 10 competencies consumers rated as important for providers to have, 8 reflected common factors: show respect, see the person holistically apart from his/her diagnosis and symptoms, listen without judgment, believe in the person's potential to recover, trust the person, care about the person, understand the person, and be accessible (Russinova et al. 2011). As the authors noted, these factors represent the traditional concept of a therapeutic alliance and forming a strong bond with the person. It can be easy to overlook the importance of such factors when individuals have severe symptoms and in-service settings that emphasize a medical model. Nevertheless, there are many opportunities to use them in public inpatient facilities.

## Treatment Planning

In the inpatient psychiatric hospital psychologists collaborate with patients and treatment team members to develop and implement treatment plans. Psychologists are involved in all aspects of treatment plan development including identifying problem areas, goals, objectives, discharge criteria, and strengths. They bring a psychological formulation to the multidisciplinary treatment planning process. Psychologists attend to developing objectives which are clear, specific, and individualized. They help plan and implement interventions to achieve goals and objectives. Psychologists are especially instrumental in overseeing the behavioral and interactional elements of treatment plans such as identifying antecedents to behaviors, ways in which staff should respond to antecedents, and reinforcement strategies.

Consistent with recovery-oriented principles, psychologists, along with other members of the treatment team, seek to involve patients in the development of treatment plans as much as possible. In the public inpatient facility this is an area in which patient involvement varies on a continuum consistent with Smith and Bartholomew's (2006) description of a *hospital* model and a *recovery* model. Both of these models apply to the state hospital setting and depend on a person's "phase of illness." The hospital model plays a central role when an individual with a mental disorder is a clear and imminent danger to self or others, and interventions such as involuntary hospitalization and "caretaking and prescriptive treatments" may be needed. Hospitals also need to promote an individual's recovery, and Smith and Bartholomew advocated progressive empowerment toward a recovery model when restrictive measures recede and autonomy increases.

In ideal circumstances individuals are motivated to make changes in the problem areas that led to their hospitalization and that will lead to a return to the community as soon as is safely possible. This might include a reduction in distressing symptoms and improved self-management of aggressive and self-injurious behaviors. In these instances all aspect of treatment planning can be very collaborative. At the other end of the continuum are situations in which individuals have very limited understanding of their mental disorder or the problems that led to their hospitalization. Unfortunately, this is the more typical case in the state psychiatric hospital. Such individuals may have little interest in developing treatment plans since they may view their hospitalization or legal charges (for those on a forensic status) as unjustified, and their only goal is immediate release from the hospital. However, the treatment team still has the responsibility to develop treatment plans consistent with hospital, legal, and regulatory requirements. Even in circumstances in which individuals are unwilling or unable to provide much input into their treatment, it might be possible to elicit their involvement in certain aspects of the plan such as suggestions for activities or items that may be used as reinforcers.

Once treatment plans have been developed, psychologists implement the plan themselves, or, more commonly, monitor and troubleshoot implementation of the plan by other staff members. This involves staff training and clarifying questions about the plan during the course of implementation. Psychologists evaluate the effectiveness of the plan, collect data, and suggest modifications based on the data and feedback from the patient and staff.

## Forensic Services

In public inpatient psychiatric hospitals, psychologists conduct evaluations of trial competency and mental state at the time of alleged offenses when questions about legal insanity are raised. For individuals who have been adjudicated incompetent to stand trial, psychologists provide restoration services. For individuals adjudicated not guilty by reason of insanity, psychologists conduct assessments to help review panels and courts make decisions about a person's disposition (e.g., continued hospitalization, release to the community), and when hospitalized, provide a range of assessment and therapeutic services. As experts recognized by courts and in statutes, psychologists have the opportunity to educate individuals in the criminal justice system who lack expertise about serious mental disorders.

The provision of psychological services to individuals on a forensic status is complicated by the increased oversight, accountability, security concerns, and stigma associated with the forensic system. These factors create tension with recovery-oriented principles (Pouncey and Lukens 2010; Simpson and Penney 2011). As noted by an expert panel convened by the National Association of State Mental Health Program Directors, "… there is a need for additional detailed guidance on how best to treat and manage persons in state psychiatric hospitals who continue to present a significant risk of violence due to a serious mental illness, substance use disorder, and/or criminal behavior in a manner that is consistent with recovery principles and practices" (Parks et al. 2014, p. 52).

Despite these added complications, individuals with SMI involved in the criminal justice system have many of the same needs as those without such involvement. As such, recovery encompasses many of the same elements including ameliorating symptoms, improving functional capabilities, developing supports, working toward desired goals, and building a satisfying life (Simpson and Penney 2011). Thus, many of the psychological services described in this chapter apply to the forensic population (Osher and Steadman 2007). For example, in forensic inpatient units at Missouri's Fulton State Hospital, a social learning program facilitated an increase in adaptive behaviors from baseline to follow-up (Newbill et al. 2011). Another proposed program for psychological services adapted the risk-needs-responsivity and the "good lives" models of treatment used with offender populations to individuals in forensic mental health settings (Gudjonsson and Young (2007).

## Training Students and Staff

The inpatient psychiatric facility provides an excellent opportunity for psychologists to train students, interns, and post-doctoral fellows in psychology; students from other disciplines; and hospital staff. In noting that the workforce "… has historically been woefully unprepared in terms of the requisite knowledge, values, and skills for working with this population…" Mueser et al. (2013, p. 54) asserted that there is a "moral imperative" to mandate training in the treatment of individuals with serious mental disorders in clinical psychology graduate programs, and that competence in working with this population should be a requirement of graduation from programs approved by the American Psychological Association (APA). In a survey of APA accredited graduate clinical psychology program training directors, 39 % of the programs did not have any faculty who identified SMI as their primary area of research, clinical practice, and/or academic interest (Reddy et al. 2010). When asked about factors that encourage or discourage students' training and education in SMI, 51 % of the respondents cited a preference by psychologists to work with clients who have "insight" and are "motivated for treatment" as factors that discouraged students. Only 41 % thought that psychologists had the relevant skills for working with individuals with SMI. More encouraging was the finding that students in 70 % of the programs had an opportunity to take a practicum that allowed at least an exposure level of supervised experience in settings that serve individuals with SMI (these settings were not only inpatient facilities, but included outpatient, residential, emergency, day treatment, rehabilitation, and crisis settings).

For students, interns, and fellows the training experience may range from exposure to serious mental disorders in the inpatient setting to assuming considerable responsibilities. At the introductory level, training may consist of observing and "shadowing" a psychologist in the hospital. At a more advanced level, students and trainees may conduct many of the psychological services described in this chapter under the supervision of a psychologist. Geczy and Cote (2002) and Hoge et al. (2000) described some of the features to incorporate in training: learning to develop a therapeutic alliance, overcoming anxiety, developing confidence, learning to provide individual and group psychotherapy, developing behavioral treatment plans, working with multidisciplinary treatment teams, learning about psychosocial rehabilitation services, working within systems of care with their bureaucracies, and learning the role of psychologists in this setting.

Many trainees may be under the impression that individuals with SMI experience a deteriorating course of illness with little hope of recovery. Furthermore, they may believe that medications are the only treatment for such disorders, and that psychologists contribute little to recovery. Psychologists in public inpatient psychiatric hospitals are in an excellent position to address the stereotypes and myths that trainees hold. They can promote clinical skills needed to work with individuals with SMI, model psychological services, and expose trainees to the range of services available to individuals with SMI.

As professionals with considerable training and experience, psychologists are called upon to provide training to students from other disciplines and hospital staff (Roe et al. 2006). Examples include basic information about mental disorders to front line staff, behavioral methods and effective ways to interact with patients (Donat et al. 1991), and in-service presentations on specialty topics. Not only do these training activities benefit students, staff, and indirectly, patients, but they can be a source of considerable professional satisfaction and enrichment for psychologists in public inpatient facilities.

## Consultation, Program Development and Leadership

In the public inpatient psychiatric hospital, psychologists serve as consultants, develop programs, and provide leadership, and in doing so can help incorporate a recovery model of care. Consultations may include in-depth assessments and treatment recommendations for exceptionally challenging cases that have confounded the efforts of treatment teams, second opinions regarding risks, and the creation of specialty treatment protocols (e.g., violence prevention, and swallowing foreign objects). Examples of program development include designing, implementing, coordinating, and evaluating the effectiveness of unit token economies, unit rules, and PSR services. In these roles psychologists collaborate with members of other disciplines, bringing their training and perspective. Psychologists serve on committees within the facility or across a state (e.g., forensic issues, seclusion/restraint reduction efforts, preparing for reviews by regulatory agencies). Leadership positions for psychologists range from being an influential and prominent member of the treatment team to the director of the facility.

## Challenges

Many of the services provided by psychologists in the inpatient psychiatric hospital as described in this chapter are consistent with recovery principles. Even more broadly, the training and professional experiences most psychologists bring to their inpatient practice are consistent with recovery principles. However, there are some tensions between recovery principles and psychological services in the inpatient psychiatric setting. Many of these are not unique to psychologists; indeed, they may be felt more keenly by members of other disciplines. In this section I discuss some of the challenges that are particularly relevant to psychologists.

### Autonomy, Choice, and Coercion

Perhaps one of the thorniest tensions in the public inpatient psychiatric hospital is balancing the autonomy of individuals with the use of coercive, restrictive, and paternalistic measures. Autonomy, self-determination, and choice are central recovery principles. However, in public psychiatric hospitals most individuals are committed involuntarily on a civil or forensic status, which is already a restriction of their freedom. This issue is further complicated by the limited insight many individuals have. As Bellack (2006) noted, "… the balance of power may need to shift toward the professional when the consumer is highly impaired and has diminished decisional capacity" (p. 441). Much of this debate is framed around the risk of harm to self and others, that is, more restrictive measure are justifiable when such risks are high (Davidson et al. 2006).

This issue is probably less pertinent to psychologists than practitioners from other disciplines because many of the services psychologists provide rely on the willing participation of the individuals they serve. For example, most formal psychological assessments (e.g., personality testing, intelligence testing) cannot be done without the person's active engagement. However, even in conducting assessments there are exceptions such as the use of clinician administered rating scales and behavioral observations, many forensic evaluations, and risk assessments. Likewise, psychotherapy, psychoeducation, and skills training require at least some engagement by patients.

Autonomy becomes more relevant for psychologists in clinical decision-making. One such area is working toward patient identified goals, another central concept of the recovery model. Examples of conflicts over goals include a person who wants immediate discharge even though he/she has been committed and is not ready for discharge (e.g., engages in and threatens aggression), and a person who wants to smoke in a tobacco-free facility. In the first example, discharge may be the ultimate goal, but often the individual views it as the immediate goal. In this situation there is agreement on the goal, but not when it will be accomplished. Another example is when an individual is unwilling to leave the hospital even though the treatment team believes the person is clinically ready, and housing, financial supports, and outpatient services are available. As an example, a middle-aged woman I worked with refused discharge until her husband, a medical doctor, came to pick her up and take her to the new home he was building for them. In reality, she had no husband, and she extended her stay in the hospital by refusing to accept available community housing. Much later, she became attracted to a male patient quite younger than herself who she regarded as her husband even though they were not married. When he was preparing for discharge, she agreed to live in the residential placement he chose. In another case, a man believed that a local government had cheated him out of a multi-million dollar service contract he bid on. As a result he thought that the government owed him a huge sum of money as compensation, and he refused discharge unless he was guaranteed a yearly income of over $100,000 and a large house.

At times, even if one wants to fulfill a person's goals, it can be difficult to know what those are. For example, a young man I worked with requested discharge from the hospital frequently, often several times a day. However, his choice of where he wanted to live often changed over the course of just a few hours. This vacillation began early in his hospitalization and went on for months before he was discharged.

As these examples show, there is a balance between autonomy and limiting choices as noted by Geller (2012) and in the following statement from SAMSHA (2011):

> Honoring self-determination, however, does not require, and is not equal to, doing whatever the person wants.... Mental health professionals are bound both by their professional ethics and by their societal obligation to act in the person's and community's best interests, even if that may be in conflict with the person's wishes at the time. When a person is incapacitated by an acute episode of psychosis, is unable to make his or her own decisions, and poses a serious and imminent risk, the recovery-oriented practitioner is equally obligated to intervene on the person's and the community's behalf.
>
> Recovery-oriented practice in this way is not contradictory to emergency intervention on the person's and community's behalf. What recovery-oriented practice requires is that such interventions be performed respectfully, in ways that ensure the dignity of the individual, with transparency, only for as long as is required by the emergent situation, and in ways that optimize the person's opportunities for exercising whatever degree of self-determination remains possible at the time. This typically requires the staff to offer the person choices, even though they may be limited to a narrow range, and to be as clear and explicit as possible with the person throughout the process about what is happening, why it is happening, and what needs to happen for the person to regain control and autonomy' (pp. 25–26).

In response to this sentiment, Davidson (2012) placed a heavy burden of responsibility on treatment providers to show that acting in conflict with a person's wishes is necessary, especially in light of a history of abusing their power simply because a person had a mental illness (e.g., lobotomies, prolonged confinement without sufficient justification).

## Diagnoses and Relief of Symptoms

To some extent advocates of recovery eschew the use of psychiatric diagnoses because it is stigmatizing, risks defining individuals as their diagnoses, and places undue emphasis on symptom relief as a treatment outcome rather than finding a meaningful life. While these are all valid concerns, accurate diagnoses and symptom relief are important in the public inpatient psychiatric facility. Accurate diagnoses can inform treatment, whether psychopharmacology or some of the psychological interventions described in this chapter, and can help the psychologist access the relevant scientific and professional literature. As an example of the importance of making accurate diagnoses, I worked with a young woman who had been committed to the hospital on a forensic status after incurring a felony charge for assaulting a police officer. She was estranged from her family, homeless, unemployed, and had no source of income. On the unit she frequently aggressed toward other patients and staff and was emotionally labile over the course of several weeks. Many members of the treatment team viewed her as having Antisocial Personality Disorder and advocated for her return to jail as soon as possible. I suggested that she had Bipolar Disorder, with or without Antisocial Personality Disorder, and recommended treatment for Bipolar Disorder. The attending psychiatrist agreed to offer a trial of a mood stabilizing medication to which she responded very well. Her aggression ceased and her mood improved dramatically. She was not prosecuted for her legal charge, and instead, with the help of the treatment team and outpatient service providers, she was discharged to a residence in the community.

With regard to the relief of symptoms as a goal of treatment, individuals admitted to public behavioral health facilities commonly experience acute symptoms. In many instances individuals experience these symptoms as distressing. Examples include hallucinations of voices making derogatory comments about the person, fear that the person's life is in danger, depression, anxiety, anger, sleep disturbance, and so on. Even when symptoms are not reported as distressing, they may underlie the reasons individuals are admitted to the hospital, especially for those on an involuntary status. In both situations, symptom relief is an important goal. Indeed, studies have found a negative correlation between symptoms and ratings of recovery by individuals with SMI (Corrigan et al. 1999; Hackman et al. 2007). Furthermore, in a Delphi study that examined the meaning of recovery as defined by individuals with lived experience, over 80 % agreed that a characteristic of recovery is when symptoms interfere less and less with daily life or do not get in the way of doing things (Law and Morrison 2014). Thus, symptom relief can be one of several treatment goals, but complete remission is not a necessary criterion for discharge.

## Hope and Discouragement

A cardinal feature of the recovery model is instilling and maintaining hope in individuals with SMI. The literature on the long-term outcome of individuals with SMI has shown that a high percentage of individuals recover, a finding that has contributed to the recovery movement. However, this same literature shows that a significant proportion of individuals do *not* recover very well. As described earlier in this chapter, the public inpatient behavioral health facility serves individuals with complex problems and needs. These individuals often have difficult to treat problems with long lengths of stay and/or repeat hospitalizations. Furthermore, psychologists and other treatment providers face criticisms of their services from patients and family members, especially from those who are angry about having been hospitalized and how they have been treated, (even prior to admission). Such criticisms and oversight by regulatory agencies perform a valuable function, namely, to stimulate the reexamination and modification of practices, policies, and procedures. Nevertheless, the lack of progress by some patients, a barrage of criticisms, and unrealistic expectations to prevent all forms of harm can lead psychologists to become discouraged. Such discouragement, could, in turn, impede psychologists' ability to convey hope to patients and search for effective services. Indeed, in a couple of studies comparing outpatient and inpatient staff, the latter were less optimistic about consumers (e.g., their ability to live in their own residences and likelihood of remaining in the mental health system for the rest of their lives) (Salyers et al. 2007; Tsai and Salyers 2008).

To prevent discouragement and to stay hopeful about individuals' recovery, it is useful to be aware of the research literature on long-term outcomes for people with SMI, to keep in mind that recovery is "nonlinear," and to recall the many successes with individuals who had poor initial prognoses. It is important to rely on one's treatment team and colleagues as a source of support, seek consultation from within and outside the facility, include consumer peers as part of the hospital workforce, and have peers who have successfully transitioned to the community available as models.

## Evidence-Based Practices (EBPs)

Many of the interventions described in this chapter are EBPs. Much has been written about EBPs in the field of psychology, and there is much debate about using them. These arguments are beyond the scope of this chapter. Instead, I focus here on their relationship to recovery-oriented practices.

As noted by Davidson et al. (2009), "… some mental health consumer advocates view the emphasis on evidence-based practices to place a further restriction on their ability to exercise choice in their care. They also are suspicious of scientific claims to offer a privileged access to truth, arguing instead for relying on first-hand experiences as at least as equally valid sources of information about the utility of psychiatric interventions" (p. 323). Similarly, Anthony et al. (2003) highlighted several limitations of evidence-based practices as they apply to recovery. These include narrowly defined outcome measures such as symptoms and rates of hospitalization, rather than ones consumers value such as having meaningful roles in society. They asserted that evidence-based practices do not take into account subjective experiences or the understanding that there are many paths to recovery. Further, many evidence-based practices undervalue the "helper-helpee" relationship, something cited as critical to recovery by individuals with lived experiences. Finally, they noted that many recovery-oriented practices draw their importance from philosophical values, not just empirical evidence.

Such criticisms led Davidson et al. (2009) to ask rhetorically whether EBPs and recovery are like oil and water (i.e., fundamentally incompatible) or oil and vinegar (i.e., concepts that can be integrated). In arguing that EBPs and recovery are indeed compatible, Davidson et al. noted that just as in other fields of medicine, patients are partners in treatment and retain the right to make informed choices (as long as they have not been deemed incompetent to make such decisions) based on, or despite, the evidence. Individual preference is part of the definition of evidence-based practices in psychology (EBPP) adopted by the American Psychological Association. According to this definition "EBPP is the integration of the best available research with clinical expertise in the context of *patient characteristics, culture, and preferences*" (APA Presidential Task Force on Evidence-Based Practice 2006, p. 280, emphasis added). In support of the compatibility of EBPs and recovery principles, others have argued that many EBPs emphasize shared decision-making and education about available interventions so that individuals can make informed choices, and they provide individuals with tools to pursue their goals (Mueser 2012; Torrey et al. 2005). Mueser (2012) went even further by asking whether services can "… be recovery oriented *without* helping individuals gain access to EBPs" (emphasis original, p. 288). He argued that "EBPs are a technology, not a value, and therefore, on their own (like computers or telephones) they are neither recovery-oriented nor antithetical to recovery" (p. 287). This is consistent with the view of SAMSHA (2011): "All of these practices [EBPs], when offered in a person-centered and empowering manner that focuses on inclusion in community life, can be viewed as recovery-oriented practices" (p. 9).

### Personal Safety

Psychologists in public psychiatric hospitals work in settings that put them at some risk of harm to themselves, albeit to a lesser extent than front line, direct care staff members and clinicians from some other disciplines. This presents an intriguing challenge in that psychologists must be vigilant to indications of imminent violence and take steps to minimize the risk of violence, while at the same time provide services in a recovery-oriented manner. It is beyond the scope of this chapter to discuss the many ways in which risks can be minimized, but some examples include forming good working relationships with patients, providing encouragement and hope, and considering how and under which conditions to provide information or take necessary actions that a person might find upsetting. While personal safety is important, psychologists will not be effective if they are so wary of violence that they severely limit their interactions with the individuals they serve.

## Conclusion

Psychologists in public inpatient psychiatric hospitals have many opportunities to provide much needed services to individuals with SMI. In this chapter, I have attempted to show how psychologists can incorporate recovery-oriented principles into their practice in these facilities, and discussed some of the challenges they face in doing so. As noted earlier, this survey of psychological services is not exhaustive, nor are all of the services described in this chapter available at all facilities. Many of these practices are consistent with the training and experience that has been a part of psychology for many years, but because most of them have not been developed specifically for individuals in public inpatient psychiatric facilities, these practices often require some adaptation. Recovery principles are easier to implement in community settings than inpatient hospitals (Tsai and Salyers 2008), and a number of tensions exist between the recovery model and clinical practice in a state psychiatric hospital. Furthermore, the meaning of recovery and how to implement it often lack clarity, which complicates efforts to adhere to recovery-oriented principles. However, recovery, both as an achievable outcome and a set of principles, can serve as a guide to the practice of psychology in inpatient psychiatric hospitals by focusing attention on how a service helps a person recover and how it aligns with recovery principles. Psychological services will evolve with additional research, policies, and debate. The prospect of such change is not only expected and consistent with the long history of treatment for individuals with SMI, but invigorating to psychologists working in this clinical setting.

## References


Addis, M. E., & Martell, C. R. (2004). *Overcoming depression one step at a time*. Oakland, CA: New Harbinger Publications.

Almvik, R., & Woods, P. (1998). The Broset violence checklist (BVC) and the prediction of inpatient violence: Some preliminary results. *Psychiatric Care, 5*, 208 211.

American Psychological Association, & Jansen, M. A. (2014). *Reframing psychology for the emerging health care environment: Recovery curriculum for people with serious mental illnesses and behavioral health disorders*. Washington, DC: American Psychological Association.

Anthony, W. (1993). Recovery from mental illness: The guiding vision of the mental health service system in the 1990s. *Psychosocial Rehabilitation Journal, 16*, 11–23.

Anthony, W., Rogers, E. S., & Farkas, M. (2003). Research on evidence-based practices: Future directions in an era of recovery. *Community Mental Health Journal, 39*, 101–114.

APA Presidential Task Force on Evidence Based Practice. (2006). Evidence-based practice in psychology. *American Psychologist, 61*, 271–285.

APA/CAPP Task Force on Serious Mental Illness and Severe Emotional Disturbance. (2007). *Catalog of clinical training opportunities: Best practices for recovery and improved outcomes for people with serious mental illness*. Retrieved from www.apa.org/practice/grid/ubdex.aspx

Bahorik, A. L., Newhill, C. E., & Eack, S. M. (2013). Characterizing the longitudinal patterns of substance use among individuals diagnosed with serious mental illness after psychiatric hospitalization. *Addition, 108*, 1259–1269.

Bartholomew, T., & Kensler, D. (2010). Illness management and recovery in state psychiatric hospitals. *American Journal of Psychiatric Rehabilitation, 13*, 105–125.

Bartholomew, T., & Zechner, M. (2014). The relationship of illness management and recovery to state hospital readmission. *The Journal of Nervous and Mental Disease, 202*, 647–650.

Beck, A. T., Rector, N. A., Stolar, N., & Grant, P. (2008). *Schizophrenia: Cognitive theory, research, and practice*. New York, NY: Guilford Press.

Beck, A. T., Rush, A. J., Shaw, B. F., & Emery, G. (1979). *Cognitive therapy of depression*. New York: Guilford Press.

Bellack, A. S. (2006). Scientific and consumer models of recovery in schizophrenia: Concordance, contrasts, and implications. *Schizophrenia Bulletin, 32*, 432–442.

Bellack, A. S., Mueser, K. T., Gingerich, S., & Agresta, J. (2004). *Social skills training for schizophrenia* (2nd ed.). New York, NY: Guilford.

Basco, Monica Ramirez, & Rush, A. J. (2005). *Cognitive behavioral therapy for bipolar disorder*. New York: Guilford Press.

Bohus, M., Haaf, B., Simms, T., Limberger, M. F., Schmahl, C., Unckel, C., et al. (2004). Effectiveness of inpatient dialectical behavioral therapy for borderline personality disorder: A controlled trial. *Behaviour Research and Therapy, 42*, 487–499.

Bohus, M., Haaf, B., Stiglmayr, C., Pohl, U., Bohme, R., & Linehan, M. (2000). Evaluation of inpatient dialectical-behavioral therapy for borderline personality disorder: A prospective study. *Behaviour Research and Therapy, 38*, 875–887.

Bolier, L., Haverman, M., Westerhof, G. J., Riper, H., Smit, F., & Bohlmeijer, E. (2013). Positive psychology interventions: A meta-analysis of randomized controlled studies. *BMC Public Health, 13*, 119–128.

Butcher, J. N., Graham, J. R., Ben-Porath, Y. S., Tellegen, A., Dahlstrom, W. G., & Kaemmer, B. (2001). *Minnesota multiphasic personality inventory-2 manual*. Minneapolis, MN: University of Minnesota Press.

Caldwell, C. B., & Gottesman, I. I. (1990). Schizophrenics kill themselves too: A review of risk factors for suicide. *Schizophrenia Bulletin, 16*, 571–589.

Center for Substance Abuse Treatment. (2005). *Substance abuse treatment for persons with co-occurring disorders.* Treatment Improvement Protocol (TIP) Series 42. DHHS Publication No. (SMA) 05-3902. Rockville, MD: Substance Abuse and Mental Health Services Administration.

Corrigan, P. W., Hess, L., & Garman, A. N. (1998). Results of a job analysis of psychologists working in state hospitals. *Journal of Clinical Psychology, 54*, 11–18.

Corrigan, P. W., Giffort, B., Rashid, F., Leary, M., & Okeke, I. (1999). Recovery as a psychological construct. *Consumer Mental Health Journal, 35*, 231–239.

Coursey, R. D., Keller, A. B., & Farrell, E. W. (1995). Individual psychotherapy and persons with serious mental illness: The clients' perspective. *Schizophrenia Bulletin, 21*, 283–301.

Davidson, L. (2012). Use of coercion in recovery-oriented care: Staying vigilant. *Psychiatric Services, 63,* 834.

Davidson, L., & Chan, K. K. S. (2014). Common factors: Evidence-based practice and recovery. *Psychiatric Services, 65*, 675–677.

Davidson, L., Drake, R. E., Schmutte, T., Dinzeo, T., & Andres-Hyman, R. (2009). Oil and water or oil and vinegar? Evidence-based medicine meets recovery. *Community Mental Health Journal, 45*, 323–332.

Davidson, L., O'Connell, M. O., Tondora, J., Styron, T., & Kangas, K. (2006). The top ten concerns about recovery encountered in mental health system transformation. *Psychiatric Services, 57*, 640–645.

Dickerson, F. B., & Lehman, A. F. (2011). Evidence-based psychotherapy for schizophrenia 2011 update. *The Journal of Nervous and Mental Disease, 199,* 520–526.

Dickerson, F. B., Tenhula, W. N., & Green-Paden, L. D. (2005). The token economy for schizophrenia: Review of the literature and recommendations for future research. *Schizophrenia Research, 75*, 405–416.

Dixon, L. B., Dickerson, F., Bellack, A. S., Bennett, M., Dickinson, D., Goldberg, R., et al. (2010). The 2009 *Schizophrenia* PORT psychosocial treatment recommendations and summary statements. *Schizophrenia Bulletin, 36*, 48–70.

Dixon, L., Perkins, D., & Calmes, C. (2009). *Guideline watch: Practice guideline for the treatment of patients with schizophrenia.* Arlington, VA: American Psychiatric Publishing.

Donat, D. C., McKeegan, G. F., & Neal, B. (1991). Training inpatient psychiatric staff in the use of behavioral methods: A program to enhance utilization. *Psychosocial Rehabilitation Journal, 15*, 69–74.

Douglas, K. S., Hart, S. D., Webster, C. D., & Belfrage, H. (2013). *HCR-20V3: Assessing risk of violence—User guide*. Burnaby, Canada: Mental Health, Law, and Policy Institute, Simon Fraser University.

Duffy, F. F., West, J. C., Wilk, J., Narrow, W. E., Hales, D., Thompson, J., et al. (2002). Mental health practitioners and trainees. In R. W. Manderscheid & M. J. Henderson (Eds.), *Mental Health, United States.* U.S. Department of Health and Human Services: Rockville, MD.

Fazel, S., Singh, J. P., Doll, H., & Grann, M. (2012). Use of risk assessment instruments to predict violence and antisocial behaviour in 73 samples involving 24,827 people: Systematic review and meta-analysis. *British Medical Journal, 345*, e4692.

Finn, S. E., & Tonsager, M. E. (1997). Information gathering and therapeutic models of assessment: Complementary paradigms. *Psychological Assessment, 9*, 374–385.

Fowler, I. L., Carr, V. J., Carter, N. T., & Lewin, T. J. (1998). Patterns of current and lifetime substance use in schizophrenia. *Schizophrenia Bulletin, 24*, 443–455.

Frueh, B. C., Grubaugh, A. L., Cusack, K., & Elhai, J. D. (2009a). Disseminating evidence based practices for adults with PTSD and severe mental illness in public sector mental health agencies. *Behavior Modification, 33*, 66–81.

Frueh, B. C., Grubaugh, A. L., Cusack, K. J., Kimble, M. O., Elhai, J. D., & Knapp, R. G. (2009b). Exposure-based cognitive-behavioral treatment of PTSD in adults with schizophrenia or schizoaffective disorder: A pilot study. *Journal of Anxiety Disorders, 23*, 665–675.

Geczy, B., & Cote, M. (2002). Developing an inpatient practicum program for patients with serious and persistent mental illness. *Professional Psychology: Research and Practice, 33*, 80–87.

Geczy, B., & Sultenfuss, J. F. (1994). Contributions of psychologists to inpatient care of persons with chronic mental illness. *Hospital & Community Psychiatry, 45*, 54–57.

Geczy, B., Sultenfuss, J. F., & Donat, D. (1990). Psychologists in state mental hospitals: Problems and recommendations. *Professional Psychology: Research and Practice, 21*, 392–397.

Geller, J. L. (2012). Patient-centered, recovery-oriented psychiatric care and treatment are not always voluntary. *Psychiatric Services, 63,* 493–495.

Gracie, A., Freeman, D., Green, S., Garety, P. A., Kuipers, E., Hardy, A., et al. (2007). The association between traumatic experience, paranoia and hallucinations: A test of the predictions of psychological models. *Acta Psychiatrica Scandanavica, 116*, 280–289.

Grant, P. M., Reisweber, J., Luther, L., Brinen, A. P., & Beck, A. T. (2014). Successfully breaking a 20-year cycle of hospitalizations with recovery-oriented cognitive therapy for schizophrenia. *Psychological Services, 11,* 125–133.

Grubaugh, A. L., Zinzow, H. M., Paul, L., Egede, L. E., & Frueh, B. C. (2011). Trauma exposure and posttraumatic stress disorder in adults with severe mental illness: A critical review. *Clinical Psychology Review, 31*, 883–899.

Gudjonsson, G. H., & Young, S. (2007). The role and scope of forensic clinical psychology in secure unit provisions: A proposed service model for psychological therapies. *The Journal of Forensic Psychiatry & Psychology, 18*, 534–556.

Gunderson, J. G., Stout, R. L., McGlashan, T. H., Shea, M. T., Morey, L. C., Grilo, C. M., et al. (2011). Ten-year course of borderline personality disorder: Psychopathology and function from the collaborative longitudinal personality disorders study. *Archives of General Psychiatry, 68*, 827–837.

Hackman, A., Brown, C., Yang, Y., Goldberg, R., Kreyenbuhl, J., & Lucksted, A. (2007). Consumer satisfaction with inpatient psychiatric treatment among persons with severe mental illness. *Community Mental Health Journal, 43*, 551–564.

Haddock, G., McCarron, J., Tarrier, N., & Faragher, E. B. (1999). Scales to measure dimensions of hallucinations and delusions: The psychotic symptom rating scales (PSYRATS). *Psychological Medicine, 29*, 879–889.

Haynes, S. N., Leisen, M. B., & Elaine, D. D. (1997). Design of individualized behavioral treatment programs using functional analytic clinical case models. *Psychological Assessment, 9*, 334–348.

Hillbrand, M., Young, J. L., & Griffith, E. E. H. (2010). Managing risk and recovery: Redefining miscibility of oil and water. *Journal of the American Academy of Psychiatry and the Law, 38*, 452–456.

Hoge, M. A., Stayner, D., & Davidson, L. (2000). Psychology internships in the treatment of severe mental illness: Implications for training in academic medical centers. *Journal of Clinical Psychology in Medical Settings, 7*, 213–222.

Howgego, I. M., Yellowlees, P., Owen, C., Meldrum, L., & Dark, F. (2003). The therapeutic alliance: The key to effective patient outcome? A descriptive review of the evidence in community mental health case management. *Australian and New Zealand Journal of Psychiatry, 37*, 169–183.

Iwata, B. A., & Dozier, C. L. (2008). Clinical application of functional analysis methodology. *Behavior Analysis in Practice, 1*, 3–9.

Jaaskelainen, E., Juola, P., Hirvonen, N., McGrath, J. J., Saha, S., Isohanni, M., et al. (2013). A systematic review and meta-analysis of recovery in schizophrenia. *Schizophrenia Bulletin, 39*, 1296–1306.

Jacobson, N. S., Dobson, K. D., Truax, P. A., Addis, M. E., Koerner, K., Gollan, J., et al. (1996). A component analysis of cognitive-behavioral treatment for depression. *Journal of Consulting and Clinical Psychology, 64*, 295–304.

Jamison, K. R. (1995). *An unquiet mind*. New York: Vintage Books.

Kay, S., Fiszbein, A., & Opler, L. A. (1987). The positive and negative syndrome scale (PANSS) for schizophrenia. *Schizophrenia Bulletin, 13*, 261–274.

Kern, R. S., Glynn, S. M., Horan, W. P., & Marder, S. R. (2009). Psychosocial treatments to promote functional recovery in schizophrenia. *Schizophrenia Bulletin, 35*, 347–361.

Kessler, R. C. (2004). The epidemiology of dual diagnosis. *Biological Psychiatry, 56*, 730–737.

Kingdon, D. G., & Turkington, D. (2008). *Cognitive therapy of schizophrenia*. New York, NY: Guilford Press.

Kopelowicz, A., Liberman, R. P., & Zarate, R. (2006). Recent advances in social skills training for schizophrenia. *Schizophrenia Bulletin, 32*, S12–S23.

Korotitsch, W. J., & Nelson-Gray, R. O. (1999). An overview of self-monitoring research in assessment and treatment. *Psychological Assessment, 11*, 415–425.

Kösters, M., Burlingame, G. M., Nachtigall, C., & Strauss, B. (2006). A meta-analytic review of the effectiveness of inpatient group psychotherapy. *Group Dynamics, 10*, 146–163.

Kroger, C., Schweiger, U., Sipos, V., Arnold, R., Kahl, K. G., Schunert, T., et al. (2006). Effectiveness of dialectical behaviour therapy for borderline personality disorder in an inpatient setting. *Behaviour Research and Therapy, 44*, 1211–1244.

Kurtz, M. M., & Mueser, K. T. (2008). A meta-analysis of controlled research on social skills training for schizophrenia. *Journal of Consulting and Clinical Psychology, 76*, 491–504.

Kurtz, M. M. (2012). Neurocognition and functional outcomes in schizophrenia. In B. A. Marcopulos & M. M. Kurtz (Eds.), *Clinical neuropsychological foundations of schizophrenia* (pp. 81–101). New York: American Academy of Neuropsychology/Psychology Press.

Kurtz, M. M., & Marcopulos, B. A. (2012). Cognition in schizophrenia. In B. A. Marcopulos & M. M. Kurtz (Eds.), *Clinical neuropsychological foundations of schizophrenia* (pp. 1–25). New York: American Academy of Neuropsychology/Psychology Press.

Lang, F. U., Kösters, M., Lang, S., Becker, T., & Jäger, M. (2013). Psychopathological long-term outcome of schizophrenia—A review. *Acta Psychiatrica Scandinavica, 127*, 173–182.

Law, H., & Morrison, A. P. (2014). Recovery in psychosis: A Delphi study with experts by experience. *Schizophrenia Bulletin, 40*, 1347–1355.

Levant, R. F., Reed, G. M., Ragusea, S. A., DiCowden, M., Murchy, M. J., Sullivna, F., et al. (2001). Envisioning and accessing new roles for professional psychology. *Professional Psychology: Research and Practice, 32*, 79–87.

Liberman, R. P. (2007). Dissemination and adoption of social skills training: Social validation of an evidence-based treatment for the mentally disabled. *Journal of Mental Health, 16*, 595–623.

Lincoln, T. M., Ziegler, M., Mehl, S., Kesting, M.-L., Lullmann, E., Westermann, S., & Rief, W. (2012). Moving from efficacy to effectiveness in cognitive behavior therapy for psychosis: A randomized clinical practice trail. *Journal of Consulting and Clinical Psychology, 80*, 674–686.

Linehan, M. M. (1993). *Cognitive-behavioral treatment of borderline personality disorder*. New York, NY: Guilford Press.

Linehan, M. M., Comtois, K. A., Murray, A. M., Brown, M. Z., Gallop, R. J., Heard, H., et al. (2006). Two-year randomized controlled trial and follow-up of dialectical behavior therapy versus therapy by experts for suicidal behaviors and borderline personality disorder. *Archives of General Psychiatry, 63*, 757–766.

Lukoff, D., Liberman, R. P., & Nuechterlien, K. H. (1986). Symptom monitoring in the rehabilitation of schizophrenic patients. *Schizophrenia Bulletin, 12*, 578–602.

Lysaker, P, H., Glynn, S. M., Wilkniss, S. M., & Silverstein, S. M. (2010). Psychotherapy and recovery from schizophrenia: A review of potential applications and need for future study. *Psychological Services, 7*, 75–91.

McGuire, A. B., Kukla, M., Green, A., Gilbride, D., Mueser, K. T., & Salyers, M. P. (2014). Illness management and recovery: A review of the literature. *Psychiatric Services, 65*, 171–179.

McGurk, S. B., Mueser, K. T., Cicerone, K. D., Silverstein, S. M., Myers, R., Bell, M., et al. (2013). Mental health system funding of cognitive enhancement interventions for schizophrenia: Summary and update of the New York Office of Mental Health expert panel and stakeholder meeting. *Psychiatric Rehabilitation Journal, 36*, 133–145.

McGurk, S. B., Twamley, E. W., Sitzer, D. I., McHugo, G. J., & Mueser, K. T. (2007). A meta-analysis of cognitive remediation in schizophrenia. *American Journal of Psychiatry, 164*, 1791–1802.

McMain, S. F., Guimond, T., Streiner, D. L., Cardish, R. J., & Links, P. S. (2012). Dialectical behavior therapy compared with general psychiatric management for borderline personality disorder: Clinical outcomes and functioning over a 2-year follow-up. *American Journal of Psychiatry, 169*, 650–661.

Medalia, A., & Belucci, D. (2012). Neuropsychologically informed interventions to treat cognitive impairment in schizophrenia. In B. A. Marcopulos & M. M. Kurtz (Eds.), *Clinical neuropsychological foundations of schizophrenia* (pp. 275–301). New York: American Academy of Neuropsychology/Psychology Press.

Meyer, G. J., Finn, S. E., Eyde, L. D., Kay, G. G., Moreland, K. L., Dies, R. R., et al. (2001). Psychological testing and psychological assessment: A review of evidence and issues. *American Psychologist, 56*, 128–165.

Michalski, D., Kohout, J., Wicherski, M., & Hart, B. (2011). 2009: Doctorate employment survey. Retrieved from http://www.apa.org/workforce/publications/09-doc-empl/?tab=1

Miklowitz, D. J. (2011). *The bipolar disorder survival guide* (2nd ed.). New York, NY: Guilford Press.

Miller, W. R., & Rollnick, S. (2013). *Motivational interviewing: Helping people change* (3rd ed.). New York: Guilford Press.

Millon, T., Grossman, S., & Millon, C. (2015). *Manual for the Millon Clinical Multiaxial Inventory-IV* (4th ed.). Minneapolis, MN: National Computer Systems.

Monahan, J., Steadman, H. J., Silver, E., Applebaum, P. S., Robbins, C., Mulvey, E. P., et al. (2001). *Rethinking risk assessment: The MacArthur study of mental disorder and violence*. New York: Oxford University Press.

Morey, L. C. (1997). *Personality assessment inventory: Professional manual* (2nd ed.). Odessa, FL: Psychological Assessment Resources.

Mueser, K. T. (2012). Evidence-based practices and recovery-oriented services: Is there a relationship? Should there be one? *Psychiatric Rehabilitation Journal, 35*, 287–288.

Mueser, K. T., Bolton, E., Carty, P. C., Bradley, M. J., Ahlgren, K. F., DiStaso, D. R., et al. (2007). The trauma recovery group: A cognitive behavioral program for post-traumatic stress disorder in persons with severe mental illness. *Community Mental Health Journal, 43*, 281–304.

Mueser, K. T., Corrigan, P. W., Hilton, D., Tanzman, B., Schaub, A., Gingerich, S., et al. (2002a). Illness management and recovery for severe mental illness: A review of the research. *Psychiatric Services, 53*, 1272–1284.

Mueser, K. T., Goodman, L. B., Trumbetta, S. L., Rosenberg, S. D., Osher, F. C., Vidaver, R., et al. (1998). Trauma and posttraumatic stress disorder in severe mental illness. *Journal of Consulting and Clinical Psychology, 66*, 493–499.

Mueser, K. T., Meyer, P. S., Penn, D. L., Clancy, R., Clancy, D. M., & Salyers, M. P. (2006). The illness management and recovery program: Rationale, development, and preliminary findings. *Schizophrenia Bulletin, 32*, S32–S43.

Mueser, K. T., Noordsy, D. L., Drake, R. E., & Fox, L. (2003a). *Integrated treatment for dual disorders*. New York: Guilford Press.

Mueser, K. T., Rosenberg, S. D., Goodman, L. A., & Trumbetta, S. L. (2002b). Trauma, PTSD, and the course of serve mental illness: An interactive model. *Schizophrenia Research, 53*, 123–143.

Mueser, K. T., Rosenberg, S. D., & Rosenberg, H. J. (2009). *Treatment of posttraumatic stress disorder in special populations*. Washington, DC: American Psychological Association.

Mueser, K. T., Rosenberg, S. D., Xie, H., Jankowski, M. K., Bolton, E. E., Lu, W., et al. (2008). A randomized controlled trial of cognitive-behavioral treatment for posttraumatic stress disorder in severe mental illness. *Journal of Consulting and Clinical Psychology, 76*, 259–271.

Mueser, K. T., Silverstein, S. M., & Farkas, M. D. (2013). Should the training of clinical psychologists require competence in the treatment and rehabilitation of individuals with a serious mental illness? *Psychiatric Rehabilitation Journal, 36*, 54–59.

Mueser, K. T., Torrey, W. C., Lynde, D., Singer, P., & Drake, R. E. (2003b). Implementing evidence-based practices for people with severe mental illness. *Behavior Modification, 27*, 387–411.

National Institute for Health and Care Excellence. (2014). *Psychosis and schizophrenia in adults: Treatment and management.* Retrieved from http://www.nice.org.uk/guidance/cg178

Newbill, W. A., Paul, G. L., Menditto, A. A., Springer, J. R., & Mehta, P. (2011). Social-learning programs facilitate an increase in adaptive behavior in a forensic mental hospital. *Behavioral Intervention, 26*, 214–230.

Norcross, J. C., Karpiak, C. P., & Santoro, S. O. (2005). Clinical psychologists across the years: The Division of Clinical Psychology from 1960 to 2003. *Journal of Clinical Psychology, 61*, 1467–1483.

O'Neill, R. E., Horner, R. H., Albin, R. W., Storey, K., & Sprague, J. R. (1997). *Functional assessment and program development: A practical handbook.* Pacific Grove, CA: Brookes/Cole Publishing Company.

Osher, F. C., & Steadman, H. J. (2007). Adapting evidence-based practices for persons with mental illness involved in the criminal justice system. *Psychiatric Services, 58*, 1472–1478.

Parks, J., Radke, A. Q., & Haupt, M. B. (2014). *The vital role of state psychiatric hospitals.* Alexandria, VA: National Association of State Mental Health Program Directors.

Parks, J., Svendsen, D., Singer, P., & Foti, M. E. (2006). *Morbidity and mortality in people with serious menal illness.* Alexandria, VA: National Association of State Mental Health Program Directors Medical Directors Council.

Paul, G. L., & Lentz, R. J. (1977). *Psychosocial treatment of chronic mental patients: Milieu versus social learning programs.* Cambridge, MA: Harvard University Press.

Posner, K., Brent, D., Lucas, C., Gould, M., Stanley, B., Fisher, P., et al. (2008). *Columbia-suicide severity rating scale.* New York, NY: The Research Foundation for Mental Hygiene.

Poston, J. M., & Hanson, W. E. (2010). Meta-analysis of psychological assessment as a therapeutic intervention. *Psychological Assessment, 22*, 203–212.

Pouncey, C. L., & Lukens, J. M. (2010). Madness versus badness: The ethical tension between the recovery movement and forensic psychiatry. *Theoretical Medicine and Bioethics, 31*, 93–105.

Prochaska, J. O., DiClemente, C. C., & Norcross, J. C. (1992). In search of how people change: Applications to addictive behavior. *American Psychologist, 47*, 1102–1114.

Reddy, F., Spaulding, W. D., Jansen, M. A., Menditto, A. A., & Pickett, S. (2010). Psychologists' roles and opportunities in rehabilitation and recovery for serious mental illness: A survey of Council of University Directors of Clinical Psychology (CUDCP) clinical psychology training and doctoral education. *Training and Education in Professional Psychology, 4*, 254–263.

Resnick, S. G., & Rosenheck, R. A. (2006). Recovery and positive psychology: Parallel themes and potential synergies. *Psychiatric Services, 57*, 120–122.

Roe, D., Yanos, P. T., & Lysaker, P. H. (2006). Overcoming barriers to increase the contribution of clinical psychologists to work with persons with severe mental illness. *Clinical Psychology: Science and Practice, 13*, 376–383.

Roncero, C., Barral, C., Grau-Lopez, L., Bacbiller, D., Szerman, N., Casas, M., & Ruiz, P. (2011). Protocols of dual diagnosis intervention in schizophrenia. *Additive Disorders & Their Treatment, 10*, 121–154.

Russinova, Z., Rogers, E. S., Ellison, M. L., & Lyass, A. (2011). Recovery promoting professional competencies: Perspectives of mental health consumers, consumer-providers, and providers. *Psychiatric Rehabilitation Journal, 34*, 177–185.

Saha, S., Chant, D., & McGrath, J. (2007). A systematic review of mortality in schizophrenia: Is the differential mortality gap worsening over time? *Archives of General Psychiatry, 64*, 1123–1131.

Salyers, M. P., Evans, L. J., Bond, G. R., & Meyer, P. S. (2004). Barriers to assessment and treatment of posttraumatic stress disorder and other trauma-related problems in people with severe mental illness: Clinician perspective. *Community Mental Health Journal, 40*, 17–31.

Salyers, M. P., McGuire, A. B., Kukla, M., Fukui, S., Lysaker, P. H., & Mueser, K. T. (2014). A randomized controlled trial of illness management and recovery, with an active control group. *Psychiatric Services, 65*, 1005–1011.

Salyers, M. P., Tsai, J., & Stultz, T. A. (2007). Measuring a recovery orientation in a hospital setting. *Psychiatric Rehabilitation Journal, 31*, 131–137.

Scott, J., Chant, D., Andrews, G., Martin, G., & McGrath, J. (2007). Association between trauma exposure and delusional experiences in a large community-based sample. *British Journal of Psychiatry, 190*, 339–343.

Schrank, B., Brownell, T., Jakaite, Z., Larkin, C., Pesola, F., Riches, S., et al. (2015). Evaluation of a positive psychotherapy group intervention for people with psychosis: Pilot randomized controlled trial. *Epidemiology & Psychiatric Services.* Available on CJO2015. doi:10.1017/S2045796015000141

Schrank, B., Brownell, T., Tylee, A., & Slade, M. (2014a). Positive psychology: An approach to supporting recovery in mental illness. *East Asian Archives of Psychiatry, 24*, 95–103.

Schrank, B., Riches, S., Coggins, T., Rashid, T., Tylee, A., & Slade, M. (2014b). WELLFOCUS PPT—A modified positive psychotherapy to improve well-being in psychosis: Study protocol for a pilot randomized controlled trial. *Trials, 15*, 203–216.

Seligman, M. E. P. (2011). *Flourish*. New York: Free Press.

Seligman, M. E. P., & Csikszentmihalyi, M. (2000). Positive psychology: An introduction. *American Psychologist, 55*, 5–14.

Seligman, M. E. P., Rashid, T., & Parks, A. C. (2006). Positive psychotherapy. *American Psychologist, 61*, 774–788.

Silverstein, S. M., Hatashita-Wong, M., Wilkniss, S., Bloch, A., Smith, T., Savitz, A., et al. (2006a). Behavioral rehabilitation of the "treatment-refractory" schizophrenia patient: Conceptual foundations, interventions, and outcome data. *Psychological Services, 3*, 145–169.

Silverstein, S. M., Spaulding, W. D., & Mendito, A. A. (2006b). *Schizophrenia*. Cambridge, MA: Hogrefe & Huber Publishers.

Simpson, A. I. F., & Penney, S. R. (2011). The recovery paradigm in forensic mental health services. *Criminal Behaviour and Mental Health, 21*, 299–306.

Sin, N. L., & Lyubomirsky, S. (2009). Enhancing well-being and alleviating depressive symptoms with positive psychology interventions: A practice-friendly meta-analysis. *Journal of Clinical Psychology, 65*, 467–487.

Singh, N. N., Matson, J. L., Lancioni, G. E., Singh, A. N., Adkins, A. D., McKeegan, G. F., & Brown, S. W. (2006). Questions about behavioral function in mental illness (QABF-MI). *Behavior Modification, 30*(6), 739–751.

Siris, S. G. (2001). Suicide and schizophrenia. *Journal of Psychopharmacology, 15*, 127–135.

Smith, G. B., Schwebel, A. I., Dunn, R. L., & McIver, S. D. (1993). The role of psychologists in the treatment, management, and prevention of chronic mental illness. *American Psychologist, 48*, 966–971.

Smtih, G. M., Ashbridge, D. M., Davis, R. H., & Steinmetz, W. (2015). Correlation between reduction of seclusion and restraint and assaults by patients in Pennsylvania's state hospitals. *Psychiatric Services, 66*, 303–309.

Smith, R. C., & Bartholomew, T. (2006). Will hospitals recover?: The implications of a recovery-orientation. *American Journal of Psychiatric Rehabilitation, 9*, 85–100.

Spaulding, W. D., Sullivan, M. E., Poland, J. S., & Ritchie, A. J. (2010). State psychiatric institutions and the left-behinds of mental health reform. *American Journal of Orthopsychiatry, 80*, 327–333.

Substance Abuse and Mental Health Services Administration. (2006). *National consensus statement on mental health recovery*. Retrieved from http://store.samhsa.gov/shin/content/SMA05-4129/SMA05-4129.pdf

Substance Abuse and Mental Health Services Administration. (2009). *Illness management and recovery: Practitioner guides and handouts. HHS Publication No. (SMA) 09-4462*. Rockville, MD: Center for Mental Health Services, Substance Abuse and Mental Health Services Administration, U.S. Department of Health and Human Services.

Substance Abuse and Mental Health Services Administration. (2011). *Recovery to practice: Frequently asked questions*. Rockville, MD: Substance Abuse and Mental Health Services Administration.

Substance Abuse and Mental Health Services Administration. (2012). *Mental health, United States, 2010. HHS Publication No. (SMA) 12-4681*. Rockville, MD: Substance Abuse and Mental Health Services Administration.

Substance Abuse and Mental Health Services Administration. (2014a). *SAMHSA's concept of trauma and guidance for a trauma-informed approach*. Rockville, MD: Substance Abuse and Mental Health Services Administration.

Substance Abuse and Mental Health Services Administration. (2014b). *Trauma-informed care in behavioral health services*. Rockville, MD: Substance Abuse and Mental Health Services Administration.

Swartz, M. S., Wagner, H. R., Swanson, J. W., Stroup, T. S., McEvoy, J. P., Canive, J., et al. (2006). Substance use in persons with schizophrenia: Baseline prevalence and correlates from the NIMH CATIE study. *Journal of Nervous and Mental Disease, 194*, 164–172.

Swenson, C. R., Sanderson, C., Dulit, R. A., & Linehan, M. M. (2001). The application of dialectical behavior therapy for patients with borderline personality disorder on inpatient units. *Psychiatric Quarterly, 72*, 307–324.

Tarasenko, M., Sullivan, M., Ritchie, A. J., & Spaulding, W. D. (2013). Effects of eliminating psychiatric rehabilitation from the secure levels of a mental-health service system. *Psychological Services, 10*, 442–451.

Taylor, T. L., Killaspy, H., Wright, C., Turton, P., White, S., Kallert, T. W., et. al. (2009). A systematic review of the international published literature relating to quality of institutional care for people with longer term mental health problems. *BioMed Central Psychiatry, 9*, 55.

Thase, M. E., Kingdon, D., & Turkington, D. (2014). The promise of cognitive behavior therapy for treatment of severe mental disorders: a review of recent developments. *World Psychiatry, 13*, 244–250.

Tsai, J., & Salyers, M. P. (2008). Recovery orientation in hospital and community settings. *Journal of Behavioral Health Services and Research, 37*, 385–399.

Torrey, W. C., Rapp, C. A., Van Tosh, L., McNabb, C. R. A., & Ralph, R. O. (2005). Recovery principles and evidence based practice: Essential ingredients of service improvement. *Community Mental Health Journal, 41*, 91–100.

Turner, D. T., van der Gaag, M., Karyotaki, E., & Cuijpers, P. (2014). Psychological interventions for psychosis: A meta-analysis of comparative outcome studies. *American Journal of Psychiatry, 171*, 523–538.

Turton, P., Wright, C., White, S., Killaspy, H., & the DEMoBinc Group. (2010). Promoting recovery in long-term institutional mental health care: An international Delphi study. *Psychiatric Services, 61*, 293–299.

Warner, R. (2010). Does the scientific evidence support the recovery model? *The Psychiatrist Online, 34*, 3–5.

Wood, K. A., Rogers, J. H., McCarthy, S. M., & Lewine, R. R. J. (1994). Psychologists in public inpatient psychiatric settings: Ethical dilemmas. *Professional Psychology: Research and Practice, 25*, 234–240.

Wright, J. H., Kingdon, D., Turkington, D., & Basco, M. R. (2008). *Cognitive-behavior therapy for severe mental illness*. Arlington, VA: American Psychiatric Publishing Inc.

Wykes, T., Huddy, V., Cellard, C., McGurk, S. R., & Czobor, P. (2011). A meta-analysis of cognitive remediation for schizophrenia: Methodology and effect sizes. *American Journal of Psychiatry, 168*, 472–485.

Wykes, T., Steel, C., Everitt, B., & Tarrier, N. (2008). Cognitive behavior therapy for schizophrenia: Effect sizes, clinical models, and methodological rigor. *Schizophrenia Bulletin, 34*, 523–537.

Young, R. C., Biggs, J. T., Ziegler, V. E., & Meyer, D. A. (1978). A rating scale for mania: Reliability, validity and sensitivity. *British Journal of Psychiatry, 133*, 429–443.

Zanarini, M. C., Frankenburg, F. R., Reich, D. B., & Fitzmaurice, G. (2012). Attainment and stability of sustained symptomatic remission and recovery among patients with borderline personality disorder and Axis II comparison subjects: A 16-year prospective follow-up study. *American Journal of Psychiatry, 169*, 476–483.

# Mental Health Nursing Services 11

Rachel E. Myers

## Introduction

The current trend in mental health systems is a strong movement toward implementation of a recovery model of care (American Nurses Association [ANA] 2014; Seed and Torkelson 2012; Substance Abuse and Mental Health Services Administration [SAMHSA] 2006). Recovery principles are rooted in the foundations of nursing practice. Components of the recovery model are consistent with the training and practice of nursing, such as providing individualized and person-centered care, viewing the individual holistically rather than narrowly defined by his/her illness or disorder, building upon the individual's strengths rather than focusing on his/her deficits, demonstrating respect, fostering hope, and enabling the individual to live a personally satisfying, meaningful life (SAMHSA 2006).

The recent emphasis on recovery supports psychiatric-mental health (PMH) nursing traditions of relationship-based care in which the focus is on the care and treatment of the individual with the disorder, and not the disorder itself. Through the use of therapeutic interpersonal skills, PMH nurses are instrumental in assisting individuals with mental disorders achieve their own recovery and wellness goals. The practice of nursing in an inpatient psychiatric hospital is particularly well suited to the mental health recovery model as nurses have the largest professional presence in this setting, often a continuous 24-hour presence (ANA 2014; Beech 2000; Turkington et al. 2006). However, the inpatient setting presents unique challenges that create tensions between recovery principles and nursing services. This chapter describes how PMH nurses can incorporate the recovery model in the provision of services in an inpatient psychiatric hospital from admission to discharge, along with some of the challenges they may face along the way.

To provide context for subsequent sections, the chapter begins with a brief description of various nursing roles, nursing's relationship to the recovery model, and the therapeutic nurse–patient relationship. This is followed by a brief description of the inpatient psychiatric hospital setting and individuals typically served in this setting. Then there is a discussion of treatment planning and the nursing process, and the vital role of the PMH nurse as an interdisciplinary treatment team member. Next, there is a discussion of some of the services nurses provide, including assessments and interventions, with an emphasis on how nurses can incorporate recovery principles into the provision of these services. The chapter concludes with a discussion of some

R.E. Myers (✉)
WellStar School of Nursing, Kennesaw State University, 520 Parliament Garden Way, MD 4102, Kennesaw, GA 30144, USA
e-mail: rmyers23@kennesaw.edu



N.N. Singh et al. (eds.), *Handbook of Recovery in Inpatient Psychiatry*,
Evidence-Based Practices in Behavioral Health, DOI 10.1007/978-3-319-40537-7_11

challenges the recovery model poses for nurses providing these services in inpatient psychiatric hospitals.

## Psychiatric-Mental Health Nursing

Psychiatric-mental health (PMH) nursing is defined as "the nursing practice specialty committed to promoting mental health through the assessment, diagnosis, and treatment of behavioral problems, mental disorders, and comorbid conditions across the lifespan" (ANA 2014, p. 19). There are two levels of practice of PMH nursing: the psychiatric-mental health registered nurse (PMH-RN), with educational preparation within a bachelor's degree, associate's degree, or a diploma program, and the psychiatric-mental health advanced practice registered nurse (PMH-APRN), with educational preparation within a master's or doctoral degree program. In addition, the PMH-APRN level has two subcategories: the psychiatric-mental health clinical nurse specialist (PMHCNS) and the psychiatric-mental health nurse practitioner (PMHNP). Nursing staff in mental health settings may also be comprised of positions other than RNs, such as licensed practical or vocational nurses, psychiatric technicians, and forensic technicians. While these other nursing staff are valuable team members that often spend substantial time with the individuals and report to the RNs, this chapter primarily focuses on the role of RNs.

The movement toward the integration of recovery principles in PMH nursing requires a paradigm shift away from a medical model, an approach that is largely inconsistent with recovery principles. The medical model has been described as not therapeutic, not empowering, and not conducive to healing, with a focus on the illness rather than the person with the illness (Chen et al. 2013; Deegan 2007; Seed and Torkelson 2012; Swarbrick 2006). In acute care and inpatient psychiatric units, PMH nurses who work primarily in a culture that emphasizes the medical model spend the majority of their time performing routine task-oriented duties such as administering medications to control or alleviate symptoms, keeping the unit safe (e.g., observing and monitoring individuals at risk), providing overly custodial care (e.g., setting strict limits or suggesting solutions instead of teaching problem-solving skills), completing excessive paperwork and other administrative duties, and attending numerous meetings (Mullen 2009; Seed and Torkelson 2012; Seed et al. 2010). While some of these duties are undeniably important, they are time consuming, narrow in scope, and often do not allow sufficient time for nurses to engage in frequent, quality interactions with individuals in order to establish a therapeutic relationship, the core of PMH nursing (Aston and Coffey 2012; Cahill et al. 2013; Mathers 2012; Mullen 2009).

In contrast to the medical model, the role of PMH nurses in the recovery model is not only to provide routine, task-oriented care and treatment, but also develop partnerships and assist individuals with their recovery goals. Examples of these goals may include renewing hope, becoming involved with meaningful activities, redefining self beyond illness, incorporating illness, managing symptoms, assuming control, becoming empowered, overcoming barriers to social inclusion, exercising citizenship, and being supported by others (Davidson et al. 2003).

Among many definitions, SAMHSA (2006) defined mental health recovery as a journey of healing and transformation, and described 10 fundamental components of recovery: hope, self-direction, individualized and person-centered, empowerment, holistic, nonlinear, strengths-based, peer support, respect, and responsibility. Regardless of the specific definition, the consensus is that recovery is what the individual does, and treatment and rehabilitation are what PMH nurses and other healthcare professionals do to facilitate the individual's journey along his/her path.

Like nursing in general, PMH nursing is both a science and an art. It is a science in that PMH nurses utilize a wide range of theories and research findings to guide their practice. They also use the nursing process as a critical thinking framework to serve as the foundation for clinical decision-making and to support evidence-based practice. When applied to PMH nursing, the nursing process involves six areas: assessment, diagnosis, outcomes identification, planning, implementation, and evaluation. PMH nurses use the nursing process to care for and treat individuals with actual or potential mental health problems, psychiatric disorders, co-occurring psychiatric and substance use disorders and risks, and co-occurring physical health problems, medical illnesses, or risks. Utilization of the nursing process in PMH is consistent with a recovery-oriented model as nurses use it to promote and foster health and safety, assess dysfunction and areas of individual strength, assist individuals to achieve their own personal recovery goals, maximize strengths, and prevent further disability.

PMH nursing is an art in that it is accomplished through interpersonal relationships, therapeutic intervention skills, and professional attributes. Examples of these attributes include self-awareness, moral integrity, and empathy, which enable PMH nurses to practice the purposeful, artful use of self in therapeutic relationships as characterized by respect, availability, hope, acceptance, advocacy, and spirituality, to name just a few. The therapeutic nurse–patient relationship concept is considered the hallmark of PMH nursing (O'Brien et al. 2013). Several characteristics define this relationship that align with recovery principles. For example, a therapeutic relationship is based on mutual respect, focused on the individual and designed to meet his/her needs, and collaborative, with both the individual and nurse contributing to growth, healing, and problem solving. The interactions are goal oriented, the goals are mutually established, and decision-making is shared. Furthermore, the relationship promotes the individual's independence to the greatest extent possible, where the nurse *works with* the individual versus *doing for* the individual (O'Brien et al. 2013).

O'Brien et al. (2013) described four qualities essential to the development of a therapeutic nurse–patient relationship. The first quality is *respect*. PMH nurses must accept individuals' beliefs and feelings with a nonjudgmental attitude, even if they differ from their own. Nurses need to also be self-aware of and examine any preconceived attitudes, beliefs, or judgments they have that may interfere with providing therapeutic care to an individual. While it is inevitable that differences will exist between PMH nurses and individuals, nurses must accept and respect these differences, attempt to understand the individual's perspective, and not impose their personal values. Nurses can demonstrate respect to individuals in numerous ways such as asking how they prefer to be addressed (e.g., first name, last name), assessing for religious or cultural factors that may influence care and treatment, being sensitive to touch and personal space, and involving individuals in decision-making and treatment planning.

The second essential quality is *trust*, which O'Brien et al. (2013) described as the foundation of all interpersonal relationships. Trust is particularly important for individuals with mental illness given their increased vulnerability, and it is essential for their PMH nurses to be honest, reliable, and dependable. Nurses must earn this trust, and it will evolve over the progression of the relationship rather than occur immediately. However, what takes a long time to build can be quickly undone by just one negative occurrence, so all nursing actions need to promote trust. Some examples include consistently following through with promises (e.g., be on time for appointments; give reinforcement for positive behaviors as agreed upon) and treating individuals fairly (e.g., in a psychosocial group, do not show unfair, subjective favoritism toward an individual).

The third significant quality is *genuineness*, or the ability for nurses to be themselves or to be real or authentic during interactions with individuals (O'Brien et al. 2013). This quality also refers to congruence between what nurses are actually feeling and their expression of these feelings. For example, if an individual shares a story about being sad and angry due to the recent death of a best friend and the PMH nurse's verbal behavior demonstrates caring and understanding but nonverbal expressions suggest apathy, this lack of genuineness could also impact the level of respect and trust in the relationship. In addition, if an individual asks the nurse something and the nurse does not know, typically there is a greater chance the individual will respect the nurse admitting his/her limitations and providing an honest, genuine response rather than providing a false response.

The fourth quality O'Brien et al. (2013) discussed as an essential characteristic of the nurse–patient relationship is *empathy*, or the ability to put oneself in another person's place and see the world as he/she does. A PMH nurse who is empathetic has an objective understanding of an individual's emotions and is sensitive to the individual's feelings without actually experiencing the emotions. Empathy helps build trust in a relationship and differs from sympathy, which is a subjective experience, involves an actual sharing of experienced emotions, and may interfere with the relationship and the nurse's ability to provide effective, supportive care, and treatment.

These four qualities—respect, trust, genuineness, and empathy—are consistent with the first three provisions of the ANA *Code of Ethics for Nurses with Interpretive Statements* (ANA 2015), which state, "the nurse practices with compassion and respect for the inherent dignity, worth, and unique attributes of every person" (p. 1), "the nurse's primary commitment is to the patient, whether an individual, family, group, community, or population" (p. 5), and "the nurse promotes, advocates for, and protects the rights, health, and safety of the patient" (p. 9), respectively. PMH nurses that adhere to these provisions help promote a therapeutic relationship with the individuals they serve and thus assist these individuals in achieving their recovery goals.

Compared to a social relationship, the professional nurse–patient relationship is purposeful, structured, and time-limited, and nurses' self-disclosure of intimate, personal information is restricted. Multiple factors contribute to the development and success of the professional relationship such as development of trust, mutually determined goals, and establishment of boundaries early in the relationship. The nurse's use of therapeutic communication techniques during all interactions, both formal and informal, is also critical, such as while conducting an assessment, engaging in an informal conversation, conducting a formal individual counseling session, or facilitating a psychosocial rehabilitation group. Examples of therapeutic communication techniques include active listening (e.g., during an assessment interview or individual counseling session), effective nonverbal techniques (e.g., appropriate facial expression, posture, and eye contact that is culturally sensitive), effective verbal techniques, and skillful communication (e.g., constructive strategies for verbally obtaining and conveying information during an interview or to encourage engagement of an individual in treatment), and assertive communication, which promotes the use of *I* versus *you* statements and allows individuals to own their feelings and communicate their wishes and needs in a respectful, nonaggressive manner (O'Brien et al. 2013).

PMH nurses practice in a variety of clinical settings across the continuum of care, including but not limited to partial hospitalization (or day treatment) and intensive outpatient programs, residential facilities, community mental health centers, assertive community treatment (ACT) teams, home healthcare, psychiatric emergency departments, and inpatient psychiatric hospitals (ANA 2014; O'Brien et al. 2013). This chapter focuses primarily on inpatient psychiatric hospitals, a setting in which the majority (two thirds) of PMH nurses work (Hanrahan 2009). Individuals admitted to inpatient psychiatric hospitals may be voluntary or involuntary (civil) commitment (i.e., court-ordered). They may also be admitted through the criminal justice system with a forensic legal status for reasons such as emergency treatment due to dangerousness to self or others, evaluation of their competency to stand trial, restoration of their competency to stand trial, or evaluation of their mental state at the time of the alleged offense (Singh et al. 2016).

Individuals served in an inpatient psychiatric hospital often have a severe mental illness (SMI), which is a mental, behavioral, or emotional disorder that substantially interferes with or limits one or more major life activities (SAMHSA 2013b). SMIs tend to last for a long time (if not a lifetime) and may be characterized by periods of relapse or reoccurrence. While many psychiatric disorders have the potential to persist and become chronic and severe, schizophrenia, major depressive disorder, and bipolar disorder tend to be most prevalent, and an individual may experience more than one mental disorder (Spaulding et al. 2016).

## Treatment Planning and Nursing Process

Individuals residing in inpatient psychiatric hospitals face many complex issues that necessitate treatment teams to take an interdisciplinary versus a multidisciplinary approach to care and treatment in order to achieve desired goals and best facilitate the individual's road to recovery. Teams that adopt a multidisciplinary approach are more clinician centered and are characterized by several disciplines working parallel to each other in silos, doing their individual pieces of the process, writing separate treatment plans, and combining the separate plans into one big plan with little to no integration (Akhavain et al. 1999; McLoughlin and Geller 2010). This approach frequently results in fragmented, redundant, complicated, confusing, and inconsistent care that lacks alignment with the recovery model. Individuals are unable to track their own progress, and team members lose focus of who is doing what and why. In contrast, teams that utilize an interdisciplinary approach are more person-centered and are depicted by disciplines that work collaboratively and cooperatively toward common goals and combine efforts to formulate one synergistic treatment plan. In comparison to the multidisciplinary approach, the interdisciplinary approach is more streamlined, simple, clear, user-friendly, and consistent and is better aligned with the recovery model as it emphasizes the importance of individuals taking significant responsibility for their own recovery by taking active ownership in their treatment and rehabilitation plan and being a dynamic participant in the team collaboration process.

PMH nurses are core members of the interdisciplinary team, along with other disciplines such as psychiatry, psychology, primary care, social work, rehabilitation services, and activity therapy (Singh et al. 2016). Although all disciplines share common knowledge and skills in some areas, each member has a unique knowledge base and skills and brings his/her own perspectives and ideas to the table that enriches the treatment team. For example, utilizing the therapeutic nurse–patient relationship as their basis, PMH nurses bring expertise in assessing an individual's capacity to engage in activities of daily living and helping the individual cope as needed (O'Brien et al. 2013). Ideally, the planned synergy that results when overlapping strengths and knowledge of the various interdisciplinary team members are tailored and matched to the needs of the individual will enhance the outcomes of care and treatment and expand the comprehensiveness of these outcomes (ANA 2014). For example, Akhavain et al.'s (1999) review of the literature suggested implementation of a collaborative team approach enhanced quality of individuals' care as evidenced by positive outcomes such as reduced mortality rates, reduced costs, and self-reported improved quality of life.

In the inpatient psychiatric hospital setting, the treatment plan serves as a blueprint or roadmap for the individual's recovery from admission to discharge (Davidson et al. 2016; Singh et al. 2016). Based on the recovery model, rehabilitation and recovery principles are typically the framework that guides development of treatment plans in inpatient psychiatric hospital settings, and the overall aims of these plans are to assist individuals in stabilization of symptoms (as indicated) and to help them obtain the skills needed to be discharged from the hospital, to experience successful community reintegration, and to have enhanced quality of life. A few modifications to these aims may be necessary in some instances such as individuals admitted with forensic status or individuals with co-occurring mental illness and developmental disabilities.

In order to be effective, treatment plans should be person-centered and focus on the individual as opposed to just on specific diseases, disorders, or deficits of the individual. They should also be tailored to the individual's needs and preferences rather than trying to fit the individual into a prewritten, cookie cutter plan. In addition, treatment plans should be meaningful to the individual and enable all team members to evaluate the attainment of goals and the effectiveness of interventions. Exact components of treatment plans vary among hospitals, but common elements typically include case formulation, diagnoses, discharge criteria and plan, discharge barriers/problems, goals and objectives, and interventions (Singh et al. 2016). In addition, while assessments are not theoretically a part of the treatment plan, they serve as the foundation for the plan's development, and reassessments must be conducted to evaluate the plan's effectiveness on a preset schedule (and more often as needed) to determine whether modifications need to be made. As core members of the interdisciplinary team, PMH nurses play a vital role in the development, implementation, and evaluation of the treatment plan.

When applied to PMH nursing, the nursing process involves six steps: assessment, diagnosis, outcomes identification, planning, implementation, and evaluation (ANA 2010, 2014). These steps essentially mirror those of the treatment planning process. Historically, inpatient psychiatric hospitals have required PMH nurses to write nursing care plans (separate from the team's treatment plan) that contain information to reflect each step in the nursing process. To be more consistent with recovery principles and the interdisciplinary approach to care and treatment, there needs to be a cultural shift away from separate nursing care plans and toward one fully integrated plan (Akhavain et al. 1999). This in no way suggests PMH nurses should stop using the nursing process as a critical thinking framework to assist individuals throughout their recovery journey.

## Nursing Assessments

Assessment is one of the PMH nurse's most important skills as it helps define the individual's actual and potential problems, and it enables the nurse and individual to establish a relationship. Although assessment is theoretically the first step in the nursing process, it is in actuality a continuous process carried out during all steps (Berman et al. 2016). The PMH-RN utilizes a systematic and ongoing method to conduct assessments and collect, organize, validate, and document comprehensive objective and subjective data in many areas, including but not limited to psychiatric, substance, physical, functional, emotional, psychosocial, cognitive, cultural, age-related, sexual, environmental, spiritual/transpersonal, and economic (ANA 2014). PMH-RN assessments also involve obtaining information about the individual's "values, preferences, knowledge of the healthcare situation, expressed needs, and recovery goals" (ANA 2014, p. 44). The PMH-APRN has an expanded scope of practice that includes additional skills such as the performance of psychiatric and mental health diagnostic evaluations and the initiation and interpretation of diagnostic tests and procedures (ANA 2014).

## Types and Functions of Assessments

PMH nurses conduct several types of assessments, including but not limited to initial, time lapsed, problem-focused, and emergency (Berman et al. 2016). Initial assessments are useful for establishing a comprehensive database for actual and potential problems and risk identification, reference, and future comparison, such as upon an individual's admission to an inpatient psychiatric hospital. The psychiatric admission nursing assessment typically consists of a biopsychosocial history, a mental status examination, and a physical assessment. PMH nurses may also conduct initial risk assessments to identify factors that place individuals at high risk for behavioral, psychiatric, and medical conditions (e.g., suicide, impaired skin integrity, falls). These risk assessments may be published scales in the literature such as the Braden Scale for Predicting Pressure Sore Risk (Bergstrom et al. 1987) or based on specific criteria determined by the hospital. In addition, nurses may also conduct screens (e.g., nutrition) to identify individuals at potential risk for a health condition (based on predetermined criteria), to trigger a more comprehensive risk assessment, and to implement immediate interventions (if clinically indicated) to keep the individual and others safe until further evaluation can be completed. Specific components of admission assessments will vary depending on factors such as the RN's scope of practice.

Time-lapsed assessments are conducted subsequent to initial assessments in order to compare the individual's current status to baseline data (Berman et al. 2016). This assessment type is particularly relevant to recovery, which is characterized as nonlinear (SAMHSA 2006). In an inpatient psychiatric hospital, individuals' progress along the road to recovery is not a step-by-step process but rather based on continual growth, occasional setback, and learning from experience. Change often occurs slowly and must be closely monitored at designated intervals, such as monthly, quarterly, and annually. Time-lapsed nursing assessments may help identify and document progress, thus instilling hope that improvement is occurring. These assessments are also helpful in detecting changes that occur more rapidly. For example, when an individual is first admitted and assessments are conducted at change of shift (and more often as indicated), progress toward stabilization of symptoms and overall functional health can be monitored.

Problem-focused assessments are an ongoing process integrated with nursing care and are conducted to determine the status of a specific problem or issue identified during a previous assessment (Berman et al. 2016). For example, if an individual has an acute change in mental status related to electrolyte abnormalities, reassessments of mental status will be conducted as often as clinically indicated until the problem is resolved. This assessment type also applies when evaluating progress toward skills training (e.g., an individual learning how to safely and effectively self-administer an insulin injection). Emergency assessments are conducted during any psychological or physiological crisis in order to identify life-threatening or new or overlooked problems. Examples include assessing suicidal tendencies or potential for violence or assessing for airway, breathing, and circulation during a cardiac arrest.

## Assessment Methods

PMH nurses use a wide array of methods to conduct the various nursing assessment types, of which the principal methods are interviews, observations, and examinations. Interviews are deliberate, purposeful conversations or communications between the nurse and individual and can serve multiple purposes such as to receive or provide information, identify problems, evaluate change, educate, or provide support, counseling or therapy. Nurses often conduct interviews when completing parts of the biopsychosocial history of the nursing admission assessment. Interviews can be structured (standardized questions) or unstructured (no standardized questions), and consist of both closed- and open-ended questions, depending on several factors such as the purpose of the interview and the needs of the individual. Often a combination of the techniques is best, and the nurse may need to adapt interview strategies based on the situation and the environment. When conducting interviews, PMH nurses should utilize therapeutic techniques described above (e.g., active listening, effective nonverbal and verbal techniques, skillful and assertive communication) that are consistent with qualities essential to development of a therapeutic nurse–patient relationship (i.e., respect, trust, genuineness, and empathy).

Nurses also gather data through observations by using their senses (sight, smell, hearing, and touch). This method not only involves noticing data but also selecting, organizing, and interpreting the data. For example, if the nurse smells foul body odor on an individual, he/she must determine what this finding is related to—poor hygiene, self-neglect, neglect by a caretaker, normal odor after physical exercise, etc. In addition, nurses conduct physical examinations using inspection, auscultation, palpation, and percussion. When doing a complete exam, nurses should utilize a systematic approach such as head-to-toe or body systems, or they may just concentrate on a particular system for problem-focused exams. Other data collection methods may include asking the individual to self-monitor, such as daily mood ratings (e.g., Tusaie 2013) and intake and output measurement.

## Sources of Data

PMH nurses obtain assessment data from both primary and secondary sources of information. The individual (primary) is usually considered the best source unless he/she is too ill, confused, or young to communicate clearly or reliably. The individual can provide subjective data no one else can offer. In inpatient psychiatric hospital settings, individuals often feel most comfortable sharing certain personal, sensitive information with the PMH nurse versus other healthcare team members because of the therapeutic relationship that develops between them due to close and frequent contact. However, it is often beneficial to also obtain data from secondary sources to not only supplement information the individual provides but to also validate or verify it in some instances, especially if there are concerns with reliability, accuracy, or completeness of information. At times individuals may also not be willing or able to provide information due to various reasons such as too ill upon admission, confusion, or paranoia of the nurse's intentions. Examples of secondary sources of data include but are not limited to family members or other support persons (e.g., friends, caregivers, shelter staff, clergy), other health professionals (e.g., verbal report from PMH nurse from another hospital; documentation of behavioral observations on a flow sheet by psychiatric technicians), past and current health records and reports (e.g., medical records, operative reports, social agency reports), laboratory and diagnostic analyses, and relevant literature (e.g., professional journals and reference texts). For individuals admitted with forensic status, the PMH nurse may also review court documents such as warrants, court orders, records from jail, and copies of previous forensic evaluations and obtain information from law enforcement officers.

## Incorporation of Recovery Principles

There are numerous ways the PMH nurse can incorporate recovery principles into the assessment process. The assessment process itself, which is continuous in nature, is consistent with recovery being *nonlinear*, such as with time-lapsed assessments described above. For most individuals with SMI, the road to recovery is long and arduous, change is slow, and many barriers and obstacles confront them. Although *hope* is internalized, PMH nurses can foster hope through actions such as providing positive reinforcement during assessments, acknowledging when even the smallest amount of progress has been made toward a goal. Hope is an individual's catalyst for recovery and is an essential motivating factor along the journey (SAMHSA 2006).

Next, the nurse should always demonstrate *respect*, which involves acceptance and appreciation of individuals, including protection of their rights and elimination of stigma and discrimination (SAMHSA 2006). For example, the nurse should always obtain consent from the individual prior to approaching family members and other support persons for assessment data (except in the case of an emergency or unless he/she is not mentally able). PMH nurses should also be both culturally sensitive and culturally competent (O'Brien et al. 2013). Cultural sensitivity refers to nurses being aware of and respecting the individual's values and lifestyles even when they differ from their own, whereas cultural competence is a broader, multidimensional concept that involves knowledge, attitude, and skills. It is important for the treatment team to assess an individual's cultural and ethnic preferences and practices and whether there are any issues that may be pertinent to his/her illness or treatment (e.g., use of complementary alternative medicine, such as healing touch or herbs, prior to admission).

In addition, nursing assessments should be *strengths-based*, which involves building upon and valuing the individual's numerous capacities, talents, resiliencies, coping abilities, and inherent worth (SAMHSA 2006). One broad example discussed above is the recent paradigm shift occurring in inpatient psychiatric hospitals, moving away from the medical model (which primarily focuses on the illness or disorder) toward a recovery model (which focuses on the individual with the illness or disorder). A more specific example that applies to PMH nursing relates to medication non-adherence. Using a strengths-based approach, instead of focusing on and trying to suppress the deviant behavior (e.g., assessing how many times individuals do not comply with practitioner orders and why they do not comply), an alternative approach may be for the PMH nurse to focus on and try to enhance the adherent behavior (e.g., assess how many times individuals take the medication as prescribed; explore with the individuals what was different the times they took the medication compared to the times they did not take it; explore what they think contributes to them taking the medication on some days but not others; explore what strategies they think may help increase the number of times they would take the medication as prescribed). Involving the individuals in discussions such as these, asking their opinions and ideas, incorporates elements of several other recovery principles such as *individualized and person-centered* and *empowerment*.

With *empowerment*, individuals have the authority to choose from a variety of options, to participate in all decisions that may affect their lives, and to speak for themselves about their needs, wants, desires, and aspirations (SAMHSA 2006). One instance of empowering individuals during the assessment process is to offer them a choice of when and where to conduct the assessment and whether they would like to have a family member or other support person present. For example, if an individual is acutely ill and unable to tolerate much contact and exploration, when at all possible, the nurse should provide him/her a choice of several brief assessment interviews instead of one long interview.

Another illustration of empowerment is to offer individuals choices related to their personal safety. For instance, PMH nurses may conduct a Personal Safety Interview with the individuals and ask them questions that elicit choices and involve them in decision-making. For example, nurses may ask the individuals how staff could help them when they noticed they were getting irritated, upset, or angry. They may also ask if they have any preferences or concerns regarding who serves them, such as gender, race, language, and culture. These examples of empowerment also demonstrate *respect* toward the individual. Still another example of how PMH nurses can empower individuals, as well as promote *responsibility* (another recovery principle, where the individual is responsible for his/her own self-care) is to teach them self-care skills and involve them in self-monitoring. For example, a PMH nurse may teach an individual newly diagnosed with diabetes how to self-monitor blood glucose and record amount of food and fluid intake at each meal. The nurse would include the individual's self-monitoring data with data from other nurses and staff when collaborating with the treatment team to evaluate overall diabetes management.

The PMH nurse can also incorporate the recovery principle of *self-direction* into nursing assessments by asking the individual to describe his/her life goals or vision of recovery, including hopes, dreams, and aspirations. Although these goals may include what the individual wishes to do while at the hospital, it is much better to assist the individual to envision life following discharge. In collaboration with the treatment team, the PMH nurse should assess life goals upon admission and then periodically revisit and revise them as the individual's psychiatric condition improves. Furthermore, psychiatric nursing assessments should reflect recovery by being comprehensive and *holistic*, examining many aspects of the individual such as physical, psychological, emotional, behavioral, functional, intellectual, social, cultural, and spiritual (ANA 2014; Berman et al. 2016; O'Brien et al. 2013). They may also include assessing resources and supports (e.g., community, family, financial), skills and strengths, and intervention needs (e.g., education, medication, therapy services), to name just a few. Specific content is determined by many factors, including content of other disciplines' assessments.

Assessments of individuals with SMI in inpatient psychiatric hospitals are multifaceted. Thus, to enhance effectiveness, treatment teams typically conduct assessments that are multidisciplinary versus interdisciplinary, where members from each discipline do their own assessments, evaluating the individual from a different perspective (Davidson et al. 2016). This approach results in several comprehensive, holistic assessments in which there is often much redundancy across disciplines. While redundancy may be useful in some instances, such as to verify reliability of information provided by the individual (e.g., chief complaint, what brought him/her to the hospital), other redundancy may be unnecessary (e.g., both the PMH-RN and psychiatrist conduct a complete mental status exam or both the PMH-RN and primary care practitioner [PCP] conduct a complete head-to-toe physical assessment). Not only is this overlap in work inefficient use of clinicians' time, but more importantly, it is not consistent with a recovery-oriented model of care.

An alternative approach to conducting some types of assessments that is more consistent with a recovery model is one of an interdisciplinary nature, in which assessments are more integrated and streamlined. This approach requires treatment team members to work collaboratively and to have role flexibility. Akhavain et al. (1999) described role flexibility as crossovers in responsibilities between members in which one discipline is not solely responsible for a task. Role flexibility can best occur when the role of each discipline is defined and understood by all members, and when there is an environment of trust and mutual respect and no inappropriate imbalances of power among members (e.g., no hierarchies based on perceived intellectual superiority). Role flexibility enhances the team's ability to provide holistic care and facilitates the use of shared knowledge and experience in a collegial atmosphere.

## Utilization of Assessment Data

Utilizing an interdisciplinary approach in a recovery model, the team comes together to analyze and synthesize all relevant assessment data from each discipline and to develop an integrated treatment plan that includes diagnoses, problems, risks, and areas of focus for care and treatment. For each assessed treatment, rehabilitation, and enrichment need included in the treatment plan, the team writes an individualized, realistic, and simple goal as well as specific objectives or steps (written in behavioral, observable, and/or measurable terms) the individual can take to accomplish the goal. As much as possible, the team should involve the individual in writing goals and objectives, and they should be written in jargon-free language he/she will understand. In inpatient psychiatric hospitals, most objectives will be learning based (i.e., related to what the individual will learn), but some may also be service-based (i.e., related to certain treatments that will be provided to the individual by staff, usually nursing). Once objectives are clearly defined, the team develops interventions that specifically indicate what staff will do to assist the individual to attain each objective (Singh et al. 2016).

## Nursing Interventions

Corresponding to the current initiative to integrate recovery-oriented practices into the delivery of mental health services, there has been an increased emphasis on evidence-based practice (ANA 2014; McLoughlin et al. 2013). Evidence-based nursing practice (EBNP) has various definitions throughout the literature, but most include that it is a problem-solving approach where nurses make practice decisions based on the best available research evidence, clinical expertise, and patient preferences (Nieswiadomy 2012; Schmidt and Brown 2012). Evidence-based findings are essential to provide quality care to individuals with mental illness and to help promote their recovery, but they are only meaningful when successfully integrated into practice.

Nurses need to conduct research to measure recovery-oriented practices in PMH nursing and evaluate effectiveness of interventions. While this research is starting to emerge, the literature is scant with only a few empirical studies that have been conducted, particularly in hospital settings (McLoughlin et al. 2013; McLoughlin and Fitzpatrick 2008).

## PMH Nursing Interventions

PMH-RNs work with individuals, families, groups, and communities to assess their mental health and other co-occurring needs, carry out each step of the nursing process, and evaluate it for effectiveness. Their practice skills are generalized, and they provide interventions such as health promotion and maintenance, intake screening and evaluation, case management, health teaching, provision of milieu therapy, counseling, and psychiatric rehabilitation. PMH-APRNs, with more specialized practice skills, assess, diagnose, and treat individuals and families with psychiatric and behavioral problems and disorders (or the potential for such) using their full scope of therapeutic skills, including prescription of medications and administration of psychotherapy (individual, group, and family) and psychoanalysis. They may also serve as consultants, educators, clinical liaison, and direct clinical supervisors. In addition, they frequently deliver primary care services, which include the diagnosis and treatment of common health problems and the provision of preventive care (ANA 2014; O'Brien et al. 2013). Both PMH-RNs and PMH-APRNs may have other duties and responsibilities than those listed here, depending on factors such as specialized training, type of license, certifications, scope of practice defined in the state Nurse Practice Act, credentialing and privileging (for PMH-APRNs), and setting worked.

## Psychopharmacological Interventions

Within their scope of practice, PMH-APRNs can implement psychopharmacological interventions, which include the prescription or recommendation of pharmacologic agents and the ordering and interpretation of laboratory and diagnostic testing (ANA 2014). Specific to psychotropic medications, while many benefits are associated with these drugs such as amelioration of symptoms and improved quality of life, the potential accompanying serious side effects such as tardive dyskinesia (TD) and extrapyramidal symptoms (EPS) raise several concerns and dilemmas, in which the benefits and risks must be weighed (O'Brien et al. 2013). As part of the recovery model, the prescribing practitioner needs to involve individuals in the decision-making process to the maximum extent possible, educating them on the options and giving them choices. This collaborative approach with the individual demonstrates respect and advocacy and has been shown to promote adherence with the prescribed regimen (Barber 2016).

While PMH-RNs cannot prescribe or order pharmacological interventions, they play an important role in their implementation. For example, with psychotropic medications, RNs not only administer the drugs but they provide education to the individuals, family/significant others, and support staff (e.g., psychiatric technicians). They also monitor closely for side effects and adverse drug reactions and immediately report problems to the practitioner. In addition, they conduct assessments to evaluate effectiveness of the medications and progress toward goals and report data to the treatment team.

Although pharmacotherapy is a well-proven treatment option for mental illness, research has shown that medication alone is often inadequate with limited efficacy. For example, medication is generally effective in treating acute episodes of mania and/or depression in bipolar disorder, but there is increasing evidence that many individuals do not achieve functional recovery with medication alone (Crowe et al. 2010). Furthermore, there often appears to be an overemphasis on medication in which medication has become the default approach in situations where other interventions could be utilized either alone or in conjunction (Mullen 2009). Therefore, consistent with a recovery orientation, psychosocial interventions are often implemented alone or in combination with psychopharmacological interventions (as clinically indicated) to optimize rehabilitation and recovery.

## Counseling and Psychotherapy

Both counseling and psychotherapy are standards of practice of PMH nursing (ANA 2014). Given that PMH-RNs are one of the largest workforces in regular contact with individuals in mental health settings (ANA 2014; Beech 2000; Turkington et al. 2006), they are well positioned to provide a wide array of counseling interventions. These interventions may be delivered in individual and group settings and include but are not limited to communication and interviewing, problem-solving activities, stress management, relaxation techniques, crisis intervention, supportive skill building and educational groups, assertiveness training, and conflict resolution (ANA 2014). PMH-APRNs may conduct individual, couples, group, and family psychotherapy. Psychotherapy is a formally structured relationship between the practitioner and the participant(s). Interventions may be brief or long term and use a range of therapy models such as psychodynamic, behavioral, cognitive, and supportive interpersonal therapies to "promote insight, produce behavioral change, maintain function, and promote recovery" (ANA 2014, p. 32).

It is critical for both PMH-RNs and PMH-APRNs to utilize effective communication strategies and techniques and the therapeutic nurse–patient relationship (as previously described) during counseling and psychotherapy interventions, respectively, so that optimal outcomes can be achieved in assisting the individual along his/her road to recovery. It is also important to research the effectiveness of these interventions in order to contribute to evidence-based nursing practice. For example, psychodynamic interpersonal therapy (PIT) is a psychological intervention that has an emerging evidence base and has demonstrated effectiveness as delivered by PMH nurses (Cahill et al. 2013; Guthrie et al. 2001; Paley et al. 2008). PIT is a model that primarily focuses on the therapeutic relationship and draws upon humanistic and interpersonal concepts (Guthrie 1999).

Cognitive-behavioral therapy (CBT) is another evidence-based intervention and is based on the idea that people's thoughts cause their behaviors and feelings versus external factors such as people, events, and situations (National Association of Cognitive-Behavioral Therapists [NACBT] 2014). CBT is a very general term and includes a range of techniques with similar characteristics. For example, CBT focuses on changing the way people think or teaching them a new way to react to people or situations. CBT incorporates several recovery principles as it involves a collaborative effort between the therapist and individual and characteristics of a therapeutic relationship, emphasizes the individual's goals, and encourages autonomy and responsibility by assigning them homework in between therapy sessions (NACBT 2014). While specialist therapists typically deliver CBT, research has shown that with proper training and supervision, PMH nurses can effectively implement cognitive-behavioral approaches (Beech 2000; Mullen 2009; Turkington et al. 2006).

## Storytelling and Narratives

Individuals with severe mental illness are vulnerable and marginalized by society (SAMHSA 2013a, b; World Health Organization [WHO] 2010). As a result, their personal stories about illness, problems in living, and recovery often get lost or rendered useless and they are unable to tell them. These individuals are often dismissed as valid sources of knowledge and instead are subjected to the knowledge of experts (Clements 2012). However, personal stories are important sources of knowledge and can help individuals know they are not alone and there is hope. PMH nurses can implement various interventions to honor and empower these individuals and help them reclaim ownership and authority over their stories to make meaning of their own illness experience and to envision recovery in their own terms. For example, individuals may verbally share a personal story during a one-to-one or group counseling/psychotherapy session. They may also write their personal narratives for others to read. Another strategy that research has shown to be effective in promoting storytelling is photovoice, a community-based participatory action research approach that involves individuals taking photographs and writing accompanying narratives or being interviewed about the content in the images (Wang and Burris 1994). These photographs and accompanying text/narratives provide rich qualitative data about individuals' experiences as they illustrate individuals' ideas, their concerns, and the realities of their lives.

Although photovoice was developed for implementation in the community and research has primarily been conducted in outpatient and community settings, it seems reasonable to expect that implementation of this arts-based approach would also have benefits in an inpatient psychiatric hospital setting. While a few modifications may need to be made (e.g., ensure no violations of privacy or confidentiality occur with taking pictures inside a hospital), using photographs and accompanying text/narratives may be an innovative strategy to explore in inpatient settings to facilitate individuals' recovery journey.

## Health Teaching and Health Promotion

Health teaching and health promotion is another standard of practice of PMH nursing (ANA 2014) and is vital for nursing care of individuals with mental illness. PMH nurses provide health teaching to individuals and their families/other support persons in both one-to-one and group settings that are related to individuals' needs, recovery goals, and situations (ANA 2014). This teaching may include a wide array of topics such as psychiatric and substance use disorders, mental health problems, treatment regimens and related self-management strategies, relapse prevention, coping skills, resources, self-care activities, problem-solving skills, conflict management, crisis management, and stress management and relaxation techniques.

Psychoeducation (or illness management) is one specific example of health teaching and health promotion PMH nurses often provide, in collaboration with other treatment team members. Psychoeducation includes information about the illness or disorder, the treatment plan, medication and other treatments prescribed (e.g., nature of each treatment, intended benefits and risks, management of side effects), and any support services or advocacy groups that may be involved (Liberman 2008; O'Brien et al. 2013). Other components that have been found to contribute to the success of psychoeducation include supportive resources during crisis periods, assistance with problem-solving skills, and emotional support (Dixon et al. 2001).

Regardless of the topic taught, health teaching and health promotion should be recovery-oriented. PMH nurses need to implement strategies that are individualized and person-centered and demonstrate respect for the individuals, taking into consideration factors such as the individuals' values, beliefs, health practices, culture, spirituality, learning needs, developmental level, language preference, socioeconomic status, and readiness and ability to learn (ANA 2014). For example, if an individual is acutely symptomatic, the nurse should keep the content of health teaching simple and offer it in brief segments, repeating it as often as necessary to ascertain learning has occurred (e.g., ask the individual to repeat back in his/her own words what was learned). With the individual's permission, the nurse should also explore the option of including family/significant others in the education to help reinforce the content and support the individual. Individuals should also be active collaborative partners with the nurse. For example, with shared decision-making, the nurse may offer the individual a choice of how he/she wishes to receive content (e.g., written materials, videos). The nurse should also seek feedback and an evaluation from the individuals regarding effectiveness of the teaching strategies utilized.

## Milieu Therapy

Milieu therapy, also a standard of practice of PMH nursing (ANA 2014), involves utilization of the environment as a therapeutic tool and is based on the belief that humans are affected by their physical, emotional, and social climate (O'Brien et al. 2013). In inpatient psychiatric hospital settings, PMH nurses play a critical role in collaborating with individuals with mental illness, their families and significant others, and other healthcare professionals to provide, structure, and maintain an environment that is safe, therapeutic, and recovery-oriented (ANA 2014). Milieu therapy includes many nursing interventions. For example, upon admission, PMH nurses orient individuals and their family to the care environment, which includes the physical environment, the roles of different healthcare providers, schedules of events pertinent to their treatment and care, how to be involved in their treatment and care, expectations regarding safe and therapeutic behaviors, and their rights and responsibilities particular to the treatment or care environment. PMH nurses also conduct ongoing assessments of the individual and use data collected to help guide and tailor interventions to provide and maintain a safe and therapeutic environment based on the individual's needs and situation at that time. For example, individuals who are acutely ill may respond best to a structured, consistent, and nonstimulating environment, whereas individuals who are well enough to be discharged may benefit most from a less structured environment that closely resembles real-life situations in the community.

PMH nurses commonly advocate that individuals be treated in the least restrictive environment necessary to maintain the safety of the individuals and others (ANA 2014). This is consistent with the recent emphasis in hospitals to reduce and ultimately eliminate use of seclusion and restraints. Upon admission, PMH nurses (in collaboration with other disciplines) should ask individuals about their past experiences with seclusion/restraint (S/R) incidents and if applicable, past successful strategies they have used to prevent or manage dangerous behavior, and what they find helpful in behavioral emergency situations that could prevent S/R from being used. S/R should only be used in emergency situations that pose an immediate risk of an individual harming him/herself, staff, or others and when lesser restrictive interventions (LRIs) are not practical or have been ineffective. LRIs may be medication administration, verbal, behavioral, recreational (e.g., physical activity), or diversionary (e.g., redirection) as well as environmental modifications to reduce stimulation (e.g., remove irritant/instigator from the area, remove individual to a quiet area or to a sensory or relaxation room).

Early intervention is critical, as soon as nursing staff notice the individual begins to act in a manner that may indicate the potential to escalate to becoming dangerous to self or others. In the event S/R must be used, PMH nurses need to do so in as much of a recovery-oriented manner as possible. For example, nurses need to protect and preserve the individual's rights, dignity, and well-being and consider how factors such as age, developmental level, cultural background, gender, and history of physical or sexual abuse may influence behavioral emergencies and affect the individual's response to S/R. Nurses should also educate the individual on the reason for S/R and the conditions necessary to remove the restrictions, involving the individual in formulating strategies to promote recovery of control and to expedite release.

## Complementary and Alternative Therapies

The overall goal of holistic nursing is to heal the whole person, and it includes the integration of complementary and alternative modalities (CAM) into clinical practice (American Holistic Nurses Association [AHNA] 2015). Complementary therapies are used together with traditional treatment modalities, whereas alternative therapies are used in place of conventional treatment (O'Brien et al. 2013). With proper training, practice, and supervision, PMH nurses can provide a variety of CAM. For example, they may give individuals a massage to promote a sense of peacefulness and relaxation or teach a yoga class. They may also deliver energy-based practices such as therapeutic touch and Reiki (see O'Brien et al. 2013). In addition, several CAM promote self-healing, self-care, and self-regulation such as breathing, centering, inner reflection, journaling, biofeedback, relaxation, and meditation. These practices enable individuals to release tension, to concentrate their attention, and to open themselves to new ideas and greater awareness for their recovery journey. Consistent with a recovery orientation, self-regulation practices greatly depend on individuals taking responsibility for their own healing and wellness versus most psychopharmacological and psychosocial interventions that are largely contingent on interventions of others.

## Psychosocial Rehabilitation Mall

Traditionally, PMH nurses in inpatient psychiatric hospitals delivered most treatment and rehabilitation interventions on individuals' living units. With a unit-based approach, interventions are often sporadic and dependent on resources of each unit (e.g., staffing), they are limited in number, variety, and individualization based on assessed needs, and the individuals often do not participate in groups and instead may do activities such as sleep in their rooms or lounge in the day room. More recently, consistent with a recovery-oriented approach, nurses and other clinical and support staff often provide treatment and rehabilitation services in a psychosocial rehabilitation (PSR) mall, or "treatment mall", where programming is centralized (Singh et al. 2016; Spaulding et al. 2016).

PSR malls are usually an off-residential location in which individuals and staff leave their units, and services are provided in large central areas with all individuals and staff combined. PSR malls have several benefits such as they help normalize the treatment and rehabilitation experience for individuals, enhance efficient use of hospital resources, and increase opportunities to individualize treatment by expanding availability of services offered to all individuals. Services should be directly linked to individuals' assessed treatment, rehabilitation, and enrichment needs and include activities designed to assist with symptom management, personal skills development, and life enrichment. A wide array of services should be offered on the mall in broad categories such as psychiatric disorders, medical, legal, community, education, and leisure that individuals can select from and attend, based on their identified needs and interests. While most services on the mall are delivered in a group format, individual therapy may be provided based on unique circumstances and needs of the individuals.

As with all interventions, services PMH nurses provide on the mall need to be recovery-oriented. For example, to the greatest extent possible, services should be delivered in the context of real-life functioning and in the rhythm of the *individual's* life, not someone else's life or a hypothetical situation or hospital context. Thus, a PSR mall needs to extend beyond the context of a place or building, and its services should be tailored to the needs of the individuals, not to the needs of the program, the staff, or the hospital. Individuals should have input and be included in decision-making processes related to the mall such as what services are offered. Services should be provided in a respectful, culturally sensitive, strengths-based environment that promotes individuals' independence, increased wellness, enhanced quality of life, and ability to thrive in the community. Milieu therapy considerations need to also be taken into account (as previously described). For example, mall spaces should look and feel as close to community living as possible, they should be safe and functional environments that are therapeutic (e.g., low noise/activity level, welcoming, supportive), and they should have the capacity to safely and effectively administer medical/nursing care. In addition, information and skills taught in the PSR mall should be reinforced in the therapeutic milieu (e.g., residential unit) when applicable and feasible, which will make them more portable upon discharge.

## Leadership

In addition to providing direct services to individuals, PMH nurses are well positioned to provide leadership interventions in inpatient psychiatric hospitals and the community at large that may indirectly affect individuals' recovery outcomes. For example, nurses may collaborate with other disciplines to assist in the development of hospital programs that help incorporate a recovery-oriented model of care. PMH nurses may also serve in hospital leadership positions ranging from being a core member of the treatment team to the facility director. In addition, nurses may serve on standing and ad hoc committees and task forces within the hospital and statewide, such as those related to performance improvement issues (e.g., reduce seclusion/restraint usage, reduce incidents of physical aggression and related injuries).

## Challenges of Incorporating Recovery Principles

It is evident that PMH nurses can incorporate recovery principles when conducting assessments and delivering an array of interventions to individuals with mental illness in inpatient psychiatric hospitals. However, in some instances, nurses may face challenges that make it difficult to provide services consistent with a recovery-oriented approach. Although many of these challenges are not unique to nursing, some may apply mostly to PMH nurses.

### Autonomy

Autonomy refers to an individual's freedom and ability to act in a self-determined manner. It represents a rational individual's right to express personal decisions independent of outside interference and to have these decisions honored (Butts and Rich 2016). While respecting one's autonomy is consistent with several recovery principles, there are some instances in inpatient psychiatric hospitals in which PMH nurses are unable to fully respect autonomy. For example, many individuals are involuntary (civil) commitment or forensic status, which by itself restricts their freedom. This restriction is further complicated by the limited insight many of them have. For individuals with forensic status, the increased oversight, accountability, security concerns, and stigma associated with the forensic system further add to the difficulty of incorporating recovery-oriented principles into nursing services (Pouncey and Lukens 2010; Simpson and Penney 2011). For example, oftentimes these individuals have restricted privileges and are on locked units with their off-unit activities limited unless accompanied by staff. They also may have less choice in their discharge goals as placement is often determined by the court system (Elm and Devine 2016). Despite these complications, individuals involved in the criminal justice system have many of the same needs as those without such involvement, and numerous nursing services can still be provided in a recovery-oriented manner. Even if nurses must limit one's autonomy, they can still provide care that is holistic, individualized, respectful, strengths-based, and hopeful (Shafer et al. 2016). For example, nurses should provide individuals with forensic status with choices when at all feasible and assist them to work on what needs to be done to gain as much autonomy back as possible (within legal restrictions).

Individuals may also have restricted autonomy related to being too unwell and experiencing acute symptoms that interfere with independent decision-making, such as upon admission or during an acute change in status. Healthcare practitioners must assess an individual's decisional capacity, or ability to consent to and refuse treatment (Butts and Rich 2016). In some instances, such as in an emergency situation where it is determined that an individual is too sick to decide on treatment, PMH nurses may have to administer a medication without an individual's consent or against his/her wishes (in accordance with a practitioner's order). This is an example of an ethical dilemma nurses face when they must strike a balance between their duty to both manage the safety of individuals and promote their independence and autonomy.

With regard to autonomy, it is important to remember that recovery is a nonlinear process, and that individuals will have continual growth with occasional setbacks along their road to recovery (SAMHSA 2006). Depending on the individual's current mental status or state, he or she may not be in a position to fully apply the recovery principles of empowerment, responsibility, or self-direction. Therefore, when it is an issue of safety and well-being, it is the responsibility of PMH nurses and other clinicians to continually assess where the individual is along the continuum and based on their findings to do more for the individual when he/she can do less, and to do less for the individual when he/she can do more (Shafer et al. 2016). In other words, nurses should direct and provide care when individuals are in acute distress and eventually transfer decision-making and self-care to the individuals when clinically appropriate and when the individual is ready (ANA 2014).

## Engagement

Another barrier PMH nurses encounter is individuals' lack of engagement in their care and treatment. In the context of recovery, engagement is the process of individuals fully participating not only in the process of treatment, but also in its content (Jackman 2014, 2016). For example, when asked questions as part of a nursing assessment interview, individuals may choose to only minimally respond (if at all) or to provide answers that lack depth or completeness. Individuals may also refuse to attend treatment team meetings, or if they do attend, they may not engage in discussions or actively partake in decisions about their plan of care. In these instances, it is essential for the nurse to capitalize on the therapeutic nurse–patient relationship he/she has built with the individual, to utilize effective communication techniques as previously described, and to provide positive reinforcement for small steps the individual makes with increasing engagement. In addition, a multitude of reasons may underlie the individual's lack of engagement, such as fear, low self-esteem, paranoia, poor motivation, loss of hope, discouragement, anger, and anxiety. It is important for the team to assess these underlying reasons, which in turn will guide additional interventions to help enhance the individual's engagement.

Individuals also often lack engagement in PSR mall groups. Their engagement is dependent upon several factors such as personal motivation, the goodness of fit between what they need and what is offered, the nature of the group, the facilitator's ability to make group process and learning interesting, boredom factor, and personal variables (Singh et al. 2016). As a group facilitator, PMH nurses can implement various strategies during the group to enhance engagement such as cold call and scaffolding. Depending on the underlying causes of lack of engagement, trained clinicians may also provide one-to-one individualized interventions to enhance group participation such as motivational interviewing and CBT.

## Conclusion

PMH nurses who work in inpatient psychiatric hospitals play a vital role as an interdisciplinary treatment team member and are well positioned to deliver a wide array of recovery-oriented services. This chapter has presented many ways nurses can incorporate recovery principles into the provision of nursing services from admission to discharge, such as when conducting assessments, facilitating PSR mall groups, delivering health teaching and health promotion, and implementing milieu therapy. The recent emphasis to transform mental health systems from a medical model to a recovery model is an opportunity for PMH nurses to return to their roots and deliver holistic care that is person-centered with a focus on the therapeutic nurse–patient relationship—the hallmark of PMH nursing.

## References


Akhavain, P., Amaral, D., Murphy, M., & Uehlinger, K. C. (1999). Collaborative practice: A nursing perspective of the psychiatric interdisciplinary treatment team. *Holistic Nursing Practice, 13*(2), 1–11.

American Holistic Nurses Association. (2015). *What is holistic nursing?* Retrieved from http://www.ahna.org/

American Nurses Association. (2010). *Nursing: Scope and standards of practice* (2nd ed.). Silver Spring, MD: Nursesbooks.org.

American Nurses Association. (2014). *Psychiatric mental health nursing: Scope and standards of practice* (2nd ed.). Silver Spring, MD: Nursesbooks.org.

American Nurses Association. (2015). *Code of ethics for nurses with interpretive statements (view-only document).* Retrieved from http://nursingworld.org/DocumentVault/Ethics_1/Code-of-Ethics-for-Nurses.html

Aston, V., & Coffey, M. (2012). Recovery: What mental health nurses and service users say about the concept of recovery. *Journal of Psychiatric and Mental Health Nursing, 19*, 257–263.

Barber, J. W. (2016). Psychiatric services. In N. N. Singh, J. W. Barber, & S. Van Sant (Eds.), *Handbook of recovery: Principles and practice in inpatient psychiatric hospitals*. New York: Springer.

Beech, B. F. (2000). The strengths and weaknesses of cognitive behavioural approaches to treating depression and their potential for wider utilization by mental health nurses. *Journal of Psychiatric and Mental Health Nursing, 7*, 343–354.

Bergstrom, N., Braden, B. J., Laguzza, A., & Holman, V. (1987). The Braden scale for predicting pressure sore risk. *Nursing Research, 36*, 205–210.

Berman, A., Snyder, S., & Frandsen, G. (2016). *Kozier & Erb's fundamentals of nursing: Concepts, process, and practice* (10th ed.). Boston, MA: Pearson.

Butts, J. B., & Rich, K. L. (2016). *Nursing ethics: Across the curriculum and into practice* (4th ed.). Burlington, MA: Jones & Bartlett Learning.

Cahill, J., Paley, G., & Hardy, G. (2013). What do patients find helpful in psychotherapy? Implications for the therapeutic relationship in mental health nursing. *Journal of Psychiatric and Mental Health Nursing, 20*, 782–791.

Chen, S. P., Krupa, T., Lysaght, R., McCay, E., & Piat, M. (2013). The development of recovery competencies for in-patient mental health providers working with people with serious mental illness. *Administration and Policy in Mental Health and Mental Health Services Research, 40*(2), 96–116.

Clements, K. (2012). Participatory action research and photovoice in a psychiatric nursing/clubhouse collaboration exploring recovery narrative. *Journal of Psychiatric and Mental Health Nursing, 19*, 785–791.

Crowe, M., Whitehead, L., Wilson, L., Carlyle, D., O'Brien, A., Inder, M., et al. (2010). Disorder-specific psychosocial interventions for bipolar disorder—A systematic review of the evidence for mental health nursing practice. *International Journal of Nursing Studies, 47*, 896–908.

Davidson, L., Carr, E., Bellamy, C., Tondora, J., Fossey, E., Styron, T., et al. (2016). Principles for recovery-oriented inpatient care. In N. N. Singh, J. W. Barber, & S. Van Sant (Eds.), *Handbook of recovery: Principles and practice in inpatient psychiatric hospitals*. New York: Springer.

Davidson, L., O'Connell, M., Sells, D., & Staeheli, M. (2003). Is there an outside to mental illness? In L. Davidson (Ed.), *Living outside mental illness: Qualitative studies of recovery in schizophrenia* (pp. 31–60). New York: New York University Press.

Deegan, P. E. (2007). The lived experience of using psychiatric medication in the recovery process and a shared decision-making program to support it. *Psychiatric Rehabilitation Journal, 31*(1), 62–69.

Dixon, L., McFarlane, W. R., Lefley, H., Lucksted, A., Cohen, M., Falloon, I., et al. (2001). Evidence-based practices for services to families of people with psychiatric disabilities. *Psychiatric Services, 52*, 903–910.

Elm, D. L., & Devine, J. L. (2016). Legal advocacy. In N. N. Singh, J. W. Barber, & S. Van Sant (Eds.), *Handbook of recovery: Principles and practice in inpatient psychiatric hospitals*. New York: Springer.

Guthrie, E. (1999). Psychodynamic interpersonal therapy. *Advances in Psychiatric Treatment, 5*, 135–145.

Guthrie, E., Kapur, N., Mackway-Jones, K., Chew-Graham, C., Moorey, J., Mendel, E., et al. (2001). Randomised controlled trial of brief psychological intervention after deliberate self poisoning. *British Medical Journal, 323*, 135–137.

Hanrahan, N. P. (2009). Analysis of the psychiatric-mental health nurse workforce in the United States. *Journal of Psychosocial Nursing and Mental Health Services, 47*(5), 34–42.

Jackman, M. M. (2014). Mindful occupational engagement. In N. N. Singh (Ed.), *Psychology of meditation* (pp. 241–278). New York: Nova Science Publishers.

Jackman, M. M. (2016). Occupational therapy services. In N. N. Singh, J. W. Barber, & S. Van Sant (Eds.), *Handbook of recovery: Principles and practice in inpatient psychiatric hospitals*. New York: Springer.

Liberman, R. P. (2008). *Recovery from disability: Manual of psychiatric rehabilitation*. Washington, DC: American Psychiatric Publishing.

Mathers, B. (2012). Acute mental health nurses: Comprehensive practitioners or specialist therapists? *Journal of Psychiatric and Mental Health Nursing, 19*, 47–52.

McLoughlin, K. A., Du Wick, A., Collazzi, C. M., & Puntil, C. (2013). Recovery-oriented practices of psychiatric-mental health nursing staff in an acute hospital setting. *Journal of the American Psychiatric Nurses Association, 19*(3), 152–159.

McLoughlin, K. A., & Fitzpatrick, J. J. (2008). Self-reports of recovery-oriented practices of mental health nurses in state mental health institutes:

Development of a measure. *Issues in Mental Health Nursing, 29*, 1051–1065.
McLoughlin, K. A., & Geller, J. L. (2010). Interdisciplinary treatment planning in inpatient settings: From myth to model. *Psychiatric Quarterly, 81*, 263–277.
Mullen, A. (2009). Mental health nurses establishing psychosocial interventions within acute inpatient settings. *International Journal of Mental Health Nursing, 18*, 83–90.
National Association of Cognitive-Behavioral Therapists. (2014). *What is CBT?* Retrieved from http://www.nacbt.org/
Nieswiadomy, R. M. (2012). *Foundations of nursing research* (6th ed.). Upper Saddle River, NJ: Pearson.
O'Brien, P. G., Kennedy, W. Z., & Ballard, K. A. (2013). *Psychiatric mental health nursing: An introduction to theory and practice* (2nd ed.). Burlington, MA: Jones & Bartlett Learning.
Paley, G., Cahill, J., Barkham, M., Shapiro, D., Jones, J., Patrick, S., et al. (2008). The effectiveness of psychodynamic-interpersonal therapy (PIT) in routine clinical practice: A benchmarking comparison. *Psychology and Psychotherapy: Theory, Research and Practice, 81*, 157–175.
Pouncey, C. L., & Lukens, J. M. (2010). Madness versus badness: The ethical tension between the recovery movement and forensic psychiatry. *Theoretical Medicine and Bioethics, 31*, 93–105.
Schmidt, N. A., & Brown, J. M. (2012). *Evidence-based practice for nurses: Appraisal and application of research* (2nd ed.). Sudbury, MA: Jones & Bartlett Learning.
Seed, M. S., & Torkelson, D. J. (2012). Beginning the recovery journey in acute psychiatric care: Using concepts from Orem's self-care deficit nursing theory. *Issues in Mental Health Nursing, 33*, 394–398.
Seed, M. S., Torkelson, D. J., & Alnatour, R. (2010). The role of the inpatient psychiatric nurse and its effect on job satisfaction. *Issues in Mental Health Nursing, 31*, 160–170.
Shafer, M. S., Staples, V., & St. George, L. (2016). Self-advocacy and empowerment. In N. N. Singh, J. Barber, & S. Van Sant (Eds.), *Recovery: Principles, research and practice in inpatient psychiatric hospitals*. New York: Springer.
Simpson, A. I. F., & Penney, S. R. (2011). The recovery paradigm in forensic mental health services. *Criminal Behaviour and Mental Health, 21*, 299–306.
Singh, N. N., Lancioni, G. E., Harris, E., & Winton, A. S. W. (2016). Inpatient treatment planning. In N. N. Singh, J. W. Barber, & S. Van Sant (Eds.), *Handbook of recovery: Principles and practice in inpatient psychiatric hospitals*. New York: Springer.
Spaulding, W. D., Montague, E., Avila, A., & Sullivan, M. E. (2016). The idea of recovery. In N. N. Singh, J. W. Barber, & S. Van Sant (Eds.), *Handbook of recovery: Principles and practice in inpatient psychiatric hospitals*. New York: Springer.
Substance Abuse and Mental Health Services Administration. (2006). *National consensus statement on mental health recovery*. Retrieved from http://store.samhsa.gov/shin/content/SMA05-4129/SMA05-4129.pdf
Substance Abuse and Mental Health Services Administration. (2013a). *Behavioral health, United States, 2012* (HHS Publication No. [SMA] 13-4797). Retrieved from http://media.samhsa.gov/data/2012BehavioralHealthUS/2012-BHUS.pdf
Substance Abuse and Mental Health Services Administration. (2013b). *Results from the 2012 national survey on drug use and health: Mental health findings* (NSDUH Series H-47, HHS Publication No. [SMA] 13-4805). Retrieved from http://www.samhsa.gov/data/sites/default/files/NSDUHmhfr2012/NSDUHmhfr2012.pdf
Swarbrick, M. (2006). A wellness approach. *Psychiatric Rehabilitation Journal, 29*(4), 311–314.
Turkington, D., Kingdon, D., Rathod, S., Hammond, K., Pelton, J., & Mehta, R. (2006). Outcomes of an effectiveness trial of cognitive-behavioural intervention by mental health nurses in schizophrenia. *British Journal of Psychiatry, 189*, 36–40.
Tusaie, K. R. (2013). Integrative management of disordered mood. In K. R. Tusaie & J. J. Fitzpatrick (Eds.), *Advanced practice psychiatric nursing: Integrating psychotherapy, psychopharmacology, and complementary and alternative approaches* (pp. 122–157). New York, NY: Springer.
Wang, C., & Burris, M. A. (1994). Empowerment through photo novella: Portraits of participation. *Health Education Quarterly, 21*, 171–186.
World Health Organization. (2010). *Mental health and development: Targeting people with mental health conditions as a vulnerable group*. Geneva: Author.

# Occupational Therapy Services 12

Monica M. Jackman

## Introduction

Contemporary definitions and diagnoses associated with mental illness are relatively new in the scope of human existence, yet throughout recorded history, philosophers, artists, and healers have written volumes on the agony caused by the mind. The profession of occupational therapy emerged in 1917 as a humanistic practice aimed at helping people who were suffering with symptoms of mental illness to the degree that they required asylum care because they were unable to function in their homes, community, and daily life routines. Occupational therapy is commonly viewed as a profession that serves to facilitate restoration and rehabilitation of lost function, i.e., occupation as an outcome of intervention. However, both founders and modern-day theorists and practitioners recognize that the potent therapeutic value of occupation lies in the transformative potential inherent in occupational engagement, i.e., occupation not only as outcome, but also as means and process.

While the popular association of the term "occupation" in the western lexicon is with pay-based vocation, occupational therapists consider an occupation to be any meaningful activity or role that occupies a person's time. Brushing teeth, grooming a pet, preparing a monthly financial budget, watching a movie with a loved one, dancing at a wedding, volunteering for a homeless shelter, and playing organized games are all examples of human occupations. Occupational science is a field of study that examines human occupation and seeks to understand how embodied occupational experiences impact human systems (Yerxa 2000). The gestalt of an individual's engagement in occupation cultivates identity, purpose, and meaning, and can impact health and well-being.

In the continuum of mental illness, there are many levels of life disruption due to mental disability, and the most severe is serious mental illness (SMI). The term SMI was initially defined in 1993 in a Federal Register report and included not only a description of the type of diagnosis, but also an indication of the degree to which the mental, emotional, or behavioral disturbance "has resulted in functional impairment which substantially interferes with or limits one or more major life activities." Since SMI is in large part characterized by degree of loss and/or deficiency of daily activity function, it follows that holistic recovery for individuals with SMI should include a focus on rehabilitation of premorbid daily activities, as well as supported discovery of new and meaningful occupations that promote mental health, wellness, and quality of life experiences. Indeed, a leading proponent of the recovery model has stated, "Psychiatry has lost much

M.M. Jackman (✉)
Little Lotus Therapy and Consulting, 3242 SW Fillmore Street, Port St. Lucie, FL 34953, USA
e-mail: mjackman2317@gmail.com


N.N. Singh et al. (eds.), *Handbook of Recovery in Inpatient Psychiatry*, Evidence-Based Practices in Behavioral Health, DOI 10.1007/978-3-319-40537-7_12

through a dwindling presence of occupational therapy and has much to gain from a resurgence of interest among occupational therapy scientists and practitioners" (Davidson 2007, p. 60).

In this chapter, I define occupation and describe its impact on mental health and wellness. I discuss the alignment between occupational therapy theory, occupational constructs, and recovery principles, and advance a holistic framework for understanding an individual as an occupational being. I then provide an overview of how occupational therapy mental health assessment can examine occupational satisfaction and value, identify meaningful personal goals, and produce baseline and subsequent measures of life function and engagement. Finally, I explore occupational therapy interventions that can support improved recovery, subjective quality of life, and occupational engagement for individuals with SMI living in residential care facilities and preparing for community transition.

## Defining Occupation: Humans as Occupational Beings

To understand how occupational therapy can support recovery for individuals with SMI, it is helpful to have a clear understanding of what occupation is and how occupation relates to the human condition both in general and, more specifically, in the lives of individuals with SMI. Occupational therapy practice began during the moral treatment movement and the subsequent mental hygiene movement, which called for reform and departure from asylum-based care of mental illness via medication, restraint, and isolation toward a new conceptualization of mental health and focus on how to help people to attain it. In the early twentieth century, a small group of physicians and health workers invested in the idea of compassionate care conceived a new type of therapy in which being occupied in daily activity could not only be supported to improve function, but also could be inherently curative. Adolph Meyer, a psychiatrist, authored a seminal work entitled "Philosophy of Occupational Therapy", which is often considered the first piece of writing to explicitly conceptualize the idea that occupation can influence one's mental health (Baum 2002).

In speaking to the role of the new occupational therapy professionals in the mental health arena, Meyer (1922) stated, "Our role consists in giving opportunities rather than prescriptions. There must be opportunities to work, opportunities to do and to plan and create, and to learn to use material" (p. 7). The link between occupation and well-being has persisted in the positive health and recovery movements that define health not in terms of absence of disease, but in light of enabling opportunity for personal growth and nurturing the strength of the human spirit to create a life worth living, even during times of adversity. Thus, a positive view of health should focus not only on symptoms of disability, but also on "knowledge of mental and physical well-being [that] requires expanding the standard litany to ask: 'What did you do today that was meaningful or fulfilling? Does your life have dignity and direction? Are you loved and cared for by another? Do you love and care for others?' These, in turn, point to interventions, not about medications or medical interventions, but about opportunities for full engagement in living." (Ryff and Singer 1998, p. 21). The idea that engagement in occupation can be not only an end goal of therapeutic intervention, but also an open-ended means to experience wellness is a cornerstone of the occupational therapy foundation.

Drawing from existential and neurobiological perspectives that have shaped the study of human occupation (i.e., occupational science), a primary assumption of this chapter is that humans are occupational beings who are intrinsically driven to engage in occupation (Wilcock 1993). Heidegger believed that man is wrought and formed by intentional action, and contemporary occupational therapy theorists share the appreciation of the importance of human action from an existential perspective, in that "it is through doing that individuals are shaped, and in turn, shape their very being in the world" (Sutton et al. 2012, p.143). Occupation differs from activity or action in that it carries and is embedded with both purpose and individualized and cultural subjective meaning, artistry, and expression.

Engagement in occupation extends beyond activity for the sake of survival or simple pleasure seeking and may be a uniquely human phenomenon. For example, all sentient beings engage in the activity of eating, yet humans engage in eating occupations as they celebrate rites of passage with parties centered around eating and drinking, take gourmet cooking classes, perform spiritual tea ceremonies, fabricate elaborate pottery and tableware, and organize food banks and charitable organizations to feed others in need. Occupations are not static mechanistic tasks, but are multidimensional transactions between person, physical environment, social milieu, and cultural contexts that are constantly influenced by changing personal motivation, purpose, meaning, and values. A holistic view of occupation considers the open dynamic system of back-and-forth interaction between intrinsic and extrinsic human factors in which engagement in an occupation affects not only the person performing it, but also the social and interpersonal network and physical environments in which it is performed, which in turn impact the individual performing the occupation.

Wilcock (2003) noted that "Because occupation is so all-embracing, and apparently, so mundane, its significance has failed to be appreciated sufficiently" (p. 157). For this reason, it is not uncommon for other members of an interdisciplinary treatment team to be unclear as to the breadth and depth that occupation encompasses. Literature and practice have indicated that the role of occupational therapists in psychiatric settings is often unclear (Harries and Caan 1994). This is particularly relevant in a clinical environment "in which traditional medical values of cure, acuity, and the sick role predominate. Physicians in such settings therefore may have greater enthusiasm for and understanding of modalities that employ physical curative agents (such as those used in physical therapy) than for occupational therapy, which relies on the person being the agent of improvement through the medium of activity that develops new skills" (Yerxa 1992, p. 82).

On the surface, it might be easy for those unfamiliar with the profession to mistake occupational therapy for activity or diversion therapy, or view occupations as basic life skills to be taught and practiced to mastery. However, the examination of human occupation in the mental health setting is complex and it extends beyond the consideration of the "doing of activities," in that it requires an individualized multifaceted perspective of the function and purpose of occupation as part of each individual's unfolding life experience. While an in-depth discussion of occupational therapy and occupational science theory and philosophy is beyond the scope of this chapter, an overview of the link between occupation and health, and a discussion of the various aspects and constructs of occupation relative to the recovery model will help us to appreciate how occupational therapy assessment and treatment differs from and complements that of other mental health clinical disciplines, and how it can be applied to support holistic treatment for individuals with SMI.

## Occupation and Health

Occupation impacts health and wellness. Wellness can be defined by the absence of negative symptoms and health conditions, and also by the presence of factors that indicate positive well-being. Reflecting on survival in brutal living conditions in the Nazi concentration camps, Frankl (1985, p. 126) wrote, "those who knew there was a task waiting for them to fulfill were most apt to survive." Occupational engagement and deprivation can be viewed as opposite ends of a spectrum in which "people are healthy or diseased in terms of the activities open to them or denied them" (Engelhardt 1977, p. 672). Indeed, prisons are designed to deprive individuals of occupational engagement as a primary form of punishment. The phenomenon of occupational deprivation via the limiting of daily routines, tool use, and autonomy of occupational engagement in the prison setting has been found to correlate with episodic psychosis, inmate rioting, and suicide (Liebling 1993; Molineaux and Whiteford 1999; Useem 1985; Whiteford 1997). Inactivity, or going from engagement in an activity to doing nothing, has been linked to negative mental health symptoms such as delusions in individuals with schizophrenia (Curson et al. 1992; Myin-Germeys et al. 2001), and increasing active engagement can aid in individual control of the intensity of psychotic symptoms (Breier and Strauss 1983). Even when psychiatric symptoms are in remission, individuals with SMI who spend less time actively engaged in non-passive occupations can have poorer measures of community function (Fervaha et al. 2014).

An alternative to measuring symptoms of disease and disability is to view wellness as one's level of subjective or psychological well-being. Subjective well-being or hedonic well-being relates to one's pursuit of pleasure and happiness, while eudaimonic well-being is more associated with living in accordance with one's personal meaning and authentic self (Ryan and Deci 2001). An exploratory qualitative study on perception and experience of well-being by Wilcock et al. (1998) found that occupation was the most common category of possible situation or environment that participants associated with well-being. Satisfaction with daily occupations has been linked to increased quality of life measures for people with schizophrenia (Aubin et al. 1999; Eklund et al. 2001). Ryff et al. (2004) described eudiamonic well-being as "purposeful life engagement [that] evokes an active, striving organism, sometimes in the face of adversity" (p. 1385), and this state of well-being has been measured with six constructs: self-acceptance; purpose in life; personal growth; positive relations with others; environmental mastery of daily life tasks; and autonomy. Eudiamonic well-being has been referred to as, "a life lived to its fullest potential" (Steger et al. 2008, p. 23); similarly, the motto of the American Occupational Therapy Association is "Occupational therapy: Living life to its fullest". Meaning in life and engagement in meaningful activities have been associated with quality of life in individuals with mental illness (Goldberg et al. 2002; Stolovy et al. 2009), and occupational engagement can function to maintain subjective well-being and mutually reinforce perceived health for individuals with SMI (Eklund et al. 2012; Rebeiro and Cook 1999).

## Occupational Therapy and the Recovery Model

The World Health Organization (2004) defined mental health as "a state of well-being in which the individual realizes his or her own abilities, can cope with the normal stresses of life, can work productively, and fruitfully, and is able to make a contribution to his or her community" (p. 12). The recovery model represents an evolution of the humane treatment movements of the late nineteenth and early twentieth centuries. The recovery philosophy mirrors the historical paradigm shift from asylum-based care to mental hygiene, in that it proceeds from a medical model of treating disease, disability, and disorders, and focuses on helping people to fully experience and engage in life, rather than merely get through it. Recovery involves "A redefinition of one's illness as only one aspect of a multidimensional sense of self capable of identifying, choosing, and pursuing, personally meaningful goals and aspirations despite continuing to suffer the effects and side effects of mental illness" (Davidson et al. 2005, p. 15).

Similarly, occupational science theorists and occupational therapists conceptualize the function of human occupation in terms of how it supports the human capacity for "doing, being, belonging, and becoming" (Wilcock 2003, 2007). Humans have occupational needs such as accomplishment, affirmation, agency, coherence, companionship, and renewal, which help them to achieve a sense of being, belonging, and becoming (Doble and Santha 2008). Both occupational therapy practice and the recovery model reflect the importance of understanding that recovery is a process and is not defined solely by outcomes. Some theorists and researchers of the recovery model have proposed a functional definition of recovery that conceptualizes recovery in terms of success with domains of daily activities (e.g., social, productive, recreation, spiritual), or includes measures of independent functioning as part of an operational definition of recovery (Harvey and Bellack 2009; Noordsy et al. 2002). Research has found engagement in meaningful occupation and independent functioning to be a dominant theme in recovery and its operational definition (Le Boutillier et al. 2011; Liberman and Kopelowicz 2005).

Onset or exacerbation of disability associated with SMI can result in suffering and changes in functional capacity. Research and theory have linked health and life satisfaction not to the degree of one's impairment, but to the ability to attain balance or congruence between an individual's capacity and goals (Pörn 1993; Reilly 1962; Yerxa 1998). A disruption in life functioning and subsequent experience of suffering requires one to reevaluate not only capacity in relation to goals, but also to formulate new occupational meaning, value, and identity in terms of new internal and external conditions to enable a healthy sense of coherence (Christiansen 1999; Persson et al. 2001). Subsequently, mental health and wellness do not occur in absence of disease and disability, but despite it. Even in the presence of psychotic symptoms, the subjective experience of recovery has been found to correlate with improved quality of life outcomes (Kukla et al. 2014). As such, well-being becomes "the sense that one's life is meaningful and purposeful,… an on-going, day-by-day-constantly unfolding phenomenon, not an end state that is once-and-for-all resolved." (Ryff and Singer 1998, p. 8). The ten constructs of recovery commonly cited in the literature are self-direction, individualized and person-centered, empowerment, holistic, nonlinear, strength-based, peer support, respect, responsibility, and hope (SAHMSA 2011).

## Self-direction, Individualized and Person-Centered, Empowerment

The individual with SMI plays the primary role in determining the course and content of treatment goals and interventions. This is advocated in both the recovery model and in occupational therapy practice (AOTA 2008; Kielhofner 2002; Kielhofner and Burke 1980; Townsend et al. 2005). The experience of SMI can be paralyzing and bring feelings of utter lack of control of symptoms (e.g., the overwhelming fear and terror of a panic attack, the groundless feeling from the betrayal of a mind that hears voices others do not) and course (e.g., symptomatic relapse during unexpected life stress, or worse, with no apparent trigger). This feeling of helplessness can be exacerbated when an individual is hospitalized and loses control of daily rhythm, contact with loved ones, previous roles, and surroundings.

The element of choice and empowerment is central to occupational justice, which is the ability of all people to engage in meaningful occupations for the purpose of cultivating health and well-being, and perceived control has been associated with increased occupational performance and well-being (Eklund 2007; Stadnyk et al. 2010). Self-determination is not only a theoretical construct that adds to the element of person-centered planning, but also a factor that can positively affect functional performance and sense of well-being. Self-concordant goals, or goals that are intrinsically driven, and are aligned with one's sense of self, can increase experiences of subjective well-being, vitality, and meaningfulness of goal attainment (McGregor and Little 1998; Nix et al. 1999; Sheldon and Elliott 1999; Sheldon and Kasser 1998). Furthermore, goals that are intrinsically motivated have a more positive effect on mental health than goals that are extrinsically motivated, for control reasons (e.g., for reward, expectation or praise) (Sheldon et al. 2004). For example, individuals in an inpatient psychiatric setting who engaged in a 6-month course of occupational therapy focused on self-chosen therapy activities exhibited more improvement in measurements of suspiciousness and preoccupation than individuals who participated in therapist-chosen activities (Hoshi et al. 2013). This may speak to the notion that self-direction and autonomy, even in acute stages of recovery, can contribute to therapeutic engagement.

While it is easy to engage in client-centered practice when the client and clinician agree on recovery goals, there must be a balance between management of risk, realistic expectations, and individual autonomy to ensure that beneficence and ethical care in practice are maintained (McColl et al. 2005; Rudnick 2002). Individuals with SMI who are in early stages of recovery may not have the insight or reality orientation to formulate realistic attainable goals commensurate with abilities or resources. In addition, individuals may be motivated by internal factors (e.g., delusions) to set goals that would result in harm to self or others. An occupation-based approach might offer an experiential alternative to verbal communication for goal formulation when an individual is not capable of logical and rational discussion. For example, rather than offering suggestions for appropriate therapy goals, an occupational therapist may introduce a variety of novel activities to provide opportunities for present-moment engagement, and then work with the individual to formulate meaningful recovery-oriented goals that align with these activities based on the interest and motivation generated by experience.

## Holism and Nonlinear Human Function

Holism and the dynamic nonlinear nature of human function and health are concepts valued by both occupational therapists and the proponents of the recovery model. Occupational scientists view individuals as occupational beings that are in a constant dynamic state of being changed and causing change, rather than an as a static amalgamation of cells, organs, body systems, and physical and behavioral symptoms. In contrast to a more mechanistic reductionist model that requires focused examination of disease and deficits, holism in occupational therapy practice can serve as a mechanism for "putting the human back together again" (Yerxa 1993, p. 4).

Given the primary assumption that people are occupational beings, it follows that it is necessary to take the same holistic and nonlinear view of occupation to truly understand how occupation impacts a person's life. This includes going beyond a conceptualization of occupation as "what" a person does to include a consideration of the "why, who, when, where, and how" of occupation (Jackman 2014). In this way, one can adopt a holistic view of an individual with SMI as an occupational being who is immersed in his or her world, rather than as a patient with deficits and diagnoses to be molded to fit into a world already defined by his or her interdisciplinary team. In the following discussion, I present a framework that supports a nonlinear view of occupation to enable a perspective of the individual as an occupational being. Examination of the human-occupation interface can offer the occupational therapist and interdisciplinary team with unique multifaceted insight to inform treatment planning.

### The *Why* of Occupation: Motivation and Value

The innate human will to act with purpose has been described from an evolutionary perspective in which, "The human brain cannot sustain purposeless living. It is not designed for that. Its systems are designed for purposive action. When that is blocked, they deteriorate, and the emotional feedback from idling those systems signals extreme discomfort and motivates the search for renewed purpose, renewed meaning" (Klinger 2012, p. 31). While activity to meet basic human needs is necessary on a primitive level, there seems to be a universal human striving for the intangible aspects associated with the purpose and value that we attach to activity. The human drive to engage in occupation is inherent and biological, and is motivated by immediate survival, social and environmental survival, and individual development, i.e., "the exercise of personal capacities to enable maintenance and development of the organism [which] is perhaps the most primary and least appreciated function of human occupation" (Wilcock 1993, p. 21).

While occupations are commonly categorized into three primary areas of work, leisure, and play, a more current perspective suggests that occupations should not be viewed categorically, but rather examined in terms of how they meet an individual's intrinsic needs for self-maintenance, expression, and fulfillment (Law et al. 1996). The Model of Human Occupation framework considers volition to be a person's primary organizing subsystem that subserves occupation and function of the human system, and one's volition is comprised of personal causation (i.e., capacity), values, and interests (Kielhofner 2002; Kielhofner and Burke 1980). Occupational value can be a precursor to experience of meaning in occupation, with the view that value can be concrete (i.e., occupation results in a necessary or desired product), symbolic (i.e., value dimension is more process based and significant at the personal, cultural, or universal level), or based in self-reward (i.e., personal enjoyment) (Persson et al. 2001). Moderate to strong correlations between occupational value and self-reported quality of life measures have been noted in individuals with long-term mental illness (Eklund et al. 2003).

Experiential opportunities for occupational engagement can influence and spark motivation, especially when an individual may be experiencing symptoms (e.g., decreased insight, cognitive dampening) that interfere with the ability to appreciate the more abstract promise of external reward consistent with of extrinsic motivation. Engagement in meaningful occupations, no matter how simple, can offer motivational benefits. For example, I have learned that if I have low mood and lack energy upon waking consistent with depression symptomology during relapse, I can immediately make my bed. By engaging in the simple occupation of bed making, I am able to commit to a decision and intention to move forward with my day, rather than retreat to bed and experience suffering in addition to pain. Through engagement in the simple task, I can gain momentum and intrinsic motivation that can result in a spillover effect to forthcoming activities. Use of an occupational therapy intervention designed to increase intrinsic motivation for individuals with SMI has resulted in improvement in intrinsic motivation and social behavior change in both individuals who were autonomy-oriented and who had motivational deficits (Wu 2001). To truly embrace a person-centered model of recovery for individuals with SMI, it is helpful to explore how occupation can influence motivation and why an individual might be moved to engage in a given occupation or role. This includes being mindful of the effects of factors that may mediate motivation, such as fluctuations in symptoms, the experience of medication side effects, changes in perceived self-efficacy, and the evolution of self-concept and identity.

### The *Who* of Occupation: Identity and Meaning

Engagement in occupation helps an individual to form a basis for identity and life meaning, and this experiential wisdom in turn influences subsequent occupational engagement and creates a feedback loop between human being and human doing. In western society, much of who we are is tied to what we do and the roles that we play. The common reference point of doing forms a basis by which people can experience shared meaning and personal understanding (Christiansen 1999). When an individual undergoes role loss as the result of disease or disability, this affects identity, and can lead to increased dysfunction and overidentification with a patient or sick role (Dickerson and Oakley 1995; Versluys 1980). For example, schizophrenia can potentially "overtake and redefine the identity of the person," and has been termed as an "I am" illness (Estroff 1989, p. 189).

When I was first diagnosed with Major Depressive Disorder in an inpatient facility and, for the course of a few subsequent relapses, the symptoms were so consuming that I identified with the disorder. As I began to experience recovery by becoming more engaged in my world and the occupations that were meaningful to me, I realized that I was not "depressed," but was a mother, therapist, friend, artist, and inventor who was feeling awful, but impermanent symptoms of a predefined condition.

Occupational identity relates to the idea that one views oneself as an occupational being, and builds identity based on occupational engagement and roles that carry personal meaning (Kielhofner 2002). Self-complexity of identity that maintains authenticity of the self in terms of autonomy and meaning has been shown to predict both improved mental health and lower levels of perceived stress (Ryan et al. 2005).

A research participant in a qualitative study that examined occupational engagement in individuals with SMI defined disengagement from occupation as, "When you're completely devoid of motivation or ability to do anything you almost feel like a nonperson. It is like you have no purpose, you have no identity, you have nothing to define yourself" (Sutton et al. 2012, p. 145). Reestablishing identity and finding meaning in life are two of the four key processes of recovery as defined by Andresen et al. (2003). Life meaning has a profound impact on one's identity and it is difficult to truly understand who someone is without examining his or her subjective life meaning. Individuals with schizophrenia have reported lower levels of life meaning than individuals who do not have a psychiatric diagnosis (Chaudhary and Sharma 1976). However, people with SMI perceive meaning as a primary component of recovery, and have reported finding life meaning through work, social interaction, social roles, pursuit of goals, spirituality, and engaging in the process of recovery itself (Andresen et al. 2003; Copic et al. 2011; Feldman and Snyder 2005; Pettie and Triolo 1999).

From an occupational perspective, occupation can be a means to develop and express personal identity and experience meaning in life (Ludwig 2004). Engagement in meaningful occupations and in occupations that are valued can impact life meaning and satisfaction (Eakman 2013; Eakman et al. 2010; Eakman and Elklund 2012), and the importance of meaning within doing in the context of occupational performance contributes to motivation and sense of well-being (Carlson et al. 1998; Doble and Santha 2008; Pentland and McColl 2008). Frankl (1985) believed that people can discover life meaning by engaging in a work or deed, by life experience or personal encounter, and by adaptation of one's attitude toward unavoidable pain and suffering. People in the process of recovery have reported finding meaning in the lived experience of mental illness (Pettie and Triolo 1999), and the recovery process has been shown to unfold in parallel with the sense of self (Davidson and Strauss 1992). Furthermore, a self-concept that builds on occupational identity formed by present-moment occupational engagement can be grounding and act as an anchor when one's mental conceptualization of self is affected by symptoms of SMI (e.g., delusions of grandeur).

Sources of life meaning as identified by the literature often contain the common thread of occupational experience. For example, Reker and Wong (1988) found that tasks to meet basic human survival needs, leisure and hobbies, creative work, interpersonal relationships, educational or vocational development, personal development, activism, altruism, values and ideals, cultural traditions, leaving a personal legacy, and religion are sources of personal meaning. Similarly, Moll et al. (2015) performed a scoping review of empirical literature examining occupation and wellness, and posited the following dimensions of distinct and meaningful occupational experience: taking care of one' s basic needs, experiencing pleasure and joy (e.g., through leisure activities); activating the body, mind and senses; connecting with others; building security and prosperity; developing capabilities and potential; developing and expressing identity; and contributing to community and society.

A qualitative study of meaningfulness and occupation in individuals with severe and persistent mental illness identified five themes of meaning in occupation: connection with others and the external environment; having enjoyment and fun; productivity and having a sense of achievement; being occupied and having routines; and maintaining health (Leufstadius et al. 2008). Understanding an individual's occupational identity and life meaning serviced through engagement in occupation can not only provide a baseline for assessment, but also inform the recovery process by ensuring that the individual is seen through his or her diagnosis. Much like motivation, one's identity is not static, but will inevitably change over the course of time and rhythm of life.

## The *When* of Occupation: Time, Temporality, and Occupational Balance

Occupation is influenced by temporal contexts, such as clock-based schedules, internal body rhythms, and habit-based routines, and also by more subjective factors such as the personal experience of time duration in occupation and the sense of the continuity of the passage of time. Yalmambirra (2000) used the term "white time" to describe the artificial control of human rhythms and routines by clocks, calendars, and time-based schedules. This phenomenon is particularly notable in residential facilities that have set schedules for sleeping and waking, eating, hygiene, daily activities, and medication administration, and thus impose institutional zeitgebers, or external controls, onto individuals' internal rhythms.

Individuals with SMI such as schizophrenia, bipolar disorder, and major depression frequently have disruptions in circadian rhythms and sleep patterns (Cohrs 2008; Jagannath et al. 2013; Manoach and Stickgold 2009; Martin et al. 2001, 2005; Wulff et al. 2012; Wulff et al. 2009), and these disruptions have been associated with decreased measures of quality of life (Hofstetter et al. 2005; Krystal et al. 2008; Ritsner et al. 2004). Fatigue and fluctuating energy levels that do not align with a preset institutional schedule can impact compliance with and engagement in daily treatment activities, even if the individual is motivated and willing to participate. Understanding an individual's rhythm of doing and sleeping can help clinicians to identify treatment modalities to impact these rhythms, to compensate for their effects, and to provide environmental and temporal modifications to support engagement until an individual's circadian rhythms and sleep patterns stabilize.

Examination of the construct of time and occupation and their relationship to function and well-being extends beyond time as a marker of life activities and awareness of differences in daily rhythms. Temporality refers to the phenomenon of time as relative and not absolute. Larson (2004) described six variations of temporality that can impact subjective response to occupational engagement: protracted duration (i.e., perceived time is longer than clock time); temporal compression (i.e., perceived time is shorter than clock time); flow (i.e., a sense of timelessness); interstitial time (i.e., waiting and future-oriented expectancy); temporal rupture (i.e., perceived time is disrupted due to life changing events and/or disturbed or altered daily routines); and synchronicity (i.e., congruence between perceived time and click time). Since the subjective perception of the passing of time can contribute to affective experiences such as pleasure, anxiety, boredom, and restlessness, this ancillary effect of engagement should be considered when working with individuals who may be prone to these symptoms. Noncompliance with group or therapeutic activities can often be attributed to SMI symptoms. However, if an individual finds a group activity or therapeutic modality to be boring or dull, this could exacerbate existing feelings of fatigue due to medication side effects, or lead to an increase in affective depressive symptoms.

Variations in temporality are affected by the nature of occupational engagement. For example, a flow experience in which time is suspended occurs when an individual is completely absorbed in an occupation. However, varied temporality and resultant subjective affect is not a purely passive experience, in that people can manipulate the perception of time by modifying the nature of occupational engagement, such as when doodling during a tedious lecture to make time seem as if it is passing faster (Flaherty 2003). Observation and probing to determine how an individual with SMI perceives time at baseline and relative to level of occupational engagement could inform treatment in terms identification of specific activities that can evoke positive subjective temporal experiences.

Individuals with schizophrenia have been found to sense time differently than can be explained by the typical environment- and activity-influenced variation in temporal perception. Research has found that in these cases, the experience of time passing does not always match the actual duration of time as measured by clock time (Freedman 1974; Kwang-Hyuk et al. 2009; Tysk 1984). This difficulty with time perception can worsen with positive symptoms and increase with cognitive demands (Petersburs et al. 2013). In addition, disruption of time continuity, which serves to provide reference to the world and a stable functional synthesis of past, present, and future, and impaired future-oriented time perception can be experienced by individuals with schizophrenia (Giersch et al. 2015; Martin et al. 2014). Deficits in one's ability to feel grounded and aware in the passing of time can be not only detrimental to engagement in daily life activities and social interaction, but also be a possible source of disorientation, anxiety, and confusion, especially when one may be living in an unfamiliar environment such as a residential or inpatient facility.

A final consideration in time and temporality of occupation is the concept of occupational balance. Occupational balance involves the perception that one is experiencing a health-giving amount and variation of occupations. Whether perceived by objective (i.e., equal distribution of actual occupations across all possible occupational domains) or subjective (i.e., congruence between ideal and actual balance of occupations) means, it has been associated with measures of well-being (Sheldon et al. 2010; Wagman et al. 2012). Life balance has been defined as "a satisfying pattern of daily activity that is healthful, meaningful, and sustainable to an individual within the context of his or her current life circumstances" (Matuska and Christiansen 2008, p. 11). Individuals with schizophrenia can have difficulty organizing daily occupations and managing time to create an occupational balance of passive and active occupations and a functional time-use framework (Bejerholm and Eklund 2004; Neville et al. 1985, Weeder 1986). In addition, life balance can be affected by one's environment if the environment is not under a person's control (Matsuka 2012).

## The *Where* of Occupation

Occupation affects and is affected by the physical, cultural, and social environments, and these contexts are considered as integral factors in occupational performance and its link to health and to functional capacity for goal attainment (American Occupational Therapy Association 2008; Dunn et al. 1994; Fidler 1996; Pörn 1993). Occupational therapists assess the physical environment to make recommendations for and adaptations to physical contextual factors (e.g., equipment, tools, physical structure and layout, furniture) to support success with occupational engagement. The physical environment can not only be manipulated to directly support occupation, but also contribute to a milieu that can indirectly impact feelings of safety, security, and well-being. For example, an individual who has difficulty integrating focal and ambient visual and auditory stimuli, or has difficulty with figure ground perception may communicate and focus better in a physical environment that is quiet and uncluttered, or benefit from use of noise canceling headphones during busy times such as shift change.

Much of the emphasis on the physical environment in inpatient settings relates to risk management, safety, and protection from harm. However, lack of control over one's physical environment, structure, surroundings, ambient stimuli, and design has been linked to feelings of helplessness and poorer mental health (Evans 2003). Conversely, improved physical design, opportunity for decoration, and available physical and recreational amenities have been shown to have a significant relationship to indicators of psychosocial adjustment, independent living, security and self-identity for individuals living in inpatient psychiatric facilities (Shumaker and Reizenstein 1982; Timko 1996). Measurement of physiological health indicators (e.g., blood pressure, pulse rate) and psychological self-report of health has revealed that people undergoing medical procedures such as blood draws prefer nature-influenced atmosphere over ambient television and more urban environmental conditions and recover from stress inducing situations faster in settings with a natural aesthetic (Ulrich et al. 1991, 2003).

The physical environment in psychiatric facilities can be manipulated to promote social interaction and decrease isolation (Holahan 1972; Holohan and Saegert 1973; Osmond 1957). In terms of human occupation, environment also includes consideration of the social context. Clark and Lawlor (2009) described the importance of examining not only the activity construct of occupation, but also the social actors who are engaged in occupations. Similar to the physical context, while individualized adaptations to the social context can directly support occupation, the social environment itself can impact subjective well-being for people with SMI. For example, DeVries and Delespaul (1989) used an experience sampling method to measure the impact of physical–social context on mental state. They found that individuals with schizophrenia living in inpatient facilities reported increased depressive symptoms when alone, a drop in self-evaluation of mental state in a crowded environment, and optimal self-evaluation of mental state when in the company of one to three people. Inpatient clinical staff provides more than prescribed treatment interventions, but they can also serve as therapeutic means via quality of their interaction and presence. Individuals with SMI have linked satisfaction with psychiatric services to social contextual variables such as staff alliance, staff empathy, and feeling comfortable when talking to staff (Howard et al. 2003). Consideration of an individual's physical and social environments can provide insight as to what types of support an individual may need to experience meaningful occupational engagement in the recovery process.

## The *How* of Occupation: Occupational Engagement

The primary goal of occupational therapy is to support and enable each person's "health and participation in life through engagement in occupation" (American Occupational Therapy Association 2008, p. 625). While early occupational therapy practice models focused more on performance, independence, and skill level, which tend to be objective and outcome dependent, the level of one's engagement in occupation is process-driven and is tied to one's subjective sense of being, presence, and fulfillment. The construct of engagement speaks to the manner of how an individual performs an occupation, and can be viewed as the degree to which an individual involves and invests him or herself in a particular task (Jackman 2014). The personal value of engagement in occupation lies not only in its purpose or outcome, but also in its resultant subjective experience (Hasselkus 2006).

Sutton et al. (2012) studied different levels of occupational engagement from the perspective of individuals in recovery from SMI, and found that various levels of engagement could offer different therapeutic benefits in response to fluctuating needs and states. For example, disengagement could foster asylum to allow for healing by removing demands of daily activity in acute stages of illness, while partial engagement offered a sense of grounding in the repetitive nature of simple tasks that created an opportunity for respite and reconnection with physical and sensory motor tasks in the present moment. Everyday engagement marked a reconnection with others, and full engagement resulted in experience of autotelic flow-type states. Participant responses collectively indicated that recovery involved not a forward progression in level of engagement, but a therapeutic freedom to move in a volitional nonlinear way between engagement states as needed.

Engagement can both be influenced by and can influence positive and negative psychiatric symptoms. Individuals with schizophrenia who reported a low overall level of engagement through time-use diaries also exhibited low measures of sense of coherence and mastery, experienced an external locus of control, and had more negative, positive, and general psychiatric symptoms (Bejerholm et al. 2006; Bejerholm and Eklund 2007). In addition, low level of occupational engagement was associated with withdrawal and low sense of meaning. A qualitative metasynthesis of studies examining occupational engagement in people with psychosis identified the following as self-reported factors that help occupational engagement: adequate challenge, assistance with self-care and domestic tasks, environment and location of the activity, fulfilling hobbies, interest, maintenance of ordinary activities of daily living, making positive lifestyle changes, presence of companion animals, previous experience with an activity, religious practices and belonging, and sufficient financial and transportation resources (Hitch et al. 2013).

## Quality of Life Reporting in People with SMI

Practitioners of both the recovery model and of occupational therapy value an individual-centered perspective on therapy goals that support the person's ability to live in a way that is meaningful, healthy, and fulfilling. When examining occupational therapy assessment and services commonly provided in mental health settings, it is important to simultaneously consider the aspects of occupation and engagement that people with SMI have indicated to be important to quality of life. Numerous researchers have employed a qualitative method of inquiry to try to understand life meaning as defined by individuals living with SMI. While review of studies related to occupational engagement and quality of life can identify themes to guide practice, these should be considered with the caveat that "meaning is contingent upon interpretation, and interpretation is never entirely detached and analytic, but is always to some extend biased by factors such as the interpreter's beliefs, language, and practices" (Zahorik and Jenison 1998, p. 82). Furthermore, subjective measures of quality of life and life satisfaction have not consistently correlated with objective measures of quality of life (Dickerson et al. 1998), possibly due in some part to the observer's effect on interpretation in conjunction with more obvious influence of confounding variables such as poor insight and cognitive difficulties.

## Assessment

Occupational therapists use comprehensive and holistic assessment to examine all factors that can influence, contribute to, hinder, and support an individual's motivation, performance, participation, and engagement in life occupations. Standardized assessment tools used for individuals with SMI can measure baseline function in terms of occupations of self-care (e.g., dressing, grooming), and instrumental activities of daily living (e.g., managing finances, shopping), as well as subjective variables such as satisfaction with daily occupations. The primary objective of assessment is to enable therapist and individual collaboration to formulate personal meaningful goals, to create an individualized occupational profile, and identify subsequent interventions and supports based on individual needs and the reason for hospitalization (American Occupational Therapy Association 2008). While standardized tests offer psychometric reassurance of validity and reliability, it is important to be aware of the impact of personal (e.g., circadian rhythms), and environmental factors (e.g., temporal context, physical environment) on the validity of assessment results, and to supplement findings with clinical observations and interviews, as functional performance and motivation may fluctuate based on medical and contextual factors.

### Self-assessment and Subjective Assessment Measures

Much emphasis in interdisciplinary assessment is placed on clinician evaluation of individual function, diagnosis, and subjective state to identify goals, needs, and interventions that will best support recovery, and balance both risk factors and quality of life outcomes. While these clinical data are crucial to treatment planning, self-assessments of performance, function, and satisfaction can provide a means for ensuring that the individual's perspective is part of the interdisciplinary team assessment. The Canadian Occupational Performance Measure (COPM; Law et al. 1991), the Satisfaction with Daily Occupations-13 (13-item version, SDO-13; Eklund et al. 2014), the Engagement in Meaningful Activities Survey (EMAS; Goldberg et al. 2002), and the Occupational Self Assessment (OSA) (Baron et al. 2006) are three assessments that elicit individual self-assessment to satisfaction and degree of meaning in daily occupations.

The COPM is a standardized semi-structured interview in which an individual identifies areas of occupation that he or she would like to improve and assigns a level of importance to each area. The individual then selects five areas that are most important and rates performance and satisfaction with these areas. Systematic review of the use of the COPM in occupational therapy literature found that it provides adequate reliability, validity, and responsiveness and has been used as a standard for comparison in psychometric studies of similar assessment tools (Carswell et al. 2004). Because the COPM is client-centered, it represents client-identified assessment domains, scoring, and areas of targeted intervention, and may not align with areas identified as important by the clinical team. Thus, if a client identifies a problem in occupation that the clinician does not observe or, conversely, if the client denies a problem that is clinically observed, the client's subjective assessment is nonetheless represented in COPM scoring and interpretation (McColl et al. 2005). However, such tools require a certain level of insight and self-awareness to present a valid client perspective (Tryssenaar et al. 1999; Waters 1995) and if an individual is having difficulty with reality orientation and/or experiencing a lack of insight to mental illness, they might be better suited for use further along in the recovery process.

The SDO-13 was developed to measure satisfaction with daily occupations in individuals with mental illness, and was designed to offer a structured, systematic, and efficient alternative to the more open-ended COPM (Eklund et al. 2014). The tool is a structured interview that measures individual satisfaction with 13 items in the areas of work/studies, leisure, home maintenance, and self-care occupations, and has satisfactory internal consistency and construct validity based on initial psychometric testing.

The Engagement in Meaningful Activities Survey (EMAS; Goldberg et al. 2002) is a 12-item survey that uses a 5-point Likert scale to measure subjective meaning in terms of self-care, identity, creativity, having a sense of accomplishment, having a feeling of competency, being valued by other people, helping other people, experiencing pleasure, having feeling of control, expressing personal values, having a sense of satisfaction, and being presented with an appropriate level of challenge. The EMAS has shown good to very good test–retest reliability, internal consistency, and convergent and predictive validity (Eakman 2011; Eakman and Eklund 2012).

## Measures of Occupational Engagement and Function

Prior to conducting a more focused assessment of function for specific occupational domains, it can be helpful to get a holistic picture of an individual's overall strengths, needs, and premorbid and current occupational functioning. The Occupational Performance History II (OPHI-II; Kielhofner et al. 2001) is an interview-based assessment that uses the following three formats for measuring occupational adaptation and function: (1) semi-structured interview that probes occupational choices, critical life events, daily routines, occupational roles, and occupational behaviors; (2) rating scales for occupational competency, occupational identity, and occupational behavior settings (i.e., environments, contexts, objects); and (3) qualitative narrative data collection related to occupational life history. Finally, the Occupational Self Assessment (OSA) (Baron et al. 2006) is a self-report tool designed to rate and assess an individual's competency and value of 21 areas of occupational performance. The OSA offers a structured rating scale format by which to support client self assessment of occupation and engage in collaborative problem solving to formulate person-centered goals. In addition to having adequate psychometric properties, a qualitative study of perceived use of the OPHI-II found that both therapists and clients in mental health settings reported value in the tool's ability to assess and appreciate an individual's lived occupational experience, and that this resultant narrative slope positively influenced intervention (Apte et al. 2005; Ennals and Fossey 2007; Kielhofner et al. 2001; Thomson 1992).

The Profile of Occupational Engagement in people with Schizophrenia (POES) provides a snapshot of an individual's current occupational engagement via the use of 24-h time-use diaries (Bejerholm et al. 2006). The POES includes nine rating scales based on the following categories of occupational engagement: daily rhythm of activity and rest, variety and range of occupations, physical environment, social context, social interplay, client interpretation, degree of meaningful occupations, routines and performance initiation (Bejerholm et al. 2006; Edgelow and Krupa 2011). If an individual is a reliable historian in terms of daily activities, this tool can provide a real-time baseline level of overall occupational function from which it assesses occupational balance and engagement and possible impact on health and life goals.

## Self-management and Activities of Daily Living

Occupation encompasses self-care (e.g., dressing, eating) and instrumental activities of daily living (e.g., medication, money management). Occupational therapy evaluation includes focused assessment of these mundane and yet vital activities that are frequently affected in individuals with SMI. Observation-based life skill batteries can be used to establish a measure of daily activity function and/or serve to predict success upon discharge to a community setting or independent living. These assessments include the Kohlman Evaluation of Living Skills, the Milwaukee Evaluation of Living skills, the Life Skills Profile, the Assessment of Motor and Process Skills (AMPS), and the Bay Area Functional Performance Assessment (Houston et al. 1989; Fisher 2003; Leonardelli 1988; Rosen et al. 1989).

The Assessment of Motor and Process Skills (AMPS) is an observation-based assessment that measures the quality of performance of 36 skills (16 motor skills and 20 process skills) necessary to perform activities of daily living (Fisher 2003). The AMPS has been shown to have good psychometric properties and good predictive validity of evidence of a client's need for assistance in the community (Bernspang and Fisher 1995; Kirkley and Fisher 1999; Merritt 2011). The Bay Area Functional Performance Measure (BAFPHE) is a test that was initially designed to measure functional occupational performance of individuals living in psychiatric hospitals (Houston et al. 1989). The assessment is comprised of a Task-Oriented Scale that includes cognitive, performance, and affective component measures, and a Social Interaction Scale, and has been shown to have satisfactory psychometric properties. In addition, the Task-Oriented Scale has been correlated with scores on the three subscales of the Weschler Adult Intelligence Scale (WAIS) and the Kohlman Evaluation of Living Skills (Thibeault and Blackmer 1987; Houston et al. 1989).

## Sensory Processing

Individuals with SMI can exhibit difficulties processing visual, auditory, and somatosensory input, and can exhibit visual motor disorganization (Brown et al. 2002; Butler and Javitt 2005; Giersch et al. 2013; Javitt 2009a, b; Lipskaya-Velikovsky et al. 2015). Tools such as the Adolescent and Adult Sensory Profile (Brown and Dunn 2002) and the Adult Sensory Processing Scale (Blanche et al. 2014) can provide a means to examine patterns in self-reported difficulties with processing and modulation of sensory information. Enhanced understanding of sensory difficulties can inform recommendations for milieu, physical environment, and sensory modalities to promote an optimal context for feelings of comfort, self-regulation, coping skills, sense of security and learning.

# Occupational Therapy Interventions

Occupational therapy as a profession encompasses a broad range of clinical specialties, and the field is relatively young in terms of empirical and evidence-based research, particularly in the area of psychosocial occupational therapy.

Evidence for many of the interventions commonly used in psychosocial occupational therapy is scarce and/or emerging, particularly in the inpatient psychiatric setting. Thus, I have expanded the literature base in the sections below to include research in community and home-based settings for individuals with SMI, and interventions that might be multidisciplinary in nature, but utilize conceptual occupation-based constructs.

## Therapeutic Use of Self

Therapeutic use of self has been defined as "practitioner's planned use of his or her personality, insights, perceptions and judgments as part of the therapeutic process" (Punwar and Peloquin 2000, p. 285). Full presence with an individual is essential to the empathic process in occupational therapy practice, and the empathic encounter should include the process of "being with" as an enactment of "doing with" (Peloquin 1995). Warmth, empathy, trust, and acceptance have been identified as occupational therapist characteristics valued by individuals with SMI, as exemplified in the following statement, "I think it's very important that any therapist displays care for their client —that they are genuinely interested, that it's not a nine to five job. You know because if somebody is showing genuine concern that's probably worth a hundred tranquillizers or antidepressants" (Blank 2004, p. 121). Embodiment of a mindful presence and attitude of nonjudgmental acceptance and respect is a primary intervention that the occupational therapist can provide to an individual who may be experiencing pain due to loss of autonomy, life role changes, anxiety, disorientation, fear, frustration, anger, or sadness due to symptoms of SMI.

## Habits, Routines, and Time-Use

In the early 1900s, habit training was introduced at John Hopkins Medical Center, and is considered by many theorists to be the first occupational therapy treatment intervention. This intervention approach proposed that for many individuals, a mental illness such as schizophrenia could result in dysfunction in daily life due to a deterioration or imbalance of occupational habits. Early occupational therapists introduced therapeutic occupations such as weaving, art, and bookbinding to clinical practice, and helped individuals to engage in purposeful daily activities. These goal-directed activities were used to help individuals learn new skills to be productive, and to gain the therapeutic benefits of a structured daily schedule. In the habit training model, insight, orientation, and awareness were not viewed as prerequisites to experiencing adaptive and healthy life habits, but rather could be nurtured when daily activities and functional habits were supported as a therapeutic means. Indeed, contemporary recovery theorists have suggested that developing new habits can precede, rather than follow, development of insight (Davidson 2007).

Individuals with SMI have indicated that everyday routines and activities are important pathways to recovery, and rhythm of life and daily activities can become impaired during acute mental crises. In addition, social rhythm disruption events have been found to predict depressive symptoms and episodes (Borg and Davidson 2008; Borg et al. 2011; Sylvia et al. 2009). As one's habits are embedded in the sociocultural and physical environment context, a thorough understanding of meaningful habits requires examination of the institutional environment as a factor that shapes habit development and adaptation (Yerxa 2002). Habits and routines are not only affected by psychiatric symptoms, but also by temporal and environmental rigidity typical of an inpatient facility with a focus on safety and restrictions, such as a forensic psychiatric setting. While measures to ensure protection from harm and violence are necessary, these safeguards can lead to lack of flexibility in establishment of meaningful routines, and potentially lead to a diminished independence in scheduling daily activities. Individuals can become dependent on the institutionalized schedule to dictate what activities they will do, and when and where they will take place.

The ability to maintain a sense of occupational balance through meaningful time-use patterns contributes to healthy life habits. Individuals living in psychiatric units and in community settings have reported engaging in predominantly passive activities, and having increased idle time, and limited and repetitive activity choices (Delespaul and DeVries 1987; Farnworth et al. 2004; Katsakou and Priebe 2007; Krupa et al. 2003; Letendre 1997; Quirk and Lelliott 2001; Quirk et al. 2006; Shattell et al. 2008; Suto and Frank 1994; Weeder 1986). This can result in an occupational imbalance characterized by having too many passive activities with little opportunity for active and meaningful engagement, especially in more restricted settings.

A qualitative occupational time-use study of individuals living in a secure forensic psychiatric unit found that individuals regarded their day-to-day routine as a series of activities to prevent boredom between meals, and verbalized that the goal of their daily routine was to "kill time" until they could return to the outside world (Farnworth et al. 2004). They subsequently experienced a disconnection from active pursuit of meaningful goals, roles, and routines, as this was a process they associated exclusively with life outside the hospital. However, these individuals reported that they found meaning and satisfaction in activities and groups that offered challenge and novelty. Similarly, in a single case qualitative study, an individual with a lived experience of psychosis described his daily routine as characterized by monotony and passive activity that made him feel like he was "wasting his life away," as he was "lazy, nonproductive, overeating, oversleeping, and not doing anything … [but] having coffee, watching TV, smoking, [doing] drugs and alcohol, or sleeping" (Legault and Rebeiro 2001, p. 94). However, he reported gains in hope and purpose when he discovered meaningful occupations to engage in, such as journaling and writing about his experience with schizophrenia, setting up art exhibits, and making patchwork quilts for the homeless (Legault and Rebeiro 2001).

Occupational therapists can adapt familiar or passive activities to create added challenge to foster interest and motivation for individuals who are experiencing boredom and are unable to find and initiate opportunities for active engagement. For example, instead of an individual simply looking through a magazine, the therapist could create a scavenger hunt of images or words to find in a set of magazines spread throughout a unit or within a group to add elements of problem solving and competition to a typically passive low challenge activity. This activity could incorporate skill building via use of a checklist that then could be applied to other life skills (e.g., grocery shopping). The occupational therapist can collaborate with group providers in a psychosocial treatment mall who are teaching skills such as court competency or social skills, that may be viewed as boring, to integrate fun and creative modalities such as games and crafts. These occupation-based modalities can add an element of novelty and meaning to inspire intrinsic motivation for active engagement.

The occupational therapist can teach an individual who is disengaged or participating in predominantly passive activities about the various levels of occupational engagement and assist him or her in identifying preferred activities of each type. In addition, the occupational therapist can collaborate with the individual to develop guidelines for when it may be appropriate to engage in identified activities based on mood, opportunity, setting, and scheduled responsibilities. Action Over Inertia (AOI) is an occupational therapy time-use intervention that was developed to help individuals with SMI experiencing impoverished daily routines predominated by passive activities (e.g., sleeping) to improve daily occupational balance and engagement (Edgelow and Krupa 2011). A pilot randomized controlled study of AOI used in an Assertive Community Treatment (ACT) setting found that following intervention, individuals in the AOI group experienced a significant decrease in daily sleeping time when compared to control group, and this decrease in sleep time resulted in increased time in active engagement.

Habituation refers to one's daily occupational patterns, roles, and routines, and can be a semi-autonomous process (Kielhofner 1980, 2002).

Daily habits and routines are not commonly a focus of explicit regard and contemplation in the therapeutic process, possibly because of the semiautonomous nature of this phenomenon. However, onset of illness or disability and resultant deterioration or loss of habits can often prompt the need for conscious attention to habits (Yerxa 2002). An occupational therapist can support an individual to explore and increase self-awareness of daily habits and routines, and provide education on building balanced, healthy and meaningful habits and routines that will support recovery.

Occupational therapists can utilize knowledge of an individual's motivation, physiological rhythms, interests, and personal goals to help identify and explore new meaningful occupations, and specific functional habits and routines that could be generalized to the outside world upon discharge. This is especially important when individual goals involve lifestyle changes. For example, Carlson et al. (1998) found that it is essential for lifestyle changes to be linked to daily routines to be successful. In a qualitative study of medication adherence, 91 % of participants reported that they used activity-based methods that were attached to existing habits and routines (e.g., putting on jewelry or turning on coffee pot in the morning just before taking medications) to prompt and cue them to take medication (Sanders and Van Oss 2013). Individuals with SMI who experience cognitive and memory impairments that impact medication adherence can benefit from individualized occupational therapy strategies that they can integrate into existing daily habits, and/or to create new routines in the context of self-management and self-care.

## Living Skills and Daily Occupational Engagement

Impairment in daily self-care and self-management is a frequent concern for individuals with schizophrenia and SMI who require hospitalization. Self-care and self-management life skills interventions are primary interventions that occupational therapists in an inpatient psychiatric setting provide (Simpson et al. 2005). Unfortunately, due to the more rigid institutional structure of inpatient settings, and often restricted material use due to risk for self-harm and danger to others, these settings can inherently provide less opportunity for individuals to engage in domestic activities of daily living. The concept of recovery can seem large, overwhelming and unattainable for people experiencing life disruption due to difficult symptoms and changes in life roles and environment, and a focus on essential and mundane self-care tasks can provide therapeutic benefits as both a process and an outcome in the acute phases of recovery. Interventions that focus on self-care activities of daily living (ADLS; e.g., grooming, dressing, eating), self-management, and instrumental activities of daily living (IADLs; e.g., medication management, transportation, meal planning and preparation) can prepare an individual for return to the community and provide a sense of meaning and domesticity to what can often feel like a sterile clinical environment.

### Self-Care

Individuals in an acute stage of SMI might not be motivated to engage in grooming activities due to decreased awareness, insight, and energy. An occupational therapist can use knowledge of the individual to customize the occupation of grooming to promote engagement by providing choices and supports that align with individual needs and interests. For example, the occupational therapist can adjust the temporal context (e.g., morning vs. evening for showering), physical environment (e.g., bedroom vs. crowded bathroom for grooming), learning methods (e.g., backward chaining, errorless learning, video modeling), as well as offer opportunities for individual decision-making (e.g., flavor of toothpaste, scent of soap) to increase intrinsic motivation, meaning, and self-efficacy.

In addition, individuals with SMI can experience physical risk during self-care activities due to medication side effects (e.g., dry mouth, extrapyramidal symptoms, orthostatic hypotension) and symptoms of disorder (impulsivity, diminished environmental awareness). This can result in the possibility of harm during mundane tasks, such as eating and ambulation. A systematic review found that dysphagia (i.e., difficulty swallowing) prevalence in individuals with mental illness ranged from 9 % to as high as 42 %, and that people with organic mental illness were 43 times more likely to die of choking or asphyxia than people in the general population (Aldridge and Taylor 2012). The occupational therapist can work with individuals who are exhibiting symptoms of dysphagia or increased risk for falls to remediate skills and identify strategies and environmental supports to improve both safety and quality of engagement during self-care tasks.

### Self-Management and Instrumental Activities of Daily Living

Life skills and psychosocial skills interventions that relate to IADLs can be provided individually or in a group setting, and can be individualized or manualized in approach. While psychosocial skills interventions that utilize modules, such as the UCLA Social and Independent Living Skills Programs (Liberman et al. 1993), can offer a structured and consistent format for teaching, skills taught in a clinical environment may not generalize to the community setting, and reviews regarding effectiveness of structured skills training programs have been mixed (Bellack 2004; Liberman et al. 1986; Pilling et al. 2002; Wallace et al. 1992).

The In Vivo Life Amplified Skills Training (IVAST) program was developed to integrate intensive case management and behavioral strategies with skills training in an effort to promote generalization and transfer of IADL skills to community living. A study of this approach found that this approach combined with skills training resulted in improved gains in social adjustment when compared to skills training alone (Glynn et al. 2002). A study by Liberman et al. (1998) compared the effects of a psychosocial skills training program (i.e., UCLA Social and Independent Living Skills Program modules for basic conversation, recreation for leisure, medication management, and symptom management) to that of a psychosocial occupational therapy intervention (i.e., art and craft modalities). Liberman et al. reported better performance of life skill function (e.g., management of personal possessions, food preparation, and money management) with the life skills intervention. However, the occupational therapy modality used in the study was a craft-based activity that did not address social skills, and thus the methodology did not allow for comparison of two intervention modalities that were targeting the same foundational skills. This observation speaks to the lack of clarity that many professionals have regarding the dynamics of occupation, the ways in which it impacts the human system, and the profession of occupational therapy itself.

While life and social skills programs that utilize a prescriptive manual can provide structure and consistency for clinicians, these programs may not allow for a more individualized view of individual occupation, i.e., examine the who, why, when, where, and how of occupation as a frame for which to reference occupational functioning. A manualized approach can teach an individual about leisure as a means for recreation as a life skill, but treatment may not include experiential opportunities to explore different activities to understand how they could be used for comfort, self-management based on level of engagement, alignment with physical functioning, and consideration of leisure access and engagement in terms of overall patterns of time-use and occupational balance. For example, an individual who is experiencing akathisia as a medication side effect can be taught to adhere to his medication regimen with training in medication management skills, but to maintain medication compliance, he may need to learn to live with the discomfort of akathisia. The occupational therapist could work with him to determine which leisure and self-management occupations can empower him to cope with physical feelings of restlessness and subsequent affective pain (e.g., running, racquetball, swimming, vacuuming, meditation), and how he can incorporate these activities into his daily routines and habits. In this way, an individual can begin to learn how occupational engagement can assist in recovery and quality of life. Finally, the occupational therapist can provide adaptations to support an individual in being better able to self-manage daily activities (e.g., visual schedule of daily activities, timer for taking medication).

## Leisure

In the western culture, leisure activity is often viewed as nonproductive, and less important than other occupations, such as work and self-management. For individuals with SMI, leisure tasks can serve as a necessary component of a balanced life. In addition to providing enrichment, engagement in leisure occupations can provide an individual with meaningful social life roles, opportunities for problem solving, means of self-regulation, and outlets for creativity and self-expression. Arts and crafts have traditionally been used by occupational therapists working in mental health settings as a means by which to engage the mind, body, and creative spirit.

During an admission in an inpatient mental health facility as a young occupational therapy intern, I was scheduled for an occupational therapy group. I remember feeling shame, anger, and helplessness, no motivation, and was having a difficult time with my new medications, which made me feel simultaneously restless and exhausted. The occupational therapist gave me a raw ceramic mug and showed me how to apply the glazes. As I painted that mug, I felt human. In retrospect, I think that through the process of transforming a blank colorless cup into my own creative work, I had planted the seed for how to initiate my own transformation. Ever since, I have found creative expression, whether through art, music, or poetry, to be an essential tool for my own ongoing recovery.

For individuals with SMI, leisure tasks can be viewed as having a temporal quality of not being as stringently bound by time or pace, and thus more conducive to enjoyment and presence. They can also serve as a means to social connection, though barriers such as limited finances, transportation, and physical disabilities could limit leisure engagement (Pieris and Craik 2004, 2006). When an individual is living in a supported environment such as a psychiatric hospital, it may be easier to access leisure activities as they are typically scheduled and facilitated by providers. An occupational therapist can work with an individual to help him to identify means and strategies to support preferred leisure engagement in terms of needs (e.g., financial and transportation), as well as modify leisure activities and/or recommend adaptations to accommodate physical or cognitive disability.

Physically active leisure has been significantly associated with lower levels of negative emotion in people with schizophrenia, and experience sampling has revealed that the bulk of leisure time is predominantly sedentary in nature in this population (McCormick et al. 2012). Engagement in active leisure occupations can benefit individuals with SMI who are at risk for health concerns due to medication side effects (e.g., weight gain), and predominance of sedentary activities (McElroy et al. 2006). Again, leisure engagement goes beyond leisure for the sake of recreation, and treatment to address leisure function should include consideration of individual motivation and meaning, as measures of leisure motivation have been found to correlate with measures of recovery (Lloyd et al. 2007).

Recovery can involve an ongoing process of coping and living despite illness symptoms, and engagement in active healthy leisure occupations can support this process. For example, an occupational therapist could use a familiar passive leisure activity, such as music listening, and teach individuals in an individual or group setting to develop playlists of songs that impact mood, motivation, and affect (e.g., songs to wake up and get going, songs that are calming). With this type of occupation-based intervention, an individual can have hands-on experience not only of engagement in the occupation itself, but also in developing an action plan for future engagement.

Leisure enhancement is an approach that involves assessment of leisure interests, education to increase awareness of leisure benefits, leisure goal setting, skill training, and supported participation (Heasman and Atwal 2004). The process of guided development of leisure action plans alone has been shown to result in the ability to maintain leisure engagement at 6-month follow-up for about half of the participants with SMI living in the community. An occupational therapist in an inpatient setting can assist individuals in small group or 1:1 sessions to develop and implement leisure action plans while in the hospital, and then perform follow-up to practice scheduling of and access to leisure occupations, with modification of leisure action plans as needed prior to discharge. Practice with the process of creating habits and routines that include active leisure engagement can be beneficial as engagement in active leisure occupations can present more of a challenge upon discharge when an individual has less accessibility to structured leisure opportunities and resources, especially when one has a goal of consistent and structured employment.

## Meaningful Employment

Productive employment is highly valued in the western culture, and vocation influences social regard and forms much of the basis for occupational identity. Indeed, as occupational beings, humans may be physiologically driven to engage in work, in that "… work is a biological necessity. Just as our muscles become flabby and degenerate if not used, so our brain slips into chaos and confusion unless we constantly use it for some work that seems worthwhile to us" (Selye 1976, p. 142). Work provides a means to a financial ends and can also provide latent effects that support health and well-being, such as a daily time structure, regular opportunity for shared experiences and social interaction, and broadening of interpersonal goals to shared goals of work place and environment (Jahoda 1981; Yerxa 1998).

Individuals with SMI who are employed have reported increased happiness and higher scores on recovery and empowerment scales, and have indicated that work provides not only financial support, but also a means to recovery and well-being (Dunn et al. 2010; Lloyd et al. 2010; Robinson et al. 2012; van Niekerk 2009). However, individuals with SMI have been found to have the lowest employment rate when compared to people in any other disability category (Bilder and Mechanic 2003). Research has shown that for individuals with SMI, factors such as fear of stigma and ability to manage medication and symptoms in the work place can hinder successful employment, while self-confidence, motivation, meaningfulness of work, work related skill competency, and access to adequate supportive resources can promote vocational recovery (Dunn et al. 2010; Fossey and Harvey 2010; Honey 2004; Killeen and O'Day 2004; Kirsh 2000; Marwaha and Johnson 2005; Woodside et al. 2006). Another important aspect of employment success is social support and connection in the workplace. Social support has been shown to mediate the relationship between work (competitive, sheltered, and unpaid) and subjective quality of life measures, even more than income derived from occupation (Rüesch et al. 2004; Woodside et al. 2006).

## Sensory and Environmental Supports

The processing and integration of sensory information helps to provide a sense of self, an understanding of the self in relationship to the environment, and the subsequent ability to filter a massive amount of information from sensory receptors to make an adaptive response and functionally interact with the external world (Ayers 1972; Javitt 2015; Javitt and Freedman 2015). Individuals with SMI can exhibit difficulty with modulation, or regulation of responses to sensory input, and processing of sensory information (Brown et al. 2002; Javitt 2009a, b, 2015; Lipskaya-Velikovsky et al. 2015). The use of supportive sensory strategies and environments can serve to empower individuals with deficits in self-control and self-regulation to self-manage arousal and emotional states (Nan Stromberg 2004; Scanlan and Novak 2015). Sensory modulation interventions and multisensory environments on acute psychiatric units designed to promote improved sensory processing and regulation have resulted in significant improvements in both subjective reports of distress and in the frequency and duration of restraint and seclusion use (Cummings et al. 2010; Lloyd et al. 2014).

In addition, history of trauma has been found to be more prevalent for individuals with SMI than for individuals in the general population. Chronic trauma can impact an individual's ability to integrate sensory, cognitive, and affective information into a meaningful and functional gestalt, and to self-modulate for self-regulation (Bebbington et al. 2004; Mueser et al. 1998; van der Kolk et al. 2005). For this reason, researchers have proposed a "bottom-up" approach that focuses on improving sensory processing and modulation as a promising means to address difficulties in dysregulation commonly seen in individuals with a history of trauma. For example, a study of a sensory integration intervention for individuals with mental illness found that a bottom-up sensory integration intervention combined with psychotherapy resulted in significant improvements in measures of trauma symptoms when compared to individuals who received psychotherapy alone (Kaiser et al. 2010).

Difficulties in sensory modulation have also been identified as possible contributors to aggression and a similar bottom-up sensory modulation approach can provide an alternative to more cognitively mediated top-down methods of de-escalation (e.g., verbal techniques) when an individual is not able to engage in these techniques due to poorly controlled autonomic arousal (Sutton et al. 2013). For example, a pilot trial of a sensory modulation intervention was conducted that involved supporting individuals to access sensory rooms on inpatient psychiatry units to identify therapeutic sensory modalities within the sensory environments. They reported that they were able to attain a calm grounded state, take comfort in an atmosphere that provoked a sense of safety, experience enhanced interpersonal connection with staff, and experience self-control, self-awareness, and emerging active self-management skills (Sutton et al. 2013). An occupational therapist can work with individuals who have experienced a history of trauma or aggression and violence to help them to identify particular patterns of sensory modulation dysfunction (e.g., tactile defensiveness, auditory sensitivity), and develop strategies and sensory modalities for coping with sensory dysregulation, which can affect all areas of daily life.

### Sleep

Sleep is restorative and essential to health and well-being, and yet there are few common sleep interventions outside of medication in the general spectrum of treatment for individuals with SMI living in an inpatient facility. People with schizophrenia have indicated that improving sleep is one of the highest priorities of treatment (Auslander and Jeste 2002). Even if not part of the symptomology of an individual's illness, or a side effect of medication, being in an unfamiliar physical and social environment can pose a challenge to the level of comfort and ease required for good sleep hygiene.

An occupational therapist can help an individual develop individualized sleep routines, habits, and environments that promote healthy sleep patterns. For example, the environment can be adapted to promote optimal level of lighting (e.g., eye mask if room cannot be darkened), calming sounds or silence (e.g., white noise, earplugs), and incorporate sensory comforts or rituals (e.g., weighted blanket, aromatherapy) that are conducive to rest, relaxation, and sleep. Education on strategies (e.g., using bed only for sleep to create a schema between bed and sleep, and not staying in bed if not sleepy) can help an individual to develop good sleep routines (Wade 2006).

### Occupational Stories

Many clinical disciplines have used the narrative process to help people facing disability and life disruption to create a life history and life story as a means of self-expression and healing. An occupational therapy perspective of the narrative life history is largely focused on the individual's telling, reflection, and understanding of her own occupational identity (Christiansen 1999; Kielhofner 2008). Occupational therapists can work with an individual to support therapeutic emplotment, a collaborative process in which the occupational therapist supports the individual to imagine possible options and scenarios for occupational engagement and identity in the continuation of the present life narrative to contribute to personal transformation (Gahnstrom-Strandqvist et al. 2004). Narrative life plots can be victimic, characterized by having little control and choice in life, or agentic, in which storytellers are active self-determined protagonists. Engagement in occupations that align with a person's goals can prompt a shift from victimic to agentic life story plots (Polkinghorne 1996).

### Spiritual Occupations

Recovery is often viewed as a process of transformation, not unlike a spiritual journey. In a study of individuals with SMI, 90 % indicated that they identified themselves as spiritual or religious (Corrigan et al. 2003). Spirituality is considered an important dimension with regard to humans as occupational beings (Christiansen 1997). Spiritual occupations, manifested at individual and community levels, have been defined as, "a variety of activities specifically imbued with spiritual meanings and effects that have been performed by human beings over many generations and across all cultures" (Kang 2003, p. 95). Occupational therapists recognize the value of addressing spirituality in evaluation and treatment, yet there exists a theory–practice gap between the awareness of its importance and its practical clinical application (Belcham 2004; Enquist et al. 1997; Farrar 2001; Johnston and Mayers 2005; Rose 1999).

In an effort to understand occupation in the spiritual context, occupational therapy researchers recruited individuals with schizophrenia to act as coresearchers in an exploratory study of spiritual practice and meaning. They found that one of the core dimensions of spirituality was that practice could be explicit (e.g., formal prayer or meditation) and/or could be ordinary activities that were imbued with spiritual meaning (Smith and Suto 2012). This finding is similar to the dualistic nature of mindfulness practice in which a person can engage in formal meditation practice, or can exercise the informal practice of being mindful during mundane activity.

Mindful occupational engagement is defined as "moment-by-moment awareness and nonjudgmental engagement in an activity, without expectation of specific outcomes" (Jackman 2014, p. 243). Mindful occupational engagement can provide an underlying spiritual context that can serve to unify and inject meaning into all areas of an individual's life, even when activities tend to be prosaic. Occupational therapists can utilize mindfulness practice as an occupation-based therapy intervention to help individuals participate and gain skills in mindfulness meditation as a primary spiritual occupation that is religious (e.g., Buddhist practice) or secular (e.g., morning meditation for stress relief). Occupational therapists can assist individuals to infuse spirituality into the seemingly mundane occupations of daily life through mindful occupational engagement. In this regard, both therapist practice of mindfulness, and therapist ability to use the practice of mindfulness as a therapeutic intervention may provide a means to more holistically address an individual as a being of body, mind, and spirit.

Finally, while the expression of spirituality can sometimes be difficult to distinguish from the symptoms of psychiatric pathology, the use of clinical reasoning and examination of the link between spiritual expression and meaningful personal and cultural occupational engagement can serve as a guide to supporting health promoting benefits of spirituality (Hess 2011). An occupational therapist can assist an individual in incorporating spiritual or religious practices into daily life in a manner that offers balance and empowerment. In addition, the occupational therapist can work with the individual in identifying means to access religious services, meditation groups, or service groups in the community.

## Conclusion

Occupational therapists can assist individuals with SMI to experience life meaning and function by supporting a journey of recovery through occupation. This chapter discussed the alignment between recovery principles and occupational therapy theory and practice. In addition, it presented a framework to examine the holistic and nonlinear nature of humans as occupational beings by moving beyond looking at *what* people do to examine the *who, why, where, when,* and *how* of occupation. Finally, the chapter reviewed occupational therapy assessments and interventions that can be used in the inpatient psychiatric setting to complement the multidisciplinary treatment effort and to help individuals learn to live life to its fullest.

## References


Aldridge, K. J., & Taylor, N. F. (2012). Dysphagia is a common and serious problem for adults with mental illness: A systematic review. *Dysphagia, 27*, 124–137.

American Occupational Therapy Association. (2008). Occupational therapy practice framework: Domain and process (2nd Ed.). *American Journal of Occupational Therapy, 62*, 625–683.

Andresen, R., Oades, L., & Caputi, P. (2003). The experience of recovery from schizophrenia: Towards an empirically validated stage model. *Australian and New Zealand Journal of Psychiatry, 37*, 586–594.

Apte, A., Kielhofner, G., Paul-Ward, A., & Braveman, B. (2005). Therapists' and clients' perceptions of the occupational performance history interview. *Occupational Therapy in Health Care, 19*(1–2), 173–192.

Aubin, G., Hachey, R., & Mercier, C. (1999). Meaning of daily activities and subjective quality of life in people with severe mental illness. *Scandinavian Journal of Occupational Therapy, 6*(2), 53–62.

Auslander, L. A., & Jeste, D. V. (2002). Perceptions of problems and needs for service among middle-aged and elderly outpatients with schizophrenia and related psychotic disorders. *Community Mental Health Journal, 38*, 391–402.

Ayres, A. (1972). *Sensory integration and learning disabilities*. Los Angeles, CA: Western Psychological Services.

Baron, K., Kielhofner, G., Iyenger, A., Goldhammer, V., & Wolenski, J. (2006). *Occupational Self Assessment Version 2.2.* Model of Human Occupation Clearinghouse.

Baum, C. (2002). Adolph Meyer's challenge: Focus on occupation in practice and in science. *OTJR: Occupation, Participation and Health, 22*(4), 130–131.

Bebbington, P. E., Bhugra, D., Brugha, T., Singleton, N., Farrell, M., Jenkins, R., et al. (2004). Psychosis, victimisation and childhood disadvantage: Evidence from the second British national survey of psychiatric morbidity. *The British Journal of Psychiatry, 185*, 220–226.

Bejerholm, U., & Eklund, M. (2004). Time use and occupational performance among persons with schizophrenia. *Occupational Therapy in Mental Health, 20*, 27–47.

Bejerholm, U., & Eklund, M. (2007). Occupational engagement in persons with schizophrenia: Relationships to self-related variables, psychopathology, and quality of life. *American Journal of Occupational Therapy, 61*, 21–32.

Bejerholm, U., Hansson, L., & Eklund, M. (2006). Profiles of occupational engagement in people with schizophrenia (POES): The development of a new instrument based on time-use diaries. *The British Journal of Occupational Therapy, 69*, 58–68.

Belcham, C. (2004). Spirituality in occupational therapy: Theory in practice? *The British Journal of Occupational Therapy, 67*, 39–46.

Bellack, A. S. (2004). Skills training for people with severe mental illness. *Psychiatric Rehabilitation Journal, 27*, 375.

Bilder, S., & Mechanic, D. (2003). Navigating the disability process: Persons with mental disorders applying for and receiving disability benefits. *Milbank Quarterly, 81*, 75–106.

Blanche, E. I., Parham, D., Chang, M., & Mallinson, T. (2014). Development of an adult sensory processing scale (ASPS). *American Journal of Occupational Therapy, 68*, 531–538.

Blank, A. (2004). Clients' experience of partnership with occupational therapists in community mental health. *The British Journal of Occupational Therapy, 67*, 118–124.

Borg, M., & Davidson, L. (2008). The nature of recovery as lived in everyday experience. *Journal of Mental Health, 17*, 129–140.

Borg, M., Karlsson, B., Lofthus, A. M., & Davidson, L. (2011). Hitting the wall: Lived experiences of mental health crises. *International Journal of Qualitative Studies on Health and Well-being, 6*(4). doi:10.3402/qhw.v6i4.7197

Breier, A., & Strauss, J. S. (1983). Self-control in psychotic disorders. *Archives of General Psychiatry, 40*, 1141–1145.

Brown, C., Cromwell, R. L., Filion, D., Dunn, W., & Tollefson, N. (2002). Sensory processing in schizophrenia: Missing and avoiding information. *Schizophrenia Research, 55*, 187–195.

Brown, C., & Dunn, W. (2002). *Adolescent-adult sensory profile: User's manual*. Tucson, AZ: Therapy Skill Builders.

Butler, P. D., & Javitt, D. C. (2005). Early-stage visual processing deficits in schizophrenia. *Current Opinion in Psychiatry, 18*, 151–157.

Carlson, M., Clark, F., & Young, B. (1998). Practical contributions of occupational science to the art of successful ageing: How to sculpt a meaningful life in older adulthood. *Journal of Occupational Science, 5*, 107–118.

Carswell, A., McColl, M. A., Baptiste, S., Law, M., Polatajko, H., & Pollock, N. (2004). The Canadian occupational performance measure: A research and

clinical literature review. *Canadian Journal of Occupational Therapy, 71*, 210–222.
Chaudhary, P., & Sharma, U. (1976). Existential frustration and mental illness: A comparative study of purpose in life in psychiatric patients and normals. *Indian Journal of Clinical Psychology, 3*, 171–174.
Christiansen, C. H. (1997). Acknowledging a spiritual dimension in occupational therapy practice. *American Journal of Occupational Therapy, 51*, 169–172.
Christiansen, C. H. (1999). Defining lives: Occupation as identity: An essay on competence, coherence, and the creation of meaning. *American Journal of Occupational Therapy, 53*, 547–558.
Clark, F., & Lawlor, M. (2009). *The making and mattering of occupational science*. Philadelphia: Lippincott Williams & Wilkins.
Cohrs, S. (2008). Sleep disturbances in patients with schizophrenia. *CNS Drugs, 22*, 939–962.
Copic, V., Deane, F. P., Crowe, T. P., & Oades, L. G. (2011). Hope, meaning and responsibility across stages of recovery for individuals living with an enduring mental illness. *The Australian Journal of Rehabilitation Counselling, 17*(2), 61–73.
Corrigan, P., McCorkle, B., Schell, B., & Kidder, K. (2003). Religion and spirituality in the lives of people with serious mental illness. *Community Mental Health Journal, 39*, 487–499.
Craik, C., & Pieris, Y. (2006). Without leisure …'it wouldn't be much of a life': The meaning of leisure for people with mental health problems. *The British Journal of Occupational Therapy, 69*, 209–216.
Cummings, K. S., Grandfield, S. A., & Coldwell, C. M. (2010). Caring with comfort rooms. Reducing seclusion and restraint use in psychiatric facilities. *Journal of Psychosocial Nursing and Mental Health Services, 48*(6), 26–30.
Curson, D. A., Pantelis, C., Ward, J., & Barnes, T. R. (1992). Institutionalism and schizophrenia 30 years on: Clinical poverty and the social environment in three British mental hospitals in 1960 compared with a fourth in 1990. *The British Journal of Psychiatry, 160*, 230–241.
Davidson, L. (2007). Habits and other anchors of everyday life that people with psychiatric disabilities may not take for granted. *OTJR: Occupation, Participation and Health, 27*(1 suppl.), 60S–68S.
Davidson, L., O'Connell, M., Tondora, J., Staeheli, M. R., & Evans, A. C. (2005). Recovery in serious mental illness: Paradigm shift or shibboleth? In L. Davidson, C. M. Harding, & L. Spaniol (Eds.), *Recovery from severe mental illnesses: Research evidence and implications for practice*. Boston, MA: Center for Psychiatric Rehabilitation, Sargent College of Health and Rehabilitation Sciences, Boston University.
Davidson, L., & Strauss, J. S. (1992). Sense of self in recovery from severe mental illness. *British Journal of Medical Psychology, 65*, 131–145.
Delespaul, P. A., & DeVries, M. W. (1987). The daily life of ambulatory chronic mental patients. *The Journal of Nervous and Mental Disease, 175*, 537–544.
DeVries, M. W., & Delespaul, P. A. (1989). Time, context, and subjective experiences in schizophrenia. *Schizophrenia Bulletin, 15*, 233–244.
Dickerson, A. E., & Oakley, F. (1995). Comparing the roles of community-living persons and patient populations. *American Journal of Occupational Therapy, 49*, 221–228.
Dickerson, F., Ringel, N., & Parente, F. (1998). Subjective quality of life in out-patients with schizophrenia: Clinical and utilization correlates. *Acta Psychiatrica Scandinavica, 98*, 124–127.
Doble, S. E., & Santha, J. C. (2008). Occupational well-being: Rethinking occupational therapy outcomes. *Canadian Journal of Occupational Therapy, 75*, 184–190.
Dunn, E. C., Wewiorski, N. J., & Rogers, E. S. (2010). A qualitative investigation of individual and contextual factors associated with vocational recovery among people with serious mental illness. *American Journal of Orthopsychiatry, 80*, 185–194.
Dunn, W., Brown, C., & McGuigan, A. (1994). The ecology of human performance: A framework for considering the effect of context. *American Journal of Occupational Therapy, 48*, 595–607.
Eakman, A. M. (2013). Relationships between meaningful activity, basic psychological needs, and meaning in life: Test of the meaningful activity and life meaning model. *OTJR: Occupation Participation and Health, 33*, 100–109.
Eakman, A. M., Carlson, M. E., & Clark, F. A. (2010). The meaningful activity participation assessment: A measure of engagement in personally valued activities. *International Journal of Aging and Human Development, 70*, 299–317.
Eakman, A. M., & Eklund, M. (2012). The relative impact of personality traits, meaningful occupation and occupational value on meaning in life and life satisfaction. *Journal of Occupational Science, 19*, 165–177.
Edgelow, M., & Krupa, T. (2011). Randomized controlled pilot study of an occupational time-use intervention for people with serious mental illness. *American Journal of Occupational Therapy, 65*, 267–276.
Eklund, M. (2007). Perceived control: How is it related to daily occupation in patients with mental illness living in the community? *American Journal of Occupational Therapy, 61*, 535–542.
Eklund, M., Backstrom, M., & Eakman, A. M. (2014). Psychometric properties and factor structure of the 13-item satisfaction with daily occupations scale when used with people with mental health problems. *Health and Quality of Life Outcomes, 12*, 191.
Eklund, M., Erlandsson, L., & Persson, D. (2003). Occupational value among individuals with long-term mental illness. *Canadian Journal of Occupational Therapy, 70*, 276–284.
Eklund, M., Hansson, L., & Bejerholm, U. (2001). Relationships between satisfaction with occupational factors and health-related variables in schizophrenia outpatients. *Social Psychiatry and Psychiatric Epidemiology, 36*, 79–85.

Eklund, M., Hermansson, A., & Håkansson, C. (2012). Meaning in life for people with schizophrenia: Does it include occupation? *Journal of Occupational Science, 19*, 93–105.

Engelhardt, H. T, Jr. (1977). Defining occupational therapy: The meaning of therapy and the virtues of occupation. *The American Journal of Occupational Therapy, 31*, 666–672.

Engquist, D. E., Short-DeGraff, M., Gliner, J., & Oltjenbruns, K. (1997). Occupational therapists' beliefs and practices with regard to spirituality and therapy. *American Journal of Occupational Therapy, 51*, 173–180.

Ennals, P., & Fossey, E. (2007). The occupational performance history interview in community mental health case management: Consumer and occupational therapist perspectives. *Australian Occupational Therapy Journal, 54*, 11–21.

Estroff, S. E. (1989). Self, identity, and subjective experiences of schizophrenia: In search of the subject. *Schizophrenia Bulletin, 15*, 189–196.

Evans, G. W. (2003). The built environment and mental health. *Journal of Urban Health, 80*, 536–555.

Farnworth, L., Nikitin, L., & Fossey, E. (2004). Being in a secure forensic psychiatric unit: Every day is the same, killing time or making the most of it. *The British Journal of Occupational Therapy, 67*, 430–438.

Farrar, J. E. (2001). Addressing spirituality and religious life in occupational therapy practice. *Physical and Occupational Therapy in Geriatrics, 18*(4), 65–85.

Feldman, D. B., & Snyder, C. R. (2005). Hope and the meaningful life: Theoretical and empirical associations between goal-directed thinking and life meaning. *Journal of Social and Clinical Psychology, 24*, 401–421.

Fervaha, G., Agid, O., McDonald, K., Foussias, G., & Remington, G. (2014). Daily activity patterns in remitted first-episode schizophrenia. *Comprehensive Psychiatry, 55*, 1182–1187.

Fidler, G. S. (1996). Life-style performance: From profile to conceptual model. *American Journal of Occupational Therapy, 50*, 139–147.

Fisher, A. G. (2003). *AMPS: Assessment of motor and process skills* (5th ed., Vol. 1). Fort Collins, CO: Three Star Press.

Flaherty, M. G. (2003). Time work: Customizing temporal experience. *Social Psychology Quarterly, 66*, 17–33.

Fossey, E. M., & Harvey, C. A. (2010). Finding and sustaining employment: A qualitative meta-synthesis of mental health consumer views. *The Canadian Journal of Occupational Therapy, 77*, 303–314.

Frankl, V. E. (1985). *Man's search for meaning*. New York: Simon and Schuster.

Freedman, B. J. (1974). The subjective experience of perceptual and cognitive disturbances in schizophrenia: A review of autobiographical accounts. *Archives of General Psychiatry, 30*, 333–340.

Gahnström-Strandqvist, K., Josephsson, S., & Tham, K. (2004). Stories of clients with mental illness: The structure of occupational therapists' interactions. *OTJR: Occupation, Participation and Health, 24*(4), 134–143.

Giersch, A., Poncelet, P. E., Capa, R. L., Martin, B., Duval, C. Z., Curzietti, M., et al. (2015). Disruption of information processing in schizophrenia: The time perspective. *Schizophrenia Research: Cognition, 56* (2), 78–83.

Giersch, A., Wilquin, H., Capa, R. L., & Delevoye-Turrell, Y. N. (2013). Combined visual and motor disorganization in patients with schizophrenia. *Frontiers in Psychology, 4*, 620.

Goldberg, B., Britnell, E. S., & Goldberg, J. (2002). The relationship between engagement in meaningful activities and quality of life in persons disabled by mental illness. *Occupational Therapy in Mental Health, 19*, 17–44.

Harvey, P. D., & Bellack, A. S. (2009). Toward a terminology for functional recovery in schizophrenia: Is functional remission a viable concept? *Schizophrenia Bulletin, 35*, 300–306.

Hasselkus, B. R. (2006). The world of everyday occupation: Real people, real lives. *American Journal of Occupational Therapy, 60*, 627–640.

Heasman, D., & Atwal, A. (2004). The active advice pilot project: Leisure enhancement and social inclusion for people with severe mental health problems. *The British Journal of Occupational Therapy, 67*, 511–514.

Hess, K. Y. (2011). A study on the discernment by occupational therapists on whether mental health service users' occupations of a spiritual nature are health seeking behaviors or manifestations of illness. Available from http://hdl.handle.net/11427/11438

Hitch, D., Pepin, G., & Stagnitti, K. (2013). Engagement in activities and occupations by people who have experienced psychosis: A metasynthesis of lived experience. *The British Journal of Occupational Therapy, 76*(2), 77–86.

Hofstetter, J. R., Lysaker, P. H., & Mayeda, A. R. (2005). Quality of sleep in patients with schizophrenia is associated with quality of life and coping. *BMC Psychiatry, 5*, 13.

Holahan, C. J. (1972). Seating patterns and patient behavior in an experimental dayroom. *Journal of Abnormal Psychology, 80*(2), 115–124.

Holahan, C. J., & Saegert, S. (1973). Behavioral and attitudinal effects of large-scale variation in the physical environment of psychiatric wards. *Journal of Abnormal Psychology, 82*, 454–462.

Honey, A. (2004). Benefits and drawbacks of employment: Perspectives of people with mental illness. *Qualitative Health Research, 14*, 381–395.

Hoshii, J., Yotsumoto, K., Tatsumi, E., Tanaka, C., Mori, T., & Hashimoto, T. (2013). Subject-chosen activities in occupational therapy for the improvement of psychiatric symptoms of inpatients with chronic schizophrenia: A controlled trial. *Clinical Rehabilitation, 27*, 638–645.

Houston, D., Williams, S. L., Bloomer, J., & Mann, W. C. (1989). The bay area functional performance

evaluation: Development and standardization. *American Journal of Occupational Therapy, 43*, 170–183.
Howard, P. B., El-Mallakh, P., Rayens, M. K., & Clark, J. J. (2003). Consumer perspectives on quality of inpatient mental health services. *Archives of Psychiatric Nursing, 17*, 205–217.
Jackman, M. M. (2014). Mindful occupational engagement. In N. N. Singh (Ed.), *Psychology of meditation* (pp. 241–278). New York: Nova Science Publishers.
Jackson, J., Carlson, M., Mandel, D., Zemke, R., & Clark, F. (1998). Occupation in lifestyle redesign: The well elderly study occupational therapy program. *American Journal of Occupational Therapy, 52*, 326–336.
Jagannath, A., Peirson, S. N., & Foster, R. G. (2013). Sleep and circadian rhythm disruption in neuropsychiatric illness. *Current Opinion in Neurobiology, 23*, 888–894.
Jahoda, M. (1981). Work, employment, and unemployment: Values, theories, and approaches in social research. *American Psychologist, 36*, 184–191.
Javitt, D. C. (2009a). When doors of perception close: Bottom-up models of disrupted cognition in schizophrenia. *Annual Review of Clinical Psychology, 5*, 249–275.
Javitt, D. C. (2009b). Sensory processing in schizophrenia: Neither simple nor intact. *Schizophrenia Bulletin, 35*, 1059–1064.
Javitt, D. C. (2015). Neurophysiological models for new treatment development in schizophrenia: Early sensory approaches. *Annals of the New York Academy of Sciences, 1344*, 92–104.
Javitt, D. C., & Freedman, R. (2015). Sensory processing dysfunction in the personal experience and neuronal machinery of schizophrenia. *American Journal of Psychiatry, 172*, 17–31.
Johnston, D., & Mayers, C. (2005). Spirituality: A review of how occupational therapists acknowledge, assess and meet spiritual needs. *The British Journal of Occupational Therapy, 68*, 386–392.
Kaiser, E. M., Gillette, C. S., & Spinazzola, J. (2010). A controlled pilot-outcome study of sensory integration (SI) in the treatment of complex adaptation to traumatic stress. *Journal of Aggression, Maltreatment and Trauma, 19*, 699–720.
Kang, C. (2003). A psychospiritual integration frame of reference for occupational therapy. Part 1: Conceptual foundations. *Australian Occupational Therapy Journal, 50*, 92–103.
Katsakou, C., & Priebe, S. (2007). Patient's experiences of involuntary hospital admission and treatment: A review of qualitative studies. *Epidemiologia e Psichiatria Sociale, 16*, 172–178.
Kielhofner, G. (2002). *A model of human occupation: Theory and application*. Philadelphia: Lippincott Williams & Wilkins.
Kielhofner, G., & Burke, J. P. (1980). A model of human occupation, part 1. Conceptual framework and content. *American Journal of Occupational Therapy, 34*, 572–581.
Kielhofner, G., Mallinson, T., Forsyth, K., & Lai, J. (2001). Psychometric properties of the second version of the occupational performance history interview (OPHI-II). *American Journal of Occupational Therapy, 55*, 260–267.
Killeen, M. B., & O'day, B. L. (2004). Challenging expectations: How individuals with psychiatric disabilities find and keep work. *Psychiatric Rehabilitation Journal, 28*, 157–163.
Kirkley, K. N., & Fisher, A. G. (1999). Alternate forms reliability of the assessment of motor and process skills. *Journal of Outcome Measurement, 3*, 53–70.
Kirsh, B. (2000). Factors associated with employment for mental health consumers. *Psychiatric Rehabilitation Journal, 24*, 13–21.
Klinger, E. (2012). The search for meaning in evolutionary goal-theory perspective. In P. T. Wong (Ed.), *The human quest for meaning: Theories, research, and applications* (pp. 23–55). New York: Routledge.
Kottorp, A., Bernspång, B., Fisher, A. G., & Bryze, K. A. (1995). IADL ability measured with the AMPS: Relation to two classification systems of mental retardation. *Scandinavian Journal of Occupational Therapy, 2*(3–4), 121–128.
Krupa, T., McLean, H., Eastabrook, S., Bonham, A., & Baksh, L. (2003). Daily time use as a measure of community adjustment for persons served by assertive community treatment teams. *American Journal of Occupational Therapy, 57*, 558–565.
Krystal, A. D., Thakur, M., & Roth, T. (2008). Sleep disturbance in psychiatric disorders: Effects on function and quality of life in mood disorders, alcoholism, and schizophrenia. *Annals of Clinical Psychiatry, 20*, 39–46.
Kukla, M., Lysaker, P. H., & Roe, D. (2014). Strong subjective recovery as a protective factor against the effects of positive symptoms on quality of life outcomes in schizophrenia. *Comprehensive Psychiatry, 55*, 1363–1368.
Larson, E. A. (2004). The time of our lives: The experience of temporality in occupation. *Canadian Journal of Occupational Therapy, 71*, 24–35.
Law, M., Cooper, B., Strong, S., Stewart, D., Rigby, P., & Letts, L. (1996). The person-environment-occupation model: A transactive approach to occupational performance. *Canadian Journal of Occupational Therapy, 63*, 9–23.
Le Boutillier, C., Leamy, M., Bird, V. J., Davidson, L., Williams, J., & Slade, M. (2011). What does recovery mean in practice? A qualitative analysis of international recovery-oriented practice guidance. *Psychiatric Services, 62*, 1470–1476.
Leamy, M., Bird, V., Le Boutillier, C., Williams, J., & Slade, M. (2011). Conceptual framework for personal recovery in mental health: Systematic review and narrative synthesis. *The British Journal of Psychiatry, 199*, 445–452.
Lee, K., Bhaker, R. S., Mysore, A., Parks, R. W., Birkett, P. B., & Woodruff, P. W. (2009). Time perception and its neuropsychological correlates in patients with

schizophrenia and in healthy volunteers. *Psychiatry Research, 166*, 174–183.

Legault, E., & Rebeiro, K. L. (2001). Occupation as means to mental health: A single-case study. *American Journal of Occupational Therapy, 55*, 90–96.

Leonardelli, C. A. (1988). *The Milwaukee evaluation of daily living skills: Evaluation in long-term psychiatric care*. Thorofare, NJ: Slack Incorporated.

Letendre, R. (1997). The everyday experience of psychiatric hospitalization: The users' viewpoint. *The International Journal of Social Psychiatry, 43*, 285–297.

Leufstadius, C., Erlandsson, L., Björkman, T., & Eklund, M. (2008). Meaningfulness in daily occupations among individuals with persistent mental illness. *Journal of Occupational Science, 15*, 27–35.

Liberman, R. P., Glynn, S., Blair, K. E., Ross, D., & Marder, S. R. (2002). In vivo amplified skills training: Promoting generalization of independent living skills for clients with schizophrenia. *Psychiatry, 65*, 137–155.

Liberman, R. P., & Kopelowicz, A. (2005). Recovery from schizophrenia: A criterion-based definition. In R. O. Ralph & P. Corrigan (Eds.), *Recovery in mental illness: Broadening our understanding of wellness* (pp. 101–129). Washington, DC: American Psychological Association.

Liberman, R. P., Mueser, K. T., Wallace, C. J., Jacobs, H. E., Eckman, T., & Massel, H. K. (1986). Training skills in the psychiatrically disabled: Learning coping and competence. *Schizophrenia Bulletin, 12*, 631–647.

Liberman, R. P., Wallace, C., Blackwell, G., Eckman, T., Vaccaro, J., & Kuehnel, T. (1993). Innovations in skills training for the seriously mentally ill: The UCLA social and independent living skills modules. *Innovations and Research, 2*, 43–59.

Liberman, R. P., Wallace, C. J., Blackwell, G., Kopelowicz, A., Vaccaro, J. V., & Mintz, J. (1998). Skills training versus psychosocial occupational therapy for persons with persistent schizophrenia. *American Journal of Psychiatry, 155*, 1087–1091.

Liebling, A. (1993). Suicides in young prisoners: A summary. *Death Studies, 17*, 381–407.

Lipskaya-Velikovsky, L., Bar-Shalita, T., & Bart, O. (2015). Sensory modulation and daily-life participation in people with schizophrenia. *Comprehensive Psychiatry, 58*, 130–137.

Lloyd, C., King, R., & Machingura, T. (2014). An investigation into the effectiveness of sensory modulation in reducing seclusion within an acute mental health unit. *Advances in Mental Health, 12*, 93–100.

Lloyd, C., King, R., McCarthy, M., & Scanlan, M. (2007). The association between leisure motivation and recovery: A pilot study. *Australian Occupational Therapy Journal, 54*, 33–41.

Lloyd, C., King, R., & Moore, L. (2010). Subjective and objective indicators of recovery in severe mental illness: A cross-sectional study. *The International Journal of Social Psychiatry, 56*, 220–229.

Ludwig, F. M. (2004). Occupation-based and occupation-centered perspectives. In K. Walker & F. M. Ludwig (Eds.), *Perspectives on theory for the practice of occupational therapy* (pp. 373–442). Austin, TX: Pro Ed.

Manoach, D. S., & Stickgold, R. (2009). Does abnormal sleep impair memory consolidation in schizophrenia? *Frontiers in Human Neuroscience, 3*, 21.

Martin, B., Wittmann, M., Franck, N., Cermolacce, M., Berna, F., & Giersch, A. (2014). Temporal structure of consciousness and minimal self in schizophrenia. *Frontiers in Psychology, 5*, 1175.

Martin, J. L., Jeste, D. V., & Ancoli-Israel, S. (2005). Older schizophrenia patients have more disrupted sleep and circadian rhythms than age-matched comparison subjects. *Journal of Psychiatric Research, 39*, 251–259.

Martin, J., Jeste, D. V., Caliguiri, M. P., Patterson, T., Heaton, R., & Ancoli-Israel, S. (2001). Actigraphic estimates of circadian rhythms and sleep/wake in older schizophrenia patients. *Schizophrenia Research, 47*, 77–86.

Marwaha, S., & Johnson, S. (2005). Views and experiences of employment among people with psychosis: A qualitative descriptive study. *The International Journal of Social Psychiatry, 51*, 302–316.

Matuska, K. M. (2012). Validity evidence of a model and measure of life balance. *OTJR: OccupationParticipation and Health, 32*, 229–237.

Matuska, K. M., & Christiansen, C. H. (2008). A proposed model of lifestyle balance. *Journal of Occupational Science, 15*, 9–19.

McColl, M. A., Law, M., Baptiste, S., Pollock, N., Carswell, A., & Polatajko, H. J. (2005). Targeted applications of the Canadian occupational performance measure. *Canadian Journal of Occupational Therapy, 72*, 298–300.

McCormick, B. P., Snethen, G., Smith, R. L., & Lysaker, P. H. (2012). Active leisure in the emotional experience of people with schizophrenia. *Therapeutic Recreation Journal, 46*, 179–190.

McElroy, S. L., Allison, D. B., & Bray, G. A. (2006). *Obesity and mental disorders*. Boca Raton, FL: CRC Press.

McGregor, I., & Little, B. R. (1998). Personal projects, happiness, and meaning: On doing well and being yourself. *Journal of Personality and Social Psychology, 74*, 494–512.

Merritt, B. K. (2011). Validity of using the assessment of motor and process skills to determine the need for assistance. *American Journal of Occupational Therapy, 65*, 643–650.

Meyer, A. (1922). The philosophy of occupation therapy. *Archives of Occupational Therapy, 1*, 1–10.

Molineux, M. L., & Whiteford, G. E. (1999). Prisons: From occupational deprivation to occupational enrichment. *Journal of Occupational Science, 6*, 124–130.
Moll, S. E., Gewurtz, R. E., Krupa, T. M., Law, M. C., Larivière, N., & Levasseur, M. (2015). "Do-live-well" A canadian framework for promoting occupation, health, and well-being. *Canadian Journal of Occupational Therapy, 82*, 9–23.
Mueser, K. T., Goodman, L. B., Trumbetta, S. L., Rosenberg, S. D., Osher, F. C., Vidaver, R., et al. (1998). Trauma and posttraumatic stress disorder in severe mental illness. *Journal of Consulting and Clinical Psychology, 66*(3), 493–499.
Myin-Germeys, I., Nicolson, N., & Delespaul, P. A. (2001). The context of delusional experiences in the daily life of patients with schizophrenia. *Psychological Medicine, 31*(03), 489–498.
Nan Stromberg, M. (2004). Sensory approaches in inpatient psychiatric settings: Innovative alternatives to seclusion and restraint. *Journal of Psychosocial Nursing and Mental Health Services, 42*(9), 34.
Neville, A., Kreisberg, A., & Kielhofner, G. (1985). Temporal dysfunction in schizophrenia. *Occupational Therapy in Mental Health, 5*, 1–19.
Nix, G. A., Ryan, R. M., Manly, J. B., & Deci, E. L. (1999). Revitalization through self-regulation: The effects of autonomous and controlled motivation on happiness and vitality. *Journal of Experimental Social Psychology, 35*, 266–284.
Noordsy, D., Torrey, W., Mueser, K., Mead, S., O'Keefe, C., & Fox, L. (2002). Recovery from severe mental illness: An intrapersonal and functional outcome definition. *International Review of Psychiatry, 14*, 318–326.
Osmond, H. (1957). Function as the basis of psychiatric ward design. *Psychiatric Services, 8*(4), 23–27.
Peloquin, S. M. (1995). The fullness of empathy: Reflections and illustrations. *American Journal of Occupational Therapy, 49*, 24–31.
Pentland, W., & McColl, M. A. (2008). Occupational integrity: Another perspective on "life balance". *Canadian Journal of Occupational Therapy, 75*(3), 135–138.
Persson, D., Erlandsson, L., Eklund, M., & Iwarsson, S. (2001). Value dimensions, meaning, and complexity in human occupation-a tentative structure for analysis. *Scandinavian Journal of Occupational Therapy, 8*, 7–18.
Peterburs, J., Nitsch, A. M., Miltner, W., & Straube, T. (2013). Impaired representation of time in schizophrenia is linked to positive symptoms and cognitive demand. *PLoS ONE, 8*(6), e67615.
Pettie, D., & Triolo, A. M. (1999). Illness as evolution: The search for identity and meaning in the recovery process. *Psychiatric Rehabilitation Journal, 22*(3), 255–262.
Pieris, Y., & Craik, C. (2004). Factors enabling and hindering participation in leisure for people with mental health problems. *The British Journal of Occupational Therapy, 67*, 240–247.
Pilling, S., Bebbington, P., Kuipers, E., Garety, P., Geddes, J., Martindale, B., et al. (2002). Psychological treatments in schizophrenia: II. Meta-analyses of randomized controlled trials of social skills training and cognitive remediation. *Psychological Medicine, 32*, 783–791.
Polatajko, H., Townsend, E., & Craik, J. (2007). Canadian model of occupational performance and engagement (CMOP-E). In E. A. Townsend & H. J. Polatajko (Eds.), *Enabling occupation II: Advancing an occupational therapy vision for health, well-being, and justice through occupation* (p. 23). Ottawa, Canada: CAOT Publications.
Polkinghorne, D. E. (1996). Transformative narratives: From victimic to agentic life plots. *American Journal of Occupational Therapy, 50*, 299–305.
Pörn, I. (1993). Health and adaptedness. *Theoretical Medicine, 14*, 295–303.
Punwar, A. J., & Peloquin, S. M. (2000). *Occupational therapy: Principles and practice*. Baltimore, MD: Lippincott Williams & Wilkins.
Quirk, A., & Lelliott, P. (2001). What do we know about life on acute psychiatric wards in the UK? A review of the research evidence. *Social Science and Medicine, 53*, 1565–1574.
Quirk, A., Lelliott, P., & Seale, C. (2006). The permeable institution: An ethnographic study of three acute psychiatric wards in london. *Social Science and Medicine, 63*(8), 2105–2117.
Rebeiro, K. L., & Cook, J. V. (1999). Opportunity, not prescription: An exploratory study of the experience of occupational engagement. *Canadian Journal of Occupational Therapy, 66*(4), 176–187.
Reilly, M. (1962). Occupational therapy can be one of the great ideas of 20th century medicine. *The American Journal of Occupational Therapy, 16*, 1–9.
Reker, G. T., & Wong, P. P. (1988). Aging as an individual process: Toward a theory of personal meaning. In J. E. Birren & V. L. Bengston (Eds.), *Emergent theories of aging* (pp. 214–246). New York, NY: Springer.
Robinson, K., Kennedy, N., & Harmon, D. (2012). Happiness: A review of evidence relevant to occupational science. *Journal of Occupational Science, 19*, 150–164.
Roley, S. S., DeLany, J. V., Barrows, C. J., Brownrigg, S., Honaker, D., Sava, D. I., et al. (2008). Occupational therapy practice framework: Domain and process. *The American Journal of Occupational Therapy, 62*, 625–683.
Rose, A. (1999). Spirituality and palliative care: The attitudes of occupational therapists. *The British Journal of Occupational Therapy, 62*, 307–312.
Rosen, A., Hadzi-Pavlovic, D., & Parker, G. (1989). The life skills profile: A measure assessing function and disability in schizophrenia. *Schizophrenia Bulletin, 15*, 325–337.
Rudnick, A. (2002). The goals of psychiatric rehabilitation: An ethical analysis. *Psychiatric Rehabilitation Journal, 25*, 310–313.

Rüesch, P., Graf, J., Meyer, P., Rössler, W., & Hell, D. (2004). Occupation, social support and quality of life in persons with schizophrenic or affective disorders. *Social Psychiatry and Psychiatric Epidemiology, 39*, 686–694.

Ryan, R. M., & Deci, E. L. (2001). On happiness and human potentials: A review of research on hedonic and eudaimonic well-being. *Annual Review of Psychology, 52*, 141–166.

Ryan, R. M., LaGuardia, J. G., & Rawsthorne, L. J. (2005). Self-complexity and the authenticity of self-aspects: Effects on well being and resilience to stressful events. *North American Journal of Psychology, 7*, 431–448.

Ryff, C. D., & Singer, B. (1998). The contours of positive human health. *Psychological Inquiry, 9*, 1–28.

Ryff, C. D., Singer, B. H., & Love, G. D. (2004). Positive health: Connecting well-being with biology. *Philosophical Transactions-Royal Society of London Series B, Biological Sciences, 359*, 1383–1394.

SAMHSA. (2011). Consensus definition of recovery in behavioral health. http://blog.samhsa.gov/2011/12/22/samhsa%E2%80%99s-definition-and-guiding-principles-of-recovery. Accessed February 1, 2015.

Sanders, M. J., & Van Oss, T. (2013). Using daily routines to promote medication adherence in older adults. *American Journal of Occupational Therapy, 67*, 91–99.

Scanlan, J. N., & Novak, T. (2015). Sensory approaches in mental health: A scoping review. *Australian Occupational Therapy Journal, 62*, 277–285.

Selye, H. (1976). *Stress without distress*. New York: Springer.

Shattell, M. M., Andes, M., & Thomas, S. P. (2008). How patients and nurses experience the acute care psychiatric environment. *Nursing Inquiry, 15*, 242–250.

Sheldon, K. M., Cummins, R., & Kamble, S. (2010). Life balance and well-being: Testing a novel conceptual and measurement approach. *Journal of Personality, 78*, 1093–1134.

Sheldon, K. M., & Elliot, A. J. (1999). Goal striving, need satisfaction, and longitudinal well-being: The self-concordance model. *Journal of Personality and Social Psychology, 76*, 482–497.

Sheldon, K. M., & Kasser, T. (1998). Pursuing personal goals: Skills enable progress, but not all progress is beneficial. *Personality and Social Psychology Bulletin, 24*, 1319–1331.

Sheldon, K. M., Ryan, R. M., Deci, E. L., & Kasser, T. (2004). The independent effects of goal contents and motives on well-being: It's both what you pursue and why you pursue it. *Personality and Social Psychology Bulletin, 30*, 475–486.

Shumaker, S. A., & Reizenstein, J. E. (1982). Environmental factors affecting inpatient stress in acute care hospitals. In G. Evans (Ed.), *Environmental stress* (pp. 179–223). Cambridge, UK: Cambridge University Press.

Simpson, A., Bowers, L., Alexander, J., Ridley, C., & Warren, J. (2005). Occupational therapy and multidisciplinary working on acute psychiatric wards: The Tompkins acute ward study. *The British Journal of Occupational Therapy, 68*, 545–552.

Smith, S., & Suto, M. J. (2012). Religious and/or spiritual practices: Extending spiritual freedom to people with schizophrenia. *Canadian Journal of Occupational Therapy, 79*(2), 77–85.

Stadnyk, R. L., Townsend, E. A., & Wilcock, A. A. (2010). Occupational justice. In C. H. Christiansen & E. A. Townsend (Eds.), *Introduction to occupation: The art and science of living* (pp. 329–358). Upper Saddle River, NJ: Pearson.

Steger, M. F., Kashdan, T. B., & Oishi, S. (2008). Being good by doing good: Daily eudaimonic activity and well-being. *Journal of Research in Personality, 42*, 22–42.

Stolovy, T., Lev-Wiesel, R., Doron, A., & Gelkopf, M. (2009). The meaning in life for hospitalized patients with schizophrenia. *The Journal of Nervous and Mental Disease, 197*, 133–135.

Suto, M., & Frank, G. (1994). Future time perspective and daily occupations of persons with chronic schizophrenia in a board and care home. *American Journal of Occupational Therapy, 48*, 7–18.

Sutton, D. J., Hocking, C. S., & Smythe, L. A. (2012). A phenomenological study of occupational engagement in recovery from mental illness. *Canadian Journal of Occupational Therapy, 79*, 142–150.

Sutton, D., Wilson, M., Van Kessel, K., & Vanderpyl, J. (2013). Optimizing arousal to manage aggression: A pilot study of sensory modulation. *International Journal of Mental Health Nursing, 22*, 500–511.

Sylvia, L. G., Alloy, L. B., Hafner, J. A., Gauger, M. C., Verdon, K., & Abramson, L. Y. (2009). Life events and social rhythms in bipolar spectrum disorders: A prospective study. *Behavior Therapy, 40*, 131–141.

Thibeault, R., & Blackmer, E. (1987). Validating a test of functional performance with psychiatric patients. *American Journal of Occupational Therapy, 41*, 515–521.

Thomson, L. K. (1992). *The Kohlman evaluation of living skills*. Rockville, MD: American Occupational Therapy Association.

Timko, C. (1996). Physical characteristics of residential psychiatric and substance abuse programs: Organizational determinants and patient outcomes. *American Journal of Community Psychology, 24*, 173–192.

Tryssenaar, J., Jones, E. J., & Lee, D. (1999). Occupational performance needs of a shelter population. *Canadian Journal of Occupational Therapy, 66*, 188–196.

Tysk, L. (1984). A longitudinal study of time estimation in psychotic disorders. *Perceptual and Motor Skills, 59*, 779–789.

Ulrich, R. S., Simons, R. F., Losito, B. D., Fiorito, E., Miles, M. A., & Zelson, M. (1991). Stress recovery during exposure to natural and urban environments. *Journal of Environmental Psychology, 11*, 201–230.

Ulrich, R. S., Simons, R. F., & Miles, M. A. (2003). Effects of environmental simulations and television on

blood donor stress. *Journal of Architectural and Planning Research, 20*, 38–47.
Useem, B. (1985). Disorganization and the New Mexico prison riot of 1980. *American Sociological Review, 50*, 677–688.
van der Kolk, B. A., Roth, S., Pelcovitz, D., Sunday, S., & Spinazzola, J. (2005). Disorders of extreme stress: The empirical foundation of a complex adaptation to trauma. *Journal of Traumatic Stress, 18*, 389–399.
van Niekerk, L. (2009). Participation in work: A source of wellness for people with psychiatric disability. *Work, 32*, 455–465.
Versluys, H. P. (1980). The remediation of role disorders through focused group work. *American Journal of Occupational Therapy, 34*, 609–614.
Wade, A. G. (2006). Sleep problems in depression: How do they impact treatment and recovery? *International Journal of Psychiatry in Clinical Practice, 10*(supl), 38–44.
Wagman, P., Håkansson, C., & Björklund, A. (2012). Occupational balance as used in occupational therapy: A concept analysis. *Scandinavian Journal of Occupational Therapy, 19*, 322–327.
Walker, K. F., & Ludwig, F. M. (2004). *Perspectives on theory for the practice of occupational therapy* (3rd ed.). Austin, TX: Pro Ed.
Wallace, C., Liberman, R., MacKain, S., Eckman, T., & Blackwell, G. (1992). The effectiveness and replicability of modules to train social and independent living skills. *American Journal of Psychiatry, 149*, 654–658.
Waters, D. (1995). Recovering from a depressive episode using the Canadian occupational performance measure. *Canadian Journal of Occupational Therapy, 62*, 278–282.
Weeder, T. C. (1986). Comparison of temporal patterns and meaningfulness of the daily activities of schizophrenic and normal adults. *Occupational Therapy in Mental Health, 6*(4), 27–48.
Whiteford, G. (1997). Occupational deprivation and incarceration. *Journal of Occupational Science, 4*(3), 126–130.
Wilcock, A. A. (1993). A theory of the human need for occupation. *Journal of Occupational Science, 1*, 17–24.
Wilcock, A. A. (2003). Occupational science: The study of humans as occupational beings. In P. Kramer, J. Hinojosa, & C. Royeen (Eds.), *Perspectives in human occupation: Participation in life* (pp. 156–180). Philadelphia, PA: Lippincott Williams & Wilkins.
Wilcock, A. A. (2007). Occupation and health: Are they one and the same? *Journal of Occupational Science, 14*, 3–8.
Wilcock, A. A., Van Der Arend, H., Darling, K., Scholz, J., Siddall, R., Snigg, C., et al. (1998). An exploratory study of people's perceptions and experiences of wellbeing. *The British Journal of Occupational Therapy, 61*(2), 75–82.
Woodside, H., Schell, L., & Allison-Hedges, J. (2006). Listening for recovery: The vocational success of people living with mental illness. *Canadian Journal of Occupational Therapy, 73*, 36–43.
World Health Organization. (2004). *Promoting mental health: concepts, emerging evidence, practice*. Geneva: Author.
Wulff, K., Dijk, D. J., Middleton, B., Foster, R. G., & Joyce, E. M. (2012). Sleep and circadian rhythm disruption in schizophrenia. *The British Journal of Psychiatry, 200*, 308–316.
Wulff, K., Porcheret, K., Cussans, E., & Foster, R. G. (2009). Sleep and circadian rhythm disturbances: Multiple genes and multiple phenotypes. *Current Opinion in Genetics & Development, 19*, 237–246.
Yalmambirra. (2000). Black time… white time: My time… your time. *Journal of Occupational Science, 7*, 133–137.
Yerxa, E. J. (1992). Some implications of occupational therapy's history for its epistemology, values, and relation to medicine. *American Journal of Occupational Therapy, 46*, 79–83.
Yerxa, E. J. (1993). Occupational science: A new source of power for participants in occupational therapy. *Journal of Occupational Science, 1*, 3–9.
Yerxa, E. J. (1998). Health and the human spirit for occupation. *American Journal of Occupational Therapy, 52*, 412–418.
Yerxa, E. J. (2000). Occupational science: A renaissance of service to humankind through knowledge. *Occupational Therapy International, 7*, 87–98.
Yerxa, E. J. (2002). Habits in context: A synthesis, with implications for research in occupational science. *OTJR: Occupation, Participation and Health, 22*(1 suppl.), 104S–110S.
Zahorik, P., & Jenison, R. L. (1998). Presence as being-in-the-world. *Presence, 7*, 78–89.

# Peer Support Services

# 13

Michael Franczak and Christina Dye

## Introduction

Few public institutions are as stereotyped—and even stigmatized—as state psychiatric inpatient hospitals. In movies, print media and the minds of the general public, psychiatric hospitals are viewed as institutions of hopelessness and a one-way ticket to a lifelong journey through mental illness. Individuals and families who have experienced an episode of care in an inpatient psychiatric ward often view their stay as life-saving, however, few are willing to speak about their experience due to the social stigma that continues to follow most people living with serious mental illnesses. Psychiatric hospitals in many ways are the public image of mental illness —tall, dark, and foreboding with barred windows and locked doors.

Surprisingly, to some observers, a quiet revolution has been spreading behind those windows and doors. Rehabilitation and recovery is beginning to replace confinement and control as common descriptors of the state hospital experience. Spurred by improvements in psychiatric medications and therapies over the past dozen years, and emerging best practices in transitions of care between inpatient facilities and community settings, hospital administrators are increasingly testing practices more fully grounded in self-determination, person-centered care and family involvement—practices that are now considered the gold standard of the mental health system.

Among the most interesting and best studied is the introduction of peer and family support services within the inpatient hospital environment. Peer support services are delivered by individuals with their own lived experience of mental health conditions. Peer services are a natural companion to the recovery movement as both are based on similar values and principles. Although peer support services have been offered in community-based mental health agencies and self-help associations for many years, the formal appearance of peer-delivered service programs in hospital settings is a relatively recent development. However, remarkable case studies of positive outcomes attributed to inpatient peer services have accumulated in a very brief period of time, including evidence of reductions in 30-day readmission rates, shorter lengths of stay and improvements in hospital staff attitudes and conduct toward clients.

At the same time the implementation of peer-delivered service programs in the very formal and structured inpatient environment has not been without challenges. Most notably, the

M. Franczak (✉)
Marc Community Resources, 924 Country Club Drive, Mesa, AZ 85201, USA
e-mail: Michael.franczak@marccr.com

C. Dye
Partners in Recovery, 924 Country Club Drive, Mesa, AZ 85201, USA



N.N. Singh et al. (eds.), *Handbook of Recovery in Inpatient Psychiatry*,
Evidence-Based Practices in Behavioral Health, DOI 10.1007/978-3-319-40537-7_13

"medical model" approach to psychiatric care that has historically exemplified the inpatient environment stands in contrast to the emphasis on person/family involvement, voice, and choice that is the hallmark of the mental health recovery movement, posing a natural tension, and resistance to change within the institutional setting. In addition, hospitals are increasingly subject to payer goals for lower costs through briefer lengths of stay and improved transitions to community services—pressures that force a reconfiguration of the clinical workflow and staffing model within psychiatric hospitals. Still, many hospitals have made notable efforts to introduce stronger person-centered and recovery-focused programming, including the introduction of person's with their own lived experience of mental health challenges as a key part of the clinical workforce.

This chapter describes the emergence and impact of peer support services and their role in supporting rehabilitation and recovery outcomes in inpatient psychiatric hospitals. Along the way, peer-delivered services are helping transform the culture of traditional mental health care—and the stigma that accompanies it—within those psychiatric institutions.

## Person-Centered Versus Institution Centered Care

While the intended purpose of inpatient psychiatric hospitalization is to secure the safety of the person and the public while medication and other treatments address the symptoms that precipitated the hospitalization, paradoxically for most individuals and their families, an episode of involuntary psychiatric hospitalization is a stressful, if not fundamentally traumatic experience. For some individuals, it may be their only experience with psychiatric hospital, while for others repeated involuntary hospitalization will be a lifelong, recurring theme. Due to the congregate nature of institutional settings, hospitals are highly regimented and require the person to obey set operating rules and protocols such as bedtime, wake up, meal time, medication administration time, phone calls and daily therapies. In this setting, loss of personal freedom limits the opportunity for the person to make any independent decisions. Even with the best intent, many of these practices are extremely difficult to change in order that the institution can safely and efficiently manage several hundred to several thousand inpatient residents each day.

The standard treatment planning process is a good example and an area where the value of adding peer- and family-delivered services has demonstrated immediate positive results. In many hospitals, treatment planning sessions are held with the hospital professional team who make all of the decisions and then invite the person to attend for a few moments at the end of the staffing without giving them any input into the decisions that were made. Another example involves scheduling treatment planning sessions on days or times in which active family members are not available to participate and then discharging the person to the family without any information regarding how they can assist in caring for their family member. Although unintentional, these "standard operating procedures" tend to de-value the person's and family member's own experience of their mental health symptoms, the supports that work for them and how they feel and function when they are well. One of the major themes of the recovery and peer movements is "Nothing about us without us." The treatment planning scenarios above are efficient and expedient for hospital operations, but they are not person-centered or recovery-oriented.

Traditional psychiatric inpatient hospitals generally operate under a "medical model" of care where the team is led by a psychiatrist who is assisted by psychiatric nurses, psychologists, social workers, and direct care staff. The psychiatrist conducts a psychiatric assessment designed to identify a diagnosis that leads to a treatment formulation that guides the team in medication management and other treatment modalities. Other disciples also conduct their specialty assessments and ideally this information is used to create an integrated individual treatment plan. Standards also require that the team develop a discharge plan that identifies the discharge criteria that the person needs to meet in order to leave the hospital setting. The standards require that discharge planning begin upon admission. More forward-thinking hospital settings have been working on developing a psychiatric rehabilitation model that includes the consideration of biological, psychological, and social factors (biopsychosocial model) in order to develop a more holistic approach to care. In this approach, the "medical model" is less evident and the treatment team usually includes the person and family members as well as a variety of professionals and in some cases peer support staff. Many hospitals are in the process of implementing this model and some have succeeded; however, the transformation is a long and challenging process and requires strong administrative support and clinical leadership.

A newer development within inpatient settings is the gradual tightening of length of time a person remains in the hospital. Cost containment goals by payers, enhancements in psychotropic medications, and increased availability of alternative pre-hospital crisis settings have significantly reduced the average length of inpatient stay over time. While this trend has the benefit of not removing the person from the community for extended periods of time, it also requires the inpatient team to act swiftly to assess, diagnose, develop a plan of care, and a discharge plan all typically within 14 days or less. Conducting comprehensive assessments, engaging the person in treatment, and working with the person's natural and professional community supports are put on an accelerated time frame that itself may limit opportunities for person and family involvement in developing the plan of care.

Person-centered care requires the person and their families become active participants in the treatment planning process. As stated earlier, many inpatient hospitals have attempted to implement a person-centered approach with varying degrees of success. The migration and transformation from a "medical model" to a "person-centered' model represents a huge cultural shift for most hospitals. Even with the best intent of the hospital, one of the major challenges is that many individuals who are admitted are significantly impaired and are unable or unwilling to actively participate in their treatment planning process. At the same time, family members are often extremely stressed and have little information on psychiatric symptoms and medications except what they have seen in the media. They also have limited or no information on other aspects of care or the community resources that are available upon discharge. A number of individuals demonstrate what Amador (2000) identified as "Anosognosia," or a lack of insight into their illness. Many individuals with this condition refuse all forms of treatment. Other individuals arrive with unstable living arrangements, homelessness, criminal justice involvement, or orders of protection. Developing an adequate discharge plan involves services beyond the typical scope of a hospital setting.

## System Transformation and Peer Support Services

Hospitals are not alone in struggling to address these forces of change. The transformation of traditional mental health system to a person-centered and recovery-oriented approach represents an international challenge. The World Health Organization's (WHO) Quality Rights Tool Kit (2012, p. 1) identified that "in many countries, the quality of care in both inpatient and outpatient facilities is poor or even harmful and can actively hinder recovery. The treatment provided is often intended to keep people and their conditions under control rather than to enhance their autonomy and improve their quality of life. People are seen as 'objects of treatment' rather than human beings with the same rights and entitlements as everybody else. They are not consulted on their care or recovery plans, in many cases receiving treatment against their wishes." While conditions have certainly improved in many developed countries, there is still a long way to go to fulfill the mission of a system that is person-centered and recovery-oriented. Fortunately, there are numerous research findings and evidence-based practices that can serve as a guide to the transformation efforts. An ongoing issue is that the incorporation and translation of research findings to clinical practice continues to be at a very slow pace.

Leamy et al. (2011) identified that orienting mental health services towards recovery will require a system transformation where professionals will need to understand that recovery is a unique personal experience rather than something a system does to the person. Creating a person-centered, recovery-oriented approach to health care requires professional staff to recognize the personal wisdom and experience that the person and their families bring to the table. In addition, the person has the right to self-determination, which includes the right to make informed decisions regarding their care and treatment. It also makes good clinical sense that when the person participates in treatment decisions with support from the professional team, it increases the likelihood that the plan will be followed.

Corrigan (2006) described self-determination as having the freedom to choose the medications and treatment activities they believe will be helpful, regardless of professional recommendations. To date, the evidence that self-determination or informed decision-making is embraced within today's healthcare system is not encouraging. Braddock et al. (1999) audiotaped 1097 encounters with physicians where 3552 clinical decisions were made. Only 9 % of decisions met their definition of completeness for informed decision-making which included the person. Basic decisions were completely informed in only 17.2 % of the cases, no intermediate decisions were completely informed, and only 1 (0.5 %) complex decision was completely informed. An assessment of the person's understanding of the decision was only made in 1.5 % of the observations.

Others have also noted the importance of the person in the decision-making process. Deegan and Drake (2006) as part of medication management and Salyers and Tsemberis (2007) as part of ACT Team protocols have identified the importance of shared decision-making as critical aspect of a person-centered, recovery-oriented approach to care. Shared decision-making is not simply a rights issue, but also critical factor in whether the person and their families or other natural supports will understand and follow the treatment plan when they leave the inpatient setting.

The emergence of formal mental health peer support services and programs over the past 15 years has been a key driver of these changes both within inpatient institutions and community mental health settings. Many states added formal peer support services over the past 20 years as a component of their comprehensive mental health and substance use service delivery system. A significant boost to the development of such programs occurred in 2006 when the Center for Medicaid and Medicare Services authorized the use of peer support service as a reimbursable Medicaid service. The resulting expansion of peer support services throughout the country has been impressive. Today most states have an active consumer movements and peer support programs. Internationally, Canada, Scotland, Australia, and New Zealand all have very active peer support initiatives.

Inpatient facilities; however, significantly lagged in adopting these practices. Oddly, peer support has been occurring naturally in inpatient treatment settings since these settings first existed. Bouchard et al. (2010) studied naturally occurring "peer support" in inpatient psychiatric units. They reported that natural peer support is a thoughtful process that involves observing, reflecting, taking supportive action, and evaluating outcomes. Supportive actions include helping with activities of daily living, sharing material goods, providing information and advice, sharing a social life, and offering emotional support. While hospital staff meticulously documented these developments as "positive social interaction" between patients and evidence of progress, they also serve as an early example of what would eventually be formalized as peer support services. Thus, while peer support has occurred naturally in hospital settings over many years, it has taken considerable time for their clinical value to be recognized and organized into an intentional program of services founded on supportive action.

## The Double Revolution: Recovery Movement and Peer Services

In order to understand the emergence of peer support services it is necessary to take a brief excursion into its roots within the recovery movement. The consumer/survivor movement can be traced to 1800s in England where the Alleged Lunatic's Friend Society was established. There were numerous other initiatives over time that developed primarily due to what was perceived as cruel conditions and the lack of the ability of individuals to control any of their care in mental health facilities. In 1908, Clifford Beers wrote an autobiography "A Mind That Found Itself," which led to the creation of the National Committee for Mental Hygiene, known today as Mental Health America. Chamberlin (1978) wrote *On Our Own: Patient Controlled Alternatives to the Mental Health System,* which became the textbook of the consumer/survivors movement. There are many excellent reviews of the consumer movement that go beyond the intended scope of this chapter. Nelson and colleagues conducted some of the most comprehensive reviews of the history of the consumer/survivor movement (Janzen et al. 2006; Nelson et al. 2006a, b, d, 2007). Another excellent review of this information that includes the psychiatric rehabilitation initiative can be found in Corrigan et al. (2008).

In support of the consumer/survivor movement, the U.S. Center for Mental Health Services began funding consumer initiatives and technical assistance centers in the 1980s. While these programs were initially developed to increase consumer voice in the mental health service system, a secondary benefit emerged. By bringing consumers together in forums and on committees, they also created collaborations that resulted in the emergence of a number of consumer-run programs. At this point, many states began creating Offices of Consumer Affairs that often reported directly to the Mental Health Commissioner. These Offices created a variety of opportunities for consumers to become involved in the state planning efforts, including advocating for the addition of more peer self-help support programs to the service array. The expansion resulted in the development of consumer drop-in centers, warm lines, and state supported consumer advisory boards across the country.

Also in the 1980s, a number of studies began to be published that demonstrated that individuals could lead fulfilling lives even with the presence of a serious mental illness. In other words, mental illness was a treatable condition, not a life sentence. The "recovery movement" was launched. On average, research has shown that 60 % of the individuals who were studied had recovered to the point of leading successful lives in their communities with minimal psychiatric symptoms (World Health Organization 1979). One of the most significant studies was a 30-year follow-up of individuals who had long-term hospitalizations in state hospitals in Vermont and Maine in the 1950s (Harding et al. 1987). The Vermont community mental health system at that time was considered to be recovery-oriented, at least as it was understood at the time, and the Maine system was considered traditional care. Using established criteria for "recovery," including having a social life indistinguishable from your neighbor, holding a job for pay or volunteering, no longer experiencing symptoms of mental illness, and no longer taking medication, Harding et al. made a memorable discovery: 63–68 % of individuals in the Vermont group met their criteria for "recovery." In the Maine group, which experienced "traditional" inpatient care, nearly half (47 %) achieved recovery as defined by the researchers. Since their study, numerous other researchers have confirmed Harding et al.'s findings that recovery is an individualized and naturally occurring process that is supported by, but not created by, the mental health treatment system.

The Harding et al. study and the others that followed proved that recovery from mental illness is possible and created the final spark that ignited the recovery movement and the peer support initiative. While many individuals achieve recovery without the assistance of peer support services, most individuals in recovery identify that a social connection with someone, a family member, friend, psychiatrist, or therapist, who believed in and supported them was a vital element in their recovery journey. The ability to provide social support appears to be one of the primary skills that peer support providers possess. Felton et al. (1995) found that individuals who were served by peer support staff reported improved social support, quality of life, a reduction in the number of major life problems, more frequent contact with their case managers and improved self-image. The availability of a social support network is often accompanied by improvements in multiple aspects of life. Hardiman and Segal (2003) examined the characteristics of peer support self-help agencies and concluded that they foster social networks leading to the experience of shared community. Peer staff provide support to the person when others are not available or not willing.

In 2010, the U.S. Substance Abuse Mental Health Service Administration (SAMHSA) launched a national dialogue to define "recovery." The final definition, shaped by advocates, care providers, families, and individuals with lived experience of recovery from mental disorders and/or substance use is as follows: "A process of change through which individuals improve their health and wellness, live a self-directed life, and strive to reach their full potential" (SAMHSA 2011, p. 1). SAMHSA (2012, p. 3) listed four dimensions of recovery: "(1) Health—Overcoming or managing one's disease(s) or symptoms—for example, abstaining from use of alcohol, illicit drugs, and non-prescribed medications if one has an addiction problem— and for everyone in recovery, making informed, healthy choices that support physical and emotional wellbeing, (2) Home—A stable and safe place to live, (3) Purpose—Meaningful daily activities, such as a job, school, volunteerism, family caretaking, or creative endeavors, and the independence, income and resources to participate in society, and (4) Community—Relationships and social networks that provide support, friendship, love, and hope." The four dimensions in many ways define the essence of peer support services and in multiple studies peer support has been found to be a major avenue for achieving the four dimensions of recovery.

## Peers, Professionals and the Power of Hope

A considerable amount of effort has been devoted to defining what peer support is and what it is not (Repper and Carter 2011). For example, Mead (2003) and Mead and MacNeil (2006) reminded us that peer support is not like clinical support, nor is it just about being friends. Peer support helps people to understand each other because they have been there, shared similar experiences, and can model for each other a willingness to learn and grow.

The President's New Freedom Commission on Mental Health (2003) laid the early foundation for formal peer service programs by emphasizing the strong link between hope and individual recovery, stating "research has validated that hope and self-determination are important factors contributing to recovery" (p.27). Years later, SAMHSA (2011) articulated more forcefully that hope can be intentionally instilled and inspired by caring friends, families and advocates, including peer providers. In their working definition of recovery, SAMHSA (2012, p. 4) stated: "Recovery emerges from hope. The belief that recovery is real provides the essential and motivating message of a better future—that people can and do overcome the internal and external challenges, barriers, and obstacles that confront them. Hope is internalized and can be fostered by peers, families, providers, allies, and others. Hope is the catalyst of the recovery process." Creating conditions that inspire hope is one of the most powerful skills that peers bring to the table. Campbell and Leaver (2003) stated that hope instilled in people recovering from mental illnesses through the dynamic exchange of peer support has the potential to foster hope and change for the mental health system.

Andresen et al. (2003) suggested that recovery comprises four key components: (1) finding and maintaining hope; (2) reestablishing a positive identity; (3) building a meaningful life, and (4) taking responsibility and control. Stratford et al. (2012) noted that recovery has hope as a keystone. Mental health practitioners have an important role in "holding the hope" for the person with mental illness, until that person is strong enough within themselves to move forward. Hope is not a boundless wish or desire; and in fact, has a probabilistic quality. We do not hope for things that are impossible. We hope for things that have some possibility of occurring. Hope looks for exemplars. Peers in recovery present a concrete exemplar. Clay (2005) reported that one of the qualities of peer support staff is that they act as role models and demonstrate that recovery is possible. If someone who has had similar experience with mental illness and now has achieved recovery, the possibility of recovery is not an unrealistic outcome. Hope is a critical motivator for what has been recently identified as "patient activation" which has been receiving significant attention in healthcare research.

SAMHSA (2009a, b, p. 10) commented further on the growing recognition of the value and role of peer providers in professional healthcare delivery, "In the medical world of today, there is scarcely a specialty where peer support is not recognized as a valuable adjunct to professional medical and social interventions. Improved outcomes are particularly notable when peer support services are provided to people with chronic conditions that require long-term self-management." In linking peer-delivered services with healthcare's new found focus on chronic disease management under the 2010 Affordable Care Act, SAMHSA (2009a, b) firmly cemented the role of peer providers as essential to healthcare of the future. Operating in a variety of new roles as "health navigators," "health coaches," and "transition specialists," peer support specialists today are leveraging the power of their personal experience to instill hope and produce real-world health outcomes that drive down costs and improve the patient experience of care—otherwise known as the Three Aims of the Affordable Care Act.

The "professionalization" of peer services through formal training, career paths and reimbursement is not without controversy. In many parts of the country, peer support is only believed to retain its "peerness" when supports are dissociated from formal mental health and addiction treatment programs. To add confusion, the growing world of children's mental health services brings with it a new type of "peer": family members of children with mental health and developmental disabilities who work with other family members experiencing challenges in navigating the system or obtaining family-centered care for their children. There is a substantial body of research on peer support and much less on family peer support. Gartner and Riessman (1982, p. 631) provided a succinct and yet complete definition of peer support: "Social emotional support, frequently coupled with instrumental support that is mutually offered or provided by persons having a mental health condition to others sharing a similar mental health condition to bring about a desired social or personal change." Family peer support could be similarly defined as social emotional support, frequently coupled with instrumental support that is offered or provided by family members to other families who share the experience of supporting a family member with a similar mental health condition to bring about a desired social or personal change.

The following core values have been recently ratified by peer supporters across the country as the core ethical guidelines for peer support practice (International Association of Peer Supporters, Inc. 2013): (1) peer support is voluntary; (2) peer supporters are hopeful; (3) peer supporters are open minded; (4) peer supporters are empathic; (5) peer supporters are respectful; (6) peer supporters facilitate change; (7) peer supporters are honest and direct; (8) peer support is mutual and reciprocal; (9) peer support is equally shared power; (10) peer support is strengths-focused; (11) peer support is transparent, and (12) peer support is person-driven.

## Outcomes of Peer Services

As with any large-scale system transformation, the introduction of peer professionals—people with their own lived experience as care-givers—sparked a veritable wave of research in studying the effects of this "disruptive innovation" on the outcomes of mental health care. Early work focused on the more obvious outcomes—the ability of peer support staff to engage individuals in their care simply because they shared the same story and experience and have "walked in their shoes." For example, Dixon et al. (1994) noted that peer staff members bring practical knowledge, street smarts, and personal experience with treatment that provide engagement skills. Davidson et al. (2006) reported that peer support workers were highly skilled and effective at engaging and communicating acceptance. They were able to increase treatment participation amongst the more disengaged in case management for consumers with comorbid mental health and alcohol and drug issues. Davidson et al. (2012) wrote that peer staff could be especially effective in engaging people into care and acting as a bridge between clients and other staff.

However to describe the value of peer services as merely the ability of peer staff to share stories and experiences is to seriously under-estimate the value of engagement within the mental healthcare system. With no-show rates hovering between 20-50 % on average at treatment facilities across the country, failure of patients to attend scheduled psychiatric appointments costs millions each year in wasted staff time while increasing the likelihood that the person will not maintain treatment gains and/or be re-hospitalized at 6- to 12-month follow-up (Schmutte et al. 2009; Sledge et al. 2008). Similar studies found that the addition of peer services early in treatment improved patient engagement with non-peer staff as well. For example, Sells et al. (2006) found that unengaged clients had more contacts with their mental health case managers when peers were part of the engagement process, compared with fewer case manager contacts when peer staff were not involved. Sells et al. (2006, p. 1184) concluded that "early in treatment, peer providers may possess distinctive skills in communicating positive regard, understanding, and acceptance to clients and a facility for increasing treatment participation among the most disengaged, leading to greater motivation for further treatment and use of peer-based community services."

Other studies focused on the effectiveness of complementary peer services on the individual's treatment goals. For example, Felton et al. (1995) found that individuals who were served by teams that included peer support specialists demonstrated greater gains in quality of life and an overall reduction in the number of major life problems. They also reported more frequent contact with their case managers and showed the largest gains in the areas of self-image, outlook, and social support.

The first substantial evidence that peer support services can be effective came from studies with peers serving as community case managers. In two studies, Solomon and Drain (1995a, b) in randomized trials of peer case management service found that peer case management teams were equally effective as non-peer teams in terms of reduced symptomology and quality of life outcomes. Chinman et al. (2000) also found that peer case management teams were equally effective as their non-peer counterparts in terms of the clinical outcomes achieved. In a randomized control trial, Clarke et al. (2000) studied assertive community treatment (ACT) teams using peers and ACT teams without peers. The study found that fewer people were hospitalized and the first hospitalization occurred later for individuals who were served by ACT teams with peers.

In a meta-review of randomized controlled studies, Pitt et al. (2013) reported that, when peer-run services were compared to those conducted by non-peer professional staff, the outcomes were equivalent. These outcomes included quality of life, depression, mental health symptoms, satisfaction with treatment, person/professional relationship, use of mental health services, hospital admissions, length of stay, and readmission.

## Unique Factors in Inpatient Settings

Psychiatric hospitals have faced a tsunami of change over the past 20 years that have significantly altered daily operations and shifted the role of the hospital within the mental health treatment community. First and foremost is the increased scrutiny paid to admission and readmission rates, as well as changes in the community standards of care that emphasizes alternatives to hospitalization, including the individual's right to self-determination and choice even within the hospital setting. The introduction of new generation antipsychotic medications that are highly effective in remediating psychiatric symptoms for a large percentage of individuals and community-based alternatives to hospitalization, such as ACT teams also played a role in reshaping the purpose of the psychiatric hospital as a short-stay setting for immediate stabilization rather than long-term rehabilitation for most patients.

Nowhere has the scrutiny on the inpatient psychiatric hospital system been more acute than in the admission, discharge and readmission process. The high cost of inpatient services, in particular, has focused the attention of Medicaid, Medicare, and managed care payers on establishing performance standards for readmission and routine monitoring for length of stay. Beginning in 2013, Medicare implemented financial penalties (reductions in per diem payments) for hospitals that exceeded inpatient readmission standards and other quality metrics. Similarly, "transitions in care" (formerly known as "Discharge Planning") has emerged as a sub-specialty area for quality and performance on its own.

The typical inpatient discharge planning process resembles two ships passing in the night. Ship A, the hospital, controls the length of stay in the facility by discharging the person when they determine that hospital services are no longer medically necessary. At the same time the hospital needs to make sure that readmission is not likely to occur by ensuring that the person has sufficient stability and is referred to appropriate community services. Ship B, a community mental health service provider, may or may not be part of the discharge planning process. The hospital needs to prevent readmissions by identifying the community services that are necessary to successfully support the person in the community, but they have no role in ensuring that the person is actually connected to the community resources. Since the hospital does not control the community resources and the community providers do not have any authority in the hospital discharge planning process, there is often significant tension between these two discrete parts of the mental health system.

In addition, mental health service funding is allocated in silos in the United States. Community providers cannot bill for services when the individual is in an inpatient setting and the hospital cannot bill when the person returns to the community. These funding silos significantly inhibit coordination of care between these settings. Organizing discharge planning sessions where the hospital and community staff both participate can be challenging. Needless to say, gaps in services are common. One of the most important predictors of readmission is whether patients attend their first appointment with a community provider. It is not uncommon to find a 30 % or greater rate of failure to appear for the first appointment. While some individuals eventually make a connection with their community providers, a sizable number fail to connect and, without ongoing treatment, remission is often inevitable. These individuals show up in emergency rooms, psychiatric inpatient settings, jails, in homeless shelters and, in some cases as mortalities.

Factors in hospital readmissions have been closely studied across multiple states and payer systems. The available research indicates that the reasons for readmission include all of the following factors: the person may be discharged prematurely without achieving functional stability; the community resources needed to support the person are either not available, not sufficient or not responsive; the person does not understand what they need to do to remain healthy; the person lacks capacity or desire to adhere to the discharge instructions upon leaving the more regimented inpatient setting; the person has an unaddressed or refuses to address a substance abuse issue; or the person's living environment does not support recovery (Hemminger 2012).

One issue that comes into play is that people who are frequently readmitted often receive discharge plans that contain the exact same locations and services that have repeatedly failed to support them in the community. Due to the rapid time frame in which the inpatient team must complete a discharge plan, the causative factors that drove the readmission are often not identified or considered when new discharge plan is developed. Even when the reasons are obvious, the hospital often has few community options to choose from that are capable of addressing the issues. If the person needs to move to a more supportive environment, those settings are often not readily available. If an ACT Team is needed to support the person, there may be a wait list for the program. Nevertheless, any approach to reduce readmissions and to support a successful community placement must address all of the factors that led to the person's initial admission and any subsequent readmission. The problem of gaps in the service array needs to be addressed by the administrators of the system of care. Inpatient hospitals and community providers need to unite to bring these gaps in care forward or the gaps and consequently high rates of readmission will continue to occur.

The discharge planning process itself has a fundamental flaw in that the person is not just leaving one level of care, but entering another. Rather than simply concluding a service, the person is transitioning between services. Research has shown that the most effective ways to reduce readmission is to provide education while the person resides in the inpatient setting, develop a discharge plan that effectively deals with the factors in the prior readmissions and provide transitional support in the community to ensure that the discharge plan is followed and readjusted if needed (Forchuk et al. 2007a, b). The goal is to connect the person with community services and supports necessary to succeed, and in each of these areas, peer services have been shown to play a beneficial role.

## Connecting the Dots: Peer Models in Inpatient Settings

Across the country many inpatient settings have begun to see the value of adding peer support and family support to their services; however, only a few have done it to the degree necessary to have the type of significant impact reported in the few randomized controlled trials that have been conducted. McGill and Patterson (1990) reported one of the earliest examples of peer support program in an inpatient setting. In this program, former patients were trained to be peer counselors in a large public sector acute psychiatric inpatient program. Due to their positive impact over a four-year period, staff that were originally skeptical changed their attitudes and began requesting that peer-run groups and services be expanded.

Several other studies have examined the role and outcomes of peers serving in inpatient settings (Chinman et al. 2001; Lawn et al. 2008; Sledge 2011). The most promising target identified issues that are the most challenging within hospital environments: the need for rapid engagement into treatment during increasingly shorter lengths of stay, effective discharge and transition planning, and readmission prevention. Others focus on education and support directed to assist the person and their family in caring through on treatment recommendations once they leave the hospital. Programs implemented to target these factors utilize peer staff that work with individuals while they are in the inpatient settings while others link the person with peer support upon discharge. Another approach attempts to bridge the inpatient-community transition process by introducing peer support services while the person is in the hospital and continuing the service when the person returns to community. Methods employed to test the effectiveness and outcomes of these interventions include randomly controlled trials, case studies, program reports, and personal accounts by peer staff and persons receiving services.

In a study that examined peer support staff who were introduced after discharge, Chinman, Weingarten, Stayner and Davidson (2001) compared peer support outpatient programs with traditional care and found a 50 % reduction in readmissions when compared to the programs where support services were not in place peer. The results support the conclusion that when individuals return to the community and receive peer support services it can reduce hospital readmissions.

Sledge et al. (2011) found that individuals who were assigned a peer support staff member had fewer hospital admissions and hospital days over a 9-month period than patients who were not assigned a peer support staff member. The average length of stay for individuals who received inpatient peer support services was 10 days as opposed to 19 days for participants without peer support and hospital admissions for individuals that received outpatient peer support were 53 % less than those without peer support.

Another group of studies examined peer supports who acted as "Bridger's" between the hospital and the community. Lawn, Smith and Hunter (2008) found that individuals who received peer support services in the hospital and when they returned to the community showed reduced admission rates and more stable community placements, fewer readmissions and reduced lengths of stay. Individuals who took part in group peer support services had a readmission rate of only 17 % compared with an expected rate of 30 %. The data suggested that peer support staff are able to connect individuals with resources both inside and outside the hospital and provide the type of hopeful engagement that maximizes treatment returns.

One of the most promising lines of research is the work of Cheryl Forchuk and her colleagues in Ontario, Canada who developed a transitional discharge model (TDM). The model strategically targets discharge planning issues and the gap between hospital and community services. Known as the "Bridge to Discharge" program, her model addressed the traditional boundaries between hospital and community settings that impede care transitions by assigning an inpatient team of professional and peer support staff work with the individual while they are in the hospital and then remain with them in the community until a therapeutic relationship (Forchuk et al. 2002) is formed with a community mental health provider. Canada does not have the same funding silos that exist in the American system, allowing for more seamless care transitions. Forchuk et al. (2005) reported that using peer support as part of the discharge process significantly reduced readmission rates and increased discharge rates. The model was tested in a randomized clinical trial involving either peer support for one year, or ongoing support from hospital staff until a therapeutic relationship was established with a community care provider. The peer group was discharged 116 days sooner than the traditional care group. The study authors also reported that individuals who received peer support demonstrated improved social support, enhanced social skills and improved social functioning.

Forchuk and Brown (1989) based the TDM model on early work on nurse–patient relationship that emphasized the importance of directed relationships in promoting health and healing (Peplau 1952). This research defined nursing as "a significant, therapeutic, interpersonal process that aims to promote a patient's health in the direction of creative, constructive, productive, personal, and community living." Forchuk and Brown expanded on Peplau's definition to include all professional staff involved with the person and then added peer support to the formulation.

Using the relationship as her framework, Forchuk et al. (2012) identified three essential elements that underlie the effectiveness of the TDM model: (1) people heal in relationships (including staff and peer relationships); (2) transitions in care are vulnerable periods for individuals with mental illness and services should be front-loaded to bridge the transition process; and (3) a network of relationships provided during transitional periods assists in sustained recovery. Forchuk et al. (2012, p. 585) summarized their findings on design components that are key to the success of the TDM approach: "… the availability of on-ward educational opportunities, presence of an accessible 'champion' for the intervention, perceived administrative support, belief in the usefulness of the intervention and in the ease of use of the intervention, and willingness to partner with outside groups. In general, active engagement and participation by staff throughout the process was critical."

Implementing the TDM involves a significant change in the relationship between hospital and community care providers as well as hospital operations. Specific strategies that facilitated the implementation of TDM within the inpatient environment include: (1) the use of educational modules for on-ward hospital staff training and peer training; (2) presence of on-site champions; and (3) supportive documentation systems. Issues identified as barriers to implementation included: (1) feeling drowned, swamped and overwhelmed; (2) death by process; (3) team dynamics; and (4) changes in champions. (Forchuk et al. (2012). In addition, they identified several actions that are critical to ensuring the person establishes a therapeutic relationship with a hospital clinical staff member before discharge and that hospital staff communicates properly, continuously, and understands their roles in the discharge process.

To emphasize the foundational role of relationships during transition, Forchuk et al. (2007a) changed the title of the TDM to transitional relationship model (TRM). To Forchuk et al. (2007a, p. 80) "therapeutic relationships include not only the nurse–client relationship but also other staff relationships, family relationships, and peer relationships. Each person needs a safety net of relationships because people are believed to heal in supportive relationships. However, traditional models of care terminate relationships at the point of hospital discharge, which is a time of vulnerability for many clients."

Forchuk et al. (2007b) also studied the transferability of the model to a facility in Scotland. Reynolds et al. (2004) implemented and evaluated the TDM on acute care psychiatric wards there and reported that the group that did not participate in the TDM model was more than two times as likely to be readmitted in the subsequent 5 months when compared to the TDM discharge group.

Hanrahan et al. (2014) used an adapted version of the TDM for older adults being released from acute care hospitals for patients with serious mental illness and medical comorbidities. The "Transitional Care Model" was delivered by a psychiatric nurse practitioner assigned within the acute setting who continued to see patients in the community. The study found that patients with immediate and pressing physical health problems were most receptive and actively utilized the service. A number of barriers were identified including communication and privacy issues making it difficult to remain engaged with persons in community mental health facilities. While the nurse practitioner was accepted and valued in the physical health arena, the psychosocial needs and relationship issues were too demanding for a single staff. The researchers concluded that a team approach including a social worker, peer provider, and consulting psychiatrist were needed for severely mentally ill patients being released from an acute physical health hospital (Solomon et al. 2014).

Similar models have been promoted in a number of locations. M-Power Advocates reported to the Massachusetts Inpatient Study Commission (2009) regarding the need to implement peer support programs designed to transition individuals from inpatient facilities. Their report stated, "One type of support for individuals transitioning out of the hospital used very successfully in New York State is a Peer Bridger Project in which a trained peer specialist provides one-to-one support to a person ready to be discharged. This relationship begins several months before the discharge date and continues for several months after discharge. This is an excellent way to address the concerns and fears a person who has been in the hospital for months or years may have about being able to make it on the outside. The Genesis Club in Worcester and the Lighthouse Clubhouse in Springfield run Peer Bridger projects under a DMH contract entitled "Peer Support in After Care." Such programs need to be expanded throughout the state" (p. 2).

Marc Community Resources has implemented a Community Transition Program utilizing trained peer support navigators to assist individuals who are being discharged from a community psychiatric inpatient setting. The peer staff engages the individual while they are in the hospital and assist them while they transition to the community using a critical time intervention model shortened to a 90 day period. The results to date (Thomas and Anderson 2015) have been encouraging. Preliminary findings from the first 75 individuals served include the following:

(1) The vast majority (65) remained in the community during the period in which they were supported, (2) a large percent of the individuals (41 % or 31 participants) were either homeless or could not return their original living environment (33 participants). (3) Many individuals have co-occurring mental health and substance abuse disorders (42.6 or 32 participants). (4) Coordination with the person's outpatient clinical team can be challenging in some cases and individuals reported that the lack of responsiveness by their teams was the main reason for their hospitalizations. (5) While the hospital staff were initially unsure how peer supports could be helpful, their attitude changed rapidly and they now see peer supports as a valuable resource.

The six participants who were re-hospitalized disengaged from both the Community Transition Program and their PNO teams soon after initial discharge and ceased all contact with both entities until they were either re-engaged upon re-hospitalization, or were located after rigorous outreach efforts. Other interesting information that has been obtained from this group is that approximately one-third of the readmissions began with a medical hospitalization. In a significant number of cases the substance abuse challenges that were prominent reason for re-hospitalization. Approximately, one-third experienced challenges with medication, i.e., some people did not want to take their medication. Approximately one-third self-discharged from the hospital and went to motels or similarly unsupportive settings whereby they soon became homeless and symptomatic.

An interesting application of the peer support model was conducted by Vijayalakshmy et al. (2006). In long-term psychiatric hospitals a small percentage of individuals resist discharge. The study described a peer support intervention that specifically addressed individuals who were reluctant to return to the community. The group utilized standard methods of rehabilitation and training with strong emphasis on validating individual needs and feelings using peer support. After 18 months of the group intervention, five of the seven group members had achieved discharge and community success.

## Bringing Peer Support to Scale in Inpatient Programs

Bluebird (2008) described a model of a peer support inpatient program that was implemented in a State Hospital setting in Delaware. In this program, the peers were not hospital employees, but were managed by an external peer-run organization that also provided the peer staff supervision. The roles of peer staff included providing support during hospitalization, providing low-level advocacy to ensure that the person's voice was heard with professional teams and that persons were treated with dignity and respect. As part of the overall plan to introduce peer services in this environment, the peer support staff were involved in all aspects of client care and operations of the hospital, ensuring that consumer voice was reflected in hospital operations and policies.

The duties assigned to peer support staff in the Delaware program were many and varied, reflecting the wide range of job functions and valued roles that peers can deliver to support effective hospital services. Staff provided one-to-one and group support, facilitated recovery groups, developed personal safety plans, provided transportation, conducted debriefings, assisted with resolving complaints, attended treatment team and admission meetings, supported crisis intervention and ran drop-in centers ("comfort rooms") as part of the hospital program.

Other facilities have developed their own approaches, such as the "Passport to Health" used at Kings County Hospital in Brooklyn, New York (Perrazo and Rodriguez 2014). Their approach employed a peer counselor who assisted the person in identifying the members of their clinical team, their diagnosis, symptoms, medications, the purpose of the medications, their daily treatment groups, their recovery goals, life goals, natural supports, and emergency contacts. Delivering instrumental support is a large component of the peer counselor job function. The counselor works with individuals by attending treatment team meetings with the person and assisting them in describing their personal goals and service preferences. The peer counselor also conducts individual and group recovery sessions designed to assist the person in developing recovery and self-management skills.

Most programs that use peer support staff in inpatient settings have similar features. Peer staff typically attempt to engage the person shortly after admission using their shared experience to establish rapport, illustrating the emotional support component of peer services. Informational support is then provided and depending on the person's response to engagement, the peer support worker can assist the person in understanding and participating in the treatment planning process and describing the services they will receive at the hospital and how they can participate in the process.

Many peer support staff who work in inpatient settings assist patients in developing a "Wellness Recovery Action Plan" or WRAP plan. WRAP is personal planning tool where individuals develop their own goals and strategies for reducing and preventing symptoms. Copeland (2007) developed the WRAP plan and it is now a widely used tool that supports person-centered and recovery-oriented planning. In a study of 519 individuals with a serious mental illness who were provided WRAP Training, Cook et al. (2011) reported that WRAP participants experienced (1) significantly greater reduction in symptom severity, (2) significantly greater improvement over time in hopefulness as assessed by the Hope Scale, and (3) enhanced improvement over time in quality of life as assessed by the World Health Organization's Quality of Life environment subscale. These results indicate that peer-delivered mental illness self-management training reduces psychiatric symptoms, enhances participants' hopefulness, and improves their quality of life over time. On psychosocial measures of hopefulness and quality of life, WRAP recipients reported not only greater improvements relative to controls, but this advantage appeared to grow over time.

Sadaaki et al. (2011) compared the results obtained between individuals who received WRAP training and a control group, and found statistically significant improvements for the WRAP trained group in psychiatric symptoms and hope after the intervention, while non-significant changes occurred in the comparison group. Their conclusion was that the evidence was promising that WRAP participation had a positive effect on psychiatric symptoms and feelings of hopefulness.

WRAP has also been found to have a dose-response relationship. Greater exposure to WRAP is predictive of improvement on psychiatric symptom severity and hopefulness for their futures when compared to individuals with less exposure (Cook et al. 2009). This study concluded that individuals need to have adequate exposure for WRAP to have a measurable impact, with participants who attended six or more recovery-oriented group sessions showing greater improvement than those attending fewer sessions. Similarly, Starnino et al. (2010) reported positive effects of their WRAP intervention with at least 75 % participation in the program. This can be challenging in inpatient settings where the lengths of stay are typically very short. Taking the analysis a step further, Falzer (2011) noted that the effectiveness of recovery-oriented programs such as WRAP might depend more on the level of participation than simply attendance.

## Benefits and Challenges

Adding peer support staff to inpatient settings has produced both positive results and identified several challenges for program implementation. For example, Salzer and Shear-Liptzin (2002) conducted thematic interviews with peer support providers and reported that peer staff themselves benefit from their roles as helpers. They noted a number of positive outcomes including improvement in their own recovery, increased feelings of social approval and self-efficacy, professional development skills and stable employment. Bradstreet and Pratt found that when peer support staff were placed on traditional clinical teams, it enhanced the team's commitment to recovery. Clinical staff reported being more aware of their use of language and becoming more aware of recovery-oriented principles. O'Hagan (2011) noted that based on interviews of staff, a significant percentage of professional staff reported that presence of peer support staff helped to create a culture change through role modeling, informal dialogue, education, and creating the conditions where some professionals felt safe to "come out" as consumers. Walker and Bryant (2013) also reported that traditional clinical staff developed increased empathy and understanding toward people in recovery as a result of working with peer support workers.

Bluebird (2008) reported that over time staff attitudes toward peer support staff became more positive, they develop more respect for patient input, began to see peer specialists as a valued role on the treatment team and became more open about sharing their own personal recovery stories. The impact on the peer specialist staff was the development of a better understanding of mental illness, higher awareness of issues people face, learning to speak up for themselves, greater confidence in speaking to medical professionals, changing their perception of some client populations and a deeper valuing of their own recovery journey.

Campbell and Leaver (2003) and Clay (2005) concurred, reporting that peer support services had the potential to be a force for positive change. Campbell and Leaver (2003) identified "Four significant forces have converged over the past century to foster peer-run support programs as they exist today for people with psychiatric problems: (1) the growth of self-help groups to address a wide range of conditions; (2) the movement of people with special needs from institutions to communities; (3) the mobilization of the consumer/survivor movement; and (4) the growing support of consumer inclusion and concepts of recovery (p. 9).

Implementing peer support within traditional psychiatric inpatient settings requires careful planning and support by agency administrators. Key challenges identified in less successful implementations tend to focus on lack of planning or clear vision of the purpose and goals of the program. When peers were introduced into inpatient settings without detailed job descriptions, clearly defined roles and without adequate staff preparation regarding the peer support function, conflict and confusion occurred. For example, Jacobson et al. (2012) conducted a review of the literature and identified that in the absence of adequately defined job descriptions and clear roles, it became challenging for peer support staff to play a meaningful role on inpatient teams. Dixon et al. (1994) found similar problems when imprecise job descriptions and inadequate structure of the peer function resulted in peer staff not being able to identify their roles. Gates and Akabas (2007) also reported role conflict and confusion when clinical and medical staff were not sufficiently prepared to work with peer support staff. Manning and Suire (1996) concluded that the lack of a clearly defined job description or role expectations was a serious impediment to realizing the full value of this service.

Meehen et al. (2002) conducted interviews with peers working in inpatient settings and identified a menu of issues that should shape planning and implementation of effective peer programs. In their review, (1) staff were not adequately trained regarding the role of peers, (2) staff used peers as tokens and discounted their contributions, (3) peers filled traditional work roles, not recovery roles, (4) staff were afraid that peers would become ill, (5) peers were overworked, and (6) peers had boundary issues. Gordon (2005) reported that the integration of peers into the workforce could be compromised by the attitudes of some mental health professionals. Hodges and Hardiman (2006) reported that some professionals, particularly those who are trained in a medical model of care, are often pessimistic about the value of peer support and are reluctant to refer or encourage consumers to participate in peer-run services.

With respect to the issue of peer staff experiencing relapse due to contact with individuals who are symptomatic, Nikkel et al. (1992) examined whether the stress and anxiety associated with exposing former consumers to patients currently receiving treatment in a hospital could cause relapse and found no evidence to suggest that the psychological wellbeing of the peer support staff suffered as a result of interacting with patients in hospital. Bluebird (2008) reported the following issues in their implementation of peer support in the Delaware state hospital program: Getting "buy-in" from staff, staff fears that peers would tell them how to do their job, some staff viewed peers as "mental patients with keys" and did not want consumers working in the hospital, boundary issues, access to some information and areas of the hospital that are restricted, pay comparison, rumors and negative comments, professional respect, power differentials, medical model of treatment, staff fears that they would let clients out of the building, and that peers would get sick and would support the person's symptoms of illness. They reported that major challenges included moving too fast, developing infrastructure, balancing training needs with work needs, getting buy-in from all staff (most are very supportive), peers conducting themselves as decision makers on treatment teams and challenging authorities.

On a positive note, peer support staff provide other traditional mental health staff the opportunity to see peers successfully functioning in productive social roles. Ockwell (2012) described how models of inpatient peer support need to be flexible to both the individual talents of peer support workers and the cultures in which they work.

## Peer Support Training

In 2007, the U.S. Center for Medicaid and Medicare Services (CMS) released a historic letter to State Medicaid Directors (Smith 2007) that authorized peer support as a reimbursable Medicaid service. Required components necessary to deliver and bill the service included a strong focus on training and clinical oversight of peer positions: "Peer support providers must complete training and certification as defined by the State. Training must provide peer support providers with a basic set of competencies necessary to perform the peer support function." This development was initially viewed with trepidation in some settings, but in fact has resulted in a significant enhancement of the peer workforce. Early on, Campbell (1990) noted that while many consumer groups demonstrated a desire to participate in the planning and delivery of services, the literature indicates that such involvement with vulnerable populations requires knowledge and skills that consumers may not already possess. While being a peer with lived experience is a basic requirement, it does not necessarily mean that the person is capable of assisting another person in their recovery process.

In our experience in Arizona (Thomas and Anderson 2015), peer supports can play many roles in the behavioral health system but there is specialized knowledge regarding accessing resources, stages of change, ethics, evidence-based practices, HIPAA, maintaining boundaries and other skills that are necessary in order to provide effective and ethical support to another person. Some individuals believe that providing additional training to peers causes them to lose their "peerness"; however, peer support staff have benefited significantly from additional education and frequently seek out advanced educational opportunities on their own. The peer support staff that we have worked with have not lost their fundamental orientation as a peer, but in fact have added additional skills to their repertoire.

When peer staff begin to work as part of a clinical team they are often confronted with rules, regulations, billing procedures and other requirements that are not familiar. For all staff entering a new position, there is an acknowledged learning curve, but eventually peers are expected to perform like all staff with respect to standard work behaviors. This requires that peer staff complete facility orientation programs and all training required by licensing, credentialing, and accrediting organizations. In some cases peer staff need to request ADA accommodations so that they can continue their own recovery process by attending services that may only occur during their work hours.

## Ingredients of Peer Support Services

What makes peer support such a unique contribution within the healthcare delivery system? SAMHSA (2009a, b), citing the work of Cobb

(1976) and Salzer (2002a), identified four types of support offered by peers: emotional, informational, instrumental, and affiliational. *Emotional support* includes demonstrating empathy, caring, or concern in order to bolster person's self-esteem and confidence. *Informational support* involves sharing knowledge and information and/or providing life or vocational skills training. *Instrumental support* includes providing concrete assistance to help others accomplish tasks. *Affiliational support* involves facilitating contacts with other people to promote learning of social and recreational skills, create community, and acquire a sense of belonging. Peer staff may exhibit each type of support within the context of their work roles, or focus on a specific type in a targeted program.

In our experience in working with peer support staff since 2001, there are several aspects of support that have special relevance in supporting recovery. Within the emotional domain peers play a special role in providing the person with hope that there can be a brighter future. Hope is a primary motivator for patient activation, which has been identified as a critical element in self-management. Ultimately, self-management is necessary to maintain recovery. No matter how often a person sees the psychiatrist, counselor, case manager, primary care provider, or peer support provider, what happens when they are not in the presence of professionals and support staff determines whether a person is living a healthy lifestyle. Decisions made on a daily basis —where to eat, whether to watch television or take a walk, whether to take prescribed medications on time and in the correct amounts—are ultimately more important than the decisions made during a treatment planning session.

Another important element of peer support services is the assistance they provide in improving a person's health literacy. Jorm (2000) hypothesized that people's symptom-management activities are influenced by their mental health literacy. This perspective is important because it leads to a greater emphasis on increasing personal vs. professional knowledge and skills about mental health, and on empowering the person experiencing disabling symptoms. Many individuals lack an understanding of their diagnosis, the available treatment options and what they have to do to remain healthy. This is as true of people managing chronic diabetes or heart conditions as those learning to live with schizophrenia.

Two of the key elements of peer support services are hope and social connectedness. Many scholars and peer professionals believe that hope is the keystone of recovery. Reynolds et al. (2004) reported that the expression and maintenance of hope for a future outside of the hospital was the central theme for many participants. They reported, "Hope was commonly found throughout many clients' comments, particularly during the early stages of the project" (p. 496).

The ability to build social support appears to be one of the primary skills that peer support providers possess. Felton et al. (1995) found that individuals who were served by peer support staff reported improved social support, quality of life, a reduction in the number of major life problems, more frequent contact with their case managers and improved self-image. The availability of a social support network is often accompanied by improvements in multiple aspects of life. Hardiman and Segal (2003) examined the characteristics of peer support self-help agencies and concluded that they foster social networks leading to the experience of shared community.

Kaplan et al. (2012) reported that those peers who participated in community activities such as parenting, employment, volunteering, college student, group membership, civic engagement, peer support, friendships, intimate relationships, and engagement in religious/spiritual activities had higher scores on the recovery, quality of life, and meaning of life measures. Younger adults had the most significant results. Coatsworth-Puspoky et al. (2006) discussed the importance of expanding the person's social network. One poignant quote from an informant clearly articulated the value added by peer support, "They've seen me at my best and at my worst and they're still my friends" (p. 496).

## Family Peer Support

There has been increased recognition that family members play a critical role in providing natural supports to individuals who experience inpatient hospitalization. Most individuals who are discharged from inpatient settings return to their family homes. The short length of the typical inpatient stay makes it challenging to involve families in formal interventions. The first priority is to provide a period of respite for the family who are typically emotionally exhausted by their efforts to care for their loved ones during the crisis that resulted in hospitalization.

The SAMHSA National Registry of Evidenced-Based Programs and Practices (2006a, b) identified family interventions as an evidence-based practice. The intervention focuses on informing families and support people about mental illness, developing coping skills, solving problems, creating social supports, and developing an alliance among consumers, practitioners, and their families or other support people. Practitioners invite five to six consumers and their families to participate in a psychoeducational group that typically meets every other week for at least 6 months. McFarlane et al. (2003) reported positive outcomes for employment, lower relapse and hospitalization rates, lower rates of negative symptoms of schizophrenia and reduced family stress. Solomon (1996) reported that when families participate in family intervention activities they gain knowledge and feel greater satisfaction with mental health treatment, experience a reduction in burden, distress, and anxiety, and improved self-efficacy and coping behaviors. Dixon et al. (2004) reported that peer support programs for families could improve their knowledge about the illness, increase confidence, and reduce caregiver burden.

Solomon (1996) described the difference between psychosocial interventions and family education programs. Psychoeducational interventions combine educational and therapeutic objectives, offering didactic material about the ill relative's disorder and therapeutic strategies to enhance the family's communication and coping skills with the goal of reducing the patient's rate of relapse. Family education differs from psychoeducation in that its primary goals are didactic and supportive rather than therapeutic. Interventions are focused on improving family members' quality of life by reducing stress and burden, and only secondarily on benefiting the ill relative.

Cuijpers (1999) conducted a meta-analysis of the impact of family interventions on the burden of relatives of psychiatric patients. Based on a review of 16 studies, family interventions were found to have a positive impact on relatives' burden, psychological distress, relationship between patient and relative, and family functioning. The analysis also revealed that, when the families participated in 12 sessions or more, the interventions had larger effects than shorter interventions. These interventions could be started while the person is in the hospital, but due to the length of the intervention, it would have to be continued after discharge.

Gingrich and Bellack (1995) reviewed a number of randomly controlled studies of formal family interventions programs and concluded that there were numerous positive effects on the course of the illness when families are included in these intervention programs. These included reductions in relapse rates, increased remission of symptoms, and reduced number of hospitalizations. The interventions included the following shared components: (1) Education was provided to patients and families about the biological nature of the illness and the principles for treatment (especially medication compliance, attention to early warning signs, reducing stress, and providing a supportive environment). (2) The family is treated as an ally by the treatment team and is discouraged from feeling guilty or to blame for the patient's illness or its course. (3) A psychoeducational workshop is conducted at the beginning of the program. (4) Regular meetings are then held with the family, ranging from weekly to monthly. (5) Support is provided by clinicians and, in most cases, by other families in a group format. (6) Families are assisted in improving their coping methods and their communication with each other. (7) Treatment teams are multidisciplinary and team members coordinate frequently with each other and outside agencies, and (8) Medication is followed closely, with rigorous attempts made to maximize compliance. In some cases family peer members played a role in these interventions, but in most cases it was a minor role.

The SAMHSA (2010a, b) Family Psychoeducation (FPE) program is an approach for partnering with consumers and families to treat serious mental illnesses. It is not a family therapy program, but rather a family support and education program where practitioners, consumers, and families work together to support recovery. Dixon et al. (2000) identified the critical ingredients of effective FPE to be (1) education about serious mental illnesses, (2) information resources, especially during periods of crises, (3) skills training and ongoing guidance about managing mental illnesses, (4) problem solving, and (5) social and emotional support.

Caplan and Caplan (2000) reported that family psychoeducation programs have the potential to extend the impact of care provision well beyond the immediate situation by activating and reinforcing both formal and informal support systems. Lukens and Mcfarlane (2004) predicted that psychoeducational interventions have far-reaching application for acute and chronic illness and other life challenges across levels of the public health, social and civic services, and/or educational systems.

There are a number of formal family psychosocial interventions that are typically conducted by professional staff and in some cases peers assist in the interventions; however, there is only one formal pure family education program that was developed by National Alliance on Mental Illness (NAMI), titled the Family to Family Program (FTF). The FTF program is a 12-week course offered by family members of adults with mental illness. Dixon et al. (2011) evaluated the effectiveness of the FTF program RTC, with one group receiving the FTF compared to a waiting list control group. The participants were interviewed at enrollment, at 3 months or after the FTF training. The study measured problem- and emotion-focused coping, subjective illness burden, and distress. The results indicated that the FTF participants had significantly greater improvements in problem-focused coping as measured by empowerment and illness knowledge. FTF participants also had significantly enhanced emotion-focused coping as measured by increased acceptance of their family member's illness, as well as reduced distress and improved problem solving.

Anderson et al. (1986) compared the satisfaction of family members participating in process versus psychoeducational groups. Families were randomly assigned to a traditional multiple family groups with a process orientation that emphasized support, destigmatization, and self-help about common problems; or to a psychoeducational multiple family groups that emphasized the provision of information about the mental illness and methods of coping with it effectively. They found a number of differences in knowledge, attitude and dyadic adjustment in the participants of both groups immediately following their respective group sessions, but there were only a few statistically significant differences between the two groups. Those who attended the psychoeducational session, however, reported significantly more satisfaction with the experience.

Pollio et al. (1998) examined the relationship between professionally prepared psychoeducation materials and the needs of the family members as identified and ranked by importance. The findings suggested that input from the family, the ill family member, and mental health providers is necessary for developing psychoeducation curricula that will meet families' needs. Professionals who design multifamily psychoeducation curricula are encouraged to incorporate enough flexibility to accommodate the specific needs of members of particular groups and to provide general information that is useful for all groups.

The Adaptive Family Tool Kit is a program that provides families with education and support (Perrazo and Rodriguez 2014). The program includes information on mental illness and diagnosis, effective treatments, the range of services available in the hospital and the community, common family reactions to illness, how these reactions are quite normal, what can be done to change the reaction, how the family can help, communicating with your loved one, how to handle crisis, aggression, identifying signs of relapse, benefits and financial support, how to care for yourself, support groups, and NAMI Programs and other resources. When working with families it is often necessary to assist them in resolving their immediate problems before educational resources and training can be attempted. Like peer support, family peer support involves family members who have lived experience in dealing with loved with mental illness. Family support partners who have this experience and have learned how to deal with and navigate what is often a very complicated and fragmented system of care, have become an extremely valuable resource. When the person leaves the hospital the family is connected with community-based agencies to continue the supports.

## Financial Impact of Peer Support Services

Given the consistency of the findings of decreased hospitalization or shortened length of hospital stay for both peer provided services and peer providers themselves, there should be financial savings to the system, as hospitalization is one of the most expensive of mental health services. There is substantial research evidence that when peer support services are combined with traditional services superior outcomes are achieved when compared to traditional mental health services only (Chinman et al. 2001; Klein et al. 1998; Lawn et al. 2008; Sledge et al. 2011).

While a number of studies have reported cost savings when peer supports deliver services in inpatient settings, at least one study that compared the total costs of both inpatient and community services found that the total cost of services decreases. Forchuk et al. (1998a, b) demonstrated savings in hospital costs of approximately $0.5M for the 14 individuals served over 1 year. In a follow-up study, Forchuk et al. (2005) reported that the intervention group left the inpatient setting an average of 116 days earlier, reducing the cost of hospitalization by $12M compared to the control group. Sledge et al. (2011) found that participants who were assigned a peer support staff member when discharged had fewer hospital admissions and hospital days over a nine-month period than patients who were not assigned a peer support staff member. There was no dollar value assigned to the cost savings.

Trachtenberg et al. (2013) reviewed six studies that reported cost savings with respect to inpatient hospital bed days. Four of the six studies (Chinman et al. 2001; Klein et al. 1998; Lawn et al. 2008; Sledge et al. 2011) showed a cost benefit in excess of the additional costs of providing peer support services. In one study, a cost benefit was positive, but was not positive when peer support services costs were added. In another study, Rivera et al. (2007) there was an increase in the costs of bed days when peers supports were added. On the basis of this evidence, they concluded that the use of peer support workers is justified on the basis of financial cost versus benefit received by the service recipients.

Simpson et al. (2014) found no significant differences between those receiving peer support and those receiving care-as-usual on two of the three main outcome measures of costs: hopelessness and loneliness. However, hope increased in both conditions with a near significant change on Beck's Hopelessness Scale in those receiving peer support. There were fewer readmissions in the peer support arm of the study, but no conclusions could be drawn from such a small sample and short follow-up period. There was also considerable attrition in this study.

In an analysis of costs across all mental service, Landers and colleagues (Landers and Zhou

2014, 2011) examined the 2003–2004 inpatient and outpatient payment claims data for 1910 individuals in Georgia who received peer support services and a randomly sampled comparison group of 3820 individuals who did not receive peer support services. The average Medicaid prescription and outpatient care costs for Georgia Medicaid beneficiaries with mental illness who received peer support services in 2003 and 2004 was higher than costs for a comparison group with mental illness who received traditional care. However, the average costs for inpatient psychiatric services, which are not covered by Georgia Medicaid, were lower among the beneficiaries receiving peer support. Overall, the average per person Medicaid and non-Medicaid costs for those who received Medicaid peer support were about $5991 higher than costs for those who did not receive peer support services.

The Georgia researchers also noted that while the overall state spending was higher for those who received peer support services, given the lack of community-based services during 2003–2004, inpatient and facility-based crisis services were the only available options. The researchers noted the finding that peer support was a significant predictor of lower nonpsychiatric inpatient costs, even after controlling for illness severity, was unexpected. They recommended further study of the connection between peer support and overall Medicaid inpatient utilization.

The caveat regarding the available array of community services in 2003–2004 makes the Georgia findings unique to that context. Since the Georgia study did not attempt to measure the quality of care or other outcomes such as quality of life or satisfaction with services for the two groups, it difficult to determine whether the costs increases are justifiable. Since one of the roles of peer support staff is to ensure that individuals are made aware of all of the resources they may need to support recovery, it would be expected that more community services would at least initially be accessed by individuals who receive peer support.

Trachtenberg et al. (2013) examined the TDM Model financial data and reported that the financial benefits of employing peer support workers do indeed exceed the costs, in some cases by a substantial margin. They also indicated, "The introduction of peer workers is a powerful way of driving a more recovery-focused approach within organizations. Just as peer workers provide hope and inspiration for services users, so they can challenge negative attitudes of staff and provide an inspiration for all members of the team. Their example demonstrates to everyone that people with mental health problems can make a valued contribution to their own and others' recovery if they are given the opportunity" (p. 5).

Given the equivocal results of the various cost-benefit analyses, future studies need to include the costs of both inpatient and outpatient services and other financial categories that are impacted by untreated mental illness, including homelessness and criminal justice. Since significant medical comorbidity also exists within the population, the scope of the review should go beyond costs of mental health services and include physical health care costs as well.

## Re-engineering the Workforce Through Peer Providers

While many observers of healthcare systems shake their heads over the 20-year gap between innovation and implementation of new practices, adoption of peer services has moved quickly to become the standard of care in most community mental health systems in the country today. Inpatient psychiatric hospitals are also beginning to test the water of peer-delivered services in larger numbers, following the success stories and implementation recommendations from early adopters of the practice. Prompted by advocates, researchers, family members and patients themselves, hospital settings are moving to embrace recovery and peer-delivered care as much for its potential to inspire hope during life's most challenging times as the clear evidence of positive outcomes produced by the service. What started as a quiet revolution in a few state hospitals is quickly becoming a movement all its own.

Georgia and Arizona were the first two states to act on the New Freedom Commission recommendations and began developing formal peer support programs in 2001. In both Georgia and Arizona, forward-thinking system administrators and legislators redesigned their state's Medicaid benefit package to allow for more recovery and rehabilitation services to be provided under the State Plan Waiver, including peer and family support services. By making peer service reimbursable, both states launched a workforce expansion and transformation that placed peer professionals in a variety of mental healthcare programs across the state.

An important first step in both Georgia and Arizona was developing formal training programs designed to give peers an understanding of the recovery process and how they can use their personal experience and "story" to assist a person in their personal recovery journey. Both states significantly expanded their peer support programs and subsequently developed peer supports to address the comorbid physical health and substance abuse issues that often co-occur with mental illness. More recently in Arizona, the Arizona Department of Health, Office of Individual and Family affairs launched a Peer Career Academy—a professional development program for the peer workforce with the goal of expanding and diversifying the roles that peers can play. By including roles within the healthcare arena, such as peer health coaching, the Academy holds promise for creating a true career path for peer providers and a vast number of different roles and job opportunities within the healthcare system (Bashor 2014).

## The Future of Health

Increasingly, the use of nontraditional peer roles is aligning mental health systems with the powerful new vision of twenty-first century healthcare articulated through the National Quality Strategy. (The U.S. Department of Health and Human Services (2011a, b, c) Report to Congress) The so-called Triple Aims of the Quality Strategy describe a future of health for the American population:

1. *Better Care*: Improve the overall quality, by making health care more patient-centered, reliable, accessible, and safe.
2. *Healthy People/Healthy Communities*: Improve the health of the US population by supporting proven interventions to address behavioral, social and, environmental determinants of health in addition to delivering higher quality care.
3. *Affordable Care*: Reduce the cost of quality health care for individuals, families, employers, and government.

To advance these aims, the National Quality Strategy focused on six priorities: (1) making care safer by reducing harm caused in the delivery of care; (2) ensuring that each person and family is engaged as partners in their care; (3) promoting effective communication and coordination of care; (4) promoting the most effective prevention and treatment practices for the leading causes of mortality; (5) working with communities to promote wide use of best practices to enable healthy living; and (6) making quality care more affordable through new health care delivery models.

Peer support services have proven to be a method that aligns with and supports the National Quality Strategies. The research is clear that peer support services have enhanced person-centered care not only by their direct application of this approach by peer support staff, but also in their ability to influence the behavior of other staff in the settings in which they work. Peer support staff have improved accessibility of care by increasing both the workforce and the types of services available in the community. The availability of Peer Respite, crisis services, drop-in centers and other options has expanded the array of options available.

Peer supports services have been able to address the behavioral, social and environmental determinants of health by using a holistic approach that not only addresses symptomatology, but also the other factors which are necessary to support recovery and resilience. Peer support services are also cost effective. However, peers need to be paid a wage that is commensurate with their education, experience and duties. Whereas peer support staff do not require advanced degrees or credentials, they often earn less than staff who are required to have these credentials. The research is undisputed in the finding that peer support staff produce outcomes that are equivalent to those of staff employed as case managers who in many cases require academic credentials. Another cost implication is that as peers become employed, they become tax-paying citizens, and reduce their reliance on SSI and SSDI funds.

Peer support services are also in line with the six priorities of the National Quality Strategies of health care. Peer supports have improved safety in inpatient settings by reducing the use of restraints in those settings. Both peer and family peer services have increased the level of person and family involvement in health care decision-making. Peer supports are often involved in spanning boundaries between providers and promote communication and coordination of care. A recent development in peer support services involves health coaching and chronic disease self-management. The expansion of peer support programs and their use in many of the new health care delivery models have made them a vital element in most healthcare systems. In fact, The Association for Behavioral Health and Wellness (2013) released a report that described several opportunities for behavioral health organizations to expand peer support services to new settings or to new responsibilities. Examples included placing peer support specialists in hospital emergency rooms to assist emergency staff in their interactions with mental health patients. Expanding the role of peer transition coaches for psychiatric hospital discharges and expanding the number of Whole Health Coaches are two additional promising strategies.

The President's New Freedom Commission on Mental Health, Achieving the Promise: Transforming Mental Health Care in America (2003) states that successfully transforming the mental health service delivery system rests on two principles. First, services and treatments must be consumer and family centered, geared to give consumers real and meaningful choices about treatment options and providers. Second, care must focus on enhancing a person's ability to successfully cope with life's challenges, on facilitating recovery, and on building resilience, and not just on managing symptoms.

In each area, peer services have demonstrated their effectiveness while supplementing more traditional models of psychiatric care. Peer support services have been effective in involving individuals and their families in their health care both by their advocacy and improvement of health literacy. These aspects of peer support have played a major role in improving what has been called "patient activation," a critical aspect of recovery and resilience. They have also significantly expanded the array of service options adding drop-in centers, working in inpatients settings, creating crisis stabilization programs and respite services. Their role in assisting the person in the recovery process by providing the necessary social supports for individuals to regain hope that life can improve, assisting the person in developing social networks and providing the guidance to obtain the necessary resources to support recovery is a significant accomplishment. The contribution of the peer workforce transcends mental health and serves as a model for the health workforce of the future.

## References


Amador, X. (2000). *I am not sick, I don't need help! How to help someone with mental illness accept treatment.* Peconic, NY: Vida Press.

Anderson, C. M., Griffin, S., Rossi, A., Pagonis, I., Holder, D. P., & Treiber, R. (1986). A comparative study of the impact of education vs. process groups for families of patients with affective disorders. *Family Process, 25*, 185–205.

Andresen, R., Oades, L., & Caputi, S. (2003). The experience of recovery from schizophrenia: Towards an empirically validated stage model. *Australian and New Zealand Journal of Psychiatry, 37*, 586–594.

Association for Behavioral Health and Wellness. (2013, January). Peer support services: A valuable component of behavioral healthcare. Available online athttp://www.abhw.org/publications/pdf/PSS%20Report.pdf

Bashor, K. (2014). Personal Communication. Office of Individual and Family Affairs. Arizona Department of Health, Division of Behavioral Health, Phoenix, Arizona.

Bluebird, G. (2008). *Paving new ground: Peers working in in-patient settings.* Alexandria, VA: National

Technical Assistance Center, National Association of State Mental Health Program Directors. Retrieved June 8, 2014 from http://www.nasmhpd.org/consumernetworking.cfm

Bouchard, L., Montreuil, M., & Gros, C. (2010). Peer support among inpatients in an adult mental health setting. *Issues in Mental Health Nursing, 31*, 589–598.

Braddock, C. H., Edwards, K. A., Hasenberg, N. M., Laidley, T. L., & Levinson, W. (1999). Informed decision-making in outpatient practice: Time to get back to basics. *Journal of the American Medical Association, 282*, 2313–2320.

Campbell, J. D. (1990). Self-esteem and the clarity of the self-concept. *Journal of Personality and Social Psychology, 59*, 538–549.

Campbell, J., & Leaver, J. (2003). *Emerging new practices in organized peer support*. Report from NTAC's National Experts Meeting, March 17–18, 2003. http://www.bu.edu/cpr/repository/documents/campbellleaver2003.pdf

Caplan, G., & Caplan, R. (2000). Principles of community psychiatry. *Community Mental Health Journal, 36*, 7–24.

Care Quality Commission. (2009). Mental health acute inpatient services survey: 2009. http://archive.cqc.org.uk/aboutcqc/howwedoit/involvingpeoplewhouseservices/patientsurveys/mentalhealthservices.cfm

Chamberlin, J. (1978). *On our own: Patient-controlled alternatives to the mental health system*. New York: Hawthorne.

Chinman, M., Rosenheck, R., Lam, J., & Davidson, L. (2000). Comparing consumer and non-consumer provided case management services for homeless persons with serious mental illness. *Journal of Nervous & Mental Disease, 188*, 446–453.

Chinman, M. J., Weingarten, R., Stayner, D., & Davidson, L. (2001). Chronicity reconsidered: Improving person-environment fit through a consumer run service. *Community Mental Health Journal, 37*, 215–229.

Clarke, G., Herinckx, H., Kinney, R., Paulson, R., Cutler, D., & Oxman, E. (2000). Psychiatric hospitalizations, arrests, emergency room visits, and homelessness of clients with serious and persistent mental illness: Findings from a randomized trial of two ACT programs vs. usual care. *Mental Health Services Research, 2*, 155–164.

Clay, S. (2005). *About us: What we have in common. On our own together: Peer programs for people with mental illness*. Nashville, TN: Vanderbilt University Press.

Coatsworth-Puspoky, R., Forchuk, C., & Ward-Griffin, C. (2006). Peer support relationships: An unexplored interpersonal process in mental health. *Journal of Psychiatric and Mental Health Nursing, 13*, 490–497.

Cobb, S. (1976). Social support as a moderator of life stress. Psychosomatic Medicine, 38, 300–314.

Cook, J. A., Copeland, M. E., Hamilton, M., Jonikas, J. A., Razzano, L. A., Floyd, C. B., et al. (2009). Initial outcomes of a mental illness self-management program based on wellness recovery action planning. *Psychiatric Services, 60*, 246–249.

Cook, J., Copeland, M. E., Hamilton, M., Razzano, L., Grey, D., Floyd, C., et al. (2011). Results of a randomized controlled trial of mental illness self-management using wellness recovery action planning. *Schizophrenia Bulletin, 38*, 881–891.

Copeland, M. E. (2007). *Wellness recovery action planning*. Retrieved January 13, 2009 from www.mentalhealthrecovery.com

Corrigan, P. W. (2006). Impact of consumer-operated services on empowerment and recovery of people with psychiatric disabilities. *Psychiatric Services, 57*, 1493–1496.

Corrigan, P., Mueser, K., Bond, G., Drake, R., & Solomon, P. (2008). *Principles and practice of psychiatric rehabilitation*. New York: Guilford Press.

Cuijpers, P. (1999). The effects of family interventions on relatives' burden: A meta-analysis. *Journal of Mental Health, 8*, 275–285.

Davidson, L., Bellamy, C., Guy, K., & Miller, R. (2012). Peer support among persons with severe mental illnesses: A review of evidence and experience. *World Psychiatry, 11*, 123–128.

Davidson, L., Chinman, M., Sells, D., & Rowe, M. (2006). Peer support among adults with serious mental illness: A report from the field. *Schizophrenia Bulletin, 32*, 443–450.

Deegan, P. E., & Drake, R. E. (2006). Shared decision-making and medication management in the recovery process: From compliance to alliance. *Psychiatric Services, 57*, 1636–1639.

Department of Health and Human Services. (2003). *New freedom commission on mental health, achieving the promise:Transforming mental health care in America.* Final report. Bethesda, MD: Author.

Dixon, L., Adams, C., & Lucksted, A. (2000). Update on family psychoeducation for schizophrenia. *Schizophrenia Bulletin, 26*, 5–20.

Dixon, L., Krauss, N., & Lehman, A. (1994). Consumers as service providers: The promise and the challenge. *Community Mental Health Journal, 30*, 615–634.

Dixon, L. B., Lucksted, A., Medoff, D., Burland, J., Stewart, B., Lehman, A., et al. (2011). Outcomes of a randomized study of a peer taught family-to family education program for mental illness. *Psychiatric Services, 62*, 591–597.

Dixon, L., Lucksted, A., Stewart, B., Burland, J., Brown, C. H., Postrado, L., et al. (2004). Outcomes of the peer-taught 12-week family-to-family education program for serious mental illnesses. *Acta Psychiactrica Scandinavica, 109*, 207–215.

Falzer, P. R. (2011). Comparing an intervention with treatment as usual. *Psychiatric Services, 62*, 807.

Felton, C. J., Stastny, P., Shern, D. L., Blanch, A., Donahue, S. A., Knight, E., & Brown, C. (1995). Consumers as peer specialists on intensive case management teams: Impact on client outcomes. *Psychiatric Services, 46*, 1037–1044.

Forchuk, C., & Brown, B. (1989). Establishing a nurse-client relationship. *Journal of Psychosocial Nursing and Mental Health Services, 27*, 30–34.
Forchuk, C., Chan, L., Schofield, R., Sircelj, M., Woodcox, V., Jewell, J., et al. (1998a). Bridging the discharge process. *Canadian Nurse, 94*, 22–26.
Forchuk, C., Hartford, K., & Blomqvist, A. (2002). *Therapeutic relationships: From hospital to community: First year results*. Ottawa: Report to the Canadian Health Services Research Foundation.
Forchuk, C., Jewell, J., Schofield, R., Sircelj, M., & Vallendor, T. (1998b). From hospital to community: Bridging therapeutic relationships. *Journal of Psychiatric and Mental Health Nursing, 5*, 197–202.
Forchuk, C., Martin, M. L., Chan, Y. L., & Jensen, E. (2005). Therapeutic relationships: From psychiatric hospital to community. *Journal of Psychiatric and Mental Health Nursing, 12*, 556–564.
Forchuk, C., Martin, M. L., Jensen, E., Ouseley, S., Sealy, P., Beal, G., et al. (2012). Integrating the transitional relationship model into clinical practice. *Archives of Psychiatric Nursing, 26*, 374–381.
Forchuk, C., Reynolds, W., Sharkey, S., Martin, M. L., & Jensen, E. (2007a). Transitional discharge based on therapeutic relationships: State of the art. *Archives of Psychiatric Nursing, 21*, 80–86.
Forchuk, C., Reynolds, W., Sharkey, S., Martin, M. L., & Jensen, E. (2007b). The transitional discharge model: Comparing implementation in Canada and Scotland. *Journal of Psychosocial Nursing and Mental Health Services, 45*, 31–38.
Gartner, A. J., & Riessman, F. (1982). Self-help and mental health. *Hospital & Community Psychiatry, 33*, 631–635.
Gates, L., & Akabas, S. (2007). Developing strategies to integrate peer providers into the staff of mental health agencies. *Administration and Policy in Mental Health and Mental Health Services Research, 34*, 293–306.
Gingerich, S. L., & Bellack, A. S. (1995). Research-based family interventions for the treatment of schizophrenia. *The Clinical Psychologist, 48*(1), 24–27.
Gordon, S. (2005). The role of the consumer in the leadership and management of mental health services. *Australasian Psychiatry: Bulletin of Royal Australian and New Zealand College of Psychiatrists, 13*, 362–365.
Hanrahan, N., Solomon, P., & Hurford, M. (2014). A pilot randomized control trial: Testing a transitional care model for acute psychiatric conditions. *Journal of the American Psychiatric Nurses Association, 20*, 315–327.
Hardiman, E. R., & Segal, S. P. (2003). Community membership and social networks in mental health self-help agencies. *Psychiatric Rehabilitation Journal, 27*, 25–33.
Harding, C. M., Brooks, G. W., Ashikaga, T., Strauss, J. S., & Breier, A. (1987). The Vermont longitudinal study of persons with severe mental illness, II: Long-term outcome of subjects who retrospectively met DSM-III criteria for schizophrenia.
Hemminger, H. (2012) *Adult inpatient psychiatric readmission data*. Maine Behavioral Health Data Forum, Maine Department of Health and Human Services.
Hodges, J., & Hardiman, E. (2006). Promoting health organizational partnerships and collaboration between consumer-run and community mental health agencies. *Administration and Policy in Mental health and Mental Health Services Research, 33*, 267–288.
International Association of Peer Supporters. (2013). *National ethical guidelines and practice guidelines for peer supporters*. Sparta, MI: Author.
Jacobson, N., Trojanowski, N., & Dewa, C. (2012). What do peer support workers do? A job description. *BMC Health Services Research, 12*, 205.
Janzen, R., Nelson, G., Trainor, J., & Ochocka, J. (2006). A longitudinal study of mental health consumer/survivor initiatives: Part IV—Benefits beyond the self? A quantitative and qualitative study of system-level activities and impacts. *Journal of Community Psychology, 34*, 285–303.
Jorm, A. F. (2000). Mental health literacy Public knowledge and beliefs about mental disorders. *The British Journal of Psychiatry, 177*, 396–401.
Kaplan, K., Salzer, M. S., & Brusilovskiy, E. (2012). Community participation as a predictor of recovery-oriented outcomes among emerging and mature adults with mental illnesses. *Psychiatric Rehabilitation Journal, 35*, 219–229.
Klein, A., Cnaan, R., & Whitecraft, J. (1998). Significance of peer social support for dually diagnosed clients: Findings from a pilot study. *Research on Social Work Practice, 8*, 529–551.
Landers, G. M., & Zhou, M. (2011). An analysis of relationships among peer support, psychiatric hospitalization and crisis stabilization. *Community Mental Health Journal, 47*, 106–112.
Landers, G. M., & Zhou, M. (2014). The impact of Medicaid peer support utilization on cost. *Medicare and Medicaid Research Review, 4*, 1.
Lawn, S., Smith, A., & Hunter, K. (2008). Mental health peer support for hospital avoidance and early discharge: An Australian example of consumer driven and operated service. *Journal of Mental Health, 17*, 498–508.
Leamy, M., Bird, V., Le Boutillier, C., Williams, J., & Slade, M. (2011). A conceptual framework for personal recovery in mental health: Systematic review and narrative synthesis. *British Journal of Psychiatry, 199*, 445–452.
Lukens, E., & McFarlane, W. (2004). Psychoeducation as evidence-based practice: Considerations for practice, research, and policy. *Brief Treatment and Crisis Intervention, 4*, 205–225.
Manning, S., & Suire, B. (1996). Consumers as employees in mental health: Bridges and roadblocks. *Psychiatric Services, 47*, 939–940.
McFarlane, W. R., Dixon, L., Lukens, E., & Lucksted, A. (2003). Family psychoeducation and schizophrenia: A review of the literature. *Journal of Marital and Family Therapy, 29*, 223–245.

McGill, C. W., & Patterson, C. J. (1990). Former patients as peer counselors on locked psychiatric inpatient units. *Patient Education and Counseling, 41*, 1017–1019.

Mead, S. (2003). Defining peer support. Available at http://www.mentalhealthpeers.com/pdfs/DefiningPeerSupport-1

Mead, S., & MacNeil, C. (2006). Peer support: What makes it unique? *International Journal of Psychosocial Rehabilitation, 10*(2), 29–37.

Meehan, T., Bergen, H., Coveney, C., & Thornton, R. (2002). Development and evaluation of a training program in peer support for former consumers. *International Journal of Mental Health Nursing, 11*, 34–39.

M-Power Testimony to the DMH Inpatient Study Commission Public Hearing Holyoke, MA. (2009).

National Alliance for Mental Illness. (1995). *Family to Family program*. New York: Author.

National Center for Education Statistics. (2006). *The health literacy of America's adults: Results from the 2003 national assessment of adult literacy*. Washington, DC: U.S. Department of Education.

Nelson, G., Ochocka, J., Janzen, R., & Trainor, J. (2006a). A longitudinal study of mental health consumer/survivor initiatives: Part I—Literature review and overview of the study. *Journal of Community Psychology, 34*, 247–260.

Nelson, G., Ochocka, J., Janzen, R., & Trainor, J. (2006b). A longitudinal study of mental health consumer/survivor initiatives: Part II—A quantitative study of impacts on new members. *Journal of Community Psychology, 34*, 261–272.

Nelson, G., Ochocka, J., Janzen, R., & Trainor, J. (2006d). Part IV—Benefits beyond the self? A quantitative and qualitative study of system-level activities and impacts. *Journal of Community Psychology, 34*, 247–260.

Nelson, G., Ochocka, J., Janzen, R., Trainor, J., Goering, P., & Lomotey, J. (2007). A longitudinal study of mental health consumer/survivor initiatives: Part V: Outcomes at 3-year follow-up. *Journal of Community Psychology, 35*, 655–665.

New Freedom Commission on Mental Health. (2003). *Achieving the promise: Transforming mental health care in America.* Final Report. Rockville, MD: Department of Health and Human Services.

Nikkel, R. E., Smith, G. D., & Edwards, D. (1992). A consumer-operated case management project. *Hospital & Community Psychiatry, 43*, 577–579.

Ockwell, C. (2012). Challenges and triumphs: Developing an inpatient peer support project. *The Journal of Mental Health Training, Education and Practice, 7*, 94–100.

O'Hagan, M. (2011). *Peer support in mental health and addiction: A background paper*. Wellington, New Zealand: Kites Trust.

Peplau, H. E. (1952). *Interpersonal relations in nursing: A conceptual framework of reference for psychodynamic nursing*. New York: Springer.

Perrazo, J., & Rodriguez, C. (2014). Personal communication. Kings County Hospital, Brooklyn, NY.

Pitt, V., Lowe, D., Hill, S., Prictor, M., Hetrick, S., Ryan, R., et al. (2013). *Consumer providers of care for adult clients of statutory mental health services*. Issue: Cochrane Database of Systematic Reviews. 3.

Pollio, D., North, C., & Douglas, A. (1998). Foster content and curriculum in psychoeducation groups for families of persons with severe mental illness. *Psychiatric Services, 49*, 816–822.

Repper, J., & Carter, T. (2011). A review of the literature on peer support in mental health services. *Journal of Mental Health, 20*, 392–411.

Reynolds, W., Lauder, W., Sharkey, S., Maciver, S., Veitch, T., & Cameron, D. (2004). The effects of a transitional discharge model for psychiatric patients. *Journal of Psychiatric and Mental Health Nursing, 11*, 82–88.

Rivera, J., Sullivan, A., Stavros, & Valenti, S. (2007). Adding consumer-providers to intensive case management: Does it improve outcome? *Psychiatric Services, 58,* 802–809.

Sadaaki, F., Starnino, V. R., Susana, M., Davidson, L., Cook, K., Rapp, C. A., et al. (2011). Effect of Wellness Recovery Action Plan (WRAP) participation on psychiatric symptoms, sense of hope, and recovery. *Psychiatric Rehabilitation Journal, 34*, 214–222.

Salyers, M., & Tsemberis, S. (2007). ACT and recovery: Integrating evidence-based practice and recovery orientation on assertive community treatment teams. *Community Mental Health Journal, 43*, 619–641.

Salzer, M. (2002a). Consumer-delivered services as a best practice in mental health care delivery and the development of practice guidelines. *Psychiatric Rehabilitation Skills, 6*, 355–383.

Salzer, M. (2002b). *Best practice guidelines for consumer-delivered services.* Unpublished paper developed for Behavioral Health Recovery Management Project. Web site: http://bhrm.org/guidelines.htm

Salzer, M., & Shear-Liptzin, S. L. (2002). Identifying consumer-provider benefits in evaluations of consumer-delivered services. *Psychiatric Rehabilitation Journal, 25*, 281–288.

Schmutte, T., Dunn, C., & Sledge, W. (2009). Characteristics of inpatients with a history of recurrent psychiatric hospitalizations: A matched-control study. *Psychiatric Services., 60*, 1683–1685.

Sells, D. L., Davidson, L., Jewell, C., Falzer, P., & Rowe, M. (2006). The treatment relationship in peer-based and regular case management for clients with severe mental illness. *Psychiatric Services, 57*, 1179–1184.

Simpson, A., Flood, C., Rowe, J., Quigley, J., Henry, S., Hall, C., et al. (2014). Results of a pilot randomized controlled trial to measure the clinical and cost effectiveness of peer support in increasing hope and quality of life in mental health patients discharged from hospital in the UK. *BMC Psychiatry, 14*, 30.

Sledge, W. H., Dunn, C. L., & Schmutte, T. (2008). Surprising predictor of rehospitalization. *Psychiatric Services., 59*, 577.

Sledge, W., Lawless, M., Sells, D., Wieland, M., O'Connell, M., & Davidson, L. (2011). Effectiveness of peer support in reducing readmissions of persons with multiple psychiatric hospitalizations. *Psychiatric Services, 62*, 541–544.

Smith, D. (2007). State medicaid directors letter #07–11. Retrieved February 20, 2008, from http://www.nasmd.org/SMD_Letters/docs/SMD_Letter_on_Peer_Support_Services.pdf

Solomon, P. (1996). Moving from psychoeducation to family education for families of adults with serious mental illness. *Psychiatric Services, 47*, 1364–1370.

Solomon, P., & Draine, J. (1995a). The efficacy of consumer case management team: 2-year outcomes of a randomized trial. *The Journal of Mental Health Administration, 22*, 135–146.

Solomon, P., & Draine, J. (1995b). One-year outcomes of a randomized trial of consumer case management. *Evaluation and Program Planning, 18*, 117–127.

Solomon, P., Hanrahan, H., Hurford, M., DeCesaris, M., & Josey, L. (2014). Lessons learned from implementing a pilot RCT of transitional care model for individuals with serious mental illness. *Archives of Psychiatric Nursing, 20*, 315–327.

Starnino, V., Mariscal, S., Hotler, M., Davidson, L., Cook, K., Fukui, S., et al. (2010). Outcomes of an illness self-management group using wellness recovery action planning. *Psychiatric Rehabilitation Journal, 34*, 57–60.

Stratford, A., Brophy, L., & Castle, D. (2012). Integrating recovery-oriented practice into psychiatric registrar training. *Australasian Psychiatry, 20*, 525–526.

Substance Abuse and Mental Health Services Administration. (2006a). *Psychoeducational multifamily groups*. Rockville, MD: Author.

Substance Abuse and Mental Health Services Administration. (2006b). *National registry of evidenced based programs and practices*. Rockville, MD: Author.

Substance Abuse and Mental Health Services Administration. (2009a). *The SAMHSA family psychoeducation*. Rockville, MD: Author.

Substance Abuse and Mental Health Services Administration. (2009b). *What are peer recovery support services*. Rockville, MD: Author.

Substance Abuse and Mental Health Services Administration. (2010a). *Peer support practices are EBPs*. Rockville, MD: Author.

Substance Abuse and Mental Health Services Administration. (2010b). *SAMHSA's working definition of recovery*. Rockville, MD: Author.

Substance Abuse and Mental Health Services Administration. (2011). *Consumer-operated services*. Rockville, MD: Author.

Substance Abuse and Mental Health Services Administration. (2012). *Equipping behavioral health systems and authorities to promote peer specialist/peer recovery coaching services*. Rockville, MD: Author.

Substance Abuse and Mental Health Services Administration. (2013). *Grantee spotlight: Peer coaches inspire success and motivate change at wellspring*. Rockville, MD: Author.

Thomas, L. & Anderson, C. (2015) Personal communication. Marc Community Resources. Community Transition Program.

Trachtenberg, M., Parsonage, M., Shepherd, G., & Boardman, J. (2013). *Peer support workers in mental health care: Is it good value for money?*. London, UK: Centre for Mental Health.

United States Department of Health & Human Services. (2011a). *Report to congress: National strategy for quality improvement in health care*. Bethesda, MD: Author.

United States Department of Health & Human Services. (2011b). *National consensus statement on mental health recovery*. Bethesda, MD: Author.

United States Department of Health and Human Services. (2011c). Report to congress. *National Quality Strategy*.

Vijayalakshmy, P., Smith, R., Schleifer, S., Morris, M., & McLennon, K. (2006) Facilitating discharge in state psychiatric institutions: A group intervention strategy. *Psychiatric Rehabilitation Journal, 29*, 183–188.

Walker, G., & Bryant, W. (2013). Peer support in adult mental health services: A meta-synthesis of qualitative findings. *Psychiatric Rehabilitation Journal, 36*, 28–34.

World Health Organization. (1979). *Schizophrenia: An international follow-up study*. New York: Wiley.

World Health Organization. (2012). *Quality Rights Tool Kit: Assessing and improving quality and human rights in mental health and social care facilities*. Geneva: Switzerland.

# Part III

# Advocacy, Resilience and Empowerment

# Self-advocacy and Empowerment

# 14

Michael S. Shafer, Vicki Staples and Lisa St. George

## Introduction

Admission to a hospital can be a stressful time for any patient and their family, friends and associates. Staff and professionals interacting with the patient can also experience stress and frustration, especially if the patient is in a heightened state of distress that manifests as anger or apathy. In addition to the disruption of familiar routines, any form of hospitalization comes with an invasion of privacy and autonomy, typically of the most personal and intimate of details. Frequently, these invasions include sharing a room with another person, restrictions placed on everything from what one eats to where one goes, to overseeing with whom one communicates. Additionally, invasive monitoring of one's bodily functions, repeated blood pressure and temperature readings, detailed accounting of urine and bowel movements can be routine during hospitalizations. Many individuals, if given the option, would avoid going to a hospital at all cost, due to the inhospitable nature of the setting.

M.S. Shafer (✉) · V. Staples
Center for Applied Behavioral Health Policy,
Arizona State University, Phoenix, AZ 85004, USA
e-mail: Michael.Shafer@asu.edu

L.St. George
Recovery Innovations International,
2701 N. 16th Street, Phoenix, AZ 85006, USA

Hospitalizations for a mental illness are more invasive and disempowering for patients and their families than hospitalizations for any other health condition. Hospitalization for a mental illness is frequently an unplanned and unscheduled event. Routinely, individuals with a mental illness are hospitalized against their will through legal procedures that vary from state to state, but which allow for forced or involuntary admissions. Contrasting the kind of care given to individuals with major physical health emergencies brought by supportive emergency medical technicians, being transported to a psychiatric hospital handcuffed and in the back of a police car, is not an uncommon experience for a person with a mental illness. During their stay in the hospital or other inpatient facility, individuals with a mental illness are likely to experience a variety of coercive measures and infringements upon their personal liberties that are unlike anything most individuals ever experience in a routine hospitalization. Such experiences may include forced medications, being physically restrained to a bed or a chair for a period of time, having personal possessions items taken from them, or experiencing isolation or seclusion, cut off from anyone else including fellow patients, hospital staff, family, and friends.

Under such circumstances, patients with a mental illness have been documented to experience a range of emotional reactions including loss of self-esteem, identity, self-control, and self-efficacy (Brophy and McDermott 2003; Danzer and Wilkus-Stone 2015; Hughes et al.



N.N. Singh et al. (eds.), *Handbook of Recovery in Inpatient Psychiatry*,
Evidence-Based Practices in Behavioral Health, DOI 10.1007/978-3-319-40537-7_14

2009; Rymaszewska 2007). Others have reported patient feelings of distress, sadness, and humiliation (Kuomanen et al. 2007), while patients have described hospitalization as depressing, unpleasant, and harmful (Olofsson and Jacobsson 2001). Such negative patient reactions are exacerbated when the patient is involuntarily hospitalized (Danzer and Wilkus-Stone 2015) and/or exposed to coercive treatment interventions, such as seclusion and restraint (Danzer and Wilkus-Stone 2015; Olofsson and Jacobsson 2001) and forced medication (Danzer and Wilkus-Stone 2015; Vuckovich and Artinian 2005). The immediate and long-term impact of these negative patient experiences upon their treatment engagement and the subsequent course of their treatment are significant, leading to a distrust of health care providers and provider systems, a disinclination to adhere to treatment protocols, or an unwillingness to seek out treatment when needed.

Given these considerations, strategies that can support patients to retain a certain degree of decision-making power and autonomy during periods of psychiatric hospitalization are essential. Maintaining as much decision-making power as possible while hospitalized reduces the degree of learned helplessness and institutionalization that patients experience. Additionally, research has demonstrated that patients' satisfaction with their psychiatric hospitalization, including those who were hospitalized against their will, can be attenuated by a variety of procedures. Patient satisfaction can be influenced by increasing (a) the information that is provided to the patient about various aspects of their hospitalization and treatment, (b) the degree to which health care providers treat the patient and family members with respect and engage them in the decision-making processes, (c) the degree to which the patient feels welcome, and comfortable, (d) the degree to which the facility operates with a set of rules and policies that are transparent and promote procedural justice and fairness, and the degree to which the facility provides a safe and structured set of activities and treatment programs, and (e) the degree to which the staff members support and relate to patients. Even in the face of involuntary hospitalization and coerced treatments, such as medication and seclusion and restraint, patients can experience both satisfaction and empowerment during their psychiatric hospitalization.

In this chapter, we contextualize the actualization of empowerment and self-advocacy among persons with a mental illness during a period of inpatient treatment and hospitalization. We begin by contextualizing the experience of psychiatric hospitalization and highlighting the common experiences of hospitalized patients that impinge upon their autonomous decision-making abilities, such as involuntary hospitalization, seclusion and restraint, and coerced treatment. Next, we provide a framework for autonomous decision-making and self-advocacy within the context of inpatient settings. This framework provides a definition of self-advocacy and empowerment, the legal basis for such rights, and a summary of research that has been conducted on strategies for promoting self-advocacy and patient empowerment. Finally, we summarize organizational and patient-level strategies that can help promote patient self-advocacy.

## Elements of Psychiatric Hospitalization that Impede Autonomous Decision-Making

The perceived or real threat to a patient's autonomy and empowered decision-making regarding their treatment are significant during their period of hospitalization. All too often, such hospitalizations occur against the wishes of the patient, and they frequently involve law enforcement along with a judicial order remanding the individual to the custody of the hospital for a specified period of time for observation and/or treatment. During this period, the individual may experience a variety of infringements against their personal liberties and decision-making capabilities along with degradation of basic human dignities. In fact, feelings of disempowerment and lack of control over their treatment is a pervasive and recurrent theme among patients hospitalized for a psychiatric condition (Katsakou et al. 2012). The three most common ways in which patients' rights and liberties are restricted during a psychiatric hospitalization include involuntary hospitalization, seclusion and restraint, and force or coerced treatment, including medication and electroconvulsive therapy (ECT).

## Involuntary Hospitalization

The involuntary hospitalization of individuals experiencing psychiatric symptoms has a long history in the Unites States and throughout the world. Despite its longstanding tradition, the practice remains highly controversial on a variety of moral and legal grounds (Dennis and Monahan 1996; Taylor and Bentley 2004), including evidence that involuntary commitments severely strain patient-provider relationships and further exacerbate an already deep reluctance to seek professional help (Danzer and Wilkus-Stone 2015; Jarrett et al. 2008).

Reported prevalence rates for involuntary admissions ranged between 4.4 and 36 % of all psychiatric hospitalizations in a comparative study of the countries comprising the European Union (Salize and Dressing 2004). The 10-year involuntary admission rate in Israel was reported to be 32 % of all psychiatric admissions for the period of 1991–2000 (Bauer et al. 2007). Most notably, a growing utilization of involuntary admissions was observed, climbing from 23.9 % of all admissions in 1991 to 38.1 % in 2000 (Bauer et al. 2007). This study also identified a variety of risk factors predicting involuntary hospitalizations, including a native-born Jewish male, aged 18–24 or 65 and older, single, less than 8 years of education, and diagnosis of schizophrenia or delusional psychosis (Bauer et al. 2007). Ironically, and unfortunately, comparable information on the rates and trends in involuntary hospitalizations in the United States is lacking (Riecher-Rossler and Rossler 1993).

A report issued by the Treatment Advocacy Center analyzed the quality of commitment laws throughout the United States, assigning letter grades to each states' quality of their inpatient commitment laws and their utilization of those laws (Stettin et al. 2014). Three forms of commitment laws were evaluated, including those governing inpatient commitments, outpatient commitment, and emergency evaluations. The evaluative scoring of the states and the various elements of involuntary commitment varied widely. However, no state received an overall grade of "A" and, in fact, 17 states were assigned an overall grade of "D" or "F". In interpreting their results, the authors noted, "...the quality of the civil commitment laws in the vast majority of states remains far below what is necessary to provide a readily accessible path to treatment and recovery for individuals with the most severe mental illnesses who are unable to seek care for themselves" (Stettin et al. 2014, p. 25).

A number of qualitative studies, the majority of which have been conducted in European countries, has captured the emotional and psychological state of these patients at the time of their commitment and, later on, at the time of their discharge. At the time of their commitment, the majority of patients who were involuntarily admitted were displaying acute psychotic symptoms, violent acts, or suicidality (Johnsen et al. 2007). Most involuntarily committed patients retrospectively described being unwell and/or at risk at the time of their admission, and acknowledging their inability to accurately assess their mental or emotional state at the time of their admission (Katsakou et al. 2012). In a qualitative study of involuntary psychiatric hospitalizations, patient's narratives revealed four overarching experiences, including: not being respected as a human being; not being involved in one's own care; receiving care that the patient perceived as meaningless or not good; and being an inferior kind of human being (Olofsson and Jacobsson 2001).

Not surprisingly, individuals who are the subject of involuntary hospitalization commitment proceedings frequently express significant feelings of distress, anger, and betrayal at the time of their commitment. Loss of self-esteem, identity, self-control, and self-efficacy as well as diminished hope in the possibility of recovery have all been reported as affective dimensions of patients' experiences from involuntary hospitalizations (Brophy and McDermott 2003; Danzer and Wilkus-Stone 2015; Hughes et al. 2009; Rymaszewska 2007). Interestingly, a consistent finding from this research is patients' retrospective acknowledgement of the appropriateness or justification for their forced treatment (Danzer and Wilkus-Stone 2015; Hopko et al. 2002; Katsakou et al. 2012). In fact, it has been reported that between 39 and 75 % of patients who were involuntarily hospitalized for their psychiatric illness reflected that their hospitalizations were appropriate (Katsakou et al. 2012).

## Seclusion and Restraint

In addition to the experience of involuntary hospitalization, seclusion and restraint can be common experiences of psychiatric hospitalization. Restraint can involve either physical, mechanical, or chemical impediment of the patient, with the latter expression also referred to as sedation. Physical restraint involves the manual or mechanical restriction of movement and physical action of the patient, including such devices as leather cuffs and belts as well as locked and secured hospital units (Kaltiala-Heino et al. 2003; Lee et al. 2003; Mayers et al. 2010). Seclusion involves the placement of the patient in a locked room from which free exit is denied, and is thought to provide containment, isolation, and sensory stimuli reduction (Kaltiala-Heino et al. 2003; Meehan et al. 2000; Mayers et al. 2010; Morrison and LeHane 1995; Wynn 2002).

The involuntary physical or chemical restraint of the psychiatric patient and/or the forced isolation or seclusion of the patient is reserved and justified in the cases of patients whose behavior is viewed to be extremely violent toward self or others, or disruptive to the therapeutic milieu. Obviously, such extreme measures are highly restrictive and seriously undermine any sense of patient autonomy or empowerment. Ironically, little research has been conducted on the relative prevalence of these practices, and there appear to be minimal safeguards in place to ensure their appropriate application.

As reported by Hendryx et al. (2010), 2–6 % of all psychiatric patients will experience seclusion or restraint during their period of hospitalization (Busch and Shore 2000), with some older research evidence suggesting that a small proportion of patients may disproportionately account for a large amount of the seclusion and restraint incidents (Hendryx et al. 2010). Larger psychiatric hospitals have reported median rates of 3.65 and 4.61 days of seclusion and restraint incidents, respectively, per 1000 patient days. For the patient experiencing seclusion, research has indicated that the average duration of each episode is approximately 17 h, and that cumulatively, such patients may experience 67 h of seclusion (Hendryx et al. 2010). Within the same study, patients were estimated to experience an average of 22.1 h of restraints per episode, and an average of 115.9 h of restraints cumulatively over the hospitalization experience. As such, research suggests that the use of seclusion and restraint, while a relatively infrequent occurrence among patients hospitalized with a psychiatric condition, tends to be clustered among a small subset of patients. Further, this research suggests that patients may be secluded or restrained upwards for a full day when it occurs.

## Coerced Treatment

Forcing or coercing a patient to receive treatment regardless of whether they have been court ordered to an inpatient facility is a highly controversial issue. Psychiatric patients may be pressured or forced to engage in programs, undergo procedures (such as electroconvulsive therapy—ECT), or take medications against their wishes. Psychological coercion in which the patient is pressured by family members or friends to comply (Kuosmanen et al. 2007; Strack et al. 2007; Strack and Schulenberg 2007). Coercive treatments have been described as intended to treat, help or cure the patient, regardless of the level of patient resistance, whereas coercive measures (i.e., seclusion and restraint) are often applied to control behavior or agitation (Kaltiala-Heino et al. 2003). Involuntary or forced medications, the most common form of coerced treatment, has been seen as unnecessarily coercive, traumatic, and even punitive (Kaltiala-Heino et al. 2003). Olofsson and Jacobsson (2001) reported that approximately 1/5 of the patients did not know the reason for being subjected to coercion.

High levels of perceived coercion were found to exacerbate the negative effects of custodial institutionalization on personality, the patient's view of their inpatient hospitalization, and preexisting hostile-dominant traits of some patients' personalities (Anestis et al. 2013; Danzer and Wilkus-Stone 2015; Georgieva et al. 2012). Patients reported experiencing fear and anger (Lucksted and Coursey 1995; Olofsson and Jacobsson 2001). The effects on the staff that use coercion are unknown (Kaltiala-Heino et al. 2003). Patients also reported that coercion and forced treatment negatively impact their relationship with the person(s) identified as initiating the pressure or force (Olofsson and Jacobsson 2001; Lucksted and Coursey 1995). Furthermore, studies indicate that the patient's legal status (i.e., voluntary versus involuntary) was not predictive of the patient's perception of being coerced (Eriksson and Westrin 1995; Lidz et al. 1995; Rogers 1993; Stender et al. 1997).

Patients who perceived less coercion tended to feel respected, treated fairly, and were more involved in decision-making processes concerning their treatment (Anestis et al. 2013; Danzer and Wilkus-Stone 2015). Programs that focus on coercion, and recognize that patients who refuse services are not a homogenous group and that there is a greater need to understand a patient's motives and reasons for the rejection, have shown success in using alternatives to coercion (Kaltiala-Heino et al. 2003).

## Legal and Ethical Standards of Patient Autonomy

A cornerstone of the community's mental health movement of the past half century in this country and others has been rights of direct service recipients to make meaningful, informed decisions about their care, their selection of providers, and the course and methods of their treatment. Emerging out of the civil rights movement of the 1960s, a variety of empowerment and self-advocacy voices began to be heard, including those of Ed Roberts and Judi Huemann that lead to the formation of the Independent Living Movement for people with physical disabilities. For people with psychiatric disabilities, the movement for patient empowerment and decision-making first began in Portland, Oregon by the likes of Dorothery Weiner, Tom Wittick, and Howard Geld. Mr. Geld, more commonly known as "Howie the Harp." The resulting manifesto of the psychiatric patient's movement was published by Chamberlain (1979) under the title, *On Our Own: Patient Controlled Alternatives to the Mental Health System.*

The growing mobilization and strength of people with physical and psychiatric disabilities set the stage for a number of legislative and judicial enactments that provide a framework for the recognition and protection of the individual rights and privileges of all Americans, regardless of their abilities and disabilities, including the Americans with Disabilities Act of 1990 (ADA), the Patient Bill of Rights of 1998, and the Olmstead v. L.C. case of 1999. Most significantly, Olmstead ruled that the unjustified segregation of persons with disabilities violated Title II of the ADA and required public entities to provide community-based services when such services are appropriate.

In 2003, the President's New Freedom Commission on Mental Health (2003) provided additional structure for the framework of a comprehensive, patient empowered mental health system in America. The Commission declared that the focus of services should be on recovery rather than symptom management, adding that the system presents barriers, which all too often add to the burden of mental illnesses for individuals, their families, and our communities. Consumers and family members are to "have access to timely and accurate information that promotes learning, self-monitoring, and accountability" and individualized plans of care developed "in full partnership with consumers and families". The partnership of personalized care outlined in the report hinges on choice of the health care professionals on the team, what and how care is to be provided, shared decision-making and providing persons with the option to agree or disagree with the treatment plan, and making available the highest quality of care and information to individuals and families, regardless of their race, gender, ethnicity, language, or place of residence. Implementing these recommendations from the President's New Freedom Commission can stimulate inpatient psychiatric facilities to become recovery-focused and person-centered. Implementing treatment planning processes that share decision-making with patients, their representatives, and the provider staff of the facility, can significantly improve patient outcomes, patient satisfaction, staff morale, while reducing critical incidents and hospital readmission.

## Strategies for Promoting Patient Autonomy and Decision-Making

A variety of strategies and approaches can facilitate the maximization of patient involvement and empowered decision-making during periods of psychiatric hospitalization. As noted in the preceding section, evidence demonstrates the value of maximizing patient decision-making and empowerment during such hospitalizations, resulting in a more satisfied patient, reduced rates of seclusion and restraint, and staff and patient injuries. Furthermore, evidence suggests that patients who experience greater decision-making and empowerment during their hospitalization are significantly less likely to be readmitted to the hospital. As health care providers face increasing scrutiny and financial penalty for patient readmissions, maximizing patient empowerment during psychiatric hospitalizations can be viewed as an insurance policy against such financial risks.

In this section, we present a variety of strategies that inpatient psychiatric facilities can take to support the decision-making and empowerment of their patients. These strategies must begin with an orientation of the hospital ward milieu that is embracing of a strengths-based, recovery-enabled approach to the care and treatment of people with psychiatric disabilities. Within this recovery culture, a variety of physical, programmatic, and provider/staff changes in policies and procedures have been shown to maximize the empowered decision-making of patients (Rider et al. 2000).

Similarly, there are strategies that patients, along with their family members and other caregivers can take to maximize their empowered authority during a psychiatric hospitalization. These strategies should be activated during periods of psychiatric stability and prior to hospitalization to ensure that a patient's informed treatment choices are duly recorded and legally recognized.

### Facility and Staff Cultural Orientation

The dichotomy of how a patient is viewed and treated by medical personnel when hospitalized on a medical/surgical unit compared to a patient with a serious mental illness who is experiencing a relapse of a chronic medical condition on an inpatient psychiatric unit provides the backdrop for the needed shifts in staff approach, cultural orientation, physical plant design, programming and policies.

Staff view patients on medical/surgical units as having a physical injury or ailment to their body. Typically, there is no blame associated with their condition nor are they shamed when they have to be readmitted for a relapse or due to complications associated with their condition. In contrast, staff view psychiatric patients on a psychiatric unit who may cycle in and out of the facility as somehow responsible for their condition. For example, the patient may be seen as malingering, attention seeking, seeking refuge, or non-adherent with medications or with treatment more generally. In reality, the patient may not have stable housing, employment, or other adequate supports and services in the community that precipitated his or her relapse.

Patients with co-occurring substance use disorders are often faced with additional stigma and may be blamed and shamed by inpatient treatment teams, community treatment staff and by family members. Co-occurring disorders can be a significant precipitator to an individual's relapse and a significant challenge to address in inpatient settings. Inpatient staff need to recognize and address the hopelessness that one feels when they have relapsed. Often substance abuse is a primary issue that prompted the need for hospitalization, yet service and discharge planning processes fail to recognize it as a coping mechanism or examine the underlying issues that need to be addressed in a holistic and recovery-oriented approach. Acute intoxication is likewise one way that individuals are frequently screened out for inpatient treatment and other services.

Reframing how patients on psychiatric units are regarded is clearly needed. Supervisors and co-workers need to hold each other accountable for creating an environment that is recovery-oriented, strength-based and patient empowered. Consistent with the President's New Freedom Commission on Mental Health (2003) report, inpatient facilities should offer patients choice of who is on their team, what and how care is to be provided, opportunities for shared decision-making, an option to agree or disagree with the treatment plan, and making available the highest quality of care and information to individuals and families.

Gordon (2005) reported that mental health professionals' attitudes toward consumers' participation in service management, planning, and involvement in their care and treatment adversely impacts consumer involvement on inpatient psychiatric units. Inpatient facilities can empower and support self-determination by using a person-centered or patient-centered planning (PCP) approach. Stewart et al. (1995) focused on six interrelated concepts in patient–centered care: (1) exploring both the disease and the illness experience; (2) understanding the whole person; (3) finding common ground regarding illness management; (4) incorporating prevention and health promotion; (5) enhancing the provider–patient relationship; and (6) being realistic about limitations and issues, such as the availability of time and resources. The interactions of these concepts include patient-as-person, clinician-as-person, shared power and responsibility, therapeutic alliance, and biopsychosocial model of health and illness.

The challenges to using a PCP approach in an inpatient setting may include the following: the patient's mental status (e.g., feelings of anger, betrayal, resentment, mistrust, lack of insight, and substance withdrawal issues); short length of stay and court time frames that require certain processes to occur in an expeditious manner; a focus on symptom reduction and discharge issues (e.g., lack of permanent housing); and family issues (e.g., availability during treatment team meetings and involvement, especially if they initiated the court ordered treatment). There are also opportunities to reduce these obstacles and facilitate the cultural shift to empowering patients and families in directing their care. Peer and family support on the units can aide in establishing rapport and bridge the transition to the community. Psychiatric rehabilitation and biopsychosocial models can be incorporated in the groups and inpatient programs. Ultimately the staff must shift their beliefs and recognize that the person is the expert in their own care and the family is a strength. Shifting power and the role of service providers to one that resembles a "consultant" who provides information, education and choice to support informed decision-making and not be a decision-maker or custodian responsible for directing and protecting the individual is critical. The PCP process itself promotes recovery, interdependence, accountability, personal responsibility, empowerment, self-advocacy and growth. Instituting a culture that supports the principles and practices of PCP starts with the executive leadership who must buy into the same philosophy.

Strength-based systems of care within hospital settings focus on the innate wisdom and strengths of individuals. While inpatient services are designed to support individuals when their symptoms put them at risk of harming themselves or others, the majority of patients are still able to communicate their preferences, hopes, and needs. When staff assume that patients are unable to offer valuable insight into who they are and what helps them, they remove the patient from being an important team member from their treatment team. Walsh and Boyle (2009) conducted focus groups to explore psychiatric inpatients' strategies for coping with a mental illness and identifying opportunities for acute inpatient psychiatric hospital services to facilitate the patient's recovery and empowerment. The main areas of concern for the patients were related to lack of information, communication, relationships, activities, self-help, patient involvement in care treatment plans, and the physical environment.

The lonely hours spent while in the hospital setting can be overwhelming and create strong feelings of hopelessness. Being able to have a connection to even one individual on the team will help the patient believe they are worthy of attention and kindness. As the relationship is created through interactive engagement, patients become invested in their care, their progress, and adherence to the plan that they have contributed to. Staff members can engage with the individuals they serve on at a human level as well as at a professional level. Further, an individual that demonstrates a firm, unending belief that recovery is possible for the patient even in the face of overwhelming illness, is identified as the most significant contributor to an individual's recovery (Detillion et al. 2004; Frankel et al. 2005).

McCann et al. (2008) examined 47 mental health professionals' attitudes towards consumer participation in two inpatient psychiatric units using the Consumer Participation and Consultant Questionnaire. They reported favorable attitudes toward participation in management such as identifying quality services and having a say in determining the delivery of services, care and treatment, and mental health planning. However, they were less supportive regarding matters that directly or indirectly related to their areas of responsibility, authority or expertise (e.g., access to medical records, prescribing medications and staff education) and expressed uncertainty whether consumer involvement would increase the stress levels among staff. Recommendations included developing guidelines for meaningful consumer participation on inpatient units, educational preparation for mental health professionals and the need for the mental health professionals to explore and discuss their own beliefs and practices regarding consumer participation.

Inpatient providers have also voiced an internal conflict between their need to protect and their desire to support a person's autonomy (Pellegrino and Thomasma 1987; Schwartz et al. 2013) and, if medicine is to achieve its goal of healing, these duties cannot remain in conflict (Pellegrino and Thomasma 1987). To support empowerment and create opportunities for patients to make decisions regarding their care, the inpatient staff and the milieu must espouse an orientation that is strengths-based and recovery-oriented in their approach to the care and treatment of people with psychiatric disabilities. Participatory dialogs is one organizational strategy that has been identified as a method to address this tension and create avenues for incorporating the principles and values of recovery to empower patients and improve inpatient care.

Participatory dialogs have been used in training mental health professionals and also in research and evaluation as a method to examine satisfaction with services. The SAMHSA (2012) guide, *Participatory Dialogues: A Guide to Organizing Interactive Discussions on Mental Health Issues among Consumers, Providers, and Family Members,* identified four goals: (a) to create better understanding and mutual respect among consumers, family members and professionals; (b) allow participants to speak from their experiences and belief systems in a safe atmosphere; (c) create partnership ventures through compromise and consensus; and (d) change attitudes and practices in the mental health system

Schwartz et al. (2013) used a provider–consumer dialog process to create positive changes in professional attitudes and consumer empowerment by exploring the tensions and personal values related to recovery in an institutional setting. This consumer–provider knowledge exchange facilitated the development of patient–staff partnerships to support a recovery-oriented model of care. One of the former patients in the Schwartz et al. (2013) study provided the following insight, attesting to the dichotomy that exists within an inpatient setting: "I discovered that the idea of consumer empowerment is difficult for the clinician, who must give up some of his or her own power and, at the same time, readjust the understanding of responsibility toward the client". Others voiced stories of feeling misunderstood and needing for their experiences to be acknowledged and not just their symptoms as exemplified by the following statement, "If you're a crazy person and you scream, all they hear is the scream … and you're pathologized for being angry and having an emotion" (p. 114). Patients reported that they felt that providers' stories took down the "shields of the profession and helped humanize the field of psychiatry" (Schwartz et al. 2003, p. 114). The researchers concluded that by naming and addressing inter- and intra-personal tensions, exploring divergence in values, openly addressing clinical concerns and risk, and including people with lived experience of mental illness in the design and delivery of services recovery-oriented care can be facilitated within institutional contexts.

Wadsworth and Epstein (1998) used a two-phased approach to build routine methods for staff at a major pubic psychiatric hospital to seek and receive consumers' evaluative feedback and collaborate with the patients to make changes to services as a result of the feedback. The first phase included a dialog to exchange experiences and thinking between staff and consumers. The second phase explored how staff–consumer feedback could be incorporated into the organizational structure and culture. The researchers found that staff were "dismayed by their own disempowerment within the service services and structure" (Wadsworth and Epstein 1998, p. 359). Based on the findings, the researchers identified four essential sites for supported dialogs to occur: (a) organizational decision-making forums, such as hospital program and management meetings, board meetings, staff selection and ethic committees, and feedback mechanisms; (b) staff–consumer dialog forums to examine beliefs, undiscussables and share thinking and assumptions; (c) consumer-only forums to provide emotional support to build on strengths to participate in such dialogs; and (d) staff-support methods, such as forums or other structures to support the staffs' needs. Emotional responses staff wanted to speak about included their fear, anxiety, rage, frustration and feeling of being treated badly. They felt these areas were forbidden to discuss, as it would dismantle their authority, and the construct between the "us"—the health professionals who are responsible, in control, competent—and "them"—the sick, emotional, dependent, incompetent and irrational patients (Wadsworth and Epstein 1998).

## Organizational Policies and Procedures

To transform services and embed a recovery philosophy of care, administrators and clinicians need to partner with patients to consider how recovery can influence an inpatient hospital's policies, practices and environments (Smith and Bartholomew 2006). Modifying the development and review process of an inpatient facility's policies and procedures to incorporate patient input is another key organization strategy that an inpatient hospital should implement to establish a recovery-oriented culture that increases avenues for patient empowerment, strengthens opportunities for self-advocacy, and supports self-determination and shared decision-making processes. Critical areas that should be examined include, but are not limited to, policies and procedures that relate to seclusion and restraint, medication management, collaborative documentation (which levels the playing the field and reduces secrecy when read to the patient), service and discharging planning, critical incidents and debriefings, and advanced directives.

Seclusion and restraint must be viewed as a treatment failure, and policy and procedures clearly need to be aligned with a "no force first" philosophy. Reductions in seclusions were found after suggesting changes in the seclusion procedure to focus on better assessment and communication (Olofsson and Jacobsson 2001) and interventions to reduce the use of seclusion and restraint have been shown to be effective (Hendryx et al. 2010). Debriefing every incident with the patient and staff involved is critical. In addition, advanced directives can reduce the number of restraints and the need for seclusion. Staff initially may be concerned with the adoption of a no force first or zero restraint approach; however, it has been found that staff injuries actually go down if properly implemented.

Medication management and the associated policies should include expectations that the patient, psychiatrist, inpatient team, peer support specialist or advocate (upon request) participate in the discussions and decisions regarding education, initiation, modification or discontinuation of prescribed medication while hospitalized and prior to discharge. When forced medications are required, the patient should be involved to the greatest extent possible. Respecting the patient's autonomy when administering involuntary medications may seem like a contradiction, although it is possible to empathetically give the patients the choice between oral and injectable medications (Danzer and Wilkus-Stone 2015; Vuckovich and Artinian 2005).

## Physical Plant and Environmental Programming

The physical structure of inpatient unit is important and can create barriers to self-advocacy among patients or it can create the kind of environment that empowers all of the people within it to engage, interact, and self-advocate. For the individuals being served on the unit, the physical barrier creates an "us versus them" environment. Patients feel separated from staff members and they see them as unreachable behind the glass.

An unexpected area that either contributes to or creates barriers against good self-advocacy for individuals who are being supported within an inpatient unit is the physical make-up of the units and the environment within them. Within a hospital setting, barriers include the nurses station being a bubble—a glassed-in enclosure surrounding an area where nurses make notes, review charts, and engage with other staff members. Nursing stations that are enclosed create both a physical and an emotional barrier for both the staff and the patients.

The staff can remain inside their bubble and never allow themselves to get to know the patients on the unit. Engaging with and taking an active role in the wellbeing of the patients can increase satisfaction with one's work, as they interact and directly support individuals from admission to hospital discharge. While the nurses remain in their bubble, the emotional barrier prevents them from easy access to the very people who need them. Remaining inaccessible within a closed space prevents the development of relationships and reduces the chance for a working alliance to develop between staff and the patients. One might think that due to the patients' severe symptoms while hospitalized, there is no chance that a working alliance could develop. However, evidence has shown that severity of symptoms does not affect the development of a therapeutic relationship and that therapeutic relationship forms the foundation for a working alliance (Horvath 1994).

While there is a need for safety in units, a balance must be struck between harsh and uninspiring surroundings and beautifully designed units that are pleasing to the eye and comforting to the soul. The idea of *healing spaces* includes the physical space, the staff demeanor being kind, respectful, and hopeful, as well as a culture of recovery in which everyone on the team believes that recovery is possible for every patient. Spaces that are quiet, and policies that ensure flexibility with family visits, support the recovery of patients and provide comfort to family members. Family members and friends must have the same access to loved ones as exists within hospitals providing physical health care. The love and support from family and friends lead to higher levels of recovery as they do for patients recovering from a host of physical health concerns. Family, friends, and peer support workers on the unit can increase the number of hopeful relationships that each patient has while in the hospital.

Having one set of standards for physical health care needs and another for psychiatric health care needs establishes stigma, and is a subtle form of discrimination. "A recurrent theme that runs through the mental health literature is the stigma attached to mental illness…" (Curtis et al. (2009). Identifying people with serious mental illness as somehow inherently dangerous or deviant has historically influenced the development of hospital environments. While many hospital environments no longer use a circular structure, it is not uncommon to see a centralized nursing station enclosed with glass from which staff can observe the activities of patients. The design that creates an observation point diminishes interaction, relationship, and thereby recovery. It is important that psychiatric hospital spaces support the privacy and independence of the patients. Supporting independence helps people to not lose touch with their life in the community. Today, the need to stay connected to the world using social media and email is important to many people. Having computers on each unit for patient use can assist in keeping them connected to their social supports.

Many studies have demonstrated the health benefits of healing spaces in a hospital setting (Francis and Glanville 2001; Ulrich 1984; Ulrich et al. 1991; Whitehouse et al. 2001). Soft furniture, open spaces and bright sunlight can improve the atmosphere of the hospital. Offering pleasant garden spaces, having indoor plants, or water features can contribute to a comforting supportive atmosphere. At the heart of the healing space is access to staff the reduction of barriers to relationships needed to support the patients to be able to practice good self-advocacy.

## Services and Treatment Programming

The inpatient milieu including psychological, physical, social, political, and spiritual components of the hospitalization experience is more than a mere predictor of patient satisfaction—it is a central experience in the patient's hospitalization and has as much potential for destruction as it does for healing and remains an important but often neglected component of psychiatric treatment (Thibeault et al. 2010). A concerted effort to provide a welcoming and compassionate environment is needed as a part of the patient's admission, introduction, and orientation to the unit.

The admission process can be overwhelming to anyone and especially to a patient who may be embarrassed, scared, distraught, experiencing severe symptoms, or brought to the hospital against their will. Staff should be patient, speak in a non-brisk manner, and recognize that an individual in an acute crisis may not be able to take in/process all the information being presented or may have trouble reading materials received in their admission packet. In order to support the person in making informed decisions regarding their care and ensure informed consent is provided, staff may need to wait until acute psychiatric symptoms that interfere with the patient's cognitive processing (e.g., thinking clearly, processing information, paying attention or remembering information) or inhibit their ability to engage in a dialog (e.g., due to intoxication, hallucinations, delusions or paranoia) have diminished. Staff should consider repeating the entire admission process at a time when the patient is able to fully process the information while also allowing ample time for the patient to ask questions. Relatives and carers accompanying the patient should also be provided information about the hospital regulations, provision of services and treatment, carer support services and the opportunity to ask questions (Walsh and Boyle 2009).

It is important to orient the patient to inpatient setting by showing them around the unit and to acquaint them with the unit's rules and protocols. Patients should be reassured that, in addition to their mental health concerns, their physical problems will be identified and addressed (Walsh and Boyle 2009). They must also be informed of their patient rights including the complaint procedure.

When appropriate, each of the members of the inpatient team should be introduced to the patient and their roles reviewed. Walsh and Boyle (2009) recommended that independent support should be provided (e.g., by an advocate, peer support specialist) and professionals (e.g., psychologists, psychotherapists, dual diagnoses experts) should be readily available.

The inpatient program needs to provide multiple activities focused on engaging the patient and offering a menu of services designed to empower and support self-determination in all aspects of care. The language used by medical staff and the services provided should be recovery-focused and it is essential for staff to continuously seeking out the person's strengths rather than concentrate only on the deficits and symptomology of the illness. Strategies to reduce patients' experiences of vulnerability and abandonment, and strengthen processes that create a sense of connectedness, engagement, and affirmation should be instituted (Thibeault et al. 2010).

Boredom in the hospital can be detrimental to the patient and there needs to be opportunities for creativity that are age appropriate. Kiosks that allow a patient to explore information at their own pace and computer-/phone-based apps on topics such as recovery, health and wellness, and services available in the community can address not only monotony in an inpatient setting but can also be educational and empowering.

Staff should also recognize that people in crisis often turn to a "higher power" or seek a spiritual connection and find healthy ways to support the individual's needs instead of judging or trying to assess if their quest is "good or bad" or a byproduct of the mental illness. Non-denominational, faith-based, spiritual and religious materials and resources should be available on the unit in addition to traditional Christian-based information.

Patients report that their relationship with the nurses and clinicians is a key aspect of the inpatient milieu, and their person-to-person interactions on the inpatient unit creates meaning for them (Thibeault et al. 2010). Lack of privacy, the presence of specific barriers to movement, and physically separate spaces for staff and patients are symbols of social separation, power imbalance, and erosion of personhood. Danzer and Wilkus-Stone (2015) found that patients were more satisfied when they experienced a hospital environment that was warm, friendly, safe, comfortable, and accommodated their individual needs based on reasonable rules and prepared them for discharge. Patients reported the needed for inpatient staff to help them settle into daily routines and get involved in structured daily activities. Activities, such as making art projects, taking walks, and playing games, were reportedly helpful for patients who were less verbal.

Another opportunity for patients to be empowered is to provide them avenues to participate in the decision process and negotiation of medications at initiation, when dosages are modified, and prior to discontinuation. Information on the reasons why a change of medication is being recommended should be provided, all concerns of the patient should be addressed, and user-friendly materials on medications also should be provided (Walsh and Boyle 2009). One study found that patients become highly reluctant and refuse medications when their autonomy is not respected during medication processes (Danzer and Wilkus-Stone 2015).

Walsh and Boyle (2009) endorsed negotiating the timing of discharge with each patient, with ample time allowed for consideration of practical arrangements regarding their returning home (e.g., taking into account patient's financial situation, issues with utilities, ensuring there is adequate food at home). Discussing with the patient a comprehensive discharge plan including involvement family, follow up services needed including support groups and outpatient mental health services. Discharge planning should start at the earliest opportunity to alleviate patients' fears and anxiety.

## Peer Support Specialists

A Peer Support Specialist can help facilitate self-advocacy of all inpatients. A peer support worker is an individual who is in recovery from mental health challenges, addiction, or a co-occurring mental health and addiction challenge. They work with individuals in a manner that validates the lived experience of having been in a psychiatric hospital or otherwise treated for mental health challenges, addiction challenges, or co-occurring challenges of mental health and addiction. Their job description includes spending time with individuals they are serving. They can talk with people help them practice what they want to say before meetings with treatment team members, support them in those meetings, and just be a good listening ear. The mutuality puts them on equal footing with those they serve and their lived experience is the key to an almost instant relationship. Another aspect of peer support is their value as an example that recovery is a fact, and once the people they are serving understand that they are in recovery, it ignites an inextinguishable spark of hope. The role, responsibilities, and outcomes of using peer support specialists inpatient psychiatric hospitals is covered in great detail by Franczak and Dye (2016) in this book.

## Psychiatric Advance Directives

Enacted in 1990, the Federal Patient Self Determination Act addresses the rights of health care users (including mental health care) to stipulate in advance how they would like to be treated by health care providers when they are incapacitated and offset the perceived imbalance between health care consumers and providers. Under this federal law, an advance directive is defined as: "A written instruction, such as a living will or durable power of attorney for health care, recognized under state law (whether statutory or as recognized by the courts of the State), relating to the provision of health care when the individual is incapacitated" (42 USC § 1395 cc(f)(3)). Although this Act did not grant additional individual rights as this is still under the authority of state law, the federal law did require policies and procedures on advanced directives be developed by hospitals and other providers (including psychiatric hospitals and other mental health providers) and healthcare plans. The right to accept or refuse medical treatment and have an advance directive and/or appoint a health care agent is mandated in state law. However, federal and state laws do not require individuals to complete any form of advance directive nor can advanced directives be required as a requisite for treatment.

The federal law also specifies mandates for entities in order to be paid under Medicare or Medicaid, including (1) written policies and certain procedures with respect to advance directives, (2) document in the patient's medical record whether or not the patient has executed an advance directive, (3) comply with all State laws regarding advance directives, (4) not condition the provision of care or otherwise discriminate against an individual based on whether or not the individual has executed an advance directive, (5) inform the individual that complaints concerning implementation of these advance directive requirements may be filed with the state agency that surveys and certifies Medicare and Medicaid providers, and (6) provide staff and community education on issues related to advance directives. These mandates encompass both medical advanced directive and psychiatric advanced directives as individuals with mental illness have equal rights under this law.

Within federal law, and most state laws, individuals are allowed to combine advance healthcare decision-making and advance mental healthcare decision-making in one document or they can establish separate advanced directives. A single care agent may be appointed to address both health and mental health care issues or two different agents may be identified. Currently, there are 25 states that have adapted specific Psychiatric Advance Directive (PAD) statues. PADs are legal documents that empower individuals to specify their wishes for future psychiatric care and appoint a proxy to make decisions should a crisis arise in which they become acutely ill, incapacitated and unable to express their desires. PADs allow individuals to plan for a crisis when they are feeling well and support the recovery process after a crisis as interventions received are those that work well and are effective as specified by individual. During times when an individual is most vulnerable to a loss of autonomy and in need of assistance, PADs maintain a person's self-determination and ensure their preferences are known and honored (Kim et al. 2007). PADs give people control over their care and treatment especially when they are not able to voice preferences due to a mental health crisis. Communication between individuals and their families, friends, healthcare professional and other professionals is enhanced and individuals are protected from unwanted, ineffective and potentially harmful interventions and treatments. PADs are valuable empowerment tools as they give people control over their recovery through their own individual voice and personal choices.

Managed care health plans are required to provide information on advanced directives at the time of enrollment and patients are asked whether they have an advanced directive or provided information on advanced directives (including psychiatric advanced directives) upon admission to a hospital. However, when a patient is unable to state whether they have an advanced directive and is unable to receive information due their mental illness, the provider should give the information to the family or surrogate instead. The provider is still required to give the information directly to the patient once they are no longer incapacitated.

PADs are a non-coercive alternative to involuntary hospitalizations that support autonomy and self-determination and reduce mandated treatment and involuntary hospitalization when a person cannot express preferences or needs. An advance instruction or a healthcare power of attorney (HCPA) may be included in the PAD. PADs are typically not developed when an individual is in a psychiatric inpatient setting and should be created when the individual is well and able to indicate his or her future treatment preferences with the understanding that they will be honored during periods of decisional incapacity.

Advance instructions may include who to contact, when to contact them, relapse factors, preferred methods for deescalating a crisis situation, preferences for medications, treatment interventions that should or should not be initiated, refusal of specific treatments (e.g., seclusion, restraint, ECT), and choice of particular hospitals or crisis facilities. Although some states limit the timeframe, typically a PAD is valid until revoked. Usually, a patient can revoke their PAD at any time unless declared incompetent or incapacitated, or they identify in the PAD that they may not revoke it at times when they are in the hospital or otherwise in a crisis. State laws vary and typically a signature of a witness or notary public is required, but most states do not mandate an attorney to sign.

Some organizations have developed formats that blend PADs with Wellness Recovery Action Plans and crisis intervention plans. Additional areas that may be addressed in a PAD include what the person enjoys doing, things that relieve stress and make the person feel better, triggers and strategies for controlling symptoms, indicators that the person is not doing well/warning signs, current medications and those to avoid, who to notify and contact information for service providers, and family members and other who the person wanted involved in their care.

The HCPA, also referred to as a healthcare agent, healthcare proxy, or durable power of attorney for health care, allows a second party to act on the individual's behalf should they becomes acutely ill and unable to make decisions about treatment. This representative makes treatment decisions on the individual's behalf (that is, using substitute judgment for the client's known preferences) when they are unable to do so (Appelbaum 2004). When possible, these decisions are to be consistent with preferences and choices outlined by the patient. The HCPA requirements may also vary from state to state, but they typically require that the individual, witnesses, or a notary public sign the document. In addition, there needs to be a signature indicating that the appointed agent appointed has accepted the responsibility to make mental health treatment decisions on behalf of the patient. The health care power of attorney and/or mental health care power of attorney may also need to be filed and registered with the Secretary of State in a form prescribed by the Secretary of State. The National Resource Center on Psychiatric Advanced Directives (http://www.nrc-pad.org) has a plethora of information on PADs, including state by state information, information for patients and consumers, health and legal professionals, and family and friends, current research and legal issues, and resources.

Providers document in the medical record whether the person was provided with information on PADs and if the advanced directive was executed. Individuals are encouraged to carry a copy of their PAD with them, share copies with service providers and family members, and have copy in a convenient location so that, in case of an emergency or crisis, they have easy access and can remember were to retrieve it from. PADs should also be included in the medical record and, with expansion of electronic medical records, organizations should be able to flag the person's file to indicate that one has been developed and shared with other service providers.

A variety of clinical outcomes may result from the use of PADs, including but not limited to treatment engagement, treatment satisfaction, treatment adherence, and working alliance. Additional benefits of PADs include increases in service utilization which can also positively impact crisis early intervention and crisis management by deescalating the crisis, identifying alternatives to hospitalization, timely notification of clinicians and family members regarding decomposition, or (if hospitalization is required) improved inpatient management strategies (Van Dorn et al. 2010).

Although advanced directives for persons with a serious mental illness date back to the 1970s, and despite the multitude of benefits of PADs, this process is still rarely used. In a survey of 193 social workers, few had knowledge of PADs, with only 5 % reported being very familiar with advanced instructions and only 15 % reported being very familiar with HCPAs for mental health (Scheyett et al. 2008). Van Dorn et al. (2010) reviewed the literature and examined four studies on the prevalence of or demand for PADs and concluded that, although individuals expressed great interest in completing PADs, the rate of completion remained low. Lack of both support and knowledge of PAD is a barrier because the majority of individuals require some level of assistance in completing them (Peto et al. 2004).

Studies have shown that although individuals with serious mental illness report great interest in completing a PAD, the low rates of completion have also been associated with illness-related barriers, consumers misunderstanding of PADs, lack of resources to complete PADs, inability to identify a proxy decision-maker, and complexity of the PAD process (e.g., having witnesses sign, documents notarized, and filing with medical record or registry). Swanson et al. (2003) described the majority of consumers (77 %) reported that they lacked the understanding of how to complete a PAD on their own. In another study, three-quarters of the 462 participants reported barriers related to the actual PAD documents and one-third indicated barriers with external support for PADs, including having no one they trusted to make decisions on their behalf (Van Dorn et al. 2006a, b).

In another study, Kim et al. (2007) found that although study participants were enthusiastic regarding the implementation of PADSs, they were concerned with clinicians' lack of knowledge of PAD. Some participants even reported being uncomfortable at even mentioning they had a PAD as they were fearful of receiving a negative response or receiving an involuntary treatment while receiving hospitalization.

The clinician's knowledge and attitude toward PADs impacts implementation and whether the patient's preferences are honored or even inquired about. Although clinical issues, including concerns with the identified treatments, have been acknowledged as a barrier, environmental issues such as the inability to access the PAD or ability to reach the HCPA during a crisis situation appear to be of more concern (Van Dorn et al. 2006a, b). Srebnik and Brodoff (2003) found that 90 % of clinicians surveyed would be more likely to support directives if a clinician endorsed the client's competence at the time the document was completed, although there is no required demonstration of competence needed when an individual completes medical advance directives.

Clinicians concerns that PADs will not allow them to treat patients aligned with community standards of care are not supported by the empirical research. Kim et al. (2007) cited two studies that reviewed over 340 completed PADs and found that none refused all treatment. Furthermore, the U.S. Court of Appeals for the 2nd Circuit struck down a state law that allowed mental health professionals to override a person's advance refusal of psychotropic medications.

Van Dorn et al. (2006a, b) reported that only 4–13 % of mental health patients receiving outpatient services had completed a PAD. In another study, the strongest predictor of the use of advanced directives was when a surrogate decision-maker was involved in the crisis. Directives were over five times more likely to be accessed for people who had repeated crises, suggesting that use increases as patients and clinicians become familiar with the crisis circumstances that trigger accessing directives. Those without a substance use diagnosis were four times more likely to have a directive accessed and individuals without prior outpatient commitment orders were six times more likely to have a directive accessed. Individuals who were identified as "higher functioning" and having fewer hospitalizations were also more like to have advanced directives accessed (Srebnik et al. 2003).

Despite these barriers, interventions to increase the completion of PADs, including a structured facilitated process using a semi-structured manualized interview and a computer-assisted program, have been successful (Kim et al. 2007). Outcomes associated with these interventions include improvement in treatment satisfaction, working alliance, competence to make treatment decisions and reductions in coercive crisis interventions including police transport and involuntary commitments (Elbogen et al. 2006; Van Dorn et al. 2006a, b). All parties involved, including inpatient and outpatient services providers, service recipients and family members, need to be educated on how to complete PADs and the positive outcomes attributable to this powerful tool that supports self-advocacy, self-determination and empowerment. As PADs become more popular, they could usher in a new era of revolution in medical decision-making, greatly increasing patient authority over medical decisions (Hoge 1994).

## Conclusion

Psychiatric hospitalization is unlike any other form of hospitalization. Individuals who experience hospitalization for their psychiatric illness are frequently hospitalized against their will and can be subjected to treatment and programming procedures to which they do not consent and/or experience radical infringements upon their decision-making authority. This chapter summarized the extent and experience of patient's psychiatric hospitalizations while offering a number of facility and patient-based strategies that can enhance patient decision-making and autonomy.

It is reasonable to assume that access to psychiatric hospitalization will increase in the future as a result of healthcare reform. Significant increases have been reported in the individuals with health insurance as a result of Medicaid expansion and the establishment of government subsidized health insurance plans. Similarly, healthcare reform has required that health plans insure parity in access and reimbursement for mental health and substance abuse treatment, consistent with coverage for medical and surgical procedures for other health conditions. As a result, it is reasonable to assume that more inpatient facilities will offer psychiatric treatment and that more individuals may have access to this form of treatment as needed. As inpatient psychiatric care access increases, it will be critical that such facilities implement the types of actions outlined in this chapter. Similarly, as more individuals obtain health insurance and gain access to care, it will be essential that they and their families establish the legal mechanisms that will ensure adherence to the patient's treatment wishes during inpatient care.

## References


Anestis, A., Daffern, M., Thomas, S., Podubinski, T., Hollander, Y., Lee, S., & Kulkarni, J. (2013). Predictors of perceived coercion in patients admitted for psychiatric hospitalization and the stability of these perceptions over time. *Psychiatry, Psychology, and the Law, 20*(4), 492–503.

Appelbaum, P. (2004). Psychiatric advance directives and the treatment of committed patients. *Psychiatric Rehabilitation, 55*(7), 751–763.

Bauer, A., Rosca, P., Grinshpoon, A., Khawaled, R., Mester, R., Yoffe, R., & Ponizovsky, A. (2007). Trends in involuntary psychiatric hospitalization in Israel 1991–2000. *International Journal of Law and Psychiatry, 30*, 60–70.

Brophy, L., & McDermott, F. (2003). What's driving involuntary treatment in the community? The social, policy, legal, and ethical context. *Australian Psychiatry, 111*, 84–90.

Busch, A. B., & Shore, M. F. (2000). Seclusion and restraint: A review of recent literature. Harvard *Review of Psychiatry, 8*, 261–270.

Chamberlain, J. (1979). *On our own: Patient controlled alternatives to the mental health system*. New York: McGraw-Hill.

Curtis, S., Gesler, W., Priebe, S., & Francis, S. (2009). New spaces of inpatient care for people with mental illness: A complex 'rebirth' of the clinic? *Health & Place, 15*(1), 340–348.

Danzer, G., & Wilkus-Stone, A. (2015). The give and take of freedom: The role of involuntary hospitalization and treatment in recovery from mental illness. *Bulletin of the Menninger Clinic, 79*, 255–280.

Dennis, D. L., & Monahan, J. (1996). *Coercion and aggressive community treatment: A new frontier in mental health law*. New York: Plenum Press.

Detillion, C. T., Craft, E., Glasper, B., Prendergast, B., & Devries, A. C. (2004). Social facilitation of wound healing. *Psychoneuroendocrinology, 29*, 1004–1011.

Elbogen, E. B., Swartz, M. S., Van Dorn, R., Swanson, J. W., Kim, M., & Scheyett, A. (2006). Clinical decision-making and views about psychiatric advance directives. *Psychiatric Services, 57*, 350–355.

Eriksson, K. I., & Westrin, C. G. (1995). Coercive measures in psychiatric care: Reports and reactions of patients and other people involved. *Acta Psychiatrica Scandinavica, 92*, 225–230.

Francis, S., & Glanville, R. (2001). *Building a 2020 vision: Future healthcare environments*. London, UK: The Nuffield Trust and RIBA Future Studies.

Franczak, M., & Dye, C. (2016). Peer support services. In N. N. Singh, J. Barber, & S. Van Sant (Eds.), *Handbook of recovery in inpatient psychiatry*. New York: Springer.

Frankel, R. M., Sung, S. H., & Hsu, J. T. (2005). Patients, doctors, and videotape: A prescription for creating optimal healing environments? *Journal of Alternative and Complementary Medicine, 11* (Supplement 1), S-31–S-39.

Georgieva, I., Mulder, C. L., & Whittington, R. (2012). Evaluation of behavioral changes and subjective distress after exposure to coercive inpatient interventions. *BMC Psychiatry, 12*, 54.

Gordon, S. (2005). The role of the consumer in the leadership and management of mental health services. *Australasian Psychiatry, 13*(4), 362–365.

Hendryx, M., Trusevich, Y., Coyle, F., Short, R., & Roll, J. (2010). The distribution and frequency of seclusion and/or restraint among psychiatric inpatients. *Journal of Behavioral Health Services and Research, 37*, 272–281.

Hoge, S. (1994). On being "too crazy" to sign into a mental hospital: The issue of consent to psychiatric hospitalization. *Bulletin of the American Academy of Psychiatry and the Law, 22*, 431–450.

Hopko, D., Averill, P., Cowan, K., & Shah, N. (2002). Self-reported and treatment outcome among non-offending involuntary inpatients. *Journal of Forensic Psychiatry, 13*(1), 88–106.

Horvath, A. (1994). Research on the alliance. In A. Horvath & L. Greenberg (Eds.), *The working alliance: Theory, research and practice* (pp. 259–286). New York: Wiley.

Hughes, R., Hayward, M., & Finlay, W. (2009). Patients' perceptions of the impact of involuntary inpatient care on self, relationships, and recovery. *Journal of Mental Health, 18*(2), 152–160.

Jarrett, M., Bowers, L., & Simpson, A. (2008). Coerced medication in psychiatric inpatient care: Literature review. *Journal of Advanced Nursing, 64*(6), 538–548.

Johnsen, L., Øysæd, H., Børnes, K., Moe, T., & Haavik, J. (2007). A systematic intervention to improve patient information routines and satisfaction in a psychiatric emergency unit. *Nordic Journal of Psychiatry, 61*, 213–218.

Kaltiala-Heino, R., Tuohimäki, C., Korkeila, J., & Lehtinen, V. (2003). Reasons for using seclusion and restraint in psychiatric inpatient care. *International Journal of Law and Psychiatry, 26*(2), 139–149.

Katsakou, C., Rose, D., Amos, T., Bowers, L., Mccabe, R., Oliver, D., et al. (2012). Psychiatric patients' views on why their involuntary hospitalization was right or wrong: A qualitative study. *Social Psychiatry and Psychiatric Epidemiology, 47*, 1169–1179.

Kim, M., Dorn, R., Scheyett, A., Elbogen, E., Swanson, J., Swartz, M., et al. (2007). Understanding the personal and clinical utility of psychiatric advance directives: A qualitative perspective. *Psychiatry: Interpersonal and Biological Processes, 70*, 19–29.

Kuosmanen, L., Hatonen, H., Malkavaara, H., Kylma, J., & Valimaki, M. (2007). Deprivation of liberty in psychiatric hospital care: The patient's perspective. *Nursing Ethics, 14*, 597–607.

Lee, S., Gray, R., Gournay, K., Wright, S., Parr, A.-M., & Sayer, J. (2003). Views of nursing staff on the use of physical restraint. *Journal of Psychiatric and Mental Health Nursing, 10*, 425–430.

Lidz, C. W., Hoge, S. K., Gardner, W., Bennet, N. S., Monahan, J., Mulvey, E. P., et al. (1995). Perceived coercion in mental hospital admission. *Archives of General Psychiatry 52,* 1034–1039.

Lucksted, A., & Coursey, R. D. (1995). Consumer perceptions of pressure and force in psychiatric treatments. *Psychiatric Services, 46*, 146–152.

Mayers, P., Keet, N., Winkler, G., & Flisher, A. (2010). Mental health service users' perceptions and experiences of sedation, seclusion and restraint. *International Journal of Social Psychiatry, 56*(1), 60–73.

McCann, T. V., Baird, J., Clark, E., & Lu, S. (2008). Mental health professionals' attitudes towards consumer participation in inpatient units. *Journal of Psychiatric and Mental Health Nursing, 15*(1), 10–16.

Meehan, T., Vermeer, C., & Windsor, C. (2000). Patients' perceptions of seclusion: A qualitative investigation. *Journal of Advanced Nursing, 31*(2), 370–377.

Morrison, P., & LeHane, M. (1995). Staffing levels and seclusion use. *Journal of Advanced Nursing, 22*(6), 1193–1202.

New Freedom Commission on Mental Health. (2003). *Achieving the promise: Transforming mental health care in America*. Rockville, MD: Author.

Olofsson, B., & Jacobsson, L. (2001). A plea for respect: Involuntarily hospitalized psychiatric patients' narratives about being subjected to coercion. *Journal of Psychiatric and Mental Health Nursing, 8*, 357–366.

Pellegrino, E. D., & Thomasma, D. C. (1987). The conflict between autonomy and beneficence in medical ethics: Proposal for a resolution. *Journal of Contemporary Health Law and Policy, 3*, 23–46.

Peto, T., Srebnik, D., Zick, E., & Russo, J. (2004). Support needed to create psychiatric advance directives. *Administration and Policy In Mental Health, 31*(5), 401–409.

Rider, A., St. George, L., & Long, M. (2000). *Peer employment training*. Unpublished training curriculum. Phoenix, AZ: RI International.

Riecher-Rossler, A., & Rossler, W. (1993). Compulsory admission of psychiatric patients: An international comparison. *Acta Psychiatrica Scandinavica, 87*, 231–236.

Rogers, A. (1993). Coercion and 'voluntary' admission: An examination of psychiatric patient views. *Behavioural Sciences and the Law, 11*, 259–267.

Rymaszewska, J. (2007). Patients' subjective quality of life during involuntary treatment in psychiatric hospitals. *BMC Psychiatry, 7*(Suppl. 1), S33.

Salize, H., & Dressing, H. (2004). Epidemiology of involuntary placement of mentally ill people across the European Union. *British Journal of Psychiatry, 184* (2), 163–168.

Scheyett, A., Kim, M., Swanson, J., Swartz, M., Elbogen, E.,Van Dorn, R., et al. (2008). Social workers' familiarity with psychiatric advance directives: Implications for education, practice, and research. *Families in Society, 89*, 228–236.

Schwartz, R., Estein, O., Komaroff, J., Lamb, J., Myers, M., Stewart, J., et al. (2013). Mental health consumers and providers dialogue in an institutional setting: A participatory approach to promoting recovery-oriented care. *Psychiatric Rehabilitation Journal, 36*(2), 113–115.

Smith, R., & Bartholomew, T. (2006). Will hospitals recover? The implications of a recovery-orientation. *American Journal of Psychiatric Rehabilitation, 9*(2), 85–100.

Srebnik, D., & Brodoff, L. (2003). Implementing psychiatric advance directives: Service provider issues and answers. *Journal of Behavioral Health Services and Research, 9*, 257–272.

Srebnik, D. S., Russo, J., Sage, J., Peto, T., & Zick, E. (2003). Interest in psychiatric advance directives among high users of crisis services and hospitalization. *Psychiatric Services, 54*, 981–986.

Stender, A. K., Hertel, C. M., Poulsen, P., Hansen, H. S., Simonsen, C., & Korner, E. A. (1997). Patienternes vurdering af tvangpå psykiatrisk afdelning. *Videnskab Og Praksis, 25*, 3947–3950.

Stettin, B., Geller, J., Ragosta, K., Cohen, K., & Ghowrwal, J. (2014). *Mental health commitment laws a survey of the states*. Treatment Advocacy Center. Accessed February 3, 2016. http://tacreports.org/storage/documents/2014-state-survey-abridged.pdf

Strack, K. M., Deal, W. P., & Schulenberg, S. E. (2007). Coercion and empowerment in the treatment of individuals with serious mental illness: A preliminary investigation. *Psychological Services, 4*(2), 96–106.

Strack, K. M., & Schulenberg, S. E. (2007). Understanding empowerment, meaning and perceived coercion in individuals with serious mental illness. *Journal of Clinical Psychology, 65*(10), 1137–1148.

Stewart, M., Brown, J. B., Weston, W. W., McWhinney, I. R., McWilliam, C. L., & Freeman, T. R. (1995). Patient centered medicine transforming the clinical method. Thousand Oaks, CA: Sage Publications.

Substance Abuse and Mental Health Services Administration. (2012). *Participatory dialogues: A Guide to organizing interactive discussions on mental health issues among consumers, providers and family members*. Rockville, MD: Author.

Swanson, J. W., Swartz, M. S., Elbogen, E. B., Wagner, R., & Burns, B. (2003). Effects of involuntary outpatient commitment on subjective quality of life in persons with severe mental illness. *Behavioral Sciences and the Law, 21*, 473–491.

Taylor, M. F., & Bentley, K. J. (2004). Changing conceptualizations of mental health and mental illness: Implications of "brain disease" and "behavioral health" for social work. *Social Work in Mental Health, 2*(4), 1–16.

Thibeault, C. A., Trudeau, K., d'Entremont, M., & Brown, T. (2010). Understanding the milieu experiences of patients on an acute inpatient psychiatric unit. *Archives of Psychiatric Nursing, 24*(4), 216–226.

Ulrich, R. S. (1984). View through a window may influence recovery from surgery. *Science, 224*, 420–421.

Ulrich, R. S., Simons, R. F., Losito, B. D., Fiorito, E., Miles, M. A., & Zelson, M. (1991). Stress recovery during exposure to natural and urban environments. *Journal of Environmental Psychology, 11*, 201–230.

Van Dorn, R. A., Elbodgen, E. B., Redich, A. D., Swanson, J. W., Swartz, M. S., & Mustillo, S. (2006a). The relationship between mandated community treatment and perceived barriers toi care in persons with severe mental illness. *International Journal of Law and Psychiatry, 29*(6), 495–506.

Van Dorn, R. A., Swartz, M. S., Elbogen, E. B., Swanson, J. W., Kim, M., Ferron, J., et al. (2006b). Clinicians' attitudes regarding barriers to the implementation of psychiatric advance directives. *Administration and Policy In Mental Health, 33*, 449–460.

Van Dorn, R. A., Scheyett, A., Swanson, J. W., & Swartz, M. S. (2010). Psychiatric advance directives and social workers: An integrative review. *Social Work, 55*(2), 157–167.

Vuckovich, P., & Artinian, B. (2005). Justifying coercion. *Nursing Ethics, 12*(4), 370–379.

Wadsworth, Y., & Epstein, M. (1998). Building in dialogue between consumers and staff in acute mental health services. *Systemic Practice and Action Research, 11*(4), 353–379.

Walsh, J., & Boyle, J. (2009). Improving acute psychiatric hospital services according to inpatient experiences. A user-led piece of research as a means to empowerment. *Issues in Mental Health Nursing, 30*(1), 31–38.

Whitehouse, S., Varni, J, W., Seid, M., Cooper-Marcus, C., Ensberg, M. J., Jacobs, J, R., et al. (2001). Evaluating a children's hospital garden environment: Utilization and consumer satisfaction. *Journal of Environmental Psychology, 21,* 301–314.

Wynn, R. (2002). Medicate, restrain or seclude? Strategies for dealing with violent and threatening behavior in a Norwegian university psychiatric hospital. *Scandinavian Journal of Caring Sciences, 16*, 287–291.

# 15 Legal Advocacy

Donna Lee Elm and Jenny L. Devine

## Introduction

Judge Learned Hand once remarked that "as a litigant I should dread a law suit beyond almost anything else short of sickness and death" (Frank 1957). What if you were in the tragic position of having chronic legal issues *and* mental health problems? Persons who are mentally ill are often burdened with both. The mentally ill are 10 times more likely to be imprisoned than receive inpatient mental health care (Murphy 2015). Approximately 20 % of state prisoners and 21 % of local jail inmates have a recent history of a mental health condition (Glaze and James 2006). Almost every patient within the walls of state forensic psychiatric hospitals is also a litigant in a criminal or civil court case involving public defenders or human rights groups. In order for these individuals to truly begin the recovery process, they must work toward *both* legal independence and mental wellness.

Each person directs his or her process of recovery uniquely. Mental health professionals utilize a myriad of tools to develop wellness for their patients, including psychotherapy and medications. Similarly, legal advocates counsel each individual client about their civil rights and develop case-specific strategies to accomplish an end goal. The legal advocate's role goes well beyond that of a guardian ad litem (who gives the client a "best interests" voice), because lawyers must attend to all legal needs of their clients even when they are not immediately aligned with their medical needs as patients. This imbues the legal process with dignity, and people flourish when they know their choices are considered and respected. Thus, the ideal of individual rights is not at all different from the ideal of recovery.

Even so, the practices of law and medicine have not always shared the same perspective. Fundamental disagreements exist between those treating illness and those protecting civil liberties (Bennion 2013). The "medical model" promotes treatment as the path to recovery, even if it is by way of involuntary hospitalizations and forced medication. The "civil rights model" advocates for the liberty of the individual to choose his or her own path to recovery, even if it includes rejecting medical treatment. Proponents of both models believe that they are improving society and the ultimate autonomy of the individual. Cannot both be correct?

Attorneys ensure the civil liberties of all individuals remain intact. In the civil and forensic mental health settings, effective legal advocacy efforts enable an individual's path to recovery by ensuring that all stakeholders meet his or her unique needs across multiple systems. Simply put, attorneys can knock down barriers to meaningful medical treatment. When the role of

D.L. Elm (✉) · J.L. Devine
Office of the Federal Defender,
Middle District of Florida, 400 N. Tampa Street,
Suite 2700, 33602 Tampa, FL, USA
e-mail: donna_elm@fd.org



N.N. Singh et al. (eds.), *Handbook of Recovery in Inpatient Psychiatry*,
Evidence-Based Practices in Behavioral Health, DOI 10.1007/978-3-319-40537-7_15

the attorney is balanced with that of the mental health professional, patients achieve the support they need for recovery because they have agency. In this context, agency is achieved through individual empowerment and intact civil rights, fostering a healthy emotional intelligence essential for the recovery process.

Using this paradigm, one can argue in a broad sense that both the "medical model" and "civil rights model" can actually work hand in hand to promote individual wellness in a free society. This chapter will focus on the particularities of the legal practice as it intersects with the practice of mental health professionals. In some cases, the treatment needs of the individual will take a backseat to the civil liberties at stake, and the necessity of these laws is explored. As is appropriate considering modern state hospital populations, the bulk of the material addresses the forensic subjects of criminal competency, restoration, and dangerousness, followed by a review of the lawyer's role in civil commitments. Attention is given to questions of recovery through the eyes of defense counsel and individuals facing chronic legal issues while saddled with mental health problems.

## Criminal Competency

### Overview of the Competency Process

In criminal competency cases, judges and (almost always) lawyers are involved. Courts are only authorized to order criminal competency evaluations when a criminal case has been filed. Hence the starting point of any competency evaluation must be the Court Order directing that it be done; it should indicate what is being sought, whether treatment or restoration is also anticipated, if additional evaluations (like insanity, restorability to competency, or dangerousness) are ordered, what the time frame to comply is, maybe whether certain testing is required, and often what form the report should take.

The primary purpose behind criminal competency placement is *expert evaluation* and not *treatment*. That is not to say that treatment is undesirable for the court system, but that treatment may be part of a secondary competency restoration process instead. In some jurisdictions (such as the federal courts), the two processes are clearly separate (18 U.S.C. § 4241(a–d)). In fact, federal defendants are often sent to different facilities for the competency evaluation and the restoration treatment. However, most states immediately initiate treatment during any evaluation placement. Practitioners involved in competency forensics should familiarize themselves with whether their jurisdiction separates treatment from evaluation.

It is important to note from the start that in competency and restoration processes, unlike most treatment protocols, recovery of good mental health is not necessarily the goal for all involved. For instance, should a defendant be found incompetent and unable to be restored, then the criminal charges will eventually be dismissed. The defense lawyer and/or the defendant may desire that outcome over a conviction, its collateral consequences, and any potential incarceration. Thus, a defendant who would otherwise normally want to gain better mental health may want to remain actively psychotic during the pendency of criminal charges.

Criminal defense attorneys have a different responsibility than treating psychiatric personnel. The lawyers' duty is to maximize their clients' *liberty*, not maximize their *health* (Uphoff 1988).[1] In other words, attorneys represent the defendants' liberty interests, not what is in their best medical interests. That is, remaining mentally ill may in fact be the best path for overall "recovery" for this defendant at this time. Hence, the goals of criminal defense may be at odds with

[1]Because liberty is the primary goal for criminal defense, the reality of the practice is that it sometimes may trump concerns that a client may be incompetent. For example, if a defendant who is obviously psychotic is offered a "time served" misdemeanor plea bargain, rather than raise incompetency (which could take 6 months in custody to resolve), the lawyer may advise the client and allow him or her to go forward with the guilty plea. As Uphoff (1988) noted, for defendants "charged with minor offenses, raising competency subjects [them] to far greater deprivation of liberty than if [they] were convicted of the crime."

the goals of the forensic treatment providers as well as the prosecution and court. This issue will be taken up again below when discussing forced medication to restore competency. That is not to say that the defense will usually try to thwart recovery; in fact, many lawyers and defendants will embrace restoration to competency so that they can return to litigation or negotiation.

The strategy decision whether to try to be found incompetent or competent is a complex one that should have been discussed between the defense lawyer and client. Treating personnel should take care not to try to advise or persuade the defendant whether to fight or go along with competency—as that is a matter of legal advice, and they would be interfering with the attorney's legal guidance as well as the defendant's Sixth Amendment right to counsel. This decision is not simple because there can be collateral consequences to being found incompetent and unrestorable as well. In some jurisdictions, there is mandatory commitment of a person found to be incompetent in a criminal case (18 U.S.C. § 4241 (d)); additionally, persons adjudicated incompetent may lose some future rights, such as the right to bear arms (18 U.S.C. § 922(d); Fla. Stat. § 790.25(1)). Moreover, some defendants have actively resisted findings of incompetence because they want to return to responsible positions once their criminal cases are behind them. Some are concerned that it will have an adverse impact on regaining custody or visitation with their children. Others simply reject it because they do not want to be considered defective or disabled by such a finding. So deciding whether to remain mentally ill (untreated), fight restoration, or try to challenge any finding of competency is a legal decision that cannot be lightly undertaken.

Certain history will lead to a decision to refer a defendant for a competency evaluation. Most commonly, a request for a competency evaluation occurs after the defense attorney or arresting law enforcement officers report that the defendant exhibits bizarre behavior. Sometimes when the defendant displays patently florid symptoms in court, the judge will order a competency examination, even absent any request by the lawyers. Competency evaluations may also arise based solely on a history of prior civil commitments and criminal incompetency or insanity findings; in an abundance of caution, referral is sometimes made simply to "rule out" incompetency at the present time.

However, a defendant's incompetency is not always immediately apparent. Highly functional individuals (especially true for those suffering from Delusional Disorders which appear reasonable because they are reality-based, or those with intellectual disabilities who have learned to try to behave normally) may not reveal underlying paranoias, delusions, or cognitive disorders for some time; alternatively, defense counsel may not be able to detect chronic psychoses until interacting with the client or investigating the client's claims for some time as well. Further, incompetency can wax and wane; the Supreme Court noted that "Mental illness … can vary over time. It interferes with an individual's functioning at different times in different ways" (*Indiana v. Edwards*, 2008). Thus, incompetency sometimes only arises well after the case is advancing, especially as the defendant's stress mounts with an imminent trial or sentencing, generating competency evaluations well into the progress of a criminal case.

## Legal Standards of Competency

The legal basis for the proposition that an incompetent defendant should not be prosecuted is the Due Process clause of the Fifth Amendment to the U.S. Constitution (*Ryan v. Gonzales*, 2013; *Cooper v. Oklahoma*, 1996). It is "fundamentally unfair" to prosecute a person whose mental illness interferes with his or her ability to understand and assist counsel in the proceedings. Evaluating doctors need to know the precise legal standard for competency in their jurisdiction before starting an evaluation. The lawyers can provide the applicable law that defines it. Note that it may differ from the common conception of competency provided below.

Virtually every jurisdiction also has statutes, rules, or regulations that govern criminal competency. Typically, state competency laws derive from the Supreme Court's federal standard from the *Dusky* case: "whether he has sufficient present ability to consult with his lawyer with a reasonable degree of rational understanding—and whether he has a rational as well as factual understanding of the proceedings against him" (*Dusky v. United States*, 1960). These are seen as two independent means of establishing competency; an individual is incompetent if he or she is either (a) unable to understand the proceedings, or (b) unable to assist counsel in his or her defense (Conn. Gen. Stat. §§ 54-56d (2012)), or of course both.

Given those options, persons may be incompetent even if they do not have a DSM-5 diagnosis. A defendant who cannot communicate due to stroke or paralysis can be incompetent, even if not suffering from any mental illness (*United States v. Calkins,* 1990; *State v. Connor*, 2014). A defendant who is developmentally disabled may be incompetent, even if he or she falls outside a neurodevelopmental diagnosis (Cal. Penal Code § 1367(d)). A person who speaks a language that cannot be translated could be incompetent.[2] Occasionally, defendants with severe or terminal medical conditions requiring considerable attention (such as advanced HIV or terminal pancreatic cancer) have been determined incompetent to assist in their defense (*United States v. Pollock*, 2014). Some jurisdictions have declared persons suffering from complete amnesia of critical events to be incompetent to assist their lawyers in defending them as well (but usually only when that is combined with other conditions to create incompetency) (*Altoonian v. Warren*, 2015; *United States v. Minter*, 2014; Tysse and Hafemeister 2006).

Insanity has different standards, but the legally significant difference between it and incompetency is that there is no constitutional right to an insanity defense, while there is a Due Process (constitutional) right to be competent.[3] This explains some of the seemingly incongruous exceptions that have been carved out of insanity defenses: what constitutes "insanity" is set by legislature or courts, whereas what constitutes "incompetency" cannot be readily cut back due to broad constitutional protections. Hence, a number of jurisdictions reject an insanity defense—no matter how psychotic the defendant was when the mental state arose from or during substance abuse (Ariz. Rev. Stat. § 13-502(a)); similarly, some reject it when the psychosis occurred during a transitory state (*i.e.*, "temporary insanity") (Ariz. Rev. Stat. § 13-502(a); Colo. Rev. Stat. § 16-8-101.5(1)); additionally, some refuse the defense when the mental abnormality constitutes "repeated criminal or otherwise antisocial conduct" (*Bethea v. United States*, 1976). Exceptions like those cannot generally be imposed on competency assessments.

Most jurisdictions take the position that competency is an objective status, not dependent on the nature of the circumstances the defendant is facing. However, others recognize that there can be differing standards of competency depending on the situation. It makes good sense that competency may be higher or more specific to waive a myriad of trial rights when pleading guilty under a plea agreement than, for instance, to be aware of being executed (Poythress et al. 2002). While evaluating professionals should verify if their jurisdiction has differing standards for incompetency depending on what the defendant is facing, following are some common competency tests where the legal undertakings make a difference:

- Competency to testify as a witness: capacity to receive accurate impressions of the facts and relate them truthfully (*State v. Kinney*, 1987).

[2]The writer represented a man who was deaf from birth. Erroneously diagnosed as profoundly mentally retarded, he was institutionalized as a very young child and never taught any language, including sign language, whatsoever. Although he was neither mentally ill nor intellectually disabled, he could not assist counsel and was found incompetent.

[3]Most present insanity standards are derived from the *M'Naghten* Rule stating that a defendant is insane when "laboring from such a defect of reason, from disease of the mind, as to not know the nature and quality of the act he was doing, or, if he did know it, that he did not know what he was doing was wrong" (*Daniel M'Naghten's* Case 1843). However, because an insanity defense is not a constitutionally protected entitlement, Idaho, Montana, Utah, and Kansas do not allow it (Applebaum 2013).

- Competency of defendant to waive *Miranda* rights and answer questions without counsel: the defendant must knowingly, intelligently, and voluntarily decide to waive *Miranda* rights (*State v. Camacho*, 1997).
- Competency to stand trial: the *Dusky* standard, "whether he has sufficient present ability to consult with his lawyer with a reasonable degree of rational understanding —and whether he has a rational as well as factual understanding of the proceedings against him" (*Dusky v. United States*, 1960).
- Competency to waive trial rights and plead guilty: in addition to the *Dusky* standard, the defendant must knowingly, intelligently, and voluntarily waive his *Miranda* and trial rights (*Jones v. Knipp*, 2013).
- Competency of a "gray area incompetent" defendant to waive the right to counsel and represent oneself at trial: a heightened standard of *Dusky* plus accounting for the borderline incompetent defendant's mental capabilities to conduct trial (*Indiana v. Edwards*, 2008).
- Competency to be sentenced: the *Dusky* standard is commonly used (*United States v. Wolfson*, 2008; N.C. Gen. Stat. § 15A-1001 (a)).
- Competency to be executed: "when, as a result of mental disease or defect, he lacks the mental capacity to understand the nature and effect of the death penalty and why it is to be carried out (*Ford v. Wainwright*, 1986; N.Y. Corr. Law § 656; Ariz. Rev. Stat. § 13-4021; Fla. Stat. § 922.07; Ga. Code § 17-10-60; Ohio Rev. Code § 2949.28; Wyo. Stat. § 7-13-901).

## Lawyers' Involvement with Competency Evaluations

Lawyers often are—and should be—involved in competency evaluations. Some forensic practitioners perceive attorneys from either side as interfering with their work, and would prefer to not deal with them. This is fair enough, as most of the population would prefer not to deal with lawyers! But generally, information from attorneys can be helpful, and sometimes the lawyer can persuade his or her client to cooperate with the evaluation or treatment.

Because one prong of the competency standard is the ability to assist counsel in legal proceedings, the competency determination must address problems the lawyer has interacting with the client. Generally, a forensic evaluator should try to discuss this relationship with the defense attorney. Admittedly, the lawyer may decline to engage, or may consider his or her interaction with the client to be "privileged" so non-disclosable. But, to the extent that lawyers are willing to discuss this with doctors, it contributes to an informed opinion.

Lawyers generally are not willing to allow the doctor to watch actual interactions between them and their clients. First, those interactions are confidential under the attorney/client privilege, and attorneys as well as their clients will seldom waive that. Second, lawyers may decline to interact with clients at all during the pendency of the evaluation, for fear of allegations that they "coached" their clients to fake symptoms (*People v. Brown*, 2014; *Matter of Foley*, 2003). Third, it is critical that lawyers not put themselves into a position where they become the evidence against their clients' liberty interests; when the strategy is to try to establish incompetency, they do not want favorable interactions with their clients to establish that the clients are competent and thereby create a conflict of interest with their client. For the same reason, defense attorneys will not want their letters, emails, or phone calls with clients to be disclosed to the evaluating physicians; it is not "hiding the ball," but rather legitimate protection of the attorney–client relationship.

## Incompetency as a Litigation Strategy

As mentioned, incompetency may in fact be the litigation strategy of choice. Having the client found incompetent and unrestorable may be the best outcome for the case, leading to dismissal of charges.[4]

Some profoundly ill individuals both were insane at the time of the offense and remain incompetent without hope of restoration, and so either option is available. But, frequently persons determined to be incompetent will have greater liberty options available to them than those determined to be insane. Hence a defendant who is committed upon a finding that he or she is incompetent, unrestorable, and dangerous is favored over one who is found not guilty by reason of insanity, placing the burden of proof on the prosecution for the former but on the defendant for the latter, and allowing greater conditions for early release to the former than the latter (18 U.S.C. § 4246(a); 18 U.S.C. § 4243(d); 18 U.S.C. § 4246 (e); 18 U.S.C. § 4243(d)). Under those circumstances, a finding of incompetency will produce a better liberty result than a finding of insanity.

On the other hand, insanity may be the goal of litigation. If the mental illness is ongoing, then a finding of incompetency could contribute substantially toward an eventual verdict of insanity. It is also not unusual to try an insanity defense "to the bench," meaning to ask the judge (rather than a jury) to decide the case; a judge who has reviewed extensive psychological records and reports from competency proceedings may already be well informed as to the defendant's mental state by the time of trial.

Competency litigation also educates the judge as to mental illness that constitutes profound mitigation for sentencing. Thus, even if the defendant will ultimately be found competent, he may want the evaluation and report to familiarize the judge familiar with these issues so that they can be weighed in when formulating the appropriate sentence.

In some states, a person who had been found incompetent in a criminal case may have a "leg up" on others when seeking to secure social services. To help the client avoid future entanglements with the authorities, a thoughtful lawyer may seek an incompetency finding so as to increase the likelihood of greater social services, which in turn will help the client remain law abiding. Moreover, a person who is found incompetent now will have a "track record" of serious mental illness for the future that precludes criminal prosecution, should that person face the proverbial "revolving door" of arrests.

Defendants do not, however, always agree with this litigation strategy. Generally, defense counsel wants to pursue the same case goals that his or her client wants (Uphoff 1988). But there are times when a lawyer is required to raise and fight for a finding of incompetency despite the client's adamant resistance. "Because the trial of an incompetent defendant necessarily is invalid as a violation of Due Process, a defense lawyer's duty to maintain the integrity of judicial proceedings requires that a trial court be advised of the defendant's possible incompetence" (*Moye v. Warden*, 2014; ABA Criminal Justice Mental Health Standards 7-4.2). This impasse arises most clearly with clients suffering from delusions, including delusions that there is nothing wrong with them (*United States v. Gillenwater*, 2013). Therefore, defense counsel may be in the untenable position of disclosing a limited amount of information conveyed by the client supposedly in confidence, so as to try to get a competency finding that the client is adamantly opposed to. The justice system prefers ruination of the attorney–client relationship, despite odds against success in competency litigation, to prosecution of an incompetent defendant.

Prosecutors likewise have a duty not to prosecute persons who are incompetent. In practice, nonetheless, they are as suspicious of claims of incompetency as they are of pleas of insanity. Unless it is facially apparent that the defendant is incompetent, they typically vigorously oppose having the defendant declared incompetent.

## Determining Competency

Although this is not a forensic how to text, a few words of caution with important implications for

[4]Competency restoration staff should also consider their own ethical conflicts raised in "regarding how, and in what ways, information could be obtained from a defendant that might not be in the defendant's best interests" (Samuel and Michaels 2011).

legal advocacy should be sounded. First, as mentioned above, because one prong of incompetency has to do with the defendant's ability to assist counsel, serious attention should be paid to examining and investigating the lawyer's interactions with his or her client. While the defense attorney may decline to discuss these matters with treatment staff, information may be available in a motion filed in court for a competency hearing and/or a transcript of what the lawyer stated in court during preliminary competency proceedings. Note that evaluating professionals should not seek to surreptitiously examine interactions between the defendant and his or her lawyer (for instance, by listening to their "legal calls" or reviewing correspondence/email between them). When seeking advice of counsel is used against a defendant, the attorney–client relationship is fractured, and the Sixth Amendment right to counsel has been poisoned.

Records of prior criminal competency matters and reports may be found in the courts rather than in traditional institutions of psychiatric medicine. Often, the lawyers can assist physicians in securing copies of those records.

Even when formal time periods are not set for the evaluation of competency and restorability, the Supreme Court held that defendants are entitled to a prompt determination of this (*Jackson v. Indiana*, 1973).

A sizeable number of criminal defendants are non-citizens. Although interpreters may assist medical staff in communicating with their patient, language translation alone may not help evaluators understand the defendant's world view and culture. It can be very beneficial, consequently, to have a network of psychological practitioners and allied professionals who hail from different countries and cultures to consult with when determining an immigrant's competency.

Often, evaluating professionals will be asked to offer multiple opinions. It is not uncommon to seek opinions on competency as well as insanity, or on restorability to competency as well as dangerousness.

Finally, much of forensic psychology focuses on trying to uncover whether the defendant is faking symptoms (Feuerstein et al. 2005). Determination if a defendant is malingering can be an important aspect of reaching a competency opinion, but it is not dispositive. The emphasis some forensic practitioners place on malingering is out of step with the rest of the mental health practice (which generally does not look for malingering to disprove a diagnosis, but instead looks for symptoms to support a diagnosis); and certainly, motives to fake mental illness outside the criminal justice system are myriad as well (Feuerstein et al. 2005).[5] A tendency to turn first to malingering would suggest a professional prejudice concerning an offender population.

Furthermore, evaluators must consider that thoroughly incompetent individuals are capable of trying to fake symptoms (*United States v. Frazier*, 2001). So just because a defendant malingers does not mean he or she must be competent (*United States v. Gigante*, 1999).

Additionally, malingering is usually defined as intentional production of false or grossly exaggerated physical or psychological symptoms (i.e., malady) for a secondary gain (Rogers 2008). Nonetheless, faking being well, when the patient is mentally ill, can be equally problematic. Professionals exploring malingering should consequently consider that it can embrace both "fake-bad" as well as "fake-good," and should attend to defendants trying to appear competent when they are not, just as they watch for the converse. There can be as many reasons to fake competency as is seen outside an offender population, especially from intellectually impaired patients (who have learned to adapt and function) as well as persons suffering from a serious Delusional Disorder.

[5]These authors claim that forensic psychology is "unique" due to motivation arising from pending criminal prosecutions. That premise has been rightfully criticized, as seasoned nonforensic practitioners well know that there are always motivations of some kind that impact the reliability of their patients' claims and symptoms. Indeed, such motivations can arise from avoiding military duty, obtaining financial compensation, and obtaining drugs—in addition to evading criminal prosecution.

## Post-incompetency Detention Process

After a competency report has been issued, the court will generally return the defendant from the therapeutic setting to the previous detention setting. If the defendant had been released to the community before the evaluation placement, then he or she would usually be released back to that same status. Departure from the hospital setting has implications for maintaining any competency that has been achieved. A defendant who is stable on a medication regimen may have to contend with irregular (or no) dosing during transportation. Furthermore, medical units in jails do not typically stock the variety of psychotropic medications that are available in psychiatric medical centers; consequently, doctors in jails may substitute other medications that may not be as efficacious. Furthermore, defendants may elect to decline treatment when in the jail setting. In addition, often the jail environment is more stressful than a therapeutic setting, so patients who are stable in psychiatric treatment facilities may decompensate under the stressors they face in detention facilities. Competency can be a fleeting state, even in the best of medical centers, and achieving competency there does not necessarily mean that it will be maintained after leaving.

One of the inherent difficulties of competency work is that psychological professionals are tasked with offering opinions on whether the defendant will be competent to proceed with trial, when all they can do is assess or render the defendant competent in a more stability-conducive medical setting. In one case, the defendant was determined to be competent 4 months before the competency hearing took place; one judge pointed out that the *Dusky* standard of competency includes "sufficient *present* ability to consult with his lawyer," and that the dated report would not necessarily reflect the defendant's *present* mental state (*United States v. Lindley*, 1985). Consequently, opinions of competency that extend beyond the psychiatric placement may not be very valid or reliable. Certainly evaluating professionals should offer a caveat that continued competency after leaving is dependent upon certain treatment/circumstances. In addition, they would best serve their patients by specifying in their reports their recommendations for continued treatment to try to maintain competency after leaving the therapeutic milieu.

Before a competency hearing is done, the lawyers may seek to explore the facts underlying and bases of the opinion. There is great utility in gathering wide-ranging information that contributes to a competency opinion (Philipsborn 2015; *United States v. Merriweather*, 2013). Bear in mind that the competency process takes place in a litigation setting, and it is not unusual for parties to contest the opinions. Hence, lawyers may want to see copies of complete medical records (including notes from support staff and security personnel), tests (including actual answers and raw test data), security camera tapes, videotaped treatment or "educational" footage (*United States v. Merriweather*, 2013), normal administrative records (such as admission, housing, movement, discipline, commissary, activities, meetings, religious practice, visitation, sick call, and personal property management), and any recorded visitation or phone calls. In rare cases, depositions will be ordered. Doctors may be asked for their CV's, medical school transcripts, and any training programs and authorities they relied upon in reaching their opinions. Treating professions should not take offense at being challenged this way, as it is part and parcel of an investigation step in the normal adversary process.

A medical opinion regarding competency is only part of what a court must consider in coming to a legal opinion regarding competency. While judges are informed by competency opinions, they may not agree with them. Moreover, there often are multiple experts offering conflicting opinions—so ultimately in those circumstances, the judge will reject someone's professional opinion regarding competency.

The judge may decide competency without a formal hearing or any testimony, but alternatively may want to hear from the doctors on the stand. Witnesses should always seek to discuss their testimony with the lawyers in advance. In the end, if the defendant is found incompetent, he or she may proceed to restoration to competency treatment, discussed further below.

## Offender Population Characteristics Relevant to Competency

**Culture:** There are some characteristics of the offender population that should be borne in mind when assessing competency. For instance, irrational ideas are not necessarily part of a psychotic process, but may instead be learned. Many persons who run afoul of the laws are not fully immersed in the predominant American culture, and may have grown up with ideas and values quite apart from the norm. The evaluator is well advised to investigate the cultural, family, and educational background of the defendant who has bizarre ideas but otherwise appears intact.

**Age:** The offender population is skewed in terms of age, with a far greater representation of younger defendants than normal. There is a clear decline of criminal conduct that tracks with age (United States Department of Justice 2003). The disproportionate number of youthful offenders is likely due to maturity lagging behind the age of majority: the full development of the human brain does not occur until approximately age 25 (Giedd 2004; Giedd and Blumenthal 1999), whereas the full legal responsibility for one's actions occurs generally at age 18. Consequently, in competency assessments of youthful adults, evaluators should consider developmental maturity issues.

**Compartmentalized Incompetency:** Some defendants may be rational about many aspects of their lives, but harbor segmented delusions, paranoias, or phobias about certain things. One of us represented a client who had delusions of being heir to the Ford Motor Company, and since these thoughts did not affect his drug case, competency was not initially raised. However, those delusions eventually intruded into the case when the defendant began to believe that the prosecution colluded with Ford to deprive him of his inheritance by falsely charging him with this crime. At that point, his paranoia impacted his competency to proceed to trial, and a competency hearing ensued. This type of fragmentation is not news to psychiatric professionals, but it has important implications for competency. Defendants who may appear rational or high functioning may harbor irrational but persistent fears about their lawyers, the prosecution, the government, or the police; deeper inquiries concerning compartmentalized delusions should be made when an intact-appearing defendant is evaluated.

**Intellectual Disability:** Although courts have held that having intellectual disabilities does not per se mean those defendants are incompetent (*Pruitt v. State*, 2005), it can clearly impact their ability to comprehend the justice system, to keep up with and grasp what is happening (often at lightning speed) in trial, and to assist counsel. Professionals should consequently delve into how these individuals function when assessing their competency. Most persons with intellectual challenges have learned to cope well and cover it up so as to secure employment or social relationships; "mentally retarded individuals use a 'cloak of competence' in an attempt to present themselves as 'normal' (or at least more capable than they actually are) as a means of avoiding the stigma of being identified as mentally retarded" (*Gumm v. Mitchell*, 2014). Extra care must therefore be taken to sort out "fake-good" attempts to portray a false sense of competency.

**Amnesia:** Due to heavy substance abuse, brain trauma, or severe psychosis, a number of defendants may genuinely experience amnesia concerning the crime (distinguished from a short-term memory disorder with chronic recall problems). Recognizing that defendants' ability to assist counsel in their defense may be truncated by retrospective amnesia, some jurisdictions allow amnesia as a basis for incompetency, concluding that "amnesia could render a defendant incompetent to stand trial under some circumstances;" on the other hand, the majority of jurisdictions have distrusted amnesia alone as a basis for incompetency (*People v. Amador*, 1988; *Morrow v. State*, 1982; *United States v. Robertson*, 2015; *Wilson v. United States*, 1968). This may be motivated by the fact that amnesia can be easily faked and all but impossible to disprove, allowing defendants an easy means of malingering incompetency (*Simon v. McCarty*, 2015). Nonetheless for those who in fact suffer from retrospective amnesia, courts may create a "legal fiction" that their lawyers can compensate for that by educating their clients as to what occurred during the crime (based on the police and witness reports). That is hardly a satisfactory corrective, as the defendant may be the only one who could give information that can generate a defense or undermine the charges.

**Multiple Personalities:** Although Dissociative Identity Disorder (DID) involving multiple personalities occurs rarely, it is not unusual for persons who have this condition to act out and attract the attention of the authorities. Those suffering from this disorder, even when highly functional, are commonly referred for competency evaluations due to their bizarre personality changes. Simple dissociation, and its attendant amnesia, does not necessarily create incompetency; in one case, the court concluded that "a splitting of defendant's mind into different directions" was not likely to interfere with trial given that he was not likely to dissociate during trial (*People v. Girk*, 2014; *United States v. Brown*, 2015). However, deciding competency when there are multiple personalities with different mental states (such as child personas or alters who are psychotic) is a far more complex undertaking. Evaluating professionals must explore which personalities are competent, which are not, and predict which of those may appear during trial. This is complicated by the speed at which these patients can switch personas (Putnam et al. 1986). Consequently, monitoring which one is present during trial, when pleading guilty, or at sentencing (if realistically possible at all) may be necessary to ensure competency during those critical stages of the criminal case; note that "sustained period of identity disruption may occur when psychosocial pressures are severe" (American Psychiatric Association 2013). Given the stressors that entering a guilty plea or trial can generate, the possibility that a substitute persona may emerge at those proceedings is not insignificant.

One fascinating case of a psychopathic killer who suffered from multiple personalities illustrates the complexities of forensic determinations with this illness. After finding the DID defendant who had committed a brutal homicide not guilty by reason of insanity, the judge committed him to the state hospital. The hospital eventually asked the judge to release him. Psychiatric staff acknowledged that he genuinely suffered from multiple personalities, but had concluded that he had been faking incompetency and insanity. Analyzing his different "alters," the state's expert concluded that several had psychotic disorders (treatable), but only one of them was psychopathic (not treatable). Because the dominant personality at that time was the psychopathic one, and it could remain dominant for years, the defendant would pose a danger if released. Consequently, he was not released from the hospital (*Ex parte Alabama Dept. of Mental Health*, 2013). Similar depths might have to be plumbed when evaluating competency of a defendant who suffers from DID involving multiple alters, including which personas are competent, which are potentially restorable to competency, and the likelihood that certain personas may take over at given junctures in the court proceedings.

## Restoration to Competency

### Restoration Process

The court order placing the defendant in a competency restoration program should spell out what the medical center is asked to try to accomplish, what reporting is needed, and what time frame is allowed for this process.

Restorative treatment can be relegated to a secondary placement, or it can be authorized during a competency evaluation. Those jurisdictions that handle it sequentially will usually conduct a hearing to determine competency before initiating restorative therapy. Although no court will fault a medical institution for offering voluntary treatment to defendants in need, whether it is expected of the evaluating facility should be spelled out in the court's order asking for the competency evaluation.

Patients returning to medical settings for competency restoration may be more psychotic than when they left. Because they have the right to be present at court proceedings, they will typically be transported to court for such purposes; they may be gone for weeks or occasionally months before returned for competency restoration. It may take that long for further expert evaluations, reports, discovery, and litigation; alternatively, the defendant's bed space in the medical center could have been assigned to the next person awaiting inpatient services, and the defendant may have to wait until bed space becomes available to return (Pemberton 2014). In any event, there can be a clinically significant time period before a defendant is returned to the medical facility for restoration to competency. Consequently, any therapeutic treatment may have been interrupted in the interim, and the restoration program could have a patient who is more psychotic than he or she was when evaluated for competency.

On the other hand, some creative institutions have allowed the defendant to stay there while appearing for the hearing by videoconference (*United States v. Baker*, 1995). This has avoided or minimized any disruption in treatment. Furthermore, some fortunate defendants will have good medical attention while incarcerated in detention centers pending the competency hearings; despite being deemed incompetent when they left, they may return fully restored due to efficacious treatment provided in the detention center.

There are cases that are effectively "doomed" for restoration, where no amount of treatment or education can correct the problem. Typically those with severe intellectual disabilities may not be restored to competency, and quite a few mental illnesses will not be sufficiently resolved within the time constraints laws allow for restoration. Similarly, those who have had no beneficial impact from previous regimens of antipsychotics will likely fare no better with yet another round of like treatment. Further, deeply disturbed individuals (such as those with developed Delusional Disorders or Dissociative Identity Disorders) may need years of therapy to restore them—time that is simply not available for these efforts. Some jurisdictions nonetheless require commitment for restoration regardless of its likelihood (18 U.S.C. § 4241(d)).

Constitutional rights impose a reasonable time frame on restoration. For example, federal courts allow 4 months whereas Washington allows only 90 days for those charged with felonies and 45 days for misdemeanors (18 U.S.C. § 4241(d)(1); Rev. Code Wash. 10.77.086(1)). Courts also place a high premium on avoiding delay in resolving criminal cases, for defendants as well as victims have rights to speedy outcomes. Hence indefinite commitment based solely on the defendant's incompetence violates the Equal Protection and Due Process clauses of the U.S. Constitution (*Jackson v. Indiana*, 1972). Nonetheless, only about half the jurisdictions set maximum periods of time for restoration (*State v. Davis*, 2008), so judges may impose their own temporal restrictions.

## Restoration Treatment

There are many paths to recovery, and many means of restoring an incompetent defendant. Historically it seems, the preferred path has been pharmacological, despite the abundance of other sound therapeutic options. Admittedly, time limitations on restoration to competency may call for a "quick fix" solution; but, practitioners involved in restoration programs should consider more creative options, especially when those do not involve serious side-effects such as sedation, slurred speech, distracting bodily movements, or a declination to assert rights and make critical decisions. In other words, because many of the drugs being favored in restoration presently may also impair competency, alternatives should be considered.

Medical centers offer a therapeutic milieu. A stable and less stressful environment in a psychological unit can have beneficial impact on a patient's recovery. Providing a safe haven, counseling, and supportive staff alone can improve any patient's condition. Its drawback is that defendants who are restored by being in a therapeutic setting may not be able to maintain competency once returned to a jail setting. On the other hand, many defendants are not detained pretrial; if they are to be returned to a home environment, then the treatment staff can work on a discharge plan with the defendant's family and outpatient providers that could provide an environment that is therapeutic in the home upon discharge.

Work and purposeful activity is beneficial to recovery as well. For that reason, many hospital settings incorporate occupational therapy and related art therapies into their treatment regimens. Aside from keeping idle hands busy and the distraction/focus that these offer, they also provide motivation for the patient to get better as patients start to want to accomplish occupational goals they are undertaking.

Educational programs can have the same productive impact of occupational and arts therapies. However, a word of caution must be sounded about some "competency restoration education" modalities. These programs started to spread in the 1990s, ostensibly as an adjunct to traditional restoration, seeking to better educate defendants as to the criminal system, its procedures, and their rights (Samuel and Michaels 2011). Based on the premise that a competent defendant must intelligently appreciate what he is facing and what will happen in his case, they seek to educate the defendant on those matters. Though this can be a helpful component of restoration, in some restoration programs "competency classes" have unfortunately become the norm and main focus of restoration rather than an adjunct to it. These programs can be criticized for merely teaching defendants to "parrot" answers to questions commonly asked by judges who are deciding whether the defendant is competent. There is little research establishing that such training programs in fact restore the ability to assist counsel and appreciate and apply judgment to critical legal decisions concerning trial; a movement may be in the offing to take into account more than the intellectual component of competency, to instead consider "the client's *appreciation* of competency-related issues as well as his *reasoning processes*—the defendant's *functional* ability" (McCoy 2011). Highly delusional defendants, individuals with paralyzing depression, floridly psychotic patients, and those with intellectual disabilities can be taught by rote learning and simple conditioning to state correct answers to a judge's inquiries such as:

Q "Do you know who your lawyer is?"
A "Yes, she is right here next to me."
Q "Do you know what a jury does?"
A "Yes, they decide if am guilty or not."
Q "Do you know what I do?"
A "Yes, you decide how much time I will get."

Yet their ability to appreciate and process what they are encountering in the justice system may remain impaired. Dr. Kathleen Ronan has posed the thoughtful question: "How do you know the defendant is not simply parroting back what you have told him rather than truly understands the legal issues and can apply them?" (McCoy 2011). Therefore, the fact that they can state correct answers to these questions should not be confused with whether they can process, understand, and use this information in making intelligent and rational decisions.

Traditional counseling or "talk therapy" may have a role to play in restoration as well. Patients in the debilitating grip of anxiety, PTSD, or depression may improve even under short-term counseling sessions with a qualified therapist (*In re N.J.M.*, 2010).

Treatment may need to escalate to harsher modalities such as antipsychotic medication—and theoretically ECT and neurosurgery (though these options have almost never been used in competency cases since the 1970s). Defendants commonly start to balk at treatment when harsher options are prescribed.

## Conflicting Goals

The goal of competency restoration as far as the court and prosecution are concerned is to restore the defendant sufficiently so that the case can proceed to trial or a plea agreement. The goal of restoration as far as the defense is concerned may align with that. However, in some cases, the best outcome of the case for the defendant may be a finding of incompetency. The defense attorney will actively fight for and protect such a finding. That is not to say that the lawyer is trying to do something underhanded—no ethical professional would advise or encourage a defendant to fake incompetency; no lawyer serious about maintaining a bar license would raise the issue of incompetence when he or she does not see any indications of incompetency. But, when there is evidence suggesting that the defendant is incompetent, the defense could reasonably conclude that the goal is a judicial finding of incompetency coupled with a finding of unrestorability.

In short, recovery (for criminal competency purposes) may involve not recovering (for best medical outcome purposes). The defense may pursue this strategy in earnest from the start of restoration. This is understandable given that the prosecution very often distrusts psychological defenses, and opposes them vigorously. Anticipating a pitched courtroom battle, the defense must plan in advance to fight for an incompetence finding.

## Treatment Decision-Making

Defendants maintain the right to decide their medical treatment unless and until a court orders otherwise. They are not utterly stripped of the right to refuse medical treatment simply because they have been arrested for a crime or found incompetent. The need to make a decision nevertheless calls into question who will render that decision; when a defendant has been deemed incompetent, his or her ability to make intelligent decisions is obviously questionable.

As a matter of law, however, a defendant is allowed to decide to reject treatment meant to restore competency (*Riggins v. Nevada*, 1992). Whether mildly incompetent or floridly psychotic, a restoration defendant's refusal of treatment must be scrupulously honored. Thus, when a defendant declines recommended treatment, the restoration program has to try alternatives acceptable to the defendant, or seek a court order (via a *Sell* hearing) to involuntarily medicate.

The more difficult problem arises when a defendant appears willing to accept treatment, but the lawyer feels that the defendant should refuse it. Unlike the above scenario, the defendant's express wishes may not decide the matter. This seeming incongruity arises because the decision to refuse treatment is a matter of preserving the legal rights guaranteed to the criminally accused, and is not based on how competent the defendant is factually to make medical decisions. Where the defense attorney has concerns that undergoing restoration treatment would harm the defendant, hurt the defendant's ability to assist in his defense, or make the defendant even less competent, the attorney can assert a refusal of treatment on behalf of the client. When that occurs, restoration staff should not go forward with the defendant's apparent voluntary acceptance of treatment until a court decides the matter. The lawyer's assertion of the right to refuse treatment suffices to trigger the *Sell* litigation needed for a judge to decide this issue.

In rare and unfortunate instances, courts have appointed a guardian ad litem to make medical decisions for an incompetent defendant (*State v. Curry*, 2009; *State v. Veale*, 2009). Defense attorneys may resist that, as guardians ad litem are not trained in criminal defense and consequently may not sufficiently understand the subtle criminal legal rights and issues that are at stake—subject matter that criminal defense specialists are experts on. Guardians ad litem may not appreciate, for instance, that although administering antipsychotic medication to an agitated psychotic individual may help him or her think more clearly, remain calmer, and enjoy a better sense of well-being, the sedative effect of these drugs could be detrimental to his or her competency to proceed with trial.

## Involuntary Treatment

We open with the proposition that involuntary treatment can be antithetical to the concept of recovery advanced in this text. Under the premises that an individual may best determine how to achieve highest functioning in his or her environment, and that self-determination is an essential factor in psychological wellness, doctors may decline to recommend forced treatment. Note that that does not mean that a judge will agree, and the court may disregard doctors' recommendations and order the defendant to comply, including involuntary administration of medication if the defendant does not.

There is no "bright line" test to determine involuntary treatment in a criminal restoration setting. Involuntary medication decisions within a non-offender population are normally decided by balancing the patients' rights to refuse treatment against health and safety (of self and others) concerns (405 I.L.C.S. 5/2-107.1). A similar balancing is done when deciding forced medication within a criminal competency setting, but there are more factors than those two to consider.

Generally, treatment can be forced onto a criminal defendant involuntarily only under two circumstances. First, if a defendant needs medication because he or she is gravely disabled or poses an imminent risk of danger to self or others, forced medication can be authorized through an administrative (hospital administration, as opposed to a criminal court) process. Some jurisdictions set forth procedures for administrative hearings in statutes or regulations, others establish it in case law. In federal courts, this is referred to as a *Harper* hearing (*Washington v. Harper*, 1990; 28 C.F.R. § 549.43). The federal courts recognize a Due Process liberty interest to not be medicated against a person's will, but that is balanced against the defendant presenting a danger to self or others, and that the medication is medically appropriate. These administrative hearings typically offer only short-term intervention. They do not authorize long-term involuntary treatment, which usually must be justified by a court order even in a noncriminal inpatient population. Because of that, these administrative hearings will not support the long-term restoration needed to return a client to get through trial. *Harper* hearings are consequently not a viable restoration strategy.

Second, if there are no such imminent dangers, defendants committed for competency or restoration have additional rights that judges must weigh before involuntary treatment is given. In addition to Due Process, their Sixth Amendment (trial) rights may be implicated by psychotropic medication (*Riggins v. Nevada*, 1992). Judges must conduct a *Sell* hearing before hospital staff can involuntarily medicate an incompetent defendant (*Sell v. United States*, 2003). According to the Supreme Court's *Sell* decision, a judge may authorize a medical center to administer involuntary treatment within the competency restoration arena, but only when a number of rights are considered. The Supreme Court in *Sell* (2003) balanced these rights in a four factor test that the government must meet: (1) there must be "important governmental interests" at stake; (2) involuntary medication must "significantly further" those important governmental interests; (3) involuntary medication must be "necessary" to further those interests; and (4) involuntary medication must be "medically appropriate." When refusal of recommended treatment occurs, medical staff must inform the judge and lawyers of this impasse, and wait for the judge to analyze these factors to determine whether treatment can be forcefully administered to the unwilling defendant.

One of the more important issues that a judge must consider in a *Sell* hearing is whether the side-effects of the anticipated medication may in fact interfere with the defendant's interaction with counsel and assistance in his defense. While physicians must be concerned with potential medical side-effects of psychoactive medications, judges must additionally be concerned with the legal impact of those side-effects. Treatment can interfere with court hearings as much as assist with them. For instance, the so-called "antipsychotic" drugs have some degree of sedative effect on the patient. A defendant whose psychosis can be controlled on Haldol may nonetheless be slow to respond, may not grasp critical testimony, may be sluggish while testifying (hesitation in answering questions could be interpreted by a jury as evidence of lying), or may sleep through part of a trial. So even though the drug corrected the underlying psychosis, it ultimately interferes with the defendant's right to defend him- or herself, and assist counsel at trial.

Additionally, the second *Sell* factor (whether the recommended treatment is in fact likely to restore the defendant to competency) is not easily established for some drugs given some diagnoses. Medications with reliable efficacious impact on certain diseases will best meet this criterion. This depends upon how well the psychoactive ingredients correct the condition causing the illness. Some drugs are well tailored to certain diseases, and may pass this *Sell* factor easily: for instance, Ritalin works reliably and dramatically well—if for short time periods—with persons having ADHD; Lithium improves many persons suffering from Bipolar disorder; and the antipsychotic drugs are effective on approximately 75 % of Schizophrenics. Other less well understood or well tailored medications, or ones being applied off-label, may be rejected during *Sell* litigation (*United States v. Holden*, 2014; Elm and Passon 2008).

Furthermore, physically forcing medication on a resistant defendant may have seriously adverse impact when he or she has certain critical symptoms. For instance, persons suffering from persecutory delusions that the government or medical institution is "out to get them" will have their "delusions" confirmed as "reality" in this process! It will be far harder to disabuse them of their paranoias after a squad in protective (identity-concealing and depersonalizing) gear physically tie them to a bed and forcefully inject a drug.[6] The experience similarly may trigger flashbacks in persons who had suffered previous trauma, contributing to the inception or worsening of PTSD. Furthermore, phobic individuals may be so terrified by this procedure that they would prefer to take their own lives rather than face it a second time (*Ferch v. Jett*, 2015). Forcefully administering treatment can thus have grave impact on both recovery and restoration in a sizeable portion of the criminal restoration population.

Because so many factors are at play in a *Sell* analysis, it is not uncommon for courts to impose restrictions on a forced medication regimen. For instance, the judge may allow it: only for a short period of time; only if the defendant willfully complies with court-ordered treatment; may specify what medication (or class of drugs) may be used; and/or may require a trial run of second generation antipsychotics (such as Geodon) first, and only progress to first generation (such as Haldol) if that is unsuccessful. The Court may also impose restrictions on what could be considered "punitive" measures. In the *Sell* case, it was apparent that Dr. Sell's noncompliance with recommended medication was being "punished" by solitary confinement, lack of freedom and normal programming within the facility, and alleged mistreatment; judges have thereafter sometimes included in their orders limitations on the type of "motivational" techniques that the facility can use to try to secure the defendant's compliance with treatment. Restoration physicians should expect judges to exercise much greater "hands on" involvement in the treatment plan after *Sell* litigation.

Defendants may also resist medication (or competency) at trial so as to demonstrate to the jury their mental state when not under treatment. This occurs rarely, but may arise when an insanity or diminished capacity defense is raised. The defense attorney may want the jury to see for themselves how insane or compromised the defendant is when not adequately medicated, so would want the defendant to remain untreated during trial. This generates a conflict between the constitutional right to an effective defense and the Due Process right to be competent when prosecuted (*Commonwealth v. Louraine*, 1983; *State v. Maryott*, 1971; *State v. Hayes*, 1978). The *Louraine* court held that the right to present an insanity defense means more than the ability to verbalize or offer an expert's testimony about it: "the jury are likely to assess the weight of the various pieces of evidence before them with reference to defendant's demeanor. Further, if the defendant appears calm and controlled at trial,

[6]No professional practicing in forensic competency or restoration should start their work without having first watched a video of the aggressive physical confrontation that occurs in forced treatment.

the jury may well discount any testimony" regarding his insanity (*Commonwealth v. Louraine*, 1983).

## Post-*Sell* Hearing

If the hospital or prosecution succeeds in securing court-ordered involuntary treatment, then the medical staff must comply whether they recommended it or not. If the treatment works, then the defendant can be returned to court for legal proceedings to resume. However, because of the numerous legal rights and concerns implicated, if treatment interventions are not showing promise, doctors should discontinue their efforts as soon as lack of improvement is apparent.

If restoration fails to render a defendant competent, then charges can eventually be dismissed. In some states, the court must dismiss some charges when the defendant is determined to likely remain incompetent; others give courts discretion whether to immediately dismiss charges. Montana and Missouri call for immediate dismissal (Mont. Code § 46-14-221(3)(b); Mo. Stat. § 522.020.11(6)); Minnesota applies that principle to misdemeanors (Minn. R. Crim. P. § 20.01(6)(b)); and Arkansas and Hawaii allow dismissal when the judge believes that so much time has elapsed that it would be "unjust" to resume a prosecution (Ark. Code § 5-2-310(C); Haw. Rev. Stat. § 704-406(3)). However, a number of jurisdictions would interpose one additional procedure before releasing an incompetent defendant: determining whether he or she would pose a danger to society.

## Dangerousness

### Dangerousness Determination Process

In some jurisdictions, the judge will seek a forensic opinion whether the defendant poses a danger if released, and may accordingly commit him or her (18 U.S.C. § 4243(b); 18 U.S.C. § 4246(b)). In anticipation of this process, some evaluating facilities offer, and some judges seek, opinions of dangerousness during competency or restorability evaluations.

Assessing risk of danger is notoriously difficult—just due to the unpredictability of human behavior alone. It becomes increasing more complex, hence less accurate, given variations in most patients' psychological conditions over time, impact of changing hospital environments and a mobile staff, vagaries of funding for treatment regimens and placement centers, and unreliability of stable placements and support upon release (*State v. Germane*, 2009; *Atchison v. Cruz*, 2011). Nevertheless, evaluating professionals may be tasked with offering their best educated judgment of a defendant's future dangerousness if released from the hospital.

These are quasi-civil/quasi-criminal commitment proceedings, and criminal commitments may have different procedures or standards than their civil counterparts (*Matter of L.W.*, 2015). Like civil commitment processes, defendants retain Due Process rights and entitlement to counsel for these proceedings. However, this process may be overseen by criminal courts, rather than civil or mental health courts.

Once an opinion of dangerousness is issued, the judge will generally hold a hearing to determine dangerousness and the need for commitment. As in competency and restoration litigation, the lawyers could seek discovery of evidence concerning dangerousness, and professional staff may be called as witnesses or experts in this litigation.

## Post-commitment Review

There have to be options to release defendants from these commitments. Analyzing them under Equal Protection, the Supreme Court concluded that committed criminal defendants should get no worse treatment than committed civil patients (*Jackson v. Indiana*, 1972). Indiana, for example, had a statutory provision for civil commitments that allowed for release when the patient was no longer gravely disabled or no longer posed a danger to self or others. The criminal statute providing for commitment of defendants found incompetent and unrestorable was, however, silent as to any potential future release. In the *Davis* case, for instance, the committed criminal defendant contended he was deprived of constitutional protections by this scheme (*State v. Davis*, 2008). The Indiana Supreme Court agreed. Accordingly, Indiana's protocol was changed to allow for release from commitment when the defendant no longer poses any danger or is no longer gravely disabled.

The United States Supreme Court has only approved involuntary commitment statutes (both civil and criminal) under the Due Process clause when they satisfy these three requirements: (1) "the confinement takes place pursuant to proper procedures and evidentiary standards;" (2) there is a finding of "dangerousness either to one's self or to others;" and (3) proof of dangerousness is "coupled … with the proof of some additional factor," such as a "mental illness" or "mental abnormality" (*Kansas v. Hendricks*, 1997). Thus, although different jurisdictions have their particularized wording and laws, they include at the least these three conditions. Some states require more of course. California, for instance, decided that in order to commit a defendant who is mentally retarded, the state must prove mental retardation, danger to self or others, and that "mental retardation was a substantial cause of serious difficulty in controlling dangerous behavior" (*People v. Cuevas*, 2013). Mental health professionals should ask the lawyers for the particular standards that apply to their opinions.

Although the focus of release hearings is often on dangerousness, defendants are entitled to release—despite posing a serious threat of danger—if their mental illness is resolved. After all, release can also be premised upon remission of the triggering mental condition (*State v. Beaver*, 2014). At that point it is the responsibility of the law enforcement system, rather than the mental health system, to control a defendant's conduct.

Each jurisdiction has its own process, allowing for review hearings periodically for the defendant to seek release, and often allowing for the hospital to ask for release (usually whenever it opines it is appropriate). Practitioners should familiarize themselves with the standards applicable in their state. Defendants are also entitled to counsel at these hearings.

### Recovery Implications

Criminal defense lawyers have an obligation to preserve their clients' liberty interests (*Humphrey v. Cady*, 1972). Recall that these lawyers may attempt to secure their clients' release even when it is clearly not in their best medical or personal interests. Defendants' release is usually conditioned upon their no longer suffering from the mental illness or defect that led to their commitment, and/or their no longer posing any danger to the community. Ironically then, the same attorneys who had been advocating that their clients were mentally ill (hence incompetent or insane), and could not be restored (so charges should be dismissed), would of necessity reverse their tactics at this juncture.

Although they try to secure their clients' release, they may also stay involved with the clients post release. After all, most defendants initially secure only conditional releases that impose a number of terms that the defendant must comply with (such as taking prescribed medication, refraining from substance abuse, remaining in a productive residence or program, and reporting to supervising social work staff). Often continued support and assistance from the lawyer helps a defendant stay on track with his or her release terms so that the defendant will not violate those conditions. The long-range goal of defense counsel at times is to free the defendant from court-ordered commitment and supervision; that is best realized by ensuring success while the client is on a conditional release plan.

## Civil Commitment

### The Roots of Modern Civil Commitment Laws

Theoretically, the modern practice of civil commitment balances individual liberty interests with the need for involuntary psychiatric treatment. In this ideal world, the courts and mental health providers practice in a Goldilocks zone providing just the right amount of Due Process and treatment toward the goal of healthy independence for all. The reality is that shifting financial and legislative priorities constantly challenge America's mental health safety net. Many state hospitals struggle daily to provide meaningful treatment and legal services to clients seeking recovery. Despite these flawed systems, it is vital for all stakeholders to contribute to the success of each patient by understanding and strategically applying involuntary treatment laws, which exist to protect citizens and promote personal and societal wellness.

The common law concept of *parens patriae*, which originally existed as a doctrine granting English royalty the inherent power and authority to "parent" the people, has survived in American jurisprudence permitting the government to protect the interests of those who cannot speak for themselves. The most common application of *parens patriae* occurs in the court's treatment of children, the elderly, the mentally ill, or others deemed incompetent to manage their own affairs (Ratliff 2000; Testa and West 2010; *Alfred L. Sapp & Son, Inc. v. Puerto Rico*, 1982; *Hawaii v. Standard Oil Co. of California*, 1972; Curtis 1976). In the context of involuntary treatment laws, *parens patriae* operates in tandem with the police powers granted to the states via the Tenth Amendment to the United States Constitution, which leaves to them expansive regulatory discretion to legislate and enforce order for the health and welfare of the masses (Arrigo 2002; Testa and West 2010). Together, these legal principles provide the underpinning for modern involuntary civil commitments. In practice, the inherent dilemma has been reaching a balance between the government's obligations to ensure the safety of the masses while preserving the civil liberties of the individual.

Faced with the perpetual question of how best to care for individuals with significant mental health issues, the United States has gradually modified its involuntary treatment laws. During the 1700s and 1800s, oversimplified statutes governed indefinite hospitalizations, which were common due to a prevailing belief system that stigmatized mental illness and presumed that the asylum benefitted every patient (Gordon 2015). Instead of offering shelter and support, the asylum eventually became known for its abuses of civil liberties (Gordon 2015; Testa and West 2010). Beginning in the 1950s, a shift toward deinstitutionalization began to occur, based in part on the efforts of mental health professionals and civil rights lawyers working in tandem for reform (Appelbaum 1997). Concurrently, pharmaceutical science gave doctors an option to manage patient care in an outpatient setting. Further, the enactment of nationwide programs like Medicare and Medicaid, which provided federal funds to support community-based treatment, prompted widespread closures of state hospitals (Gordon 2015; Testa and West 2010).

Hand in hand with this deinstitutionalization shift came the development of the "dangerousness paradigm." In the civil commitment setting, this new legal standard was prescribed by the Supreme Court in *O'Connor v. Donaldson* (1975): "a State cannot constitutionally confine without more a nondangerous individual who is capable of surviving safely in freedom by himself or with the help of willing and responsible family members or friends." The Supreme Court made clear that the state must show at least one of the following three justifications for civil commitment: danger to self or others, inability to care for oneself, or the necessity of treatment to cure a mental illness (*O'Connor v. Donaldson*, 1975). These parameters remain the underpinning of almost every involuntary treatment commitment law today.

Since this major shift in American mental health policy, problems have continued to plague the nation's mentally ill. The positive growth of community-based treatment providers seen in the early days of deinstitutionalization faltered as state and federal spending shifted to a decentralized model in the 1980s, which impaired the development of comprehensive modern mental health services (Gordon 2015; McGuan 2009). Scores of mentally ill Americans have since been funneled into the prison system (Gordon 2015;

McGuan 2009; Testa and West 2010). For others caught in the revolving door of involuntary commitments, meaningful mental health treatment with individualized recovery in the least restrictive setting remains an elusive goal.

Recently, perceived problems with the "dangerousness" legal framework have led to an uptick in the demand for further reform of the civil commitment system. The change is toward a focus on a "need for treatment" standard and increased use of outpatient treatment (Gordon 2015; McGuan 2009; Stettin et al. 2014). Some of these proposals are promising, and many have been spearheaded by mental health professionals and lawyers alike. Even so, the current state of the law in almost every state continues to use "dangerousness" language, and therefore all practitioners must remain educated in these standards and work within them to promote health and wellness for their patients.

## Inpatient Civil Commitment: Elements, Definitions, and Due Process

Since the *Donaldson* case, the Supreme Court has been quite laissez-faire in the arena of civil commitments. Even so, certain important precedent has been set by the highest court, which continues to dictate state legislation and civil commitment procedure. Four years after the groundbreaking *Donaldson* decision, in *Addington v. Texas* (1979), the Supreme Court raised the standard of proof for all involuntary treatment commitments from "preponderance of the evidence," to "clear and convincing evidence." Thus, the Court required greater proof (of dangerousness or grave disability) before allowing a judge to deprive an individual of his or her liberty interests by commitment. In 1982, the Supreme Court made clear in *Youngblood v. Romero* (1982) that every person has a protected interest in freedom from confinement and personal restraint, requiring Due Process before that civil liberty is restrained by involuntary commitment.

Every state allows for involuntary commitments of individuals who suffer from a diagnosable mental health disorder and are a danger to themselves or others. Not all statutes read similarly, nor are they used uniformly across the nation (Brooks 2007; Treatment Advocacy Center 2011). Commonly, involuntary treatment laws include the following legal elements: the individual is currently suffering from a diagnosable mental health disorder (DSM-5) *and as a result of this disorder*; the individual is a danger to herself or others, *or* the individual is gravely disabled, *and* the individual is unwilling or unable to be voluntarily treated, *and* Assisted Outpatient Treatment ("AOT") is inadequate to address the immediate risk. These statutory elements are legal and not medical in nature. State laws or court opinions define, for example, "dangerousness" or "grave disability;" these terms are not intended to be flexible, nor are they subject to interpretation by mental health professionals on a case-by-case basis. These standards exist to promote uniformity, fairness, and integrity to the process due each patient every time he or she is facing commitment proceedings.

To understand these legal elements, definitions, and commitment practices, it is useful to focus on one particular state's Involuntary Treatment Act. The state of Washington has a well-developed system for handling civil commitments that is typical of others found across the country. Washington prefers that an individual receive the least restrictive means of treatment possible, and allows for AOT orders when appropriate (Rev. Code Wash. 71.05.012; Rev. Code Wash. 71.05.145). Where inpatient commitment is sought, the state must prove that the individual (a) has a mental disorder and, as a result of that mental disorder, (b) is gravely disabled, or (c) presents a likelihood of serious harm to themselves, others, or property (Rev. Code Wash. 71.05.153; Rev. Code Wash. 71.05.240). Washington's definition of "mental disorder" encompasses "any organic, mental, or emotional impairment which has substantial adverse effects on a person's cognitive or volitional functions" (Rev. Code Wash. 71.05.020(26)). Therefore, it includes, but is not limited to, the following: depression, schizophrenia, bipolar disorder, dementia, developmental disabilities, and traumatic brain injury (Rev. Code Wash. 71.05.040).

The presence of a "mental disorder" alone cannot result in an involuntary commitment (*In re LaBelle*, 1986). It must be sufficiently serious to impair cognitive or volitional functioning, resulting in presenting as gravely disabled or dangerous. Washington's "gravely disabled" standard is met when the state can prove by clear and convincing evidence that, as a result of the person's mental disorder, the person is: (a) in danger of serious physical harm resulting from a failure to provide for his or her essential human needs or health or safety; or (b) manifesting severe deterioration in routine functioning evidenced by repeated and escalating loss of cognitive or volitional control over his or her actions and not receiving such care as is essential for his or her health or safety (Rev. Code Wash. 71.05.020(17)). Gravely disabled persons may display the following examples of behavior occurring as a result of a diagnosable mental condition and its symptoms: individuals who are starving themselves; individuals who are allowing medical conditions to become unmanageable; individuals who are on reckless spending sprees or losing their homes; individuals who are not perceiving reality or orienting themselves to time, place, and person; or individuals who have lost cognitive functioning or cannot remember or retain information. These persons may suffer from dementia and Alzheimer's, have been inflicted with traumatic brain injury, or are catatonic. They can be gravely disabled under other medical conditions as well, so long as those fit within the parameters of the DSM-5, and the problematic behavior is a result of those symptoms.

Even though these gravely disabled cases can include some factually very disturbing situations, civil commitment remains a significant deprivation of liberty that is not to be taken lightly. Even when the patient is nonresponsive, if a civil commitment lawyer believes that the alleged grave disability does not meet the above elements, or that the individual can be cared for by family and friends in a less restrictive setting, the lawyer will actively contest commitment. In most states, the simple fact that a person may need treatment is not grounds for involuntary commitment (Brooks 2007). Additionally, just because a person may make questionable choices should not result in loss of liberty. The concerning behavior must not be a lifestyle choice, but rather a result of such deteriorated thinking based on the underlying mental condition so as to render the person incapable of making rational decisions (*In re LaBelle*, 1986). This standard may seem cruel as it results in the release of people whose condition may be improved by treatment, but the *Donaldson* (1975) opinion made clear that no one should be confined against their will if they can live free in adequate safety.

The presence of a mental disorder alone also does not establish dangerousness. Unlike the gravely disabled standard, which relies on a danger of harm due to *passive* behavior, this provision relies on that danger from *active* conduct by the patient (*In re LaBelle*, 1986). The individual must present with a likelihood of serious harm. Washington's dangerousness standard is met when the state can prove by clear and convincing evidence that as a result of the person's mental disorder, there is a substantial risk that: (a) physical harm will be inflicted by an individual upon his or her own person, as evidenced by threats or attempts to commit suicide or inflict physical harm on oneself; (b) physical harm will be inflicted by an individual upon another person, as evidenced by behavior which has caused such harm or which places another person or persons in reasonable fear of sustaining such harm; (c) physical harm will be inflicted by an individual upon the property of others, as evidenced by behavior which has caused substantial loss or damage to the property of others; or (d) the individual has threatened the physical safety of another and has a history of one or more violent acts (Rev. Code Wash. 71.05.020(25)).

Recent and tangible factual evidence of these elements must be present, which often includes suicidal or homicidal threats, or criminal acting out (where law enforcement benevolently decided the better course would be commitment rather than arrest). This may mean that the evidence of the problematic behavior used to determine commitment is often established by some non-medical assessment by a lay person or police; these lay witnesses are not trained mental health professionals, and their evidence consequently may not be the most useful information for proving dangerousness or grave disability. Hence, many states allow courts to also consider the individual's recent history when determining dangerousness, including information from recent civil commitments or treating physicians (Rev. Code Wash. 71.05.012).

If the person is likely to be arrested if released from the involuntary treatment hold, lawyers will often attempt to convince the patient to agree to the civil commitment in lieu of facing criminal charges. However, if the individual is likely to face freedom should they be released from the hold, these dangerousness commitments can often result in contested hearings with testimony not unlike criminal trials.

It should be noted that even in the civil, nonforensic arena, people face significant social stigma and collateral consequences if involuntarily civilly committed. Even a short 14-day commitment can cost people their jobs or housing, or displace them from a comforting schedule of activities or interaction with friends and family, which may be invaluable to that person. Involuntary commitment also carries potential future criminal consequences, for example, in some jurisdictions those who were committed can be arrested if they later possess a firearm (18 U.S.C. §922(g)(4)). Therefore, although the individual could benefit from treatment, he or she may vigorously contest commitment for reasons far beyond those contemplated by mental health professionals. Again, it is the lawyer's job to advocate for liberty, which may or may not always be in line with an individual's path to recovery.

Once a mental health professional has identified an individual who meets commitment criteria, the involuntary treatment process begins with an initial detention. In Washington, this is a 72-hour hold period that cannot last longer without patient consent or a court order (Rev. Code Wash. 71.05.180; Rev. Code Wash. 71.05.240). Though some individuals never need more than the three-day hospitalization, so do not see legal advocates, most persons in initial detention are moving into the commitment process, so end up with counsel. The court appoints a lawyer to represent any individual facing a 14-day (or longer) civil commitment (Rev. Code Wash. 71.05.150(2)(c)). The attorney visits the client and advises him or her of Due Process rights and what to expect in this process. Often, the lawyer will seek information about the circumstances surrounding the current detention, as well as the individual's background and life circumstances. It should be noted that attorneys are often referred to by the apt title of "counselors at law," and the civil commitment legal practice involves a lot of active listening and redirection, professional interactions commonly associated with therapeutic "counseling." If the client is able to communicate a decision regarding commitment, he or she will either consent to it or request a contested hearing (Rev. Code Wash. 71.05.240). When the client is unable to speak for him- or herself, the attorney must request the appointment of a guardian ad litem to speak for the client. This should be minimized, as even the most disabled patients should guide their own legal representation if they can communicate at all (*In re Detention of J.S.*, 2007).

The legal representation of persons facing civil commitment is both necessary and important. Because Due Process is a constitutional mandate, it behooves mental health professionals to assist lawyers, even when they are on opposite sides of commitment litigation. To that end, hospital and treatment center staff should consider the following: (1) providing confidential areas for attorney–client visits that are also safe and accessible by security; (2) accommodating lawyers when they request access to medical records and copy machines; and (3) engaging in candid conversations with legal advocates about relevant recovery topics, including social services, and community resources, and other long-term plans for the client beyond the narrow four corners of the commitment petition. In the end, even when medical staff "loses" a commitment hearing, the patient's rights were protected, and the doctors will have contributed to devising the best outpatient treatment plan for their patient.

All is not adversarial in the civil commitment setting. When the client chooses to comply with treatment, the legal advocate may be more willing to work hand in hand with the mental health professional. But, before this can occur, attorneys need to be able to safely and timely assess the client's legal situation. Staff efforts to hamper this process would only create more litigation; cooperation with discovery for the lawyer may thus avoid a pitched court battle. Additionally, because civil commitment cases move quickly, lawyers do not have time to mediate any conflict with staff before they are expected to competently advise the client and appear in court. Consequently, when lawyers have easy access to clients and records in a safe and confidential environment, they have more time to work with treating doctors, family, and community support systems to further the recovery needs of the patient.

When the client wants to fight commitment, or when conciliatory efforts fail, the court holds an evidentiary hearing and makes findings of fact and law determining whether the person is released or hospitalized. In Washington, a 90-day petition for inpatient treatment is available for individuals who continue to meet commitment standards even after the initial period of detention, and still cannot be served by less restrictive conditions in the community (Rev. Code Wash. 71.05.300). At this stage, Due Process is heightened, and so a jury trial may be requested. For these trials, legal advocates can also hire their own experts (Rev. Code Wash. 71.05.300). Further 180-day proceedings are rare and have somewhat different procedures, such as excluding commitments for individuals who are a harm to self (Rev. Code Wash. 71.05.320(2)).

## Patient Rights

Once committed, patients continue to have rights, which are codified in state law and the federal mental health patient's Bill of Rights (42 U.S.C. § 9501; Rev. Code Wash. 71.05.220). Relevant to this topic is the patients' continuing rights to the following:

- appropriate treatment and services in a setting most supportive of their personal liberty, which should only be restricted to the extent necessary consistent with all relevant laws and court orders;
- regular review of their individualized treatment plan to include reassessment of whether inpatient treatment is necessary;
- patient participation with that treatment plan with accessible explanations thereof;
- protection from certain treatment modalities, including experimentation, unless permitted by law;
- freedom from restraints and seclusion unless in an emergent well-documented situation;
- humane conditions of confinement, including privacy and confidentiality with access to records and visitors with limited exceptions;
- grievance procedures for patients to self-advocate without fear of retaliation; and
- referrals to case-appropriate community professionals upon discharge.

While these standards are all exercised in slightly different ways throughout the nation's hospitals, they must be posted in the wards where patients can access and review them (42 U.S.C. § 9501(3)(D)). The monumental *Donaldson* (1975) case arose not only in response to the lack of Due Process at the commitment stage, but also due to Donaldson's subsequent 15-year restraint with virtually no liberties within the facility itself. The Court was shocked by the continual denial (without explanation) of Donaldson's repeated requests for ground privileges, occupational training, and opportunities to discuss his treatment plan. Patient rights are an integral piece of the commitment process, without which the fundamental ideals of treatment toward recovery crumble.

Involuntary medication in civil commitments continues to present challenges. While the law regulating involuntary medication of a criminal defendant is well defined in the forensic context, it is less well developed in the civil context. "Forced meds" in the civil commitment setting is not governed by any Supreme Court case, and so there is a great variation in how different states handle it. Nonetheless, all must at least overcome the "compelling state interest" standard (Hinton and Forrest 2007). Generally in Washington, patients have a right to refuse antipsychotic medicine unless the failure to medicate is determined to result in a likelihood of serious harm or substantial deterioration and there is no less intrusive course of treatment (Rev. Code Wash. 71.05.210; Rev. Code Wash. 71.05.215; Rev. Code Wash. 71.05.217). ECT may only be administered upon a court order after full Due Process and proof shown by clear and convincing evidence that it is necessary (Rev. Code Wash. 71.05.217; *In re Schuoler*, 1986).

## Beyond the "Dangerousness" Standard

After *Donaldson* (1975), many states constructed narrow statutes including specific language tracking the Supreme Court opinion. However, exceptions exist, such as in Arizona, which has a "need-for-treatment" standard as opposed to the typical "danger to self or others" requirement (Ariz. Rev. Stat. § 36-540(A)). Commitment will be ordered in Arizona even when a person can still meet basic survival needs and exhibits no violent or suicidal tendencies if they are found to be "persistently or acutely disabled" (Ariz. Rev. Stat. § 36-501(31)). This is defined as a severe mental disorder meeting the following criteria:

- If not treated has a substantial probability of causing the person to suffer or continue to suffer severe and abnormal mental, emotional, or physical harm that significantly impairs judgment, reason, behavior, or capacity to recognize reality.
- Substantially impairs the person's capacity to make an informed decision regarding treatment and this impairment causes the person to be incapable of understanding and expressing an understanding of the advantages and disadvantages of accepting treatment and understanding and expressing an understanding of the alternatives to the particular treatment offered after the advantages, disadvantages, and alternatives are explained to that person.
- Has a reasonable prospect of being treatable.

Thus, immanency and dangerousness are not required in Arizona, which casts a broader net and impacts the liberty interests of more individuals. This type of statutory language has been widely advocated for by mental health professionals—and for good reason from their perspective—as it may serve to protect more people and treat patients before actual harm or an arrest occurs. However, if history is any indication, the shift back to an over-reliance on *parens patriae* and the police powers of the states to involuntarily commit people only because they need treatment can result in a myriad of civil liberties abuses that the Supreme Court has specifically precluded. A measured approach is needed to ensure that Due Process and patient rights remain intact, while the abuses of the past are not repeated and relitigated in an infinite loop.

The emerging push to better utilize "assisted outpatient treatment" laws or "AOT" is perhaps less polarizing to civil libertarians and mental health providers. New York's "Kendra's Law" is an AOT statute backed by a state mandate for counties to "operate, direct and supervise an AOT program" (N.Y. Mental Hyg. Law § 9.60). Thus, involuntary treatment courts in New York have far more less restrictive options when fashioning commitment orders because AOT is funded and available. This assists new patients as well as individuals reintegrating into society after a lengthier inpatient commitment. While AOT impacts civil liberties (because discharged patients are still under court orders mandating treatment, and violation may result in returning to hospital placement), the restraints on freedom of movement, privacy, and other constitutional concerns are mitigated in this setting. In Washington, individuals facing violation of their AOT have the same right to notice, hearing, and counsel as a person facing initial commitment (Rev. Code. Wash. 71.05.230; Rev. Code. Wash. 71.05.240). Thus, AOT provides an opportunity for greater liberty while ensuring that Due

Process remains intact should the individual's mental state worsen.

Whether or not a state has a "dangerousness" or "need-for-treatment" statute, or is utilizing their AOT laws to their fullest extent, the mental health community faces challenging populations who need treatment, but do not fully meet the definitions for the "severe mental disease or defect" requirement. These individuals include persons suffering from personality disorders, eating disorders, and disorders involving addiction (Testa and West 2010). The DSM-5 may resolve some of these concerns by removing the "Axis II" label and relying more heavily on the impact of symptoms. Mental health professionals should expect to see litigation regarding those DSM-5 changes over the coming years, if not already in some localities.

## The Goals of Civil Commitment

Despite the frequent adversarial relationship of lawyers and mental health professionals in civil commitment courts, these two groups also have a history of working together on systemic change. In fact, the ultimate goals of mental health professionals and lawyers in the involuntary treatment setting are not so different (Rev. Code. Wash. 71.05.010). Mental health advocates have always looked to put an end to the inappropriate, indefinite commitment of the mentally ill; legal advocates have worked to try to find the best treatment options for clients as well. Mental health providers aim to provide prompt evaluation and short-term treatment of patients; lawyers want to provide effective advocacy quickly so as to avoid continuances and unnecessary involuntary detentions. Mental health advocates often hope to safeguard individual rights of patients just as much as lawyers, and extend those sensitivities into the realm of forced medications and controversial treatment modalities. Hospitals want to provide continuity of care and attorneys want to maintain communication with clients, mental health professionals, and family to accomplish their client's unique end goal. Mental health advocates are actively promoting and encouraging community-based care, just as lawyers advocate for the recovery path of the client's choosing. Mental health professionals are interested in protecting the public safety; civil commitment lawyers are always educating the client on both short-and long-term impacts of legal decisions while enabling choices leading the client away from future involuntary detention in hospitals or jails. In all of these ways, these two groups have more in common than it may seem at first glance.

## Conclusion

Despite efforts in the latter half of the twentieth century to shift mental health treatment into the community, more than 200 state hospitals remain open and serve a diverse patient population (Fisher et al. 2009). All of these patients have a constitutionally protected interest in their liberty and specific Due Process rights associated with their detention. Doubtless they also have medical needs that must be addressed before reaching a state of wellness. Doctors and lawyers may have different roles to play in the lives of these patients, but everyone is working toward an overarching goal of recovery in a free society.

The modern Hippocratic Oath (Miles 2004) champions the circumvention of "those twin traps of overtreatment and therapeutic nihilism," and urges "that warmth, sympathy, and understanding may outweigh the surgeon's knife or the chemist's drug." The Oath encourages seeking assistance "when the skills of another are needed for a patient's recovery," reminds that illness "may affect the person's family and economic stability," and inspires a sense of social responsibility "with special obligations to all my fellow human beings." Similarly, the Preamble to the American Bar Association's Model Rules of Professional Conduct (ABA Model Rules of Professional Conduct, Preamble (1), (6)) states that "[a] lawyer, as a member of the legal profession, is a representative of clients, an officer of the legal system and a public citizen having special responsibility for the quality of justice." It continues:

> As a public citizen, a lawyer should seek improvement of the law, access to the legal system, the administration of justice and the quality of service rendered by the legal profession. In addition, a lawyer should further the public's understanding of and confidence in the rule of law and the justice system because legal institutions in a constitutional democracy depend on popular participation and support to maintain their authority. A lawyer should be mindful of deficiencies in the administration of justice and of the fact that the poor, and sometimes persons who are not poor, cannot afford adequate legal assistance. Therefore, all lawyers should devote professional time and resources and use civic influence to ensure equal access to our system of justice for all those who because of economic or social barriers cannot afford or secure adequate legal counsel.

Collectively, these professional vows and guidelines are inspiring and complimentary. Together, mental health providers and legal advocates can mold a genuine yet practical vision of a mental health system providing justice and a path to recovery for all.

**Acknowledgment** The authors are deeply indebted to the research contributions of Carlos Cruz, a Stetson University College of Law student, in gathering materials for this publication.

## Statutes

18 U.S.C. § 922
18 U.S.C. § 4241
18 U.S.C. § 4243
18 U.S.C. § 4246
28 C.F.R. § 549.43
42 U.S.C. § 9501
405 I.L.C.S. 5/2-107
ABA Criminal Justice Mental Health Standards
ABA Model Rules of Professional Responsibility
Ariz. Rev. Stat. § 13-502
Ariz. Rev. Stat. § 13-4021
Ariz. Rev. Stat. § 36-501
Ariz. Rev. Stat. § 36-540
Ark. Code § 5-2-310
Cal. Penal Code § 1367
Colo. Rev. Stat. § 16-8-101.5
Conn. Gen. Stat. §§ 54-56d
Fla. Stat. § 790.25
Fla. Stat. § 922.07
Ga. Code § 17-10-60
Haw. Rev. Stat. § 704-406
Minn. R. Crim. P. § 20.01
Mo. Stat. § 522.020.11
Mont. Code § 46-14-221
N.C. Gen. Stat. § 15A-1001
N.Y. Corr. Law § 656
N.Y. Mental Hygiene Law § 9.60
Ohio Rev. Code § 2949.28
Rev. Code Wash. 10.77.086
Rev. Code Wash. 71.05.010
Rev. Code Wash. 71.05.012
Rev. Code Wash. 71.05.020
Rev. Code Wash. 71.05.040
Rev. Code Wash. 71.05.145
Rev. Code Wash. 71.05.150
Rev. Code Wash. 71.05.153
Rev. Code Wash. 71.05.180
Rev. Code Wash. 71.05.210
Rev. Code Wash. 71.05.215
Rev. Code Wash. 71.05.217
Rev. Code Wash. 71.05.220
Rev. Code Wash. 71.05.230
Rev. Code Wash. 71.05.240
Rev. Code Wash. 71.05.300
Rev. Code Wash. 71.05.320
Wyo. Stat. § 7-13-901

## Cases

*Addington v. Texas*, 441 U.S. 418 (1979).
*Alfred L. Snapp & Son, Inc. v. Puerto Rico*, 458 U.S. 592 (1982).
*Altoonian v. Warren*, 2015 WL 1345378 (E.D. Mich. 2015).
*Atchison v. Cruz*, 2011 WL 783096 (E.D. Mich. 2011).
*Bethea v. United States*, 365 A.2d 64 (D.C. 1976).

*Commonwealth v. Louraine*, 390 Mass. 28 (1983).
*Cooper v. Oklahoma*, 517 U.S. 348 (1996).
*Daniel M'Naghten's* Case (1843) 8 ER 718.
*Dusky v. United States*, 362 U.S. 402 (1960).
*Ex parte Alabama Dept. of Mental Health,* 146 So.3d 413 (Ala. 2013).
*Faretta v. California*, 422 U.S. 806 (1975).
*Ferch v. Jett*, 2015 WL 251766 (D. Minn. 2015).
*Ford v. Wainwright*, 477 U.S. 399 (1986).
*Godinez v. Moran*, 509 U.S. 389 (1993).
*Gumm v. Mitchell*, 775 F. 3d 345 (6th Cir. 2014).
*Hawaii v. Standard Oil Co. of California*, 405 U.S. 251 (1972).
*Hubbard v. State*, 31 S.W. 3d 25 (Mo. App. 2000).
*Humphrey v. Cady*, 405 U.S. 504 (1972).
*In re Detention of J.S.*, 159 P.3d 435 (2007).
*In re LaBelle*, 107 Wash.2d 196 (1986).
*In re N.J.M.,* 2010 WL 4621877 (Ohio App. 2010).
*In re Schuoler*, 106 Wash.2d 500 (1986).
*Indiana v. Edwards,* 554 U.S. 164 (2008).
*Jackson v. Indiana*, 406 U.S. 715 (1972).
*Jones v. Knipp*, 2013 WL 6145245 (E.D. Cal. 2013).
*Kansas v. Hendricks*, 521 U.S. 346 (1997).
*Matter of Foley*, 439 Mass. 324 (2003).
*Matter of L.W.*, 2015 WL 135571 (Tex. App. 2015).
*Morrow v. State*, 293 Md. 247 (1982).
*Moye v. Warden*, 2014 WL 1674172 (Conn. Super. 2014).
*O'Connor v. Donaldson*, 422 U.S. 563 (1975).
*People v. Amador,* 200 Cal. App.3d 1449 (1988).
*People v. Brown*, 2014 WL 2836000 (Ill. App. 2014).
*People v. Cuevas*, 160 Cal. Rptr.3d 773 (Cal. App. 2013).
*People v. Girk,* 2014 WL 2510503 (Cal. App. 2014).
*Pruitt v. State*, 834 N.E. 2d 90 (Ind. 2005).
*Riggins v. Nevada*, 504 U.S. 127 (1992).
*Ryan v. Gonzales*, 133 S. Ct. 696 (2013).
*Sell v. United States*, 539 U.S. 166 (2003).
*Simon v. McCarty*, 2014 WL 7338860 (E.D. N.Y. 2015).
*State v. Beaver*, 184 Wash. App. 235 (Wash. 2014).
*State v. Camacho*, 561 N.W.2d 160 (Minn. 1997).
*State v. Connor*, 152 Conn. App. 780 (2014).
*State v. Curry*, 186 Vt. 623 (2009).
*State v. Davis*, 898 N.E.2d 281 (Ind. 2008).
*State v. Germane*, 971 A.2d 555 (R.I. 2009).
*State v. Hayes*, 118 N.H. 458 (1978).
*State v. Kinney*, 35 Ohio App.3d 84 (1987).
*State v. Maestas*, 299 P.3d 892 (Utah 2012).
*State v. Maryott,* 6 Wash. App. 96 (1971).
*State v. Veale*, 158 N.H. 632 (2009).
*United States v. Baker*, 45 F.3d 837 (4th Cir. 1995).
*United States v. Benson*, 2015 WL 1064738 (N. D. Cal. 2015).
*United States v. Brown*, 2015 WL 1573365 (E.D. Pa. 2015).
*United States v. Calkins,* 906 F.2d 1240 (8th Cir. 1990).
*United States v. Frazier*, 255 F. Supp. 2d 27 (D. Conn. 2001).
*United States v. Gigante*, 166 F.3d 175 (2nd Cir. 1999).
*United States v. Gillenwater*, 717 F.3d 1070 (9th Cir. 2013).
*United States v. Holden*, 53 Conn. Super. 290 (2014).
*United States v. Lindley*, 774 F.2d 993 (9th Cir. 1985).
*United States v. Merriweather*, 921 F. Supp. 2d 1265 (N.D. Ala. 2013).
*United States v. Minter*, 45 F. Supp. 3d 1390 (N.D. Ga. 2014).
*United States v. Pollock*, 2014 WL 5782778 (M.D. Fla. 2014).
*United States v. Robertson*, 2015 WL 520220 (E.D.N.Y. 2015).
*United States v. Wolfson*, 616 F. Supp. 2d 398 (S.D.N.Y. 2008).
*Washington v. Harper,* 494 U.S. 210 (1990).
*Wilson v. United States*, 391 F.2d 460 (D.C. Cir. 1968).
*Youngblood v. Romero*, 457 U.S. 307 (1982).

## References


American Psychiatric Association. (2013). *The diagnostic and statistical manual of mental disorders* (5th ed). Washington, D.C.

Appelbaum, P. (1997). Almost a revolution: An international perspective on the law of civil commitment. *Journal of the American Academy of Psychiatry and Law, 25*, 135.

Applebaum, P. (2013). Law and psychiatry: Does the constitution require an insanity defense? *Psychology, 64*(10), 943–945.

Arrigo, B. A. (2002). *Punishing the mentally ill: A critical analysis of law and psychiatry*. Albany, NY: State University of New York Press.

Bennion, E. (2013). A right to remain psychotic? A new standard for involuntary treatment in light of current science. *Loyola of Los Angeles Law Review, 47*, 251.

Brooks, R. A. (2007). Psychiatrists' opinions about involuntary civil commitment: Results of a national survey. *Journal of the American Academy of Psychiatry and Law, 35*(2), 221–223.

Curtis, G. P. (1976). The checkered career of parens patriae: The state as parent or tyrant? *DePaul Law Review, 25*, 895.

Elm, D., & Passon, D. (2008). Forced medication after U. S. v. Sell: Fighting your client's "war on drugs." *The Champion*, 32.

Feuerstein, S., Fortunati, F., Southwick, S., Temporini, H., & Morgan, C. (2005). Malingering and forensic psychiatry. *Psychiatry (Edgemont), 2*(12), 25–28.

Fisher, W. H., Geller, J. L., & Pandiani, J. A. (2009). The changing role of the state psychiatric hospital. *Health Affairs, 28*, 3676–3684.

Frank, J. N. (1957). Some reflections on judge learned hand. *Faculty Scholarship Series*, Paper 4099 (Yale Law School).

Giedd, J. N. (2004). Structural magnetic resonance imaging of the adolescent brain. *Annals of the New York Academy of Sciences, 1021*, 77–85.

Giedd, J. N., & Blumethal, J. (1999). Brain development during childhood and adolescence: A longitudinal MRI study. *Nature Neuroscience, 2*(10), 861–863.

Glaze, L. E., & James, D. J. (2006). *Mental Health Problems of Prison and Jail Inmates*. Bureau of Justice Statistics Special Report. U.S. Department of Justice, Office of Justice Programs Washington, D.C. Retrieved from http://bjs.ojp.usdoj.gov/content/pub/pdf/mhppji.pdf

Gordon, S. (2015). The danger zone: How the dangerousness standard in civil commitment proceedings harms people with serious mental illness. *Utah Law Review*.

Hinton, J., & Forrest, R. (2007). Involuntary non-emergent psychotropic medication. *Journal of the American Academy of Psychiatry and Law, 35*(3), 398.

McCoy, D. (2011). The psychology of litigation. *Forensic Psych Pages*. Retrieved from http://www.forensicpsychpages.com/competency_restoration.htm

McGuan, E. A. (2009). New standards for the involuntary commitment of the mentally ill: "Danger" redefined. *Marquette Elder's Advisor, 11*, 188.

Miles, S. H. (2004). *The hippocratic oath and the ethics of medicine*. Oxford: Oxford University Press.

Murphy, T. (2015). Another provision of helping families in mental health crisis act advances in the house (Press release). Retrieved from http://murphy.house.gov/latest-news/another-provision-of-helping-families-in-mental-health-crisis-act-advances-in-the-house/

Pemberton, P. (2014). Mentally ill defendants languish in jail from lack of hospital space. *The Tribune*. Retrieved from http://www.sanluisobispo.com/2014/01/04/2862256_mentally-ill-defendants-legal.html?rh=1

Philipsborn, J. (2015). Selected competence-related rulings: Useful lessons in approaches to the analysis of competence to stand trial. *The Champion*, 50.

Poythress, N., Monhan, J., Bonnie, R., Otto, R. K., & Hoge, S. K. (2002). *Adjudicative competence: The MacArthur studies*. New York: Kluwer/Plenum.

Putnam, F. W., Guroff, J. J., Silberman, E. K., Barban, L., & Post, R. M. (1986). The clinical phenomenology of multiple personality disorder: A review of 100 recent cases. *Journal of Clinical Psychiatry, 47*, 285–293.

Ratliff, J. (2000). Parens patriae: An overview. *Tulane Law Review, 74*, 1847.

Rogers, R. (2008). *Clinical assessment of malingering and deception* (3rd ed.). New York: Guilford Press.

Samuel, S., & Michaels, T. (2011). Competency restoration. In E. Drogin, F. Dattilio, R. Sadoff, & T. Gutheil (Eds.), *Handbook of forensic assessment: Psychological and psychiatric perspectives*. New York: John Wiley.

Stettin, B., Geller, J., Ragosta, K., Cohen, K., & Ghowrwal, J. (2014). *Mental health commitment laws: A survey of the states*. Arlington, VA: Treatment Advocacy Center.

Testa, M., & West, S. G. (2010). Civil commitment in the United States. *Psychiatry, 7*, 30.

Treatment Advocacy Center. (2011). *State standards charts for assisted treatment: Civil commitment criteria and initiation procedures by state*. Arlington, VA: Author.

Tysse, J. E., & Hafemeister, T. L. (2006). Amnesia and the determination of competency to stand trial. *Developments in Mental Health Law, 25*, 65.

United States Department of Justice. (2003). *Uniform crime reports: Age-specific arrest rates and race-specific arrest rates for selected offenses, 1993–2001*. Washington, DC: Author.

Uphoff, R. (1988). The role of the criminal defense lawyer in representing the mentally impaired defendant: Zealous advocate or officer of the court? *Wisconsin Law Review*, 65–109.

# 16 Stigma and Recovery

Kathy Bashor, Susan Junck, Colleen McGregor and Cheryl Anderson

## Introduction

One of the strongest deterrents to seeking mental healthcare is the stigma associated with mental illness in our society. Johnstone (2001, p. 201) stated, "People suffering from mental illness and other mental health problems are among the most stigmatized, discriminated against, marginalized, disadvantaged and vulnerable members of our society." Stigma is a pernicious form of discrimination that has broad effects on the lives of those seeking treatment, their families, and caregivers. One in four of us will personally experience mental illness in our lifetime. We are all likely to deal with mental illness at some point in our life journey, whether with a family member, a loved one, a friend or professional colleague, neighbor, or with ourselves. The effects of stigma on an individual, their families and their friends can be overwhelming (Wahl 1999; Wahl and Harman 1989). As individuals living with mental illness experience the full brunt of the disease, their loved ones experience the ramifications of the disease, right along with them. Denial, anger, fear and sadness are just a few of the emotions experienced by individuals with mental illness—the experience is much like being on an emotional roller coaster. The difficulties associated with living with mental illness are magnified by one's experience with rejection and discrimination, which are consequences of stigma.

Deegan (1993) and Reidy (1993) provided their personal experience with stigma and how it impacts self-esteem, empowerment, hope, and sense of recovery. Accompanying the roller coaster of emotions, people who have intimately experienced mental illness encounter various challenges that complicate their lives caused by the stigma that surrounds mental illness, such as lack of social support, housing, employment, that negatively impact their mental health treatment (Borinstein 1992; Corrigan 2004; Link and Phelan 2001; Link et al. 1997; Overton and Medina 2008). Furthermore, mental illness knows no boundaries and, like any other illness, does not discriminate based on race or ethnicity. The stigma of mental illness affects all ethnic groups and cultures and it is necessary to understand that culture has a direct impact on the stigma attached to mental illness. In fact, in certain cultures individuals are less likely to seek

K. Bashor (✉) · S. Junck
Office of Individual and Family Affairs, AZ Health Care Cost Containment System (AHCCCS), 701 E. Jefferson St., Phoenix, AZ 85034, USA
e-mail: Kathy.Bashor@azahcccs.gov

S. Junck
e-mail: Susan.Junck@azahcccs.gov

C. McGregor
Regional Behavioral Health Authority, Mercy Maricopa Integrated Care, 4350 E. Cotton Center Blvd., Phoenix, AZ, USA

C. Anderson
Marc Community Resources, 924 Country Club Drive, Mesa, AZ 85201, USA



N.N. Singh et al. (eds.), *Handbook of Recovery in Inpatient Psychiatry*,
Evidence-Based Practices in Behavioral Health, DOI 10.1007/978-3-319-40537-7_16

mental health treatment based on their cultural beliefs surrounding mental illness, such as Latinos, Asians, and African Americans (Anglin et al. 2006). Discrimination, prejudice, and stigma also have a negative impact that may lead to mental health issues in minority populations. Kidd et al. (2011) described the powerful impact of prejudice and social stress, and its impact on the mental health of lesbian, gay, and bisexual populations. Likewise, Williams and Williams-Morris (2000) identified how racism affects the mental health of African Americans.

The Surgeon General (2015) reported that more than 43 million adults in our country struggled with mental illness in the past year. Half meet the criteria for a diagnosable mental health condition at some point in their lives; one quarter by the age of 14, and more than 20 million adults have an alcohol or drug abuse problem. Yet, in spite of how common mental illness and addiction are in our families and in our communities, prejudice and barriers to accessing care still keep too many people from getting the treatment they need. Earlier, Kessler et al. (2005) reported that researchers have noted there is a worldwide epidemic of individuals with psychiatric problems not seeking treatment.

One of the main barriers to seeking and accessing care is the stigma that occurs when one reports or is identified as having a mental illness. While most people who experience a mental illness do not have to enter an inpatient hospital setting, those who do, experience the most potent form of stigma. The individual, their families, and friends all are affected by the experience. The person can be traumatized by the sudden lack of independence, will likely remember many aspects of the experience and may need to identify it on a variety of applications for licensure, health care, housing, and/or employment. While the American with Disabilities Act (ADA) has prevented many of these overt forms of discrimination, stigma plays a subtler role and creates discriminatory practice that are not under the control of ADA regulations. This is one of the reasons that the Surgeon General identified stigma as one of the most pressing issues affecting public health. There is nothing shameful about having mental illness and there is nothing weak about reaching out for help; however, no other medical condition experiences the degree of stigma that mental health experiences.

Stigma has the harmful consequence of diminishing motivation to enroll and participate in many forms of treatment. Aakre et al. (2015, p. 125) identified that "when the individual receives a mental health diagnosis and/or identifies as a person with a mental health condition, these stereotypes become personally relevant. This puts the person at risk for 'self-concurrence', or believing that the stigmatizing attitudes are true of him or herself. This is self-stigma." Self-stigma is a major deterrent to seeking behavioral health care and is based on the negative attitude that many individuals have regarding the likelihood of improvement or the "I am so damaged that I can't he helped." In a survey conducted by the American Psychological Association (Miller et al. 2006), 76 % of potential consumers had low confidence in the expected outcomes of services. The self-stigmatizing attitude has been nurtured by portrayals of mental health services by the media, in the workplace, school settings and by the very professionals who provide care. The attitude that "therapist's know best" have made many consumers feel helpless and that improvement, if it is to occur at all, is long drawn-out arcane process based only on the skills of the therapist (Corrigan et al. 2009). Self-stigma results in negative judgments we levy against ourselves based on devalued group identities (Scheyett 2005). This attitude is in conflict with what research has indicated to be the most important predictor of successful outcome: engagement and participation in treatment (Orlinsky et al. 1994).

Myers described two forms of stigma. According to Myers, enacted stigma is exterior and refers to discrimination against people with a psychiatric illness because of their perceived unacceptability or inferiority. Felt stigma is interior and refers to both the fear of enacted stigma and a feeling of shame associated with having a mental illness. Myers described enacted stigma as systemic, including the lack of parity in health insurance coverage, employment discrimination, housing discrimination, and denial of insurance coverage for preexisting conditions. Felt stigma is how the shame and guilt that the person experiences can impact the person's willingness to seek or remain in treatment, or to reveal issues to their treatment professionals.

The cognitive and emotional reactions to stigma resemble the effects that have been duplicated in behavioral research studies on the phenomenon of learned helplessness (Seligman 1977). Learned helplessness is the person's inability to see any effective solution to an environmental stressor. It is caused by a series of experiences in which the person learns that nothing they do matters to change the stressful situation and the belief that your actions will be futile. Learned helplessness can be prevented if, before the experience with helplessness occurs, the person learns that his/her actions can make a difference. Unremitting learned helplessness can lead to hopelessness and depression.

A major problem in combating stigma is the lack of public awareness of the advances made in the field of psychiatry and behavioral health over the past several decades. Too often, perceptions are guided by the media which portrays psychiatric inpatient hospitals as "snake pits" or that all patients are undergoing intensive, five-day-a week psychoanalysis or experience arcane treatments, such as lobotomies. Vast ignorance continues to exist in society with respect to the advances made in psychiatry and other mental health fields, which coupled with the pervasive stigma attached to having a mental illness prevent people from recognizing, seeking, and receiving the help they need (Fung et al. 2010). Further complicating matters is the myth that the American character should embody one of strength and self-reliance and being able to take care of ourselves. This false perception continues to take precedence over the concept that mental illness is a biological illness that is treatable and not self-induced (Fink and Tasman 1992).

The way that mental illness is portrayed in the media and the entertainment industry has significantly contributed to stigma. Stigma (like beauty) is in the eye of the beholder, and a body of evidence supports the concepts of stereotypes of mental illness (Byrne 1997, 2000; Philo 1997; Townsend 1979). Goffman (1961, 1963) described the difference between a normal and a stigmatized person as a question of perspective, not reality. Public (or social) stigma is the awareness of stereotypes that the public and society holds about people who are living with mental illnesses. In movies, this often means portraying characters with mental illness as physically violent and unpredictable. A salient example is the 1978 movie, *Halloween*, in which the villain is a patient who escaped from a mental institution and terrorizes everyone he encounters. Public stigma also involves prejudice, or ascribing to stereotypes that foster negative emotional reactions, such as fear and avoidance. With the rapid evolution of media, it has become a powerful tool for most of us to learn, to understand, to seek advice, and obtain knowledge.

Research has shown that many people get their only information about mental illness from the mass media (Wahl et al. 2002). What they see and hear influences their thoughts and opinions. Mental Health America (1999; formerly the National Mental Health Association) reported that, according to a survey for the Screen Actors' Guild, characters in prime time television portrayed as having a mental illness are depicted as the most dangerous of all demographic groups: 60 % were shown to be involved in crime or violence. Most news accounts portray people with mental illness as dangerous. The vast majority of news stories on mental illness either focus on other negative characteristics related to people with the disorder (e.g., unpredictability and unsociability) or on medical treatments. Absent are positive stories that highlight recovery of many persons with even the most serious of mental illnesses (Wahl et al. 2002).

Inaccurate and stereotypical representations of mental illness also exist in other entertainment media, including music, novels, and cartoons (Wahl 1995). The media can perpetuate stigma, giving the public narrowly focused stories based on stereotypes; however, the media can also be a useful means to challenge and replace these stereotypes. Contrary to what is often portrayed in the media, people with psychiatric disabilities are far more likely to be victims than perpetrators of violent crime (Appleby et al. 2001). In spite of this, Watson et al. (2004) reported that police and correctional officers often have attitudes that people with mental illness are dangerous. Researchers at North Carolina State University and Duke University found that people with severe mental illnesses—schizophrenia, bipolar disorder, or psychosis—are two and half times more likely to be attacked, raped, or mugged than the general population (Hiday 2006; Hiday et al. 1999, 2001, 2002; Phelan et al. 2000; Townsend 1979). Partially due to the media, many people associate individuals with mental illness with psychopathic or what is now known as sociopathic personality disorder. This condition represents only 1.2 % of individuals with mental illness. In fact, the vast majority of criminal acts are committed by individuals who display instrumental criminal acts, designed to obtain money or revenge (Mulvey 1994).

Over time, the media has slowly become conscious of these harmful portrayals. In 2013, the Associated Press added an entry on mental illness to its *Stylebook* to help journalists write about mental illness fairly and accurately. And, in recent years, Hinshaw (2005, 2006), Hinshaw and Cicchetti (2000), Hinshaw and Stier (2008) noted, screenwriters have made an effort to portray more humanized characterizations of individuals with mental illness. For example, Carrie Mathison on Showtime's *Homeland* who has bipolar disorder, Bradley Cooper's character in *Silver Linings Playbook* and John Nash, the Nobel Prize-winning economist, with schizophrenia in *A Beautiful Mind.* In each case, the portrayals are more realistic and hopeful, and show that individuals can attain valued lives.

What we do know today is that stigma is not a new problem. Stigmatization of people with mental illness has continued throughout history in the United States (Araujo and Borrell 2006) and can be traced as far back as ancient Greece. The word originated from markings or brandings placed on Greek slaves to clearly separate them from the common, free man. Goffman (1961, 1963), an early scholar, defined stigma "a mark of disgrace." This perception of individuals with mental illness reduced their value as human beings and labeled them as being "less than" in society. In ancient civilizations, mental illness was thought to have been caused by supernatural forces serving, largely, as a punishment for sins. These afflicted individuals were allowed to live free as part of society, just as long as they were not dangerous.

Today, while progress has been made, from a societal as well as system perspective regarding the views, acceptance and treatment of people with mental illness, much work still remains to demystify perceptions, engage with and educate the general public and health care professionals, and build capacity for complete inclusion. Efforts to combat stigma are focused on reinstilling hope, supporting resiliency, and providing dignity to those who have been and continue to be deprived the right to fully participate in society (Corrigan and Watson 2002). These principles can be realized is inpatient settings when staffs have appropriate training and supervision.

## The Dynamics of Stigmatization

Stigma and discrimination associated with mental illness is an epidemic that impacts peoples' lives in a chronic and severely debilitating manner. People who suffer from mental illness are challenged doubly. On the one hand, they struggle with the symptoms and disabilities that result from the disease. On the other, they are challenged by the stereotypes and prejudice that result from misconceptions about mental illness. As a result of both, people with mental illness are robbed of the opportunities that define a quality life: good jobs, safe housing, satisfactory health care, and affiliation with a diverse group of people. Although research has gone far to understand the impact of diseases, it has only recently begun to explain stigma in mental illness (Brohan et al. 2010). Much work yet needs to be done to fully understand the breadth and scope of prejudice against people with mental illness. Fortunately or unfortunately, social psychologists and sociologists have been studying phenomena related to stigma for several decades and what is known is that stigma is often internalized by individuals, and is even fostered by some health care professionals (Reavley et al. 2014; Stuber et al. 2014). This ethics-laden issue acts as a barrier to individuals who may seek or engage in treatment services.

The report *Respect Costs Nothing* is a survey that was conducted to identify how people with experience of mental illness have faced discrimination and the impact such discrimination has had on their lives (Mental Health Foundation, 2004). Respondents to this survey identified discrimination associated with mental illness in all aspects of their lives. The report highlights that fear of further discrimination often prevents people from participating in many activities. In addition, internalizing stereotypes about mental illness discourages people from pursuing dreams or goals. Lucksted and Drapalski (2015) described the pervasive effects of stigma, as "Much like breathing in polluted air, it is very hard to not take in at least pieces of societal prejudices like racism, sexism, classism, homophobia, and mental illness stigmatization" (p. 99).

The impact of stigma is twofold, public stigma, which is the reaction that the general population has to people with mental illness and self-stigma, the prejudice which people with mental illness turn against themselves. Both public and self-stigma may be understood in terms of three components: stereotypes, prejudice, and discrimination. Stigma about mental illness seems to be widely endorsed by the general public in the Western world. Studies suggest that the majority of citizens in the United States (Link 1987) and many Western European nations (Bhugra 1989) have stigmatizing attitudes about mental illness. Furthermore, stigmatizing views about mental illness are not limited to uninformed members of the general public; even well-trained professionals from most mental health disciplines subscribe to stereotypes about mental illness (Keane 1990, 1991).

Several themes describe misconceptions about mental illness and corresponding stigmatizing attitudes. Media presentations typically portray those with mental illness in three ways: people with mental illness are homicidal maniacs who need to be feared; they have childlike perceptions of the world; or they are responsible for their illness because they have weak character (Gabbard and Gabbard 1992). Results of two independent factor analyses of survey responses of more than 2000 English and American citizen's parallel the Gabbards' observations (Brockington et al. 1993). The survey revealed that the public had the following perceptions of people with a mental illness: (a) fear and exclusion—persons with severe mental illness should be feared and, therefore, be kept out of most communities; (b) authoritarianism—persons with severe mental illness are irresponsible, so life decisions should be made by others; and (c) benevolence—persons with severe mental illness are childlike and need to be protected.

Although stigmatizing attitudes are not limited to mental illness, the public appears to disapprove of persons with psychiatric disabilities significantly more than persons with related physical illness (Corrigan et al. 2000). Severe mental illness has been likened to drug addiction, prostitution, and criminality (Albrecht et al. 1982). Unlike physical disabilities, persons with mental illness are perceived by the public to be in control of their disabilities and responsible for causing them (Corrigan et al. 2000). Furthermore, research respondents are less likely to pity persons with mental illness, instead reacting to psychiatric disability with anger and believing that help is not deserved (Socall and Holtgraves 1992). The behavioral impact (or discrimination) that results from public stigma have been examined in many studies and has shown that the public will withhold help to some minority groups because of corresponding stigma (Weiner et al. 1988). A more extreme form of this behavior is social avoidance, where the public strives to not interact with people with mental illness altogether and it takes four forms: withholding help, avoidance, coercive treatment, and segregated institutions.

People with psychiatric disabilities living in a society that widely endorses stigmatizing ideas, internalize these ideas and believe that they are less valued because of their psychiatric disorder. Self-esteem suffers, as does confidence in one's future (Allport 1979). Given this research, models of self-stigma need to account for the deleterious effects of prejudice on an individual's conception of him or herself. However, research suggests that, instead of being diminished by the stigma, many persons become righteously angry because of the prejudice that they have experienced (Chamberlin 1998). This kind of reaction empowers people to change their roles in the mental health system, becoming more active participants in their treatment plan and often pushing for improvements in the quality of services (Corrigan et al. 2000).

Low self-esteem versus righteous anger describes a fundamental paradox in self-stigma (Corrigan et al. 2000). Models that explain the experience of self-stigma need to account for some persons whose sense of self is harmed by social stigma versus others who are energized by, and forcefully react to the injustice (Corrigan 2004, 2011; Corrigan et al. 2000, 2002, 2009, 2013; Corrigan and Lundin 2001; Corrigan and Penn 1999; Corrigan and Rao 2012). In addition, there is yet a third group that needs to be considered in describing the impact of stigma on the self. The sense of self for many persons with mental illness is neither hurt, nor energized, by social stigma, instead showing a seeming indifference to it altogether.

## Attitudes Toward Mental Illness and the Power of Stigma

An issue that people consider before consulting a mental health professional, or encouraging someone else to do so, is the stigma many people experience by reporting that they are in "therapy." When people engage in counseling or therapy from a psychiatrist or psychologist, they have to realize that they may have to answer challenging questions when they are posed on a job application or interview, applications for occupational or professional licensure, a driver's license, applications for health or life insurance, and/or questions posed on school and college applications such as, "Have you ever had psychiatric or psychological therapy?" When a person applies for a job, or an occupational licensure or driver's license, or for an insurance policy, or admission to an educational program, or even better—wants to serve our country as a member of a jury or to enter the military, will often be required to answer questions about their health status. When people answer such questions, candidly and honestly, admitting to having received psychiatric or psychological help, the result all too often will be loss of important opportunities.

Answering "yes" to such questions often results in rejection for employment, licensure, admissions, acceptance, denial, and even services to one's country. Sometimes the person will be forced to ask their therapist to file a report when they apply for a license, become insured, or required by Child Protective Services to reunite a family. If, on the other hand, the person conceals their experience of psychiatric or psychological therapy by answering "no," thereafter they will have to worry, and for good reason, that they will be found out and the "cover-up" revealed (Corrigan et al. 2012).

Many people who would benefit from mental health services opt not to pursue them or fail to fully participate once they have begun. Not surprisingly, Swarbrick and Roe (2011) identified the adverse impact that stigma has on the persons willingness to take psychotropic medications. Stigma yields two kinds of harm that may impede treatment participation: It diminishes self-esteem and robs people of social opportunities. Although the quality and effectiveness of mental health treatments and services has improved greatly over the past 50 years, many people who might benefit from these services choose not to obtain them, or do not fully adhere to the treatment regimens once they are begun (Fung et al. 2010). Stigma is one of several reasons why people make choices to avoid the label of mental illness that results when people are associated with mental health care (Livingston and Boyd 2010).

Stigma and discrimination continue to be a reality in the lives of people suffering from mental illness and prove to be one of the greatest barriers to regaining a normal lifestyle and overall health. Negative attitudes about mental illness often underlie stigma, which in turn, can cause people affected to deny symptoms, delay treatment, be excluded from employment, housing or relationships, and interfere with recovery. Furthermore, these societal attitudes that view symptoms of psychopathology as threatening and uncomfortable are frequently the catalysts that foster stigma and discrimination toward people with mental health problems. Such reactions are common when people are brave enough to admit they have a mental health problem, and they can often lead to various forms of exclusion or discrimination, either within social circles, the workplace or in the military. Hoge et al. (2006) reported that the percentage of military personnel experiencing mental health concerns who utilize behavioral health services could be as low as 23 %. Gould et al. (2010), Kim et al. (2010), Ben-Zeev et al. (2012) and the Mental Health Advisory Team (2009) identified stigma as the most prominent reason that military personnel do not seek mental health care.

## Where Did the Stigma of Mental Illness Begin?

Stigma is not a new problem and has a history that dates back to the age of what were called asylums. While these asylums no longer exist in their previous form, they represent society's efforts to deal with mental illness in what they thought was a humane approach by segregating people with mental illness from others. While long-term segregation is no longer the general approach, there continues to be a social separation between those with mental illness and others. The separation no longer needs a physical location; it now consists of a mental attitude known as stigma.

## Mental Illness and the Age of the Asylum: A Historical Perspective

The public mental health system is experiencing new challenges in a rapidly changing environment. Health care reform, economic restraint, complex civil commitment laws, and the need to ensure civil rights have placed pressures on the capacity and adequacy of state psychiatric inpatient hospitals. Today, most people with mental illness are served successfully in community settings; however, at times, those with the most serious mental illness need inpatient care provided in community outpatient or community inpatient psychiatric hospitals. While there is no broad consensus on what the role community inpatient psychiatric hospitals play in the continuum of care, the National Association of State Mental Health Program Directors (NASMHPD 2014) reported that psychiatric inpatient hospitals, including state psychiatric hospitals, play a vital role in the continuum of recovery services.

In order to fully understand the effects of stigma on individuals with mental illness, we need to examine the roles that psychiatric inpatient hospitals have played in the past and present. It is important to have an understanding of the history and the context of the mental health system in the United States, and to understand how and why state and community psychiatric inpatient hospitals function as they do in the present day. State psychiatric hospitals were originally established to reform how persons with mental illness received care. It was done with humanitarian motives. In colonial times, persons who were considered "demented" were placed in local jails or almshouse if no relative, loved one, or neighbor could care for them. With limited funding and oversight, these environments became riddled with abuse and neglect.

In the 1840s, and during the time period known as the *Age of Asylums* in the US, Dorthea

Dix, a schoolteacher from Cambridge, Massachusetts and an advocate for better treatment for people with mental illnesses, helped establish the construction of asylums. Dix led a movement to establish a national policy for caring for persons with mental illness and for federal lands to be set aside across the county dedicated to asylums as outlined in the 12–225,000 Acre Bill. The movement emphasized the need for humane care based on compassion and moral treatment, rather than ridding the person of demonic possession through corporal punishment. Care would be provided in asylums rather than housing people in jails, poorhouses, or having them live on the streets. Dix testified before the legislature in 1844 to the conditions individuals with mental illness suffered living in inhumane conditions, often without heat, water, bathrooms, and bound by chains. The stigma of being mentally ill was such an unfavorable quality that society did not feel it necessary to treat these individuals humanely.

Madness was seen as a domestic problem to be taken care of by families or parishes. If families could not care for their loved ones, they were sent to other family members for private seclusion. Further, due to the shame and stigma of having a family member with mental illness, many families hid their mentally ill relative in cellars and cages, or were abandoned altogether. During this time, society practiced social distancing by separating individuals from their families who bore the "mark of disgrace." The effect on individuals with mental illness was deep, with an increase in the number of asylums. Care for individuals with mental illness transferred from families to asylums and further distanced people from the natural supports of their families.

Individuals living in asylums were taken care of by people who were often poorly trained and, in some cases, unsympathetic to mental illness. Further, asylums were not a place of treatment for individuals who were suffering from mental illness, but merely a place to house the mentally ill, keeping them isolated and out of mainstream society. The living conditions in asylums were deplorable, with no sanitation, no engagement with the outside world, and food was often sparse. If individuals were given treatment for their afflictions, it followed the best practices of the times, which included bloodletting and ice cold baths. It was not until later that treatment options expanded to include shock therapy and lobotomies. Individuals and their families had neither voice nor choice in their treatment.

While the legislation Dorthea Dix advocated for passed the House and Senate in 1854, President Franklin Pierce vetoed the bill stating that the responsibility for care of persons with mental illness should be placed on the states, not the federal government. States were left to rely on state tax dollars to fund these facilities. Despite this veto, Dix's advocacy led to the establishment of 32 psychiatric inpatient hospitals in 18 states. The implications of this veto and placement of this responsibility on states have had long lasting fiscal and philosophical effects that are still felt today.

## The Deinstitutionalization Movement

Beginning in the 1950s, there was an effort throughout the United States to remove long-term patients from psychiatric facilities and place them in community-based treatment programs. The impetus of this *deinstitutionalization* movement came from a convergence of several social forces. First, with the successes in treating soldiers traumatized by their experiences in World War II, psychiatrists became optimistic about their ability to effectively treat mental disorders outside of hospital settings. Second, there was a growing feeling that the abusive conditions found in most state psychiatric hospitals, and the negative effects of long-term institutionalization, were at least as harmful as the chronic mental illness itself. Many came to believe that the civil rights of people with mental illness were being violated. Third, fiscal conservatives in the government were concerned with the enormous expense of caring for patients in large institutions. Finally, in 1954, the discovery of chlorpromazine (Thorazine), the first effective anti-psychotic medication, made it reasonably possible to manage the care of persons with chronic mental illness outside the hospital. All together, these forces brought about a dramatic shift in admission and discharge practices at state and county psychiatric hospitals.

While this initiative could have had a positive impact on stigma in the community, the services that were needed to treat these individuals were not readily available, leading many to homelessness and jails (Butterfield 1998). The net effect was an increase in the community's perception that individuals with serious mental illness could not adapt to the community and needed to be isolated in segregated settings. While improvements have occurred in the availability of some services, there continues to be gaps that pose significant barriers to community integration.

According to Jencks (1994) the deinstitutionalization movement in the United States has been an utter disaster. Jencks (1994) reported that good care is expensive, whether it takes place in a hospital or in the community and deinstitutionalization saves big money only when it is followed by gross neglect. Furthermore, Jencks added the term deinstitutionalization, as it is applied in the United States, is a misnomer and a more accurate way to describe what took place would be *dehospitalization*. Long-term patients were discharged, while short-term inpatient care increased. Care for those suffering from chronic, serious mental illness did not change, but rather just the patterns of care. For many patients, they were merely reinstitutionalized and placed back in settings such as nursing homes and board-and-care facilities while others were relegated to temporary shelters and single-room occupancy (SROs) hotels (Jencks 1994). Perhaps the worst development of this time period would be the criminalization of mental illness and the front row seat the criminal justice system had taken on replacing the old state hospitals (Lamb and Weinberger 1998). Citing jail as possibly "our most enduring asylum," Briar (1983) noted that, "when traditional pathways of care are blocked, the local jail becomes the recycling station for some deinstitutionalized persons. Like the old asylums, the jail increasingly functions as the one place in town where troubled persons can be deposited by law enforcement and not be turned away."

In addition, since the 1980s, homelessness and criminalization amongst persons with serious mental illness has become increasingly prevalent and has been cited as a significant consequence of the gaps in policy shift from institutional to community-based care. Studies demonstrate that persons with serious mental illness are ten to twenty times more likely than the general population to be at risk for homelessness (Sharfstein 2000). For example, Steadman et al. (2009) found rates of current serious mental illness for recently booked jail inmates were 14.5 % for men and 31.0 % for women across the jails and study phases. These percentages further reinforce the substantial prevalence of inmates entering incarceration with serious mental illnesses (Sharfstein and Dickerson 2009).

The 1950s were also overshadowed by an ununiformed public perception of mental illness. Social scientists began to address questions concerning lay persons' understanding of mental illness and how they reacted to people who suffered from mental illness. The results were disheartening in that the studies revealed an uninformed public orientation toward mental illness and a social fabric that was inundated with negative stereotypes, fears, and rejection (Phelan et al. 2000). Indeed, based on interviews with over 3000 Americans, Star (1952, 1955, 1957) concluded that there was a strong tendency for people to equate mental illness with psychosis and to view other kinds of emotional, behavioral, or personality problems in nonmental health terms as "an emotional or character difference of a non-problematic sort" (Star 1952, p. 7).

Further, it was because mental illness was defined in such narrow and extreme terms that the public feared, rejected, and devalued people with mental illnesses (Crocetti et al. 1973; Gove 1982). Regardless of the source of these negative attitudes, their presence was well documented. Nunnally (1961, p. 46), for example, found that people were more likely to apply a broad range of negative adjectives such as "dangerous," "dirty," "worthless," "bad," "weak," and "ignorant" to a person labeled as "insane" or "neurotic" than to an "average" person. Similarly, Star (1952, 1955) found that many Americans, in using their own words to describe their understanding of the term mental illness, included characteristics such as dangerousness and unpredictability. Cumming and Cumming (1955), in their study of two communities in Saskatchewan, found that most people preferred to avoid close personal contact with someone who had been mentally ill and that the researchers' efforts to change those attitudes were met with anxiety and hostility. Not surprisingly, Yarrow et al. (1955) found that fear of stigma was a serious concern for wives of psychiatric patients.

The public's negative orientation toward mental illness also extended to the professionals who treated it. Nunnally (1961) found that the public evaluated professionals who treat mental disorders significantly more negatively than those who treat physical disorders. Star (1957) found that the idea of consulting a psychiatrist enjoyed little public endorsement, with few people knowing anyone who had met with a psychiatrist or who they thought might be helped by a psychiatrist. As one respondent bluntly put it: "I don't think I'd have to go to anybody to tell me I was crazy to just hold my hand and talk to me for twenty dollars an hour. If they didn't have any more sense than to go to a psychiatrist they ought to be put in a nut house" (Star 1957, p. 3). Jennings et al. (2015) concluded, "When individuals perceive that others would view them negatively for seeking treatment, they may endorse similar stigmatizing beliefs toward themselves, and subsequently prefer handling problems on their own rather than seek treatment. Thus, heightened stigma may make individuals feel that they should handle problems themselves rather than seeking professional help."

These findings were discouraging to mental health professionals and researchers for several reasons. They implied that public education efforts regarding mental illness had produced little effect. They implied that persons identified as mentally ill might suffer extreme rejection and stigmatization. In addition, they implied that many people would fail to seek mental health treatment that might benefit them.

According to the groundbreaking first Surgeon General's Report on Mental Health (1999), in the 1950s, the public viewed mental illness as a stigmatized condition and displayed an unscientific understanding of mental illness. Survey respondents typically were not able to identify individuals as mentally ill when presented with vignettes of individuals who would have been said to be mentally ill according to the professional standards of the day. The public was not particularly skilled at distinguishing mental illness from ordinary unhappiness and worry, and tended to see only extreme forms of behavior (i.e., psychosis) as mental illness. Mental illness carried great social stigma, especially linked with fear of unpredictable and violent behavior. With the advent of new pharmaceuticals that made it possible to moderate the extreme behavior of many who were institutionalized, it was thought that allowing patients to leave and be treated in the community would be more humane. Unfortunately without the necessary community resources, this hope was not realized.

## The Community Mental Health Centers

The history of the consumer/survivor movement began in the 1960s, when President Kennedy signed the Community Mental Health Center Act and moved people with mental illness out of institutions and into community settings. The intention of the act was to deinstitutionalize people with mental illness and place them into community settings where they could receive local services. These community mental health centers developed as an important part of our mental health system and formed an important core of a growing community mental health movement. However, they were never adequately funded and so were never able to provide community-based mental health care for all those who had been deinstitutionalized. Deinstitutionalization reduced the population of state and county mental hospitals from a high of about 560,000 in 1955 to well below 100,000 by the 1990s. While deinstitutionalization eliminated over 90 % of former state psychiatric hospital beds, an adequate community-based mental health system has not been created, even today (Sigurdson 2000).

On July 30, 1965 Medicare, a federal single payer system for those over 65 and, after 1972 for those with a disability, was created. Its companion program Medicaid was also created to cover long-term care for the elderly and others, and care for mothers and children who met income guidelines. Unfortunately, to this day, Medicare discriminates against mental health coverage, charging 50 % co-pay for mental health care while charging 20 % co-pay for medical and surgical care. In addition, there was no Medicare coverage for pharmaceutical care outside the hospital setting for the first four decades of the program. As Medicaid moved to a managed care model, additional challenges emerged in serving this population. Limits on the number of psychiatric appointments and lengths of stay in hospital settings continue to exist.

The continued growth of a wide variety of pharmaceuticals led to an increased reliance on pharmaceutical care rather than hospital care for mental health as well as medical and surgical care. After the failed 1992 national health care reform effort, managed care became the standard way to organize care, including mental health care. This business model of mental health treatment helped further medicalize mental health care by disconnecting it from support services. The rise in reliance on pharmaceutical care, combined with managed care led to a decrease in other forms of therapy and support for those who were deinstitutionalized. In fact, it would not be an understatement to say that pharmaceutical companies took on a growing role in defining care options. In mental health, this lead to the colloquialism, "off his meds," to refer to someone who was exhibiting symptoms of psychiatric illness.

In speeches to medical societies in the 1940s and 1950s, Bill Wilson, the founder of Alcoholics Anonymous, noted the important role played by leading psychiatrists in the development of AA. Yet, there developed a split between the treatment of mental illness and the treatment of substance abuse and addiction. The varying stigma associated with these two sets of disorders, and the public's and the health care community's failure to understand their interrelationship, lead to a situation where patients with co-occurring mental illness and substance abuse or addiction were bounced back and forth between these systems because neither system was fully able to treat both disorders. This is now changing due to the new brain science that is clarifying the underlying disease processes at work and making possible the identification of effective dual-diagnosis treatments.

After the Vietnam War, military veterans fought for years to gain the recognition of the diagnosis of posttraumatic stress disorder, PTSD, as a diagnosable and treatable mental health disorder. Later it was recognized that PTSD could also affect other sufferers of trauma, sexual assault, and torture. During the conflicts in Iraq and Afghanistan, it was recognized that combat and operational stress are treatable disorders and that their immediate treatment can lower rates of PTSD in warriors who experience the stress of life in the combat zone. In addition, military health care providers are seeing the importance of traumatic brain injury (TBI) and this is leading to the recognition of the importance of treatment of this disorder throughout the health care system, and a reduction in the stigma that our wounded warriors felt when they returned home.

Consumer movements, like those that lead to the recognition of PTSD, have also grown up with a number of other mental health disorders. Consumer organizations, and organizations of family members of those with mental illness, have played an important role in recent years in raising awareness among policy maker and health care leaders in the need to treat mental illness. The consumer/survivor movement continues to advocate for many of these same consumer rights, such as (a) An individual's rights to safe medication and other treatment, (b) Being given the facts needed to make informed choices about one's own care, (c) The right to choose the care one receives, and (d) The right to be heard in the development of government policy and programs.

## The Consumer–Survivor Movement

One set of initiatives that has addressed stigma has been the development of the consumer–survivor movement. Their efforts to inform the public about the mental illness, their insistence on equal rights and their advocacy for appropriate services has had a positive impact on reducing stigma. These groups have called attention to erroneous media portrayals of mental illness, health insurance inequalities, inhumane practices, and inadequate community care.

The consumer/survivor movement started in the 1970s in response to decades of inadequate care in hospitals and the community. During this time, state hospitals across the country were being closed and people who were released began meeting in groups to share feelings of anger about the abusive treatment they experienced while they were there, and their need for independent living. Eventually these groups coalesced with the common desire for personal freedom and radical system change, and a liberation movement began (Zinman 2009). The groups that were part of this movement developed key principles. Members were against forced treatment, against inhumane treatment such as certain medications, lobotomy, and electroconvulsive therapy, against the medical model, and in favor of consumer involvement in every aspect of the mental health system. The groups' members, who described themselves as "psychiatric inmates," were primarily located on the east and west coasts.

The groups had militant names like Network against Psychiatric Assault, Insane Liberation Front, and Mental Patient Liberation Front. Group members developed a communication vehicle called "Madness Network News," and held the annual "Conference on Human Rights and Against Psychiatric Oppression" at campgrounds and college campuses.

Since the 1970s, there has been fierce debate over whether deinstitutionalization has been a direct cause of homelessness among persons with chronic mental illness who comprise only about one-quarter to one-third of the entire homeless population. Although the deinstitutionalization process began in the mid-1950, a disproportionate number of mentally ill persons only began to appear among the homeless population in the mid-1970. This lag of twenty years makes it impossible to claim that deinstitutionalization was the sole cause of homelessness among persons with chronic mental illness. The prevalence of housing and employment discrimination made it impossible for many people discharged from hospitals to overcome poverty, one of the primary factors in homelessness.

Second, as originally planned, deinstitutionalization was to take place in conjunction with the establishment of community mental health programs that would take on the responsibility for the treatment of persons with chronic mental illness. President Kennedy signed the Community Mental Health Center Act in October 1963, which allocated federal funds to community clinics if they provided a full range of services, including outpatient, inpatient, and crisis services to persons with mental illness. However, these comprehensive community mental health centers were never adequately developed, and neither were the supportive services (e.g., housing and rehabilitation programs) that are necessary for maintaining individuals in the community. Thus, neglect in the community took the place of abuse in the asylum and stigma continued to grow as the community witnessed more individuals with serious mental illness living in the community without the services they needed.

## The Self-help/Peer Support Movement

In the 1980s, the groups became more streamlined and its members began the process of reentering the world that they felt had previously betrayed them. The mental health system began funding self-help//peer-support programs and drop-in centers, such as On Our Own in Baltimore started in 1981, Berkeley Drop-In Center in 1985, Ruby Rogers Drop-In Center in Cambridge, Massachusetts in 1985, and Oakland Independence Support Center in 1986. The federal National Institute of Mental Health Community Support Program funded consumer/survivor-run programs. Statewide consumer-run organizations, such as the California Network of Mental Health Clients, began in 1983. Rights protection organizations were developed and there were gains in protective legislation.

More consumers/survivors began to sit on decision-making bodies.

## Client-Run Systems Change

The 1990s saw the fruition of changes sought in the mental health system in the previous decade with consumers being employed in the mental health system and in self-help programs, including in management level jobs. Growth emerged in self-help/peer-support programs with system-level funding from federal sources, which resulted in the establishment of two consumer/survivor-run technical assistance centers supporting self-help programs (Allen et al. 2010). During this time the consumer/survivor involvement was noticeable at most levels of the mental health system, and client-run research began. The same principles as the earlier days were expressed in positive terms, such as self-determination and choice, rights protections, stigma and discrimination reduction, holistic services, self-help/peer-support programs, involvement in every aspect of the mental health system—"Nothing about us without us"—and the concept of recovery, which encompasses all of the above.

Important developments in mental health occurred during the 1980s and 1990s to include the growth and impact of self-advocacy service recipient movement (Sledge et al. 2011). This critical movement in social justice began with the establishment of self-help groups and further expanded and formalized in the 1990s toward organized advocacy, peer-services, and roles and services within the state and in federal initiatives (Steadman et al. 2009). The 1999 Surgeon General's Report on Mental Health and the 2003 President's New Freedom Commission Report on Mental Health sought service recipient input and found that, "nearly every consumer of mental health service expressed the need to fully participate in his or her plan for recovery. Service recipients and families told the Commission that having hope and the opportunity to regain control of their lives were vital" (Susser et al. 1997).

Another development during this period was the amendment of the American with Disabilities Act (1990). The United States Congress found that "(1) physical or mental disabilities in no way diminish a person's right to fully participate in all aspects of society, yet many people with physical or mental disabilities have been precluded from doing so because of discrimination; others who have a record of a disability or are regarded as having a disability also have been subjected to discrimination; (2) historically, society has tended to isolate and segregate individuals with disabilities, and, despite some improvements, such forms of discrimination against individuals with disabilities continue to be a serious and pervasive social problem; (3) discrimination against individuals with disabilities persists in such critical areas as employment, housing, public accommodations, education, transportation, communication, recreation, institutionalization, health services, voting, and access to public services; (4) unlike individuals who have experienced discrimination on the basis of race, color, sex, national origin, religion, or age, individuals who have experienced discrimination on the basis of disability have often had no legal recourse to redress such discrimination; (5) individuals with disabilities continually encounter various forms of discrimination, including outright intentional exclusion, the discriminatory effects of architectural, transportation, and communication barriers, overprotective rules and policies, failure to make modifications to existing facilities and practices, exclusionary qualification standards and criteria, segregation, and relegation to lesser services, programs, activities, benefits, jobs, or other opportunities; and (6) the continuing existence of unfair and unnecessary discrimination and prejudice denies people with disabilities the opportunity to compete on an equal basis and to pursue those opportunities for which our free society is justifiably famous, and costs the United States billions of dollars in unnecessary expenses resulting from dependency and nonproductivity" (Sect. 12010).

In most recent history, the Mental Health Parity and Addiction Equity Act of 2008 reflects reduced discrimination against people with mental illness with the understanding that financial and treatment requirements for mental illness and substance use disorders can be no more restrictive than those of medical or surgical benefits. Further, the passage of the Affordable Care Act (ACA) of 2010 may help expand access to mental health services. However, the Health Information Technology for Economic and Clinical Health (HITECH) Act of 2009 does not include psychiatric hospitals and community mental health centers as eligible recipients for the Electronic Health Records (EHRs) stimulus payments that general hospitals can receive. Further, there was a growing understanding of the relationship between children's and adult mental health and the effects of early childhood trauma on the person's entire adult life.

## The Decade for Recovery, Wellness and the Mental Health Services Act

In the 2000s, systems culture change has occurred at all levels of the mental health system as a result of consumer/survivor involvement. The *Mental Health Services Act* (MHSA) has consumer/survivor values embedded throughout, such as voluntary promotion of self-help/peer support programs, involvement of consumers/survivors at all levels of the mental health system, inclusion of consumers/survivors to train the mental health work force, and promotion of recovery as a goal. The Substance Abuse and Mental Health Services Administration's (SAMHSA 2012) *National Consensus Statement on Mental Health Recovery* reflects basic consumer/survivor principles. Generally speaking, consumer/survivor-run programs and peer support are essential components of most mental health programs (Zinman 2009).

Many people never get to hear or experience the message that people with mental illnesses can and do recover. Staff who work in inpatient psychiatric settings are particularly challenged to see individuals who they have served living successfully in the community. Mental illness is an illness, just like diabetes and any other chronic diseases. People with mental illnesses can recover and go on to lead happy, healthy, productive lives. They contribute to society and make the world a better place. People can often benefit from medication, rehabilitation, therapy, self-help or a combination of these.

One of the most important factors in recovery is the understanding and acceptance of family and friends and the community. The experience of support from friends, family, and professionals combat stigma by creating hope. The evocation of hope can be the most important and central element of recovery by proactively addressing situations that can be changed in a positive manner. Related to this is an acceptance of situations that cannot reasonably be altered despite one's efforts. Measures of hope have been found to correlate with a broad range of positive outcomes. Summarizing this literature, Snyder concluded that "high hope persons have a greater number of goals, have more difficult goals, have greater happiness and less distress, have superior coping skills, recover better from physical injury, and report less burnout at work." In fact, inspiring hope is the practitioner's first duty to the client and major contribution to treatment.

## Promising Developments in Mental Health

Many promising developments emerged during the twenty-first century and psychiatric treatment has become highly specific by diagnosis or age groups, enabling treatment to be more individualized with more emphasis on choice. Service recipients and family members have become more educated, informed, engaged, and involved in shared decision-making. Particularly since 1990, advances in brain science, brain scans, growing understanding of brain biochemistry, advances in psychological therapy, electrical brain stimulation, and the role of the genome in brain development and functioning are bringing important new understandings to health care providers, policy makers, and the public. The concept of recovery has become more infused philosophically into care, and peer-supported services have increased, contributing to the recovery process for people with serious mental illness.

In addition, evidence-based practices have emerged and treatment and options continually improve. The U.S. Supreme Court's Olmstead decision and the American Disabilities Act have also been important developments that underscore people living and being treated in the community wherever possible and at a fraction of state psychiatric hospital care costs. The recognition that mental health is integral to overall well-being has begun to drive the integration of mental health, addiction, and primary health care with an increased focus on overall health and wellness for people with mental illness. Furthermore, harmful, inhumane practices such as seclusion and restraints are being reduced and facilities are being held accountable for those practices. Frank and Glied (2008) have attributed improvements in the care for mental illness to people with mental illness being able to receive disability income and housing supports, greater care options and choice, newer medications that are easier to tolerate and prescribed appropriately, and more people with serious mental illness being treated successfully by primary care physicians.

## Capacity Building for Recovery

### Changing the Culture and Building the Continuum of Recovery Supports

Stigma and discrimination manifest themselves in many ways, and these barriers will need to be eliminated or significantly reduced for individuals seeking behavioral health care and gaining access to comprehensive care. Stigma needs to be eliminated not only toward individuals with mental health or substance abuse service needs, but also across professional groups, such as between primary care providers and behavioral health providers.

Inpatient psychiatric hospitals are a vital part of the continuum of care and should operate as recovery-oriented and integrated facilities with connections to a robust set of community support services. The conditions in psychiatric hospitals and the need for humane treatment, however, have been an underlying theme driving reform over history. Since the late 1990s, the NASMHPDs has focused on national efforts to reduce coercive environments and practices to change the culture of violence that has existed in many inpatient psychiatric hospitals. Through such changes, many inpatient psychiatric hospitals have significantly altered their culture and reduced the use of seclusion and restraints.

Changing the environment, climate, and culture of the inpatient psychiatric hospitals are paramount to providing effective care. The culture of the psychiatric hospitals should be recovery-oriented, trauma-informed, culturally and linguistically competent and appropriate, transparent, hopeful, respectful, holistic, peer infused and supported, and driven by meeting the needs of the people served in inpatient psychiatric hospitals while addressing and maintaining the utmost in safety for the people being served, staff, and the community. Such cultures can create environments where those individuals being served heal and staff thrives.

Regardless of the reason for being admitted to the hospital or a person's behavior in the hospital, all people being served in inpatient psychiatric hospitals should be considered to be in the process of recovery and the focus should be to engage the person in their care and empower them to participate in making decisions about their care, with the ultimate goal of helping each person manage his or her own illness. This approach is similar to treating people with other chronic health care conditions, such as diabetes, high blood pressure, or congestive heart failure.

Inpatient psychiatric hospitals and the services provided should be respectful, person-centered, and recovery-oriented. Recipients of services should be integral in the process of recovery and should be served in the most integrated and least restrictive environment possible. This paradigm shift in thought and practice is complicated, however, by the fact that states and other key stakeholders have varying definitions of recovery. In response to the need for defining this important and fundamental concept, the SAMHSA (2012) developed a working definition of recovery that includes the following guiding principles:

*Recovery emerges from hope.* The belief that recovery is real provides the essential and motivating message of a better future—that people can and do overcome internal and external challenges, barriers, and obstacles that confront them. Hope is internalized and can be fostered by peers, families, providers, allies, and others. Hope is the catalyst of the recovery process.

*Recovery is person-driven.* Self-determination and self-direction are the foundations for recovery as individuals define their own life goals and design their unique path(s) toward those goals. Individuals optimize their autonomy and independence to the greatest extent possible by leading, controlling, and exercising choice over the services and supports that assist their recovery and resilience. In doing so, they are empowered and provided the resources to make informed decisions, initiate recovery, build their strengths, and gain or regain control over their lives.

*Recovery occurs via many pathways.* Individuals are unique with distinct needs, strengths, preferences, goals, culture, and backgrounds, including trauma experiences that affect and determine their pathway(s) to recovery. Recovery is built on the multiple capacities, strengths, talents, coping abilities, resources, and inherent value of each individual. Recovery pathways are highly personalized. They may include professional clinical treatment, use of medications, support from families and in schools, faith-based approaches, peer support, and other approaches. Recovery is nonlinear, characterized by continual growth and improved functioning that may involve setbacks. Because setbacks are a natural, though not inevitable, part of the recovery process, it is essential to foster resilience for all individuals and families. In some cases, creating a supportive environment can enable recovery pathways. This is especially true for children, who may not have the legal or developmental capacity to set their own course.

*Recovery is holistic.* Recovery encompasses an individual's whole life, including mind, body, spirit, and community. This includes addressing self-care practices, family, housing, employment, education, clinical treatment for mental disorders and substance use disorders, services and supports, primary healthcare, oral healthcare, complementary and alternative services, faith, spirituality, creativity, social networks, transportation, and community participation. The array of services and supports available should be comprehensive, integrated, and coordinated.

*Recovery is supported by peers and allies.* Mutual support and mutual aid groups, including shared experiential knowledge and skills, as well as social learning, play an invaluable role in recovery. Peers encourage, engage other peers, and provide each other with a vital sense of belonging, supportive relationships, valued roles, and community. Through helping others and giving back to the community, one helps oneself. Peer-operated supports and services provide important resources to assist people along their journeys of recovery and wellness. Professionals can also play an important role in the recovery process by providing clinical treatment and other services that support individuals in their chosen recovery path. While peers and allies play an important role for many in recovery, their role for children and youth may be slightly different. Peer support for families are very important for children with behavioral health problems and can also play a supportive role for youth in recovery.

*Recovery is supported through relationship and social networks.* An important factor in the recovery process is the presence and involvement of people who believe in the person's ability to recover, who offer hope, support, and encouragement, and who also suggest strategies and resources for change. Family members, peers, providers, faith groups, community members, and other allies form vital support networks. Through these relationships, people leave unhealthy and/or unfulfilling life roles behind and engage in new roles (e.g., partner, caregiver, friend, student, and employee) that led to a greater sense of belonging, personhood, empowerment, autonomy, social inclusion, and community participation.

*Recovery is culturally based and influenced.* Culture and cultural background in all of its diverse representations including values, traditions, and beliefs are keys in determining a person's journey and unique pathway to recover. Services should be culturally grounded, attuned, sensitive, congruent, and competent, as well as personalized to meet each individual's unique needs.

*Recovery is supported by addressing trauma.* The experience of trauma, such as physical or sexual abuse, domestic violence, war, and disaster, is often a precursor to or associated with alcohol and drug use, mental health problems, and related issues. Services and supports should be trauma-informed to foster physical and emotional safety and trust, as well as promote choice, empowerment, and collaboration.

*Recovery involves individual, family, and community strengths and responsibility.* Individuals, families, and communities have strengths and resources that serve as a foundation for recovery. In addition, individuals have a personal responsibility for their own self-care and journeys of recovery. Individuals should be supported in speaking for themselves. Families and significant others have responsibilities to support their loved ones, especially for children and youth in recovery. Communities have responsibilities to provide opportunities and resources to address discrimination and to foster social inclusion and recovery. Individuals in recovery also have a social responsibility and should have the ability to join with peers to speak collectively about their strengths, needs, wants, desires, and aspirations.

*Recovery is based on respect.* Community, systems, and societal acceptance and appreciation for people affected by mental health and substance use problems, including protecting their rights and eliminating discrimination, are crucial in achieving recovery. There is a need to acknowledge that taking steps toward recovery may require great courage. Self-acceptance, developing a positive meaningful sense of identity, and regaining belief in one's self are particularly important.

## Conclusion

There are a number of ways in which inpatient psychiatric facilities can support the reduction of stigma. Creating an environment that supports recovery principles identified by SAMHSA is a significant first step. Another is involving peers in recovery in the hospital workforce. Peer support services are an integral part of assisting in individual's recovery process and need to be made available to all service recipients in inpatient psychiatric hospitals. Peer support specialists and care coordinators should be made an equal member of the treatment team.

It is important to note the fact that an inpatient psychiatric hospital is not a person's home. The focus of inpatient psychiatric hospitals needs to be on assimilating individuals back into the community quickly when they no longer meet inpatient criteria. Cultivating and fostering partnerships among inpatient psychiatric hospital personnel, service recipients, and community service providers is vital in the assimilation back to community and should be an on-going process that is integral to the individuals transition and discharge plan, and includes the community services that would be most helpful to the individuals transition back to community life. Leadership and a well-trained, professional and paraprofessional workforce are paramount in ensuring comprehensive, high quality care is timely, appropriate, and accessible to individuals who receive care in a state psychiatric hospital and the continuum care remains intact upon discharge and re-assimilation back into the community (Salgado et al. 2010).

There are also a number of specific programs that have been developed to combat stigma. Corrigan (2011) described a number of methods that are effective in marketing campaigns. Yanos et al. (2011, 2012) have introduced narrative enhancement and cognitive therapy techniques that are used in groups to treat internalized stigma. Russinova et al. (2014) developed a peer-run antistigma photovoice intervention. Many of these techniques could be used in inpatient settings for individuals.

The National Alliance of Mental Illness (NAMI), an organization at the forefront of advancing mental health in this country, can be a major resource for hospitals and patients within hospital settings. NAMI has a plethora of supports, services, and treatment options for individuals who have to contend with a serious mental illness. Across the country, NAMI has thousands of trained volunteers that bring peer-led programs to a wide variety of hospital and community settings. With the unique understanding of people with lived experience of mental illness, these programs and support groups provide free education, skills training, and support.

## References


Aakre, J., Klingaman, E., & Docherty, N. (2015). The relationship between stigma sentiments and self-identity of individuals with schizophrenia. *Psychiatric Rehabilitation Journal, 38*(2), 125–131.

Albrecht, G., Walker, V., & Levy, J. (1982). Social distance from the stigmatized: A test of two theories. *Social Science Medicine, 16*, 1319–1327.

Allen, J., Parks, J., & Radke, A. (2010). *Consumer involvement with state mental health agencies*. Alexandria, VA: National Association of State Mental Health Program Directors.

Allport, G. (1979). *The nature of prejudice*. New York, NY: Doubleday.

Americans with Disabilities Act. (1990). Public Law 101-336.

Anglin, D., Link, B., & Phelan, J. (2006). Racial differences in stigmatizing attitudes toward people with mental illness. *Psychiatric Services, 57*(6), 857–862.

Appleby, L., Mortensen, P. B., Dunn, G., & Hiroeh, U. (2001). Death by homicide, suicide, and other unnatural causes in people with mental illness: a population-based study. *The Lancet, 358*, 2110–2112.

Araujo, B., & Borrell, L. (2006). Understanding the link between discrimination, mental health outcomes, and life chances among Latinos. *Hispanic Journal of Behavioral Sciences, 28*, 245–266.

Associated Press. (2013). *Stylebook*. Philadelphia, PA: Associated Press.

Ben-Zeev, D., Corrigan, P. W., Brin, T. W., & Langford, L. (2012). Stigma of mental illness and service use in the military. *Journal of Mental Health, 21*, 264–273.

Bhugra, D. (1989). Attitudes towards mental illness: A review of the literature. *Acta Psychiatrica Scandinavica, 80*, 1–12.

Borinstein, A. (1992). Public attitudes toward persons with mental illness. *Health Affairs, 11*, 3186–3196.

Briar, K. H. (1983). Jails: Neglected asylums. *Social Casework, 64*, 387–393.

Brockington, I., Hall, P., & Levings, J. (1993). The community's tolerance of the mentally ill. *British Journal of Psychiatry, 162*, 93–99.

Brohan, E., Elgie, R., Sartorius, N., Thomicroft, G., & The GAMIAN Europe Study Group. (2010). Self-stigma, empowerment and perceived discrimination among people with schizophrenia in 14 European countries: The GAMIAN-Europe study. *Schizophrenia Research, I22*, 232–238.

Butterfield, F. (1998, March 5). Asylums behind bars: A special report; prisons replace hospitals for the nation's mentally ill. *New York Times*. Retrieved from http://www.nami.org/update/980305.html

Byrne, P. (1997). Psychiatric stigma: Past, passing and to come. *Journal of the Royal Society of Medicine, 90*, 618–621.

Byrne, P. (2000). Stigma of mental illness and ways of diminishing it. *Advances in Psychiatry Treatment, 6*, 65–72.

Chamberlin, J. (1998). Citizenship rights and psychiatric disability. *Psychiatric Rehabilitation Journal, 21*, 405–408.

Corrigan, P. (2004). How stigma interferes with mental health care. *American Psychologist, 59*, 614–625.

Corrigan, P. W. (2011). Strategic stigma change (SSC): Five principles for social marketing campaigns to reduce stigma. *Psychiatric Services, 62*, 824–826.

Corrigan, P. W., Kosyluk, K. A., & Rilsch, N. (2013). Reducing self-stigma by coming out proud. *American Journal of Public Health, 103*, 794–800.

Corrigan, P. W., Larson, J. E., & Rilsch, N. (2009). Self-stigma and the "why try" effect: Impact on life goals and evidence-based practices. *World Psychiatry, 8*, 75–81.

Corrigan, P. W., & Lundin, R. K. (2001). *Don't call me nuts! Coping with the stigma of mental illness*. Tinley Park, IL: Recovery Press.

Corrigan, P. W., & Penn, D. L. (1999). Lessons from social psychology on discrediting psychiatric stigma. *American Psychologist, 54*, 765–776.

Corrigan, P. W., & Rao, D. (2012). On the self-stigma of mental illness: Stages, disclosure, and strategies for change. *Canadian Journal of Psychiatry, 57*, 464–469.

Corrigan, P., River, L. P., Lundin, R. K., Wasowski, K. U., Campion, J., Mathisen, J., et al. (2000). Stigmatizing attributions about mental illness. *Journal of Community Psychology, 28*, 91–103.

Corrigan, P. W., Rowan, D., Green, A., Lundin, R., River, P., Uphoff-Wasowski, K., et al. (2002). Challenging two mental illness stigmas: Personal responsibility and dangerousness. *Schizophrenia Bulletin, 28*, 293–310.

Corrigan, P., & Watson, A. (2002). The paradox of self-stigma and mental illness. *Clinical Psychology: Science and Practice, 9*, 35–53.

Crocetti, G., Spiro, H., & Siassi, I. (1973). *Contemporary attitudes towards mental illness*. Pittsburgh, PA: University of Pittsburgh Press.

Cumming, J., & Cumming, E. (1955). Mental health education in a Canadian community. In B. D. Paul (Ed.), *Health, culture and community*. New York: Russell Sage Foundation.

Deegan, P. E. (1993). Recovering our sense of value after being labeled mentally ill. *Journal of Psychosocial Nursing and Mental Health Services, 31*, 7–11.

Department of Health and Human Services. (1999). *Mental health: A report of the surgeon general*. Bethesda, MD: Substance Abuse and Mental health Services Administration, Center for Mental Health Services, National Institutes of Health, National Institute of Mental Health.

Department of Health and Human Services. (2015). *Mental health: A report of the surgeon general*. Bethesda, MD: Substance Abuse and Mental health Services Administration, Center for Mental Health Services, National Institutes of Health, National Institute of Mental Health.

Fink, P., & Tasman, A. (1992). *Stigma and mental illness*. Washington, DC: American Psychiatric Press.

Frank, R., & Glied, S. A. (2008). *Better but not well: Mental health policy in the United States since 1950*. Baltimore, MD: Johns Hopkins University Press.

Fung, K. M., Tsang, H. W., & Chan, F. (2010). Self-stigma, stages of change and psychosocial treatment adherence among Chinese people with schizophrenia: A path analysis. *Social Psychiatry and Psychiatric Epidemiology, 45*, 561–568.

Gabbard, G., & Gabbard, K. (1992). Cinematic stereotypes contributing to the stigmatization of psychiatrists. In P. J. Fink & A. Tasman (Eds.), *Stigma and mental illness* (pp. 113–126). Washington, DC: American Psychiatric Press.

Goffman, E. (1961). *Asylums: Essays on the social situation of mental patients and their inmates*. New York, NY: Anchor Books.

Goffman, E. (1963). *Stigma: Notes on the management of spoiled identity*. New York, NY: Simon & Schuster.

Gould, M., Adler, A., Zamorski, M., Castro, C., Hanily, N., Steele, N., & Greenberg, N. (2010). Do stigma and other perceived barriers to mental health care differ across Armed Forces? *Journal of the Royal Society of Medicine, 103*, 148–156.

Gove, W. (1982). Labeling theory's explanation of mental illness: An update of recent evidence. *Deviant Behavior, 34*, 307–327.

Hiday, V. A. (2006). Putting community risk in perspective: A look at correlations, causes and controls. *International Journal of Law and Psychiatry, 29*, 316–331.

Hiday, V. A., Swanson, J. W., Swartz, M. S., Borum, R., & Wagner, H. R. (1999). Criminal victimization of persons with severe mental illness. *Psychiatric Services, 50*, 62–68.

Hiday, V. A., Swanson, J. W., Swartz, M. S., Borum, R., & Wagner, H. R. (2001). Victimization: A link between mental illness and violence? *International Journal of Law and Psychiatry, 24*, 559–572.

Hiday, V. A., Swartz, M. S., Swanson, J. W., Borum, R., & Wagner, H. R. (2002). Impact of outpatient commitment on victimization of people with severe mental illness. *American Journal of Psychiatry, 8*, 1403–1411.

Hinshaw, S. P. (2005). The stigmatization of mental illness in children and parents: Developmental issues, family concerns, and research needs. *Journal of Child Psychology and Psychiatry, 46*, 714–734.

Hinshaw, S. P. (2006). Stigma and mental illness: Developmental issues. In D. Cicchetti & D. Cohen (Eds.), *Developmental psychopathology* (2nd ed., Vol. 3, pp. 841–881). New York: Wiley.

Hinshaw, S. P., & Cicchetti, D. (2000). Stigma and mental disorder: Conceptions of illness, public attitudes, personal disclosure, and social policy. *Development and Psychopathology, 12*(04), 555–598.

Hinshaw, S. P., & Stier, A. (2008). Stigma in relation to mental disorders. *Annual Review of Clinical Psychology, 4*, 269–293.

Hoge, C. W., Auchterlonie, J. L., & Milliken, C. S. (2006). Mental health problems, use of mental health services, and attrition from military service after returning from deployment to Iraq or Afghanistan. *Journal of the American Medical Association, 295*, 1023–1032.

Jencks, C. (1994). *The homeless*. Cambridge, MA: Harvard University Press.

Jennings, K., Cheung, J., Britt, T., Goguen, K., Jeffirs, S., Peasley, A., & Lee, A. (2015). How are perceived stigma, self-stigma, and self-reliance related to treatment-seeking? A three-path model. *Psychiatric Rehabilitation Journal, 38*(2), 109–116. http://psycnet.apa.org/psycinfo/2015-14530-001/

Johnstone, M. (2001). Stigma, social justice and the rights of the mentally ill: Challenging the status quo. *Australian and New Zealand Journal of Mental Health Nursing, 10*, 200–209.

Keane, M. (1990). Contemporary beliefs about mental illness among medical students: Implications for education and practice. *Academic Psychiatry, 14*, 172–177.

Keane, M. (1991). Acceptance vs. rejection: Nursing students' attitudes about mental illness. *Perspectives in Psychiatric Care, 27*, 13–18.

Kennedy, J. (1962). Special message to the Congress on protecting the consumer interest. Retrieved from http://www.presidency.ucsb.edu/ws/?pid=9108

Kessler, R., Demler, O., Frank, R., Olfson, M., Pincus, H., Walters, E., & Zaslavsky, A. (2005). Prevalence and treatment of mental disorders, 1990 to 2003. *The New England Journal of Medicine, 352*, 2515–2523.

Kidd, S., Veltman, A., Gately, C., Chan, K., & Cohen, J. (2011). Lesbian, gay, and transgender persons with severe mental illness: Negotiating wellness in the context of multiple sources of stigma. *American Journal of Psychiatric Rehabilitation, 14*, 13–39.

Kim, P., Thomas, J., Wille, J., Castro, C., & Hoge, C. (2010). Stigma, barriers to care, and use of mental health services among active duty and National Guard soldiers after combat. *Psychiatric Services, 61*, 582–588.

Lamb, H. R., & Weinberger, L. E. (1998). Persons with severe mental illness in jails and prisons: A review. *Psychiatric Services, 49*(4), 483–492.

Link, G. (1987). Understanding labeling effects in the area of mental disorders: An assessment of the effects of expectations of rejection. *American Sociological Review, 52*, 96–112.

Link, G., & Phelan, J. (2001). Conceptualizing stigma. *Annual Review of Sociology, 27*, 363–385.

Link, G., Struening, E., Rahav, M., Phelan, J., & Nuttbrock, L. (1997). On stigma and its consequences: Evidence from a longitudinal study of men with dual diagnoses of mental illness and substance abuse. *Journal of Health and Social Behavior, 38*, 177–190.

Livingston, J., & Boyd, J. (2010). Correlates and consequences of internalized stigma for people with mental illness: A systematic review and meta-analysis. *Social Science and Medicine, 71*, 2150–2161.

Lucksted, A., & Drapalski, A. (2015). Self-stigma regarding mental illness: Definition, impact and relationship to societal stigma. *Psychiatric Rehabilitation Journal, 38*(2), 99–102.

Mental Health Advisory Team. (2009). *Operation Iraqi Freedom 07–09*. Washington, DC: Office of the Surgeon, Multi-National Corps Iraq & Office of the Surgeon General, United States Army Medical Command.

Mental Health America. (1999). *American opinions on mental health issues*. Alexandria, VA: Author.

Miller, S., Duncan, B., Brown, J., Sorrell, R., & Chalk, M. (2006). Using formal client feedback to improve retention and outcome: Making ongoing, real-time assessment feasible. *Journal of Brief Therapy, 5*(1), 5–22.

Mulvey, E. P. (1994). Assessing the evidence of a link between mental illness and violence. *Hospital and Community Psychiatry, 45*, 663–668.

NASMHPD. (2014). *The vital role of state psychiatric hospitals*. Alexandria, VA: NASMHPD Publications.

New Freedom Commission on Mental Health. (2003). *Achieving the promise: Transforming mental health care in America.* Final Report. Rockville, MD: Department of Health and Human Services.

Nunnally, J. C. (1961). *Popular conceptions of mental health*. New York: Holt, Rinehart and Winston.

Orlinsky, D., Grawe, K., & Parks, B. (1994). Process and outcome in psychotherapy. In A. Bergin & S. Garfield (Eds.), *Handbook of psychotherapy and behavior change* (4th ed.). New York, NY: Wiley.

Overton, L., & Medina, L. (2008). The stigma of mental illness. *Journal of Counseling and Development, 86*, 143–151.

Phelan, J., Link, G., Stueve, A., & Pescosolido, B. (2000). Public conceptions of mental illness in 1950 and 1996: What is mental illness and is it to be feared? *Journal of Health and Social Behavior, 41*, 188–207.

Philo, G. (1997). Changing media representations of mental health. *Psychiatric Bulletin, 21*, 171–172.

Reavley, N. J., Mackinnon, A. J., Morgan, A. J., & Jonn, A. F. (2014). Stigmatizing attitudes towards people with mental disorders: A comparison of Australian health professionals with the general community. *Australian and New Zealand Journal of Psychiatry, 48*, 433–441.

Reidy, D. E. (1993). *Stigma is social death: Mental health consumers/survivors talk about stigma in their lives*. Holyoke, MA: Education for Community Initiatives.

Russinova, Z., Rogers, E. S., Gagne, C., Bloch, P., Drake, K. M., & Mueser, K. T. (2014). A randomized controlled trial of a peer-run antistigma photovoice intervention. *Psychiatric Services, 65*, 242–246.

Salgado, J. D., Deane, F. P., Crowe, T. P., & Oades, L. G. (2010). Hope and improvements in mental health service providers' recovery attitudes following training. *Journal of Mental Health (Abingdon, England), 19*, 243–248.

Substance Abuse and Mental Health Services Administration. (2010). *SAMHSA's working definition of recovery*. Rockville, MD: Author.

Substance Abuse and Mental Health Services Administration. (2014). *Eight dimensions of wellness*. Rockville, MD: Author.

Scheyett, A. (2005). The mark of madness: Stigma, serious mental illnesses, and social work. *Social Work in Mental Health, 3*, 79–97.

Seligman, M. (1977). Helplessness. In B. Wolman (Ed.), *International encyclopedia of psychology, psychiatry, psychoanalysis, and neurology*. New York, NY: Human Sciences Press.

Sharfstein, S. (2000). Whatever happened to community mental health? *Psychiatric Services, 51*(5), 616–620.

Sharfstein, S., & Dickerson, F. (2009). Hospital psychiatry for the twenty-first century. *Health Affairs, 28*(3), 685–688.

Sigurdson, C. (2000). Mad, the bad and the abandoned: The mentally ill in prisons and jails. *Corrections Today, 62*(7), 70–78.

Sledge, W., Lawless, M., Sells, D., Wiedland, M., O'Connell, M., & Davidson, L. (2011). Effectiveness of peer support in reducing readmissions of persons with multiple psychiatric hospitalizations. *Psychiatric Services, 62*(5), 541–544.

Socall, D., & Holtgraves, T. (1992). Attitudes toward the mentally ill: The effects of label and beliefs. *Sociology Quarterly, 33*, 435–445.

Star, S. (1952). *What the public thinks about mental health and mental illness*. Chicago, IL: National Opinion Research Center.

Star, S. (1955). *The public's ideas about mental illness*. Chicago, IL: National Opinion Research Center.

Star, S. (1957). *The place of psychiatry in popular thinking*. Chicago: National Opinion Research Center.

Steadman, H. C., Osher, O. F., Robbins, P. C., Case, B., & Samuels, S. (2009). Prevalence of serious mental illness among jail inmates. *Psychiatric Services, 60*(6), 761–765.

Stuber, J. P., Rocha, A., Christian, A., & Link, B. G. (2014). Conceptions of mental illness: Attitudes of mental health professionals and the general public. *Psychiatric Services, 65*, 490–497.

Susser, E., Valencia, E., Conovor, S., Felix, A., Tsai, W., & Wyatt, R. (1997). Preventing reoccurring homelessness among mentally ill men: a "critical time" intervention after discharge from a shelter. *American Journal of Public Health, 87*(2), 256–262.

Swarbrick, M., & Roe, D. (2011). Experiences and motives relative to psychiatric medication choice. *Psychiatric Rehabilitation Journal, 35*, 45–50.

Townsend, P. (1979). *Poverty in the United Kingdom*. London, UK: Allen Lane.

US Congress. (1963). Community Mental Health Center Act (Public Law 88-164).

US Congress. (2008). Mental Health Parity and Addiction Equity Act (Public Law 110-343).

US Congress. (2009). Health Information Technology for Economic and Clinical Health (HITECH) Act (Public Law 111-5).

Wahl, O. (1995). *Media madness: Public images of mental illness*. New Brunswick, NJ: Rutgers University Press.

Wahl, O. (1999). Mental health consumers' experiences of stigma. *Schizophrenia Bulletin, 25*(3), 467–478.

Wahl, O., & Harman, F. (1989). Family views of stigma. *Schizophrenia Bulletin, 5*(1), 131–139.

Wahl, O. E., Wood, A., & Richards, R. (2002). Newspaper coverage of mental illness: Is it changing? *Psychiatric Rehabilitation Skills, 6*, 9–31.

Watson, A. C., Corrigan, P. W., & Ottati, V. (2004). Police officers' attitudes toward and decisions about persons with mental illness. *Psychiatric Services, 55*, 49–53.

Weiner, B., Perry, R. P., & Magnusson, J. (1998). An attributional analysis of reactions to stigmas. *Journal of Personality and Social Psychology, 55*, 738–748. http://www.ncbi.nlm.nih.gov/pubmed/2974883

Williams, D. R., & Williams-Morris, R. (2000). Racism and mental health: The African American experience. *Ethnicity and Health, 5*, 243–268.

Yanos, P. T., Roe, D., & Lysaker, P. H. (2011). Narrative enhancement and cognitive therapy: A new group-based treatment for internalized stigma among persons with severe mental illness. *International Journal of Group Psychotherapy, 61*, 516–595.

Yanos, P. T., Roe, D., West, M. L., Smith, S. M., & Lysaker, P. H. (2012). Group-based treatment for internalized stigma among persons with severe mental illness: Findings from a randomized controlled trial. *Psychological Services, 9*, 248–258.

Yarrow, M., Clausen, J., & Robbins, P. (1955). The social meaning of mental illness. *Journal of Social Issues, 11* (4), 33–48.

Zinman, S. (2009). *The history of the mental health consumer/survivor movement*. Presentation sponsored by SAMHSA's Resource Center to Promote Acceptance, Dignity and Social Inclusion associated with Mental Health.

# Enhancing Resilience and Sustaining Recovery

17

Michael Franczak, Doug Barshter, John W. Reich, Martha Kent and Alex J. Zautra

## Introduction

People who suffer the devastating and long-term consequences of serious mental illnesses were historically viewed as permanently and irreversibly impaired. Over the last several decades, recovery from serious mental illness has become accepted as a realistic process and a desired outcome for individuals who have experienced a serious mental illness. The national mood and understanding by policymakers, practitioners, advocates, and people in various services has shifted dramatically away from the maintenance and symptom management approach. Both inpatient and community-based services are now focused on providing people with skills, social connectedness, and hope to build a happy and successful life while coping with the very symptoms that previously incapacitated them. To be sure, the process can be long and arduous, but new medications, methodologies, and evidence-based practices have repeatedly demonstrated that individuals can live independent, successful, and happy lives in their communities when the person is given the opportunity to learn new skills and balance those with the cyclical nature of his/her mental illness. Should the person encounter a "rough spot," practitioners and supports are available and accessible to assist and maintain hope while the person deals with the difficulties at hand, such as recurrent symptoms, physical and emotional stress, confusion, fear of failure, and the impact of discrimination and/or stigma.

While the philosophical approach to preventing and treating mental illness has changed, the recovery principles require helping a person with mental illness maintain his/her recovery throughout his/her lifetime. A person who has embraced his/her personal recovery journey must continue this journey regardless of the environment, the experiences and the daily stress of being a productive member of a community. The individual must wake up every day and cope with all he/she encounters. The individual must build and maintain new skills. He or she must adjust current skills and knowledge to deal with unexpected life changes. The person must also seek and utilize current or new resources and draw upon people who can and will support the individual's recovery effort. This is commonly called "resilience" and it is fundamental to every person when confronted by a challenge and/or traumatic event. The media are rife with examples of people who have overcome seemingly insurmountable odds to lead productive and happy lives. What is their secret? Research has revealed that each person has an

M. Franczak (✉) · D. Barshter
Marc Community Resources, 924 Country Club Drive, Mesa, AZ 85201, USA
e-mail: Michael.franczak@marccr.com

J.W. Reich · A.J. Zautra
Department of Psychology, Arizona State University, Tempe, AZ, USA

M. Kent
Phoenix Veterans Affairs Health, Phoenix, AZ, USA


N.N. Singh et al. (eds.), *Handbook of Recovery in Inpatient Psychiatry*,
Evidence-Based Practices in Behavioral Health, DOI 10.1007/978-3-319-40537-7_17

innate ability to respond to stress and act to stabilize the situation and his/her life, despite trauma and the limitations imposed by a drastically altered life. In many cases, the person develops new skills and resources to overcome his/her limitations and resume a happy, productive life.

Someone in recovery will have to respond to many situations, all of which have the potential to disrupt the daily routine and/or push the person toward a relapse. Stress causes a person to undertake actions to reduce and/or ameliorate the stress. Sometimes the actions are successful; other times the actions fall short. Resilience is the ability to overcome the disabling aspects of mental illness and find ways to sustain recovery over time. Each person draws upon a bank of skills that assist the person to overcome the adversity. These "asset accounts" are places where the person metaphorically deposits resources to draw upon at a later date. The asset bank accounts focus on the following domains: biological, psychological, social, and spiritual (Franczak and Moore 2014). Taken together they provide the individual with internal resources that are unique and accessible at all times. Research shows that resilience can be promoted by specific interventions leading to a positive evaluation of one's self, a sense of continued growth and development, the belief that life is purposeful and meaningful, the possession of quality relations with others, the capacity to effectively manage one's life, and a sense of self-determination (Fava and Tomba 2009). It can be built and/or replenished as the person continues in recovery and masters techniques to help overcome adversity.

While the President's New Freedom Commission on Mental Health (2003) report and the Substance Abuse Mental Health Services (SAMHSA 2010) definitions of recovery mention the concept of resilience they do not provide any elaboration on the concept or describe how recovery and resilience are related. While there is an extensive and growing body of research on both recovery and resilience, they appear in different literature streams that do not seem to merge in any cogent fashion. Many of the articles on recovery appear in psychosocial rehabilitation journals while the body of research on resilience appears in a wide variety of academic journals and textbooks. In the resilience area, Reich et al. (2010), Kent et al. (2014), Masten (2014), and Reich (2015) have collected, summarized, and analyzed an extensive body of research on resilience that is relevant to assisting the development of the individual's skills to self-manage their health care and life in general.

In this chapter, we describe the difference between recovery and resilience. We explore the importance of creating supports and services that support both recovery and resilience, the relationship between the concepts of recovery and resilience and those of locus of control, self-efficacy, and self-management which include health literacy and health activation, and we consider the role the inpatient hospital can play in supporting both recovery and resilience. The difference between the concepts of recovery and resilience is clearly articulated in a document prepared as part of the St. Luke's Health Initiatives (Hughes 2003). Hughes described the current health care approach as one having the ultimate goal as recovery. This approach "proceeds through diagnosis and treatment based on science, evidence and best practices. Illness, pathology, needs and deficiencies are identified, treatment and services are provided and patients are restored to health" (Hughes 2003, p. 5). The current process is designed to effectively promote recovery from illness or injury. Resilience on the other hand is described as the "harmonious integration of mind, body and spirit within a responsive community" (Hughes 2003, p. 6). Resilience implies growth and sustainability that makes the person stronger and more capable of dealing with the next stressful event that is bound to occur. Zautra et al. (2010a) broadly defined resilience as "an outcome of successful adaptation to adversity" (p. 4). Resilience necessarily implies exposure to an adverse event, illness, injury or threat, and includes two major components: *recovery* and *sustainability* (Zautra 2009; Zautra et al. 2010a). While recovery is necessary for resilience, it is not sufficient for long-term sustainability and growth.

Another difference between recovery and resilience in the mental health arena is that the original concept of recovery primarily addressed recovery from substance abuse and mental illness, while resilience addresses a more holistic healing and health care delivery process. Decades earlier, the World Health Organization (1948) defined health as a complete state of physical, mental, and social well-being, and not merely the absence of disease or infirmity. In July 2006, the Medical Directors Council of the Association of Mental Health Directors released a report titled *Morbidity and Mortality in People with Serious Mental Illness* (National Association of State Mental Health Program Directors 2006) that detailed how people with serious mental illness served by our public mental health systems die, on average, at least 25 years earlier than the general population. The report further indicated that the mortality and morbidity were due to conditions that could have been effectively treated if the person had received and participated in the physical health services that were available.

Based on these findings, SAMHSA (2014b) expanded the recovery concept to include wellness that covered a more inclusive and holistic view of health. SAMHSA defined health and wellness not as the absence of disease, illness, or stress, but the presence of purpose in life, active involvement in satisfying work and play, joyful relationships, a healthy body and living environment, and happiness. Swarbrick (2006) developed a health and wellness model that SAMHSA adapted and includes these eight dimensions of wellness

1. Emotional: Coping effectively with life and creating satisfying relationships.
2. Environmental: Occupying pleasant and stimulating environments.
3. Financial: Being satisfied with current and future financial situations.
4. Intellectual: Recognizing creative abilities and finding ways to expand knowledge and skills.
5. Occupational: Getting personal satisfaction and enrichment from one's work.
6. Physical: Recognizing the need for physical activity, healthy foods, and sleep.
7. Social: Developing a sense of connection and belonging, and having a well-developed support system.
8. Spiritual: Expanding our sense of purpose and meaning in life.

Since the report was released, the question of how to address these additional dimensions of health and wellness has been at the forefront of many public mental health systems. One common approach has been to integrate the physical and mental health care systems so that individuals do not have to navigate distinct provider systems to obtain care for their mind and body. There is no identified gold standard or best approach to integration, but there are many experiments occurring across the country that may yield effective models. When a person enters an inpatient hospital setting, he/she is typically in a setting that provides integrated care where both the mental and physical conditions that are in need of care are identified. In fact, this may be the most integrated treatment he/she will ever receive. When he/she leaves the facility, the responsibility for developing and maintaining healthy behavior ultimately rests with the person, the support of the outpatient clinical team and the person's natural support network. This is particularly challenging for individuals who are discharged from psychiatric hospital settings where many individuals may have gained stability of their positive symptoms, but many retain residual negative symptoms and cognitive deficits (Mosolov et al. 2012). Nevertheless, the hospital treatment team can begin identifying and addressing the issues, skills, and abilities that eventually will improve the person's abilities to understand and actively manage his/her own health care. During the discharge planning process, the hospital treatment team needs to ensure that the resources that can support the person to continue their recovery journey are identified. In many cases, the person is not capable of navigating the typically complex community behavioral health system without the support of advocates, family members, and skilled navigators (Franczak 2013).

While health systems can attempt to communicate, coordinate, collaborate, and integrate, the individual needs to become an informed and active participant in his/her health care. Duncan (2005) reported that five decades of scientific studies identified the client as the single most potent factor, contributing to a positive health outcome. Individuals have to develop what Bandura (1982) called self-efficacy or what the health field currently calls self-management. How to assist and support individuals has been the goal of many of the investigators who have been involved in recovery and resiliency research as well as those involved in health care reform. Manderscheid (2014) noted that there are several competing concepts, such as "self-management," "engagement," and "health-activation," but none of these labels adequately describes the full range of skills being practiced by those who have developed this capacity. People who have lived and experienced their own recovery and wellness, and who have had to protect their own resiliency when confronted with stress, trauma, and symptom reoccurrence, have learned the skills we describe in this chapter. Health-activated people are at the forefront of a new social movement. They are able to implement their own recovery and wellness so effectively because they have learned and honed specific skills that increase their subsequent resiliency.

When providing peer support training to individuals with a serious mental illness, we have found a clear difference between those individuals who have been able to attain the notable goal of recovery from those who are able to demonstrate what the literature has described as resilience (Franczak and Barshter 2015). In both cases, the person typically shows a reduction in positive psychiatric symptoms, but individuals who demonstrate resilience also exhibit self-efficacy and mastery of their chronic condition, and demonstrate improvements in their negative psychiatric symptoms as well. Resilient individuals exhibit growth in a number of emotional, cognitive, and social areas and are generally more aware of the subtleties of their chronic illnesses, understand triggers, and signs of remission, know the most effective treatments for their specific condition and, most importantly, become more active participants in their own care and daily decisions to manage their illness. They also demonstrate mastery of their emotional reactions to stressful events. For resilient individuals stressful events are handled as part of daily life and the human experience and do not typically cause significant ongoing distress or symptom remission. For resilient individuals there is growth from the experience that is used to manage their chronic illness, maintain functional behaviors, and develop healthy social relationships in the face of the everyday stressors we all experience. We believe that while recovery is certainly a significant milestone that needs to be celebrated, building resilience should be the ultimate goal of supports and services.

Bonanno (2004) described recovery as a gradual return to pre-event levels of functioning, whereas sustainable recovery (resilience) is the capacity to quickly regain equilibrium following a potentially traumatic event with little to no disruption in functioning. While Bonanno (2004) believed that resilience is different from recovery, Luthar et al. (2000) proposed that recovery is a domain of resiliency. Based on our experience, recovery appears to be a stage of resilience and, as stated previously, necessary for resilience but not sufficient. Some individuals who attain recovery from mental illness or substance abuse never attain resilience, but can lead functional lives using ongoing system and family supports (Franczak and Dye 2004). For these individuals, remissions may be more likely, depending upon the level of stress in their environment and the supports they have in the community. There may be long periods without symptomatology or functional impairments. For others, recovery can be fleeting and is constantly being challenged by having to deal with stressful events. The environment in which the person lives plays a major role in supporting recovery and resilience. Many of the current assessments (e.g., ASAM, LOCUS, and CALOCUS) have a dimension that measures what is termed "recovery oriented environments," which is used to identify the extent to which the environment is supportive of the person's recovery. Many environments are not supportive and some are clearly toxic.

## Stress and Trauma

One issue that resilience research has identified is the role of stress on physical and mental health, well-being, quality of life, recovery, and resilience. According to the American Psychological Association (2015) there are indisputable data showing that stress has a profound effect on health status and longevity. For example, Schneiderman et al. (2005) found that when stress is unremitting, the long-term effects can damage health and, moreover, the relationship between psychosocial stress and disease is affected by the nature, number, and persistence of the stressors, as well as by the individual's biological vulnerability, psychosocial resources, and learned patterns of coping. Among the many factors that create stress, two that are frequent for individuals with mental illness are trauma and illness. When the illness is a chronic condition or the trauma is unresolved, stress can be unremitting.

The World Health Organization (WHO 2005) identified chronic disease as conditions of ill health that accompany the individual for a long period of time, produce incapacity, or residual disability caused by irreversible pathological alterations, demand rehabilitation, and follow-up over a long time, and may present periods of improvement and periods of worsening in acute stages. A more recent definition by Goodman et al. (2013) identified chronic conditions as those that last a year or more, require ongoing medical attention and/or limit activities of daily living such as physical medical conditions, behavioral health problems, and developmental disabilities. Many forms of mental illness and substance abuse are chronic health conditions of a cyclic nature that require continual attention in order to identify and mitigate the potential for remission and relapse.

The frequency of chronic illness in the general population is startling. The California Health Care Foundation (2015) estimated 11.4 million adults in California (41 %) have one or more of five chronic health conditions. Of the 11.4 million with chronic health conditions, 8.2 million (30 % of all adults in the state) have just one condition, 2.6 million (9 %) have two, and 0.6 million (2 %) have three to five chronic conditions. Serious psychological distress affected 2.2 million (7.9 %). In addition, a significant number of individuals with a serious mental illness also have multiple physical health chronic conditions (Alegría et al. 2003; Parks et al. 2006). Persons with mental illness are more likely than others to suffer from physical health problems, including chronic diseases such as diabetes, cardiovascular disease, obesity, asthma, epilepsy, and cancer (Freeman et al. 2010; Glasgow et al. 2002; Leucht and Burkard 2007). Recently Cook et al. (2015) undertook health screenings on 457 adults with serious mental illnesses for eight common medical comorbidities and health risk factors. They also collected data on self-reported health competencies, medical conditions, and health service utilization. Compared to non-institutionalized US adults, markedly higher proportions screened positive for obesity (60 %), hypertension (32 %), diabetes (14 %), smoking (44 %), nicotine dependence (62 %), alcohol abuse (17 %), drug abuse (11 %), and coronary heart disease (10 %). As a result, the life expectancy of those with serious mental illness is roughly 25 years less than that of the average individual (Parks et al. 2006). This is partially due to the fact that many individuals with mental illness have unhealthy lifestyles (Brown et al. 1999).

Understandably, the costs for patients with a number of chronic conditions have caught the attention of government funding agencies and health care insurers (Ehrlich et al. 2010). In 2008, spending for patients with two chronic conditions averaged $13,146 per patient per year, twice as much as for those with only one condition ($6573 per patient per year). At $27,763 per patient per year, spending on patients with three or more chronic conditions was four times the level of spending for patients with one chronic condition. Parekh (2011) reported that individuals with chronic diseases take only 50 % of the prescribed doses of medications and not follow referral advice, and 75 % do not keep follow-up on appointments.

One of the factors that impacts cost is whether the person actively works to manage their chronic conditions. Hibbard et al. (2013) found that patients with the lowest health activation levels had predicted average health care costs that were 8 % higher in the first year and 21 % higher in the first half of the second year than the costs of patients with the highest activation levels. The Center for Advancing Health (2010) reported that advances in medicine, technology, and health care services promise increases in the length and quality of life for many Americans. However, obtaining the benefit of these advances to prevent, manage, and cure disease depends increasingly on individuals' energy, knowledge and skills, regardless of whether they are sick or well. This situation is partially due to the failure of the treatment team in engaging the person in care planning. Bohanske and Franczak (2010) described the extensive research evidence supporting the critical role that the person receiving care plays in achieving positive health outcomes. Moreover, many models of care fail to realize or take advantage of this finding by not fully engaging the person in treatment planning. This may change as the Center for Medicare and Medicaid Innovation (2011) announced that supporting patient engagement efforts will be factors in scoring applications for Accountable Care Organizations (ACOs). Understanding how the health care system can increase recovery and cultivate engagement, encourage self-management and resilience, even in the presence of a chronic condition, has become a more pressing issue because organizations that deliver inpatient services will be facing financial disincentives.

Another issue confronting individuals with serious mental illness is that the majority have experienced trauma in their past and, for some, on a recurring basis (SAMHSA 2014a). Spitzer et al. (2009) found that traumatic stress increased the risk for mental illness and also increased the symptom severity of mental illness. This increased impact of the trauma is the result of both the event itself and how the person experiences the event. In some cases, trauma exacerbates behavioral dysfunction and ultimately compromises community functioning, happiness and success. In severe situations, traumatic events may be a contributing factor to hospitalization and chronic illness long after the traumatic event took place. Inpatient psychiatric hospital recidivism can often be linked to the reliving of the thoughts and emotions related to the traumatic events.

Elliott et al. (2005) recognized the importance of positive adaptation and resilience. Elliot identified that "trauma informed care embraces a per-spective that highlights adaptation over symptoms and resilience over pathology" (p. 467). Trauma-informed care has become an approach that is closely allied with recovery and resiliency practices for people having serious mental health conditions (SAMHSA 2014a). Trauma-informed care focuses on helping the person recognize the traumatic event(s) and understand how past trauma can negatively impact many aspects of a person's emotions, thoughts, values and world view, and community integration and wellness. Trauma-informed care assists the person in addressing the debilitating aftereffects of trauma and help the person cope with the social, psychological, and biological realities of his/her life. New skills are developed and old, unsuccessful coping mechanisms are discarded. Trauma-informed care can assist the individual by utilizing his/her strengths and assets to build resilience and maintain hope. It includes helping the person to understand the role that trauma has played in his/her life, how he/she has coped with the trauma and how it has impacted current thinking or behavior. It provides the person with new self-care options, opportunities to form new relationships and networks, and reinforces the notion that the person is the expert in managing his/her own life.

## Personal Mastery, Locus of Control, and Resilience: One Size Does Not Fit All

Personal mastery is one mechanism an individual can use to develop resilience. Reich (2015) observed, "well-being can be positively influenced by being in more control of your life and less distressed if you give up trying to control the uncontrollable. Humans are highly adaptable, and switching to accommodation and acceptance is a systematic pathway to achieving your goals even when the world puts up what might otherwise seem uncontrollable" (p. 259). One issue critical to building resilience is that "one size does not fit all." For some individuals, it is based on having the person control of all the stressful events that are experienced. For others, it is the ability to accept the circumstances that cannot be changed and to move on. For yet others, it is having the social support of others that strengthens their resilience. Extensive research and clinical practice have consistently shown that a key to this ability is the importance of the individual's belief in his/her ability to control the events that affect his/her life. The concept of *perceived control* (or its numerous variants) has been succinctly captured by Rodin (1986, p. 141): "Perceived control refers to the expectations of being able to participate in making decisions and engaging in actions in order to obtain desirable consequences and avoid unfavorable ones."

Since the inception of the locus of control concept by Rotter (1966), this way of thinking about human adaptation has infused entire areas of the social sciences. Treated either as a stable character trait or as a process of dealing with life events, the evidence is overwhelming in showing that having this personal belief is related to higher levels of mental and physical health. Conversely, individuals who believe that they cannot control the events and outcomes of their lives are at risk for such conditions as depression, anxiety, and low levels of activation, such as learned helplessness (but see below). Both facets of control would appear on the face of it to have valuable insights into models of therapeutic intervention and specifically training principles of self-management. In fact, the largest body of research and practice on perceived control is found in the health care field.

Research has shown that people who have high perceived control beliefs, "internals" (in the language of this research) engage in greater levels of health-enhancing activities (exercise, illness prevention activities, and information gathering), and report fewer activity limitations due to health issues. In fact, they report better health—they have fewer heart conditions, they are more successful in lowering cigarette consumption and sustaining that reduction, and they have lower incidence of PTSD, and tended to live longer as shown in one national survey in German adults. In addiction treatment studies, people in alcohol treatment programs tend to score higher on the "external" control dimension compared to carefully matched controls not in treatment. Even among casual drinkers, those who scored higher on external control drank more than people who scored higher on control. Externally scoring alcoholics in treatment reported higher levels of depression than internally scoring participants.

On the other hand, more complex research designs have been able to examine the relationship between one's control beliefs and environments judged as more controlling versus more open. Thus, in a study of the effectiveness of psychotherapy, Kilman et al. (1975) showed that high external people responded well to highly structured therapy regimens, while higher internal people responded with more avoidance and were less cooperative in structured therapy. Brownell (1982) showed that internals performed more effectively in an experimental task when their participation was important to the task, whereas externals performed more effectively when the structure was outside of them in the experimental arrangements and when their own control was less important.

This entire issue concerning the match between the person's control beliefs and the openness or structuredness of that person's environment, the so-called Person X Environment congruence issue, is a relatively understudied subject in the practice literature. It requires us to think about how controlling or flexible we are in adapting to our own environment. It opens up entirely new ways to think about treatment and support. While the evidence described above leads one to assume that believing in one's ability to control one's world leads to better mental and physical health, nevertheless that model may not fit all situations well. For example, in the world of therapy and treatment for addictions, the usual care model is one in which "patients" are "helped" to recover. The implication of this model is that patients will get "better" if they are induced to develop a greater sense of personal mastery. But helping them do this, in fact, may not be helpful. For example, some people may not respond positively to therapeutic attempts to have them adopt higher levels of independence because the self-reliance encouragement may not fit with their own personal control and mastery beliefs. This also suggests the possibility that there is a downside to control. For example, some people may respond positively to being encouraged to rely on external forces, such as other people rather than themselves, at least for some temporary period in their life. Getting people to adopt taking medications for their improvement may in fact just be encouraging reliance on external rather than internal personal forces.

Inpatient psychiatric hospitals are highly controlled environments where some individuals (externals) will respond quickly to the structure while others (internals) may not respond as well. Upon discharge, those individuals with high perceived control would theoretically be the persons in charge of their health care while those individuals who rely on external control would need a support network to assist them in making decisions. In many cases, sufficient supports are not available for many individuals who leave hospital settings. For people who rely on external control, unless the person is both health literate and health activated, the likelihood of changing unhealthy behaviors is slim unless they are enrolled in programs that effectively engage, educate, and support the person. For individuals who rely on internal controls, unless they have higher healthy literacy and are health activated, change is also unlikely.

The question of relying on other people was pursued in two studies of rheumatoid arthritis patients (Reich and Zautra 1995a, b). Married couples responded to questionnaire items asking about the extent to which the spouse of the patients encouraged their wives to be independent ("Told her she should make her own decisions," "Encouraged her to be more self-reliant") or to be more reliant on him ("Suggested that she be more reliant on others," "Suggested that she let others take more responsibility for solving her problems"). Participants also responded to a standardized measure of personal control beliefs as well as outcome measures of adjustment and well-being. The results showed that patients with high levels of personal control beliefs showed no statistical relationship between their spouses' behavior and their outcomes; internal control beliefs reduced one's sensitivity to the behavior of the spouse. However, those with low levels of personal control beliefs (i.e., the externals) were more highly responsive to their spouses. They reported poorer levels of well-being if their spouses had been encouraging independence, especially if they were older and in poor health. Conversely, if they were younger and or in relatively better health, then independence encouragement had more positive effects on their well-being. Dependence encouragement in fact had positive effects on adjustment for patients who had recently experienced a downturn in their health, but negative effects if they had experienced their illness for a longer period of time, presumably because they had more time to adjust to the stresses of their illness.

This pattern of results was also found in a sample of cardiac patients and spousal caregiving. Helgeson (1993) found that spousal protectiveness had positive benefits at the initial stages of illness, but in later stages of recovery and adjustment, it tended to have negative effects. So, encouraging independence or dependence may have both positive and negative consequences depending on the "fit" of the personal control beliefs of the person and the social environment's treatment of control issues. This model has not been tested in samples of mental health or addiction "patients" nor in mental health or addiction treatment studies, so its generalizability is unknown at this point, but it seems promising to attempt to examine more extensively in Person X Environment fit situations.

The notion that dependence may have positive effects despite what we know about the value of higher levels of believing in one's own control may well provide useful insight into the Alcoholics Anonymous (AA) model of recovery. Among other beliefs and actions, the AA model requires that a participant admit to a lack of control over his/her alcoholism, addiction, or compulsion and to recognize a higher power that can restore sanity. Both of these seem to directly violate the principles of control supported so consistently in the research and clinical practice literature—that one can gain from asserting one's personal control. Although there are a number of questions about the effectiveness of AA, millions attest to its effectiveness and have been doing so for decades.

The seeming logical inconsistency with regard to internal and external control can be resolved by expanding the definition of "control." Rothbaum et al. (1984) have carefully pointed out that in fact control has various facets or components. The kind of internal control, internality, we have described here is what they label as "primary control." They characterize primary control as "bringing the world into line with our needs." But this has to be contrasted with "secondary control," or bringing "oneself into line with your world." Thus, in the AA model, to bring yourself into line with the realization that you cannot control your addiction and that you can willingly give yourself over to a higher power is in itself a form of control; it reflects your self-chosen willingness to give over control to a supportive external agent, a shift to secondary control. In this sense of personal control, then, acceptance of the uncontrollable would appear to be a valuable first step in attaining a better sense of control in one's own life. The resolution of the seeming contradiction between the AA model and the personal control beliefs model is not a deep contradiction. The resolution simply requires an expansion of our understanding of control beliefs, per se. This model of the resolution of the seeming contradiction has not been tested extensively; however, the power of secondary control per se as a form of acceptance as prescribed in the AA model is a useful expansion of our thinking. It does explicitly suggest the power of employing both primary and secondary control ways of thinking and how people can successfully guide their own adjustment to the stresses in their lives.

While many of the studies in this tradition tend to be questionnaire/survey based, one coherent body of research on intervention studies tested a number of techniques that enhance personal control beliefs. Most of these studies employed what might be called psychoeducational techniques. Investigators typically involve presenting participants with educational materials that explain personal control concepts and offer suggestions as to how to employ them in their own personal daily lives. The classic studies (e.g., Rodin and Langer 1977; Schulz and Hanusa 1978) involved nursing home residents. Other approaches engaged community-residing adults. These studies investigated control principles and control-enhancing activities in which they compared outcome results against closely matched comparison samples that did not receive control-enhancing instructions. In the dozen studies in this tradition, the evidence consistently shows improvement in a wide range of outcome variables (Reich 2015). Only a few of these studies assessed preexisting beliefs in personal control. Of these, Reich and Zautra (1990) showed that those with external beliefs were more likely to report improved mental health following the control-enhancing treatment.

These intervention studies are useful for revealing a key aspect of therapeutic treatment effects, namely, they suggest that greater attention should be paid to control beliefs versus control-related actions. Mazzucchelli et al. (2010) performed a meta-analysis of 20 studies that related different measures of life satisfaction with a set of behavioral intervention techniques, which are commonly used in therapeutic treatments. The key technique was behavioral activation (BA) techniques. When compared to other treatment conditions, BA was significantly related to a number of measures of positive well-being. In a similar approach, Jacobson et al. (1996, 2001) compared the effectiveness of various components of standard cognitive behavior therapy (CBT), perhaps the most empirically well-supported therapy in contemporary practice. Separate experimental treatments showed that the behavioral activation component (BA) was just as effective on a number of outcome variables as the full CBT treatment. Indeed, BA was shown to be the key component in the overall effectiveness of CBT. Thus, having clients do such simple tasks as monitoring daily activities and completing daily tasks is considerably less costly and more efficient than the full CBT treatment in achieving equal degrees of treatment success. What remains to be shown is that BA is also infused with personal control beliefs. Many aspects of our daily activities directly impact our personal control beliefs, while other aspects of daily activities are responses to externally arising causes beyond our own control. These aspects of activation of control beliefs are in need of much deeper exploration. This is especially relevant to the therapeutic situation, which is especially under the control of the therapist and/or the therapeutic situation. The evidence so far suggests that there is value in infusing personal control principles into our current models of therapeutic models and resilience-building efforts with patients. Current interest in teaching the principles of self-management should be able to gain from expanding the focus incorporating both internal and external control principles.

The evidence is powerful in suggesting the value of this approach, but studies have revealed that the issue is a complex one. There are important differences in the specific definitions and characterizations of the concept of personal control itself and evidence shows that it is critical to employ and Person X Environment model of how the person's particular beliefs match, or do not match, the controlling events in that person's environment. Therapy is an environment, and mental illness, alcohol and drug addictions define complex parameters within which control beliefs, internal or external, exert their effects.

## The Evidence for Resilience

The term resilience was originally used in engineering where metals are subject to stress in order to determine the force required to bend or break the metal. Resilience as a mental health concept was popularized by studies of children who had experienced adverse conditions and yet had no enduring developmental, emotional, psychological, or functional impairments (Felitti et al. 1998). Masten (2014) described resilience as "ordinary magic" that occurs naturally and is based on ordinary resources and processes. Masten et al. (1990) and Masten (2014) defined resilience as the "the capacity of a dynamic system to adapt successfully to disturbances that threaten system function, viability or development" (p. 10). The occurrence of trauma or the emergence and ongoing presence of chronic medical or psychiatric illness are expressions of disturbances that disrupt the adaptive system.

Evidence taken from personal accounts of people confronted with traumatic situations, yet surviving and growing from them, repeatedly points to innate actions that some people engage into overcome adversity and move forward in their lives (Kent et al. 2014). Research also suggests that every person must experience a certain optimal dose of stress in order to develop resilience and adaptive responses. Fortunately or unfortunately, the world provides us with a host of daily opportunities for stress. There are countless examples of children who were raised in extreme poverty, wartime conditions, and so on, who grew up showing no negative effects from the extreme conditions they experienced. The ability to overcome extreme doses of adverse events can be promoted and learned. However, to some extent overcoming adversity is dependent upon a person's attachment relationships (Masten 2014). Having a strong sense of attachment and support is a key to a person's ability to overcome trauma and stress. This may take the form of a family member, mentor, teacher, clergyman, or others who can be supportive in times of need.

There is extensive evidence that building resiliency skills can improve health outcomes. For example, Cal et al. (2015) conducted a review of the literature on resilience and chronic disease published during the 20 years from June 1993 to June 2013. The review reported a negative relationship between resilience and depression, anxiety, incapacitation, and somatization. The review also demonstrated an inverse correlation between resilience scores and the progression of illness (i.e., activity of the disease, control of glycemic level, and severity of depression), and an association between resilience and quality of life as well as health promotional behaviors. The authors concluded that resilience was directly related to health outcomes, and that it was necessary to develop preventive interventions that fostered protective factors for resilience to be developed that could improve health outcomes. Connor and Davidson (2003) reported that when there was an increase in resilience, it was associated with greater treatment improvements in primary care outpatients, general psychiatric outpatients, and in patients treated for generalized anxiety disorder and posttraumatic stress disorder.

Historically, inpatient treatment focused on symptom abatement as the primary criterion for managing and discharging a patient. The advent of shorter hospital stays, whole person healthcare and person-centered care have shifted the focus of treatment to assisting the patient to manage both the symptoms and care planning for his/her life outside of the institution (Vijayalakshmy et al. 2006). Unfortunately, when a patient is discharged from a hospital, there is a high likelihood that he/she will experience stress simply by returning to a situation that may have, at least in part, led to the hospital stay. How the person anticipates, reacts to and overcomes that stress may determine future recidivism and/or community tenure.

New approaches involve the patient, the entire treatment team and other stakeholders in a proactive group planning process to build and execute treatment and discharge planning. Psychiatric rehabilitation practices buttress this approach—engaging the person in a shared process, recognizing the person as the primary decision-maker about his/her healthcare and giving the person choices that are based upon his/her assets, abilities, and social supports (Palmer-Erbs and Anthony 1995). By providing the person with skills, abilities, and resources to use following discharge, successful transitions to the community can be achieved. The new approach recognizes that recovery is possible and that inpatient treatment should be geared to support this as an outcome.

While the process of recovery is designed to return a person from a state of illness to homeostasis or equilibrium, resilience is a process that sustains homeostasis and builds strength to endure and overcome the next stressor or cycle of a chronic illness (Zautra and Franczak 2014). Resilience is more than regaining homeostasis, as there is evidence demonstrated by new learning, growth, and development resulting from adversity. This resilience process allows the individual to be transformed by going through the adverse experience (Zautra et al. 2010b). Sterling and Eyer (1988) introduced the concept of allostasis or the ability of an organism to maintain stability under changing conditions. This concept is particularly pertinent when we experience stress. Wingfield (2003) described allostasis as a fundamental process through which organisms actively adjust to both predictable and unpredictable events. Resilience has been similarly defined as a construct that describes the person's capacity to respond positively to adverse situations, even when these pose a potential risk to his/her health or development (Luthar et al. 2000). Individuals who deal with trauma or chronic illness live with frequent stress and expend considerable energy on maintaining or recovering homeostasis or achieving allostasis. However, there is a physical cost to allostatis. Allostatic load refers to the cumulative cost to the body of allostasis. Allostatic overload refers to a state in which serious physical or mental pathology that can occur when allostasis is not relieved (Sterling 2004). For individuals who do not have the skills, abilities or resources to reduce, eliminate or adapt to stress, their allostatic load can reach critical levels. Many individuals with a serious mental illness have not developed the adaptive skills to deal with stress in healthy ways and often resort to smoking, excessive drinking and eating, illegal drugs, and other high-risk behaviors to reduce the anxiety caused by stress. These same individuals often lack social supports that for most people are an important source of relief from stressful events.

The result of high allostatic load may contribute to a number of physical and mental illnesses and eventually lead to physical or mental health hospitalization.

## Building Resilience

While some individuals experience Masten's (2014) "ordinary magic," the question of whether it is possible to build resilience in individuals that are not so fortunate has been the subject of extensive scientific research. When the individual has available skills, abilities, supports and resources, allostasis can be achieved without the strain of allostatic load. But what are the skills, abilities, supports, and resources that characterize resilient individuals? Skodol (2010) described a resilient individual as a person who has a strong sense of self, as evidenced by self-esteem, self-confidence, self-efficacy, self-understanding, a positive future orientation. The resilient individual has the ability to manage negative behaviors and emotionally believes in his/her abilities to effectively manage life's challenges and situations. This conception of a resilient person is very similar to someone who has developed self-management skills, a concept described in the physical health literature.

Folkman and Lazarus (1985) suggested that building resiliency skills requires strengthening the person's ability to develop self-management skills in order to cope with and master the stressful events in life that we all experience. Von Korff et al. (1997) stated that providers needed to assure that individuals receive behaviorally sophisticated self-management support that gives priority to increasing patients' confidence and skills so that they can be the ultimate manager of their illness. In order to manage their own health care, individuals need knowledge, skills, abilities, and the motivation to do so.

Zautra et al. (2010b) found that sustainable resilience capacities were not developed in a short period, but are built over time, and require time and a focus (often a refocus) on strengths not weaknesses, and rest on improved self-organization, self-control (mastery), and social connection. Reich and Zautra (1981) reported that with increases in well-being, individuals could cope more effectively with future negative experiences. While this development may be undertaken alone, in many cases, it involves a reliance on others through social support networks (Demos 1989).

A variety of programs have emerged that promote the skills noted above. For example, the Stanford Chronic Disease Self-Management Program, the SAMHSA Illness Management and Recovery Toolkit, a variation of the SAMHSA Whole Health Action Management program, Mindfulness Training and the Social Intelligence program can be used. While each individual program does not deal with all of the potential resiliency skills identified by research, in combination, they address the majority of them. In addition, having a variety of programs allows individuals to select a program that best fits their learning style. This would be in line with the Person X Environment fit issue discussed earlier. These programs can all be adapted for use in inpatient settings.

We have identified two abilities that are critical for resilience and self-management—the ability to understand health care issues and the motivation to act on this knowledge to develop healthy lifestyle habits. Hibbard et al. (2013) proposed that the role of an effective self-manager required a high level of knowledge, skill, and confidence. Two areas that have received particular attention are the individual's ability to understand health information, or health literacy, and the motivation to use the information to take action and how these two skills interact (Smith et al. 2013). Having the health knowledge without taking action is inadequate and taking action without knowledge is purposeless. A famous quote from Wolfgang Goethe (Saunders 1906) captures this linkage very well "Knowing is not enough, we must apply. Willing is not enough, we must do." The ability to grow and mobilize biological, psychological, social, and spiritual assets is a key to recovery and resilience, and a key ability to sustaining wellness after discharge from an inpatient unit. Increasing a patient's ability to understand health information and supporting the person in using resiliency skills when stress and/or symptoms arise can augment inpatient care.

**Health Literacy**: Basic knowledge about medical conditions and its treatment approaches are fundamental to being an active participant in care (Peerson and Saunders 2009; Salyers et al. 2009; Institute of medicine 2004a, b). The relationship between poor literacy skills and health status is now well recognized (Nutbeam 2008). Nielsen-Bohlman et al. (2004) defined health literacy as the degree to which individuals can obtain, process, and understand the basic health information and services they need in order to make appropriate health decisions. Furthermore, these investigators also indicated that health literacy also depends upon the skills, preferences, and expectations of health information providers including the doctors, nurses, administrators, home health workers, the media, and many others. Ultimately, literacy develops from a convergence of education, health services, and social and cultural factors that bring together research and practice from diverse fields. The World Health Organization (WHO 2005) defined health literacy as the cognitive and social skills that determine the motivation and ability of individuals to gain access to, understand, and use information in ways that promote and maintain good health. This definition includes motivation, abilities, and skills as essential elements of helping the individual to develop and sustain healthy behaviors.

Kirsch et al. (1993) reported on the results of the National Assessment of Adult Literacy Survey in which only 12 % of adults have proficient health literacy. Slightly more than nine out of ten adults lacked the skills needed to manage their health and prevent disease. Fourteen percent of adults (30 million people) had levels that were below basic health literacy. Low literacy was linked to poor health outcomes, such as higher rates of emergency rooms and hospitalization and less frequent use of preventive service leading to higher healthcare costs (Baker 2006; Baker et al. 2002; Howard et al 2005). Many individuals with a serious mental illness fell in the category of low health literacy, with some due to the cognitive impairments caused by the illness, some others due to poor overall literacy, and yet others due to refusal to accept their illness (Dickerson et al. 2005).

When they asked patients to repeat back what the physician told them, Schillinger et al. (2004) found that 50 % gave inaccurate responses. When asked to "Describe how your physician wanted you to take this medication," 50 % of the patients could not repeat the instructions. Crane (1997) conducted an exit interview with 314 patients treated and released from an emergency room, with instructions from their health care professional. Crane reported that of 314 patients treated and released from an emergency room, only 59 % correctly repeated the instructions they received from their health care professional. Spanish speaking patients scored significantly lower on all questions. In the Medicare program, Williams and Heller (2007) found that only about 30 % of older people reported feeling that they possessed both the motivation and skills to participate fully in their care.

In another study, Hibbard et al. (2007) evaluated whether individuals could understand and were motivated to make health changes. They reported that while 23 % of respondents had adopted new behaviors related to their health care, they were not confident they could maintain them in the face of stress or a crisis. The responses of the remaining 77 % ranged from thinking they could remain passive recipients of care (12 %) to not having basic facts or being able to understand their recommended regimens (29 %) to having some facts, but lacking the confidence and skills to act on them (36 %).

Bodenheimer et al. (2002) found that education alone was generally not sufficient for effective patient self-management of chronic disease due to the challenges individuals experienced in applying the information they acquired in the context of their daily living and the barriers to care they experienced. Increased training in problem solving and coping skills appears to be necessary. While inpatient treatment settings can provide significant education regarding the illness and how the individual can identify triggers and early warning signs of remission, acting on this knowledge requires another aspect of self-management.

Efforts to improve health literacy have led to the conclusion that health information has to be reduced from a technical level to the literacy level of the person receiving the information and it has to be repeated and confirmed with the person on each encounter (Glasgow et al. 2003; Osborne 2004; Pignone et al. 2005; Seubert 2009). Professionals in inpatient settings need to incorporate these findings in their provision of mental health services.

**Patient Activation**: Karoly (2010) proposed that resilience or successful adjustment to adversity could be written in the language of goal-guided self-regulation. He suggested that resilience could be seen as the effective operation of self-regulatory processes under conditions of stress or transition or, alternatively, as the result of especially well-developed self-regulatory functions under stressful circumstances. A very similar concept is Patient Activation in which individual takes action to improve his/her health particularly when health is challenged by an illness. Von Korff et al. (1997) and Wagner (1998) found that chronic care management programs needed to develop interventions that assisted patients with acquiring knowledge, skills, motivation, and confidence to make effective decisions to manage their health.

Hibbard and colleagues (2008, 2009, 2010) recognized that individuals were increasingly being asked to manage their health by making daily decisions that affect their health outcomes. Individuals are required to make many daily choices about leading a healthy lifestyle. Many individuals, particularly those with a serious mental illness, ignore their physical health and never or rarely see their physical health care provider except in emergency rooms. Others may see their health care provider a few times a year, receive health care advice and then take or leave it. Alegría et al. (2008) found that patients who received activation and empowerment interventions were over twice as likely to be retained in treatment and over three times as likely to have scheduled at least one visit during the 6-month follow-up period. Similarly, intervention participants demonstrated 29 % higher attendance at scheduled visits than comparison patients. Hibbard et al. (2013) found that patients with higher health activation scores had nine out of thirteen better health outcomes, including better clinical indicators, more healthy behaviors, and greater use of preventive screening tests—as well as lower health care costs when measured two years later. Hibbard et al. (2013) found that patients with the lowest activation levels had predicted average costs that were 8 % higher in the base year and 21 % higher in the first half of the next year than the costs of patients with the highest activation levels, both significant differences.

Hibbard et al. (2004, 2005) and Green et al. (2010) developed the Patient Activation Measure (PAM) which measures the person's role in the care process and the knowledge, skills and confidence they need to manage his/her health. Research has shown that PAM scores correlate with health outcomes and costs over time, and changes in assessed activation detected by PAM lead to expected changes in outcomes and costs (Mosen et al. 2007). Furthermore, individuals who are more active in their health care have better outcomes and measurable cost savings than individuals who are less active (Greene and Hibbard 2011). Hibbard et al. (2007) have characterized patient activation as a developmental process that consists of four stages: the provider believing that the patient's role in care is important; the person having the confidence and the knowledge necessary to take action; the person taking action to maintain and improve his/her health; and the person staying the course even under the stress of adverse life conditions.

How to activate patients to change poor health behavior that worsen chronic conditions and deteriorate health in general has been the subject of considerable research. Much of the activation research and development of interventions are based on the work of Bandura (1982). The concept of self-efficacy is defined as the belief people hold about their capabilities to perform specific behaviors and their ability to exercise influence over events that affect their lives. Self-efficacy beliefs determine how people feel, think, motivate themselves, and behave. Self-efficacy is a core element of self-management. Self-management and self-management support are now considered evidenced-based practices in primary health care and are an essential ingredient of the Chronic Care Model (Glasgow et al. 2002, 2003; Wagner 1998). Bodenheimer et al. (2002) described self-management support as the means by which individual practitioners and the broader health care system support patients in self-management. The Institute of Medicine (2003) defined self-management support as the systematic provision of education and supportive interventions by health care staff to increase patients' skills and confidence in managing their health problems, including regular assessment of progress and problems, goal setting, and problem solving.

Self-management includes the tasks that individuals must undertake to live well with one or more chronic conditions. These tasks include having the confidence to deal with medical management, role management, and emotional management of their conditions. The IOM (2003) endorses the completion of a patient-generated "action plan" as a key feature of a self-management program. This process assists in developing short-term goals (1–2 weeks) to help patients initiate changes and achieve success in managing their condition effectively. They further identified that the key to good action planning is that the planned actions are generated by the patient, and not the provider. One approach that has been used in the mental health and substance abuse field to improve self-management has been the use of psychiatric rehabilitation.

## Psychiatric Rehabilitation Principles and Practices

Inpatient treatment has historically focused on symptom abatement as the primary criterion for managing and discharging a patient. The development of self-management skills is not considered a formal element of discharge planning; however, many teams have undoubtedly speculated about whether a patient had the skills, abilities, or supports to follow through on the treatments team's recommendations. In many cases, treatment team members are very accurate in their impressions of whether someone has the self-management skills necessary to live effectively with a chronic illness. Public psychiatric inpatient settings are frequently seen as the treatment setting of last resort for people who have not responded adequately to services available in the community or private sector (Salyers et al. 2007). The advent of shorter hospital stays, financial penalties for frequent readmissions, whole person health care and person-centered care has shifted the focus of treatment. Beginning in the 1990s, some hospitals initiated new approaches to assist the hospitalized person in managing both the symptoms and planning for his/her life outside of the facility (Bopp et al. 1996; Vijayalakshmy et al. 2006).

Tools have been developed to measure the application of recovery-oriented practices in inpatient settings (O'Connell et al. 2005). The Recovery Self-Assessment (RSA) has been used to assess the recovery promoting aspects of the environment. The score is based on the perceptions of providers, people in services, and significant others. Salyers et al. (2007) used the RSA to compare recovery attitudes in community settings to those of an inpatient facility. They found that, as expected, inpatient staff members generally scored lower than staff members of community-based organizations. However, recovery practices have made their way into inpatient treatment systems, and are providing the patient with flexibility and encouragement to engage in the development of skills that can be translated into success in his/her postdischarge world. Shorter hospital stays have brought about a realization that a discharged patient has not completed his/her treatment when they leave the hospital, but needs to continue recovery, master skills, and use knowledge to overcome the limitations of a behavioral health disorder. This is a model of community-based recovery and the field of psychiatric rehabilitation is aimed at providing the former patient with hope and the mastery of skills for the challenges of community living. Individuals who achieve recovery have taken the first step to develop resilience. Continuing the journey involves developing or fine-tuning a number of skills that support dealing with the stresses that exists in the dynamic environment of our typical communities.

The preparation for self-management of symptoms while overcoming daily challenges can begin while the person is still in the hospital. New approaches involve the patient, the entire treatment team, and other stakeholders in a group planning process that builds and executes proactive discharge. Engaging the person in his/her care is a shared process that recognizes the person as the primary decision-maker about his/her healthcare and provides choices that are based upon his/her assets and abilities (Palmer-Erbs and Anthony 1995), as well as providing the person with resources to use following discharge. For some individuals (externals), the involvement of others can be an extremely important element of the planning process. Helplessness and hopelessness are overcome with a sense of accomplishment, challenge, and commitment to change the circumstances that had led to a hospital admission. In the language of resilience, this means the development of skills, assets, and supports to lessen allostatic load.

In the 1970s, psychosocial rehabilitation became a field of study within the behavioral health field (Anthony and Farkas 2009). It captured the principles that practices be consistent with the research findings on self-management, recovery, and resilience. These principles have been employed throughout the world in structuring program services. In addition, the principles include the provision that patients be provided with health care information and receive support for patient activation. During the late 1970s, professional organizations and universities began to codify the following principles for the development and delivery of services. A sample of the principles relevant to self-management and resilience are listed below

**Principle 1**: Psychiatric rehabilitation practitioners convey hope and respect; practitioners believe that all individuals have the capacity for learning and growth.

**Principle 2**: Psychiatric rehabilitation practitioners recognize that culture is central to recovery, and strive to ensure that all services are culturally relevant to individuals receiving services.

**Principle 3**: Psychiatric rehabilitation practitioners engage in the processes of informed and shared decision-making and facilitate partnerships with other persons identified by the recipient of services.

**Principle 4**: Psychiatric rehabilitation practices build on the strengths and capabilities of individuals

**Principle 5**: Psychiatric rehabilitation practices are person-centered and address the unique needs of individuals, in ways that are consistent with the individuals' values, hopes and aspirations.

**Principle 7**: Psychiatric rehabilitation practices promote self-determination and empowerment. All individuals have the right to make their own decisions, including decisions about the types of services and supports they receive.

**Principle 8**: Psychiatric rehabilitation practices facilitate the development of personal support networks by utilizing natural supports within communities, peer support initiatives, and self- and mutual-help groups.

**Principle 9**: Psychiatric rehabilitation practices strive to help individuals improve the quality of all aspects of their lives including social, occupational, educational, residential, intellectual, spiritual, and financial.

**Principle 10**: Psychiatric rehabilitation practices promote health and wellness and they encourage individuals to develop and use individualized wellness plans.

Over time, additional documents elaborated on the principles as the systems of care changed and innovative approaches emerged (Anthony and Farkas 2009). They emphasized the importance of maximizing individual choice, engagement, hope, the management of symptoms, and build self-management skills.

The practice of psychiatric rehabilitation and the process of recovery and building resilience are based on the belief that every person who suffers a behavioral health disorder has the innate ability and capacity to move beyond the disorder and reestablish his/her life within a community of choice. This fundamental principle upholds the idea that practitioners, support staff members and family are required to "do with, not for." In other words, the practitioner works in partnership with the person, utilizing practices to support the individual's skill building, resource management, assessment and planning, advocacy and networking in a proactive, shared process. This model is predicated upon the belief that the person is the best person to manage his/her recovery journey and that the building of resilience is best completed within the local community. Indeed, this model holds that the person is the one who defines the process and the outcome. This journey is not made without challenges and setbacks. In fact, failure is a necessary element in the journey that represents an opportunity for growth. This is ultimately how a person's resilience is grows, adapts, is tested and supported.

As hospitals become aware of and accept recovery principles and practices, the primary obstacle to implementing them is staff member attitudes and skills (Anthony and Farkas 2009). Staff members are at a significant disadvantage in observing individuals living successfully in the community. Staffs only see these individuals at the worst stage of an illness and rarely get to see those individuals who have achieved recovery and resilience. The ability of staff to modify traditional ways of thinking about inpatient treatment and to adjust traditional treatment methods to account for the unique qualities of each person is required for successful treatment during hospital stay and following discharge (Pollard et al. 2008). Psychosocial educational model can provide lasting benefits for psychiatric patients, in symptom management, reduction of psychiatric hospital readmission rates, and improved quality of life. These principles were introduced into inpatient settings through the creation of "treatment malls."

**Treatment Malls**: Concepts such as treatment malls have demonstrated that even in the most restrictive inpatient environments, patients can be engaged in shared decision-making even in the most restrictive inpatient environments (Webster et al. 2005). Treatment malls offer an array of group activities that engage the patients and all staff members in dialog, planning, and brainstorming with a focus on the person's unique attributes and abilities to overcome stress and adversity. Treatment malls provide a self-directed learning experience that meets the person-centered needs of the participants (Ballard 2008). Individuals move into and out of units, classes, and activities with the guidance of staff members who encourage and mobilize the person. Activities are designed to replicate, to the greatest extent possible, real-life and community-based events and settings. The treatment mall is designed to improve a person's activation, provide new information, resources, improve his/her participation in activities of choice while inpatient and postdischarge.

There are limitations in the treatment mall concept. The greatest challenges are the curriculum that is often homemade, not updated routinely, and often do not use evidence-based practices. In many cases, it is difficult to discern the intent of the program or its efficacy. Moreover, people who have long hospital stays get the same program for months. In short, programs people continuously enter and leave the program in ways that interfere with monitoring progress and addressing specific needs of the individual, such that it leads to boredom and poor attendance. In addition, it is difficult to organize the treatment mall activities due to the short lengths of stay that many individuals experience, the fact that individuals are admitted to the facility and enrolled in the program on an ongoing basis making to it difficult to follow a progressive curriculum in a group format. Addressing the person's specific needs in a structured program can also be difficult, and measuring and reporting progress to the team can also be challenging.

Several hospitals have developed treatment mall programs and have adjusted their operations and workforce to provide recovery-oriented services. Although the data are still being collected some general themes have emerged (Forgeron 2009). For example, staff members must be adequately trained and must actively support recovery-oriented services. Patients should have choice, encouragement, and positive feedback to generate hope, positive self-regard, and empowerment. Daily interactions between patients and staff members are focused on optimizing the patient's strengths and aspirations. The inpatient hospital must minimize reliance on the traditional hospital unit and be able to promote the need for patients to move about within the facility to access preferred services and activities. Services address those aspects of daily life that support community success and tenure—housing, vocational training, social contact, physical health management, self-advocacy and communication, legal matters and family support, among others. Preliminary outcome data point to a decrease in recidivism among former patients who complete the various treatment modalities. The positive outcomes are enhanced when recovery-oriented activities are continued in community-based services (Kauffman 2000; Webster et al. 2005).

## Community Programs that Promote Recovery and Resilience

Several community programs provide and promote recovery programs. For example, Marc Community Resources, in Mesa, Arizona has implemented several programs that are designed to increase the resilience of the participants. Although Marc is a community-based program, they serve many individuals who were recently discharged from hospital settings. The programs and protocols that they provide can easily be adapted to inpatient settings. Of course, they have been most fortunate in developing a relationship with the Resiliency Solutions Group at the Arizona State University and their leading researchers in the resilience field.

The Marc resilience model is based on the following overarching bank account metaphor (Franczak and Moore 2014). Analogous to bank accounts, individuals develop and store assets and capital in physical, psychological, social, and spiritual accounts. In the physical account, individuals add value by having good nutrition, exercise, practicing good hygiene, developing health literacy, maintain a healthy weight, avoiding smoking, and so on. Individuals also inherit or lose physical capital through genetics. Excessive drinking, smoking, overeating, poor nutrition, and other unhealthy behaviors withdraw capital from their physical account. In the psychological account, people build capital by developing problem solving or coping skills, building, and maintaining self-esteem, using stress reduction techniques, using their gifts and strengths, and finding meaning in daily life. Withdrawals from accounts occur when problems are seen as personal pervasive failures that lead to a loss of self-esteem, and the individual experiences helplessness or hopelessness. In the social account, people build capital by interacting with others and the community, developing and maintaining friendships, and in volunteering and enjoying the rich diversity in the people around them. Capital is withdrawn when people isolate, avoid contact with friends and family, and see social situations and the community as something to be avoided. In the spiritual account value is by creating a sense of purpose. According to Dingle (2014) spirituality grounds people, gives meaning, and can tie our suffering into the greater good of all. Spirituality is a means that can transform physical/emotional "defeats" into successes and tie the person to community, culture, and the self. Spirituality manifests our human nature: we are more than our cognitions, we are more than our biology, we are more than our social supports, we belong to something greater, and we stand for something more. This quote by de Chardin (1999), "We are not human beings in search of spirituality, we are spiritual beings in search of humanity" highlights the importance of spirituality in the quality of our life.

Similar to today's bank accounts, the physical, psychological, social, and spiritual accounts are linked so that withdrawals or deposits in one account can affect the others. For example, when we lose a close relationship with a family member or friend, it can influence our psychological and our physical accounts. We may have lost someone who was important to our self-esteem. We can become troubled by how we can regain the person's attention. Depending on the severity of the loss, we may lose sleep over the matter or change our eating habits or engage in other unhealthy habits, such as over eating or drinking. When a chronic physical illness is diagnosed our self-esteem and problem-solving abilities may be taxed to their limit while we try to understand how this illness will impact our daily well-being. We may begin to avoid contact with family and friends, as we deal with the stress of this life change.

This model of resilience depends on using each of these accounts to both restore and sustain our ability to accept and embrace the "new normal." This approach inquires not only about whether the program helped repair damage and speed recovery from hurt, but whether those helped now know more about what to do, should they be hurt again. We all know that the world contains numerous challenges that often emerge when we least expect them. A resilient person has developed the adaptive skills to identify challenges and to adjust problem-solving methods to new or novel situations. The resilient individual uses assets and capital from all of their accounts to successfully navigate new challenges. It is important to have a balanced set of assets, as reliance on a single category of asset will create challenge when we have a significant withdrawal from that asset. For example, when we have a significant challenge to our health, the biological account may be tapped out. If we do not have assets in the other categories, we have a limited array of skills to use to retain our resilience.

In order to assist individuals in building assets in their biological, psychological, social, and spiritual accounts, service providers can use a variety of available evidence-based programs that are designed to assist the individual in making deposits into their accounts. For example, the Marc Community Resources currently use the Stanford Chronic Disease Self-Management program, the SAMHSA Illness Management program, the WHAM program (modified), Mindfulness-based interventions, and Social Intelligence programs. Other programs, such as the GRIT program, can also be utilized. These programs are tailored to the needs and preferences of the person, and can also be used in inpatient settings. Staff members receive basic training in stages of change (Prochaska and DiClemente 1986), motivational interviewing (Miller and Rollnick 2012; Rollnick et al. 1992, 2007), behavioral activation (Lewinsohn 1975), and specific training in the program methodologies. Fidelity testing is also conducted to ensure that personnel implement the protocols with consistency.

## Holistic Health and Wellness Programs

### Stanford Chronic Disease Self-Management Program (CDSMP)

The CDSMP is a hands-on psychoeducational and practical method to build psychobiological, social, and spiritual assets. The CDSMP or Healthy Living Workshop is a 6-week self-management workshop that meets once a week, for two and a half hours. The 6-week period can be adjusted to suit inpatient settings. Two trained peer leaders facilitate each workshop by using an established curriculum developed by Lorig (1999, 2006). The peer leaders receive four days of initial training and are then observed by a trained instructor in order to ensure fidelity to the program model. The workshops are interactive and encourage discussion.

CDSMP addresses both health literacy and health activation. Materials cover chronic illnesses and issues that may impact a life of quality that is lived with an illness. Each person then develops an individualized plan to manage his/her particular chronic condition and reports back on his/her progress at each session. Barriers to progress are identified, and methods to overcome these are considered. The program is available in English, Spanish (Tomando Control de su Salud), and a wide variety of other languages. In an inpatient setting, the workshop scheduling may need to be adjusted to meet short and long lengths of stay. The length of the session may also need to be modified when working with individuals who have cognitive impairments or are unable to sustain attention for long periods of time. With these slight accommodations, the formal CDSMP is applicable to individuals with a serious mental illness. Druss et al. (2010) have developed the HARP that a modified version of the CDSMP to be used specifically with individuals with mental illness.

The CDSMP workshop topics include identifying and managing symptoms, goal setting, action plans, managing stress, problem solving, dealing with difficult emotions, nutrition, understanding medications, making informed treatment decisions, increasing strength and stamina through better fitness, and using your mind to manage symptoms. CDSMP is based on three underlying assumptions: (1) regardless of the chronic condition, people have similar problems and concerns and face similar challenges; (2) people can learn the skills needed to better manage their disease and the day-to-day issues they face; and (3) people who understand and take control of their condition will be healthier and happier (Lorig et al. 1994).

The Center for Disease Control and Prevention (2010) has reviewed the findings of the Stanford Chronic Disease Self-Management Program (CDSP) with respect to physical, emotional and health-related quality of life, and health care utilization and costs. It has concluded that CDSMP: (1) has strong beneficial effects on physical and emotional outcomes, and health-related quality of life; (2) consistently results in greater energy/reduced fatigue, more exercise, fewer social role limitations, better psychological well-being, enhanced partnerships with physicians, improved health status, and greater self-efficacy; (3) reduces healthcare expenditures (Lorig et al. 1999, 2001); (4) is effective across socioeconomic and educational levels; (5) is used with various ethnic groups in the US and internationally; and (6) reduces healthcare expenditures sufficiently to pay for itself within the first year (Lorig et al. 1999, 2001).

Goldberg et al. (2013) developed a variation of the Chronic Disease Management Program called "Living Well" that is tailored for individuals with mental illness. They found that participants showed significant post-intervention improvements across a range of attitudinal (self-efficacy and patient activation), behavioral (illness self-management techniques), and functional (physical and emotional well-being and general health functioning) outcomes. They also found evidence of continued improvement in health-related locus of control and reports of healthy eating and physical activity and a notable decrease in use of the emergency room for medical care.

## Whole Health Action Management Program (WHAM)

The Whole Health Action Management Program (WHAM) (SAMHSA 2002), published by SAMHSA-HRSA Center for Integrated Health solutions (www.integration.samhsa.gov), is another program that has proven useful in assisting people with behavioral health difficulties to self-manage their healthcare. This program is based on recovery principles and practices, and it uses peer workers to engage and work with the participants. The structured curriculum trains people to manage chronic physical health conditions and mental health concerns to achieve whole health. It includes training skills in health literacy and health activation. Peer support workers facilitate discussions among health care service recipients in an active process to modify negative behavior and attitudes that undermine health. WHAM builds on the person's strengths and assets to enhance positive emotions, attitudes, and activities that impact both physical and mental health outcomes. The curriculum is designed to assist the person in formulating a whole health goal for self-management. It incorporates ten health and resiliency factors: stress management; healthy eating; physical activity; restful sleep; service to others; support network; optimism based on positive expectations; cognitive skills to avoid negative thinking; spiritual beliefs and practices; and a sense of meaning and purpose.

The second component of WHAM is designed to maximize mind–body resiliency. Individuals are engaged in a series of discussions and activities to strengthen their abilities to rise above the debilitating aspects of chronic disease. Included are hands-on activities and psychological approaches to improve relaxation, reduce stress, and minimize negative self-talk and use spiritual strength. WHAM has identified five keys to whole health success: person-centered goal setting; weekly action planning; creating a daily/weekly personal log; one-to-one peer support; and weekly peer support group.

WHAM has demonstrated that people who are supported in managing their self-care on an ongoing basis are less likely to relapse and are better able to cope with the cyclical nature of a chronic disorder. There are limitations to implementing the WHAM program in an inpatient setting. The use of paraprofessional peer workers is considered fundamental to this model. While the use of peers in an inpatient setting is not available in some locations, there is no reason why it cannot be.

## Illness Management and Recovery (IMR)

The Illness Management and Recovery (IMR) is another evidence-based practice endorsed by SAMHSA. This practice actively engages people who are in recovery in a process of teaching information and training skills that include psychoeducation, motivation, cognitive behavioral strategies, behavioral restructuring for medication adherence, relapse prevention, coping strategies for stress reduction, and managing persistent symptoms. Toolkit workbooks are provided to services and practitioners. A computer-based version of IMR has been developed and pilot tested recently (Wright-Berryman et al. 2013). Moemi et al. (2013) have adapted the tool for international use and computerized tools are also available and offer the computer savvy easy access to IMR information.

Preliminary data from these programs suggest that patients in a recovery-oriented settings are more actively engaged and participate more frequently and fully while hospitalized than in traditional settings. Implementation of evidence-based practices such as IMR requires a significant front-end cost, mainly in the training of personnel and application of new training modalities and materials. After start-up, costs are similar to those of traditional inpatient facilities. There are demands on personnel in transitioning to recovery models. The practices involve staff members and patients alike in some anxiety-provoking changes in behavior, daily scheduling, daily tasks, and documentation of services. The anxiety and stress of implementing a treatment mall or IMR program is largely felt at the front end while the facility is redesigned, the staff members are trained, and new materials and activities are developed and initiated. Patients do not exhibit any increase in violence or disruptive behaviors during this period. For example, violence actually decreased among a forensic population in a study that compared a treatment mall approach to a civil-committed population using a traditional model of treatment. (Holland et al. 2005).

## Resilience-Building Models and Activities

### Mindfulness

The practice of mindfulness provides a flexible tool that can be used in various settings to help people overcome the debilitating effects of chronic disorders. Mindfulness is the nonjudgmental awareness of thoughts, feelings and perceptions in the present moment. It has significant positive effects on health and wellness, on pain reduction, psychiatric and psychological distress, and stress-related symptoms (Shapiro and Carlson 2009). The methods of mindfulness originated in Eastern wisdom traditions. Mindfulness has attracted current psychological research and is increasingly used in cognitive behavioral strategies for health and wellness and for personal transformation (Didonna 2009). Thirty years of research have demonstrated that mindfulness-based stress reduction effectively reduces medical, psychiatric, and psychological symptoms across a wide range target behaviors (Singh et al. 2008). Although mindfulness-based approaches vary in their components, they typically include one or more of the following: a personal meditation practice based on concentration and/or contemplative meditation exercises, behavioral practices (e.g., loving kindness, compassion, and generosity), cognitive strategies (e.g., reflection on the transitory nature of events and the emptiness of self), and empathic strategies (e.g., happiness and accepting suffering). All of these techniques are viewed collectively as elements of training the mind. Although research is beginning to explore the mechanisms by which mindfulness works, it is thought that its effects are mediated through attention regulation, body awareness, emotion regulation, and change in perspective on the self (Hölzel et al. 2011).

Mindfulness-based approaches have resulted in a proliferation of research that attest to replicable clinical findings across disorders and settings. The effectiveness of mindfulness is demonstrated across a range of clinical and nonclinical issues: psychiatric disorders (personality disorders, eating disorders, addictive behaviors, PTSD, psychosis, and OCD, depression), physical health and wellness (e.g., pain, obesity, smoking, and migraines), medical problems (e.g., cancer, heart disease, diabetes, and hypertension), and behavioral issues (e.g., parenting, aggression, and fear) (Didonna 2009).

Kabat-Zinn (1990, 2003) introduced Mindfulness-Based Stress Reduction (MBSR) to the clinical community at the University of Massachusetts Medical School's Stress Reduction Clinic. This program has served as a model for many others. This program is based on a form of meditation known as mindfulness. The standard MBSR course consists of eight weekly two and a half hours classes and a full-day retreat. The program components can include guided instruction in mindfulness meditation practices, gentle stretching, and mindful yoga, group dialog and mindful communication exercises to enhance awareness in everyday life, individually tailored instructions, daily assignments, and practice materials.

Participants can also be taught mindfulness observation of thoughts, a standard mindfulness procedure for observing thoughts, and the language used to express thoughts Participants are taught that they are not their thoughts and that their desires are merely transient thoughts that can be used to observe "desire" thoughts and let them go. Participants are taught a four-part series of mindfulness procedures that enable them to disengage from their thoughts. The mindfulness procedures require (1) a focus on successive thoughts, (2) to observe the beginning, middle, and end of each thought, (3) observe thoughts as clouds ("thought clouds") and passing through awareness, and (4) observe desires as thought clouds without (a) pushing the thoughts away, (b) engaging with the thoughts, or (c) becoming emotionally attached to the thoughts.

## Social Intelligence

As social animals, humans seek and utilize social assets throughout their lives. Many inpatient settings foster less than ideal social skills that do not translate well to outside setting. Many people discharged from a hospital have few skills in self-advocacy, clear communication, assertiveness and social integration. The Social Intelligence (SI) Institute assists individuals, organizations, and communities develop healthy human connection and counter detachment, disengagement and disregard of one another. A past, punctuated by painful social interactions and a current style of self-serving defensiveness and distrust often preclude dialog. Social conflict ensues as people fail to humanize their interactions. Thus polarized, individuals and communities struggle to find themselves and get beyond the loneliness within and lack of empathic concern for others. The SI Institute provides a new narrative framework beyond self-interest, a narrative not of "me" but "we," which embraces the value of understanding one another, and of acting with others in mind to nourish healthy relationships. The training programs are designed to guide participants to more thoughtful reflection about their own needs, a greater understanding of the complexity of their social worlds, and increased flexibility in adapting to their social difficulties by program activities.

Individuals of all ages facing difficult life transitions, and those who care for them, can benefit from the curriculum. Individuals with serious mental illness and/or substance abuse disorders often have challenges in relating to others. Their struggles to connect in positive ways to family, friends, and coworkers have often included mistreatment and bias. Professional and nonprofessional caregivers may benefit from SI training to support capacities for empathetic concern and continued job satisfaction in helping others.

The program is based on four fundamental principles: (1) neuroplasticity—the capacity for change at any age; (2) individual uniqueness—no two people are alike, each deserves to be understood fully and without stereotypes; (3) awareness of unconscious automatic processes that often dominate social interactions; and (4) humanization—people are not objects or a collection of body parts but are sentient beings deserving of attention. Based on these principles, training can lead to higher levels of social maturity in personal and professional life.

SI training is a ten-hour program that can be completed individually or in groups with facilitation. The basic program consists of 7 modules that are covered over 42 sessions.

**Module 1**: **Neuroplasticity**. This module addresses brain development and the life-long capacity to form new neuro-connections that guide future social relations. (6 lessons)

**Module 2**: **The Unconscious and Unconscious Brain Mechanisms**. This module describes how the brain processes information about the self and others and by how it is guided by individual schemas and cognitive biases. Greater awareness of the utility and fallibility of these ways of thinking and how to improve the understanding of ourselves and others. (8 lessons)

**Module 3**: **Mind Reading**. The foundation for this module is the ability to identify the feelings and thoughts of another person, and to respond to those feelings and thoughts in appropriate ways. (7 lessons)

**Module 4**: **Them**. This module addresses how thoughts and behavior toward others are shaped by the brain's automatic categorization and by the groups to which we belong. We instinctively display favoritism toward those who are like us, and biases toward those who are different. (8 lessons)

**Module 5**: **Face-to-face Conversations**. This module focuses on the ebb and flow of smooth social interactions and the fundamental importance of getting outside of our own heads and connecting with other people. (7 lessons)

**Module 6**: **The Past**. This module addresses how our backgrounds and past experiences influence the ability to form quality relationships, to feel comfortable with others, and to love and be loved. (4 lessons)

**Module 7**: **SI is about Choice**. This module shows that we are not destined to repeat old patterns of relating. We can consciously choose to change ways of relating through both awareness and effort. (1 lesson)

The SI Institute is dedicated to making the program accessible to audiences around the world using latest technology to present the training online with highly educational and engaging videos, sets of reflective questions in order to increased self-awareness, hands-on activities to try out concepts, and actions to practice and build new habits.

A recent study showed that individuals who completed the SI course through the Social Intelligence Institute improved on a number of key indicators of social and emotional intelligence, including improved social skills and social information processing, increased sensitivity to others' emotion and perspective taking, and improved empathy, self-monitoring, and psychological well-being (Zautra et al. 2015a, b). The Social Intelligence Institute has tested the SI training program in several settings that included individuals with serious mental illnesses and peer counselors. The SI program enhanced students' sensitivity to others and increased confidence in their ability to successfully navigate social relations. In addition, trainees reported that the materials were very helpful in both their professional and personal lives.

## Goal-Directed Resilience in Training (GRIT)

For persons with serious mental illnesses, the most common effects of long-term stress are seen in recurrent inpatient hospitalization and poor community survival. The Goal-directed Resilience in Training (GRIT) model has demonstrated positive impact on people who have experienced trauma and stress that resulted from widely different life events (Kent and Davis 2014; Kent et al. 2014, 2015). There are two overarching strengths that assist people during and after these events: (1) approach or engagement in their situations in ways that keep the person well, and (2) social relatedness or connection with other people. Approach/engagement covers experiences of interest, curiosity, appreciation, and noticing beauty. Social relatedness consists of experiences of empathy, compassion, appreciation, and noticing beauty. These two basic strengths were extrapolated from real-life examples of people who experienced severe trauma and overcame it. The GRIT model consists of four modules that aim to transform past pain and suffering [Module (1) Rebuilding Approach/Engagement; Module (2) Rebuilding Social Connectedness, Bonds, Affiliation; Module (3) Transforming Distress and Trauma with Resilience Skills; and Module (4) Building a Good Life].

The program starts by asking participants to set aside their most painful or distressing experience. These will be encountered later. Participants are encouraged to identify and explore an episode in which they are cherished or loved or they cherished or loved someone or something else. Participants are to turn to this episode when they are distressed during the course of the program, to help them be calm and be able to do the work of the program. The two core resilience skills are then applied to participants' lives. The approach/engagement module covers experiences that demonstrate interest, curiosity, appreciation, and noticing beauty. Participants are asked to find examples of these in their own lives, particularly childhood and early adulthood. They are asked to notice the responses of their five senses during episodes of interest, curiosity, and other expressions of engagement. This allows them to reexperience at emotional, cognitive, physiological levels these engagement experiences. Social connectedness module covers experiences of empathy, compassion, helping, friendship, and love. Participants are again asked to identify social connection experiences of empathy, helping, friendship, and love from their lives, with an emphasis on childhood and early adulthood. They are asked to reexperience them and note the responses of their five senses. In the transformation module, these strengths are applied to distress, trauma and pain by facing them with engagement (interest, curiosity, etc.) and/or social relatedness (empathy, helping, etc.). In the last module participants apply the skills of engagement and social relatedness to building a good life for themselves, a life that contains engagement and social connection and has expanded beyond distress and trauma. Thus, the person learns new skills to overcome pain and suffering, and concurrently explores new engagement and social environments. Classroom activities and homework assignments seek to expand the person's awareness of and reexperience of resilience skills, and provide opportunities to learn how to apply the new skills to overcome distress and to lead a richer and fuller life. GRIT ends with incorporating new learning into a design for a good life for each participant.

## Conclusion

The growing emphasis on reducing health care costs, reducing inpatient hospital utilization, length of stay, and decreasing readmission, as well as increasing health and wellness in community settings has sharpened the focus on preventive and wellness-based treatment methodologies. While recovery- and resilience-based treatments have flourished in many community mental health centers, and are promoted through national policy and research initiatives, inpatient services have been challenged to adopt new techniques. The hesitancy lies at multiple levels including: the cost of retooling inpatient units; the cost of identifying, recruiting and training the hospital workforce; overcoming fear and uncertainty among health care workers and the fact that they are working with individuals who are highly symptomatic upon admission. All these obstacles notwithstanding, current thought increasingly points to the need to import some of the recovery/resilience theories and practices into inpatient settings.

There is an abundance of data and rationale for incorporating resilience-oriented activities to patients in inpatient settings as a means to assist them in becoming more actively involved in their treatment and wellness. Traumatic experiences, debilitating symptoms, and long-term reactions to stress significantly undermine the best efforts of many patients. Nevertheless, many find a way to overcome these limitations through resiliency skill building, practicing skills, and developing new internal and external resources. Although a person may learn many new skills as part of his/her recovery, it is incumbent upon the person and his/her health care workers that they become comfortable and conversant with the language of resilience and wellness within a long-term perspective.

Health literacy is a necessity for it allows a person in treatment to better understand and communicate needs, preferences, strengths, and abilities as part of an ongoing process to plan for a healthy lifestyle and improve happiness over the long term. Health activation is another essential ingredient to this new approach as it points to the person's willingness and abilities to mobilize resources, make key decisions and understand consequences of actions taken by both the person in services and the key practitioners in his/her life.

Hope is another ingredient that is essential to successfully navigating one's path toward community living and a healthy lifestyle. The patient must have a firm belief that his/her life will improve, that he/she can overcome the debilitating effect of a major mental illness and that the simple act of trying to get well is, in itself, uplifting. Enhancing and using one's resilience assets is essential to this process and an exploration of these assets with the patient is a key to mobilizing them in the inpatient unit and preparing them for discharge.

Several practices and techniques can be used to build a person's resilience and recovery before he/she leaves the inpatient setting. Some of these are emerging or evidence-based practices endorsed by policymakers and funding sources. Others are basic intervention strategies designed to improve communication, increase self-awareness, build hope and improve communication with practitioners and others. Ultimately, a person's lifestyle choices and health often revolve around making choices and moving forward. In addition to stabilizing the positive symptoms of mental illness, supporting the development of self-management skills is one of the most important activities that hospitals can offer the person. Introducing these choices and assisting a person to make healthy choices before leaving a hospital is aimed at optimizing the patient's transition back into the community and improving the likelihood that the person will remain relatively healthy, happy and independent for the rest of his/her life.

## References


Alegría, M., Jackson, J., Kessler, R., & Takeuchi, D. (2003). *National comorbidity survey replication*. Ann Arbor, MI: Interuniversity Consortium for Political and Social Research.

Alegría, M., Polo, A., Gao, S., Santana, L., Rothstein, D., Jimenez, A., et al. (2008). Evaluation of a patient activation and empowerment intervention in mental health care. *Medical Care, 46*(3), 247–256.

American Psychological Association. (2015). *Stress in America: Paying with our health*. Washington DC: Author.

Anthony, W., & Farkas, M. (2009). *A primer on the psychiatric rehabilitation process*. Boston, MA: Boston University Center for Psychiatric Rehabilitation.

Baker, D. (2006). The meaning and the measure of health literacy. *Journal General Internal Medicine, 21*, 878–883.

Baker, D., Gazmararian, J., Williams, M., Scott, T., Parker, R., Green, D., et al. (2002). Functional health literacy and the risk of hospital admission among Medicare managed care enrollees. *American Journal of Public Health, 92*(8), 1278–1283.

Ballard, F. (2008). Benefits of psychosocial rehabilitation programming in a treatment mall. *Journal of Psychosocial Nursing Mental Health Services, 46*(2), 26–32.

Bandura, A. (1982). Self-efficacy mechanism in human agency. *American Psychologist, 37*(2), 122–147.

Bodenheimer, T., Lorig, K., Holman, H., & Grumbach, K. (2002). Patient self-management of chronic disease in primary care. *Journal of the American Medical Association, 288*(19), 2469–2475.

Bohanske, R., & Franczak, M. (2010). Transforming public behavioral health care: a case example of consumer-directed, recovery and common factors. In B. Duncan, S. Miller, B. Wampold, & M. Hubble (Eds.), *The heart and soul of change: Delivering what works in therapy* (2nd ed., pp. 299–322). Washington, DC: American Psychological Association.

Bonanno, G. (2004). Loss, trauma and human resilience: Have we underestimated the human capacity to thrive after extremely aversive event? *American Psychologist, 59*, 20–28.

Bopp, J., Ribble, D., Cassidy, J., & Markoff, R. (1996). Re-engineering the state hospital to promote rehabilitation and recovery. *Psychiatric Services, 47*, 697–701.

Brown, S., Birtwistle, J., Roe, L., & Thompson, C. (1999). The unhealthy lifestyle of people with schizophrenia. *Psychological Medicine, 29*(3), 697–701.

Brownell, P. (1982). The effects of personality-situation congruence in a managerial context: Locus of control and budgetary participation. *Journal of Personality and Social Psychology, 42*, 753–763.

Cal, S., de Sa, L., Glustak, M., & Santiago, M. (2015). Resilience in chronic diseases: A systematic review. *Cogent Psychology, 2*, 1024928.

California Health Care Foundation. (2015). *Californians with the top chronic conditions: 11 million and counting*. Oakland, CA: Author.

Center for Advancing Health. (2010). *A new definition of patient engagement: What is engagement and why is it important?*. Washington, DC: Author.

Center for Medicare and Medicaid Innovation. (2011). *Pioneer Accountable Care Organization (ACO) model request for application*. Baltimore, MD: Author.

Centers for Disease Control and Prevention. (2010). *Chronic diseases and health promotion*. Atlanta, GA: Author.

Connor, K., & Davidson, J. (2003). Development of a new resilience scale: The Connor-Davidson Resilience Scale (CD-RISC). *Depression and Anxiety, 18*, 76–82.

Cook, J., Razzano, L., Swarbrick, M., Jonikas, J., Yost, C., Burke, L., et al. (2015). Health risks and changes in self-efficacy following community health screening of adults with serious mental illnesses. *PLoS ONE, 10* (4), e0123552.

Crane, J. (1997). Patient comprehension of doctor-patient communication on discharge from the emergency department. *Journal of Emergency Medicine, 1*, 1–7.

de Chardin, T. (1999). *The human phenomenon*. Sussex, UK: Sussex Academic Press.

Demos, E. (1989). Resiliency in infancy. In T. Dugan & R. Cole (Eds.), *The child of our times: Studies in the development of resiliency* (pp. 3–22). Philadelphia: Brunner/Mazel.

Dickerson, F., Goldberg, R., Brown, C., Kreyenbuhl, J., Wohlheiter, K., Fang, L., et al. (2005). Diabetes knowledge among persons with serious mental illness and type 2 diabetes. *Psychosomatics, 46*(5), 418–424.

Didonna, F. (2009). *Clinical handbook of mindfulness*. New York, NY: Springer.

Dingle, S. (2014). Spirituality and resilience. In, *Presentation at the Exploring Resiliency Conference*. Phoenix, AZ: ASU Center for Applied Behavioral Health Policy.

Druss, B., Zhao, L., von Essenwein, S., Bona, J., Fricks, L., Jenkins-Tucker, S., et al. (2010). The Health and Recovery Peer (HARP) program: A peer-led intervention to improve medical self-management for persons with serious mental illness. *Schizophrenia Research, 118*, 264–270.

Duncan, B. (2005). *What's right with you debunking dysfunction and changing your life*. Deerfield Beach, FL: Health Communications.

Ehrlich, E., Kofke-Egger, H., & Udow-Phillips, M. (2010). *Health care cost drivers: Chronic disease, comorbidity, and health risk factors in the US and Michigan*. Ann Arbor, MI: Center for Healthcare Research and Transformation.

Elliott, D. E., Bjelajac, P., Fallot, R. D., Markoff, L. S., & Reed, B. G. (2005). Trauma-informed or trauma-denied: Principles and implementation of trauma-informed services for women. *Journal of Community Psychology, 33*, 461–477.

Fava, G., & Tomba, E. (2009). Increasing psychological well-being and resilience by psychotherapeutic methods. *Journal of Personality, 77*(6), 1903–1934.

Felitti, V., Anda, R., Nordenberg, D., Williamson, D., Spitz, A., Edwards, V., et al. (1998). Relationship of childhood abuse and household dysfunction to many of the leading causes of death in adults: The Adverse Childhood Experiences (ACE) study. *American Journal of Preventive Medicine, 14*(4), 245–258.

Folkman, S., & Lazarus, R, S. (1985). If it changes it must be a process: Study of emotion and coping during three stages of a college examination. *Journal of Personality and Social Psychology, 48*, 150–170

Forgeron, E. (2009). There is preliminary evidence on the effect of treatment mall on individuals with chronic mental illness. *Mental Health CATS*. Paper 6. http://commons.pacificu.edu/otmh/6

Franczak, M. (2013). Communication, coordination and collaboration in community behavioral health. In D. Mailer & K. Langsam (Eds.), *Community mental health practice* (pp. 19–35). Westport, CT: Praeger.

Franczak, M., & Barshter, D. (2015). *Building resiliency: Strategies for promoting well-being across the life span*. Phoenix, AZ: ASU Center for Applied Behavioral Health Policy.

Franczak, M., & Dye, C. (2004). *Mental illness and substance abuse: Making matters worse*. Tucson, AZ: Michael Berren, Publisher.

Franczak, M., & Moore, J. (2014). Building your resilience assets. In, *Presentation at the Exploring Resiliency Conference*. Phoenix, AZ: ASU Center for Applied Behavioral Health Policy.

Freeman E. J., Colpe L. J., Strine T. W., Dhingra, S., McGuire, L. C., Elam-Evans, L. D., et al. (2010). Public health surveillance for mental health. *Preventing Chronic Disease, 7*. http://www.cdc.gov/pcd/issues/2010/jan/09_0126.htm

Glasgow, R., Davis, C., Funnell, M., & Beck, A. (2003). Implementing practical interventions to support chronic illness self-management. *Joint Commission Journal on Quality and Safety, 29*(11), 563–574.

Glasgow, R., Funnell, M., Bonomi, A., Davis, C., Beckham, V., & Wagner, E. (2002). Self management aspects for the improving chronic illness care breakthrough series: Implementation with diabetes and heart failure teams. *Annals of Behavioral Medicine, 24*(2), 80–87.

Goldberg, W., Dickerson, F., Lucksted, A., Brown, C., Weber, E., Tenhula, W., et al. (2013). Living well: An intervention to improve self-management of medical illness for individuals with serious mental illness. *Psychiatric Services, 64*, 51–57.

Goodman, R., Posner, S., Huang, E., Parekh, A., & Koh, H. (2013). Defining and measuring chronic conditions: Imperatives for research, policy, program, and practice. *Preventing Chronic Disease, 10*, 120239.

Green, C., Perrin, N., Polen, M., Leo, M., Hibbard, J., & Tusler, M. (2010). Development of the patient activation measure for mental health. *Administration Policy Mental Health, 37*(4), 327–333.

Greene, J., & Hibbard, J. (2011). Why does patient activation matter? An examination of the relationship between patient activation and health-related outcomes. *Journal of General Internal Medicine, 27*(5), 520–526.

Helgeson, V. S. (1993). The onset of chronic illness: Its effect on the patient-spouse relationship. *Journal of Social and Clinical Psychology, 12*, 406–428.

Hibbard, J., & Cunningham, P. (2008). How engaged are consumers in their health and health care, and why does it matter? *Research Briefs, 8*, 1–9.

Hibbard, J., Greene, J., & Overton, V. (2013). Patients with lower activation associated with higher costs: Delivery systems should know their patients' scores. *Health Affairs*, *32,* 216–222.

Hibbard, J., Greene, J., & Tusler, M. (2009). Improving the outcomes of disease management by tailoring care to the patient's level of activation. *American Journal of Managed Care, 15*, 353–360.

Hibbard, J., & Mahoney, E. (2010). Toward a theory of patient and consumer activation. *Patient Educational Counseling, 78*, 377–381.

Hibbard, J., Mahoney, E., Stock, R., & Tusler, M. (2007). Do increases in patient activation results in improved self-management behaviors? *Health Services Research, 42*, 1443–1463.

Hibbard, J., Mahoney, E., & Tusler, M. (2005). Development and testing of a short form of the patient activation measure. *Health Services Research, 40*, 1918–1930.

Hibbard, J., Stockard, J., Mahoney, E., & Tusler, M. (2004). Development of the Patient Activation Measure (PAM): Conceptualizing and measuring activation in patients and consumers. *Health Services Research, 39*, 1005–1026.

Holland, J., Vidoni-Clark, C., Prandoni, J., Fain, M., Richardson, E., & Montalbano, P. (2005). Moving beyond ward based treatment: A public mental health hospital's transition to a treatment mall. *Psychiatric Rehabilitation Journal, 28*, 295–297.

Hölzel, B., Carmody, J., Vangel, M., Congleton, C., Yerramsetti, S., Gard, T., et al. (2011). Mindfulness practice leads to increases in regional brain gray matter density. *Psychiatry Research, 191*, 36–43.

Howard, D., Gazmararian, J., & Parker, R. (2005). The impact of low health literacy on the medical costs of Medicare managed care enrollees. *The American Journal of Medicine, 118*, 371–377.

Hughes, R. (2003). *Resilience: Health in a new key*. Phoenix, AZ: St. Luke's Health Initiative.

Institute of Medicine (IOM). (2003). *Priority areas for national action: Transforming health care quality*. Washington, DC: National Academy Press.

Institute of Medicine (IOM). (2004a). *Committee on the crossing the quality chasm: Next steps toward a new health care system patient self-management support*. Washington, DC: National Academies Press.

Institute of Medicine (IOM). (2004b). *Health literacy: A prescription to end confusion*. Washington, DC: National Academy Press.

Jacobson, N., Dobson, K., Truax, P., Addis, M., Koerner, K., Gollan, J., et al. (1996). A component analysis of cognitive-behavioral treatment for depression. *Journal of Consulting and Clinical Psychology, 64*, 295–304.

Jacobson, N., Martell, C., & Dimidjian, S. (2001). Behavioral activation for depression: Returning to contextual roots. *Clinical Psychology: Science and Practice, 8*, 255–270.

Kabat-Zinn, J. (1990). *Full catastrophe living: Using the wisdom of your body and mind to face stress, pain and illness*. New York, NY: Delacorte.

Kabat-Zinn, J. (2003). Mindfulness-based interventions in context: Past, present, and future. *Clinical Psychology: Science and Practice, 10*, 144–156.

Karoly, P. (2010). Psychopathology as dysfunctional self-regulation. In J. Reich, A. Zautra, & J. Hall (Eds.), *Handbook of adult resilience* (pp. 146–170). New York, NY: Guilford Press.

Kauffman, D. (2000). The effects of a treatment mall on patients with dual diagnosis. *NADD Bulletin, 3*(2).

Kent, M., & Davis, M. C. (2014). Resilience training for action and agency to stress and trauma: Becoming the hero of your life. In M. Kent, M. C. Davis, & J. W. Reich (Eds.), *The resilience handbook: Approaches to stress and trauma/* (pp. 227–244). New York: Routledge.

Kent, M., Davis, M., & Reich, J. (2014). *The resilience handbook: Approaches to stress and trauma*. New York: Routledge.

Kent, M., Rivers, C. T., & Wrenn, G. (2015). Goal-Directed Resilience in Training (GRIT): A biopsychosocial model of self-regulation, executive functions, and personal growth (eudaimonia) in evocative contexts of PTSD, obesity, and chronic pain. *Behavioral Sciences, 5*, 1–38.

Kilman, P. R., Albert, B. M., & Sotile, W. M. (1975). Relationship between locus of control, structure of therapy, and outcomes. *Journal of Consulting and Clinical Psychology, 43*, 588.

Kirsch, I. S., Jungeblut, A., Jenkins, L., & Kolstad, A. (1993). *Adult literacy in America: A first look at the results of the national adult literacy survey (NALS)*. Washington, DC: National Center for Education Statistics, U.S. Department of Education.

Leucht, S., & Burkard, T. (2007). *Physical illness and schizophrenia: A review of the evidence*. New York: Cambridge University Press.

Lewinsohn, P. (1975). The behavioral study and treatment of depression. In M. Hersen, R. M., Eisler, & P. M. Miller (Eds.), *Progress in behavior modification* (Vol. 1, pp. 19–65). New York: Academic Press.

Lorig, K. (1999). *Chronic disease self-management leader's manual*. Palo Alto, CA: Stanford Patient Education Research Center.

Lorig, K. (2006). *Chronic disease self-management leader's manual*. Palo Alto, CA: Stanford Patient Education Research Center.

Lorig, K., Holman, H., Sobel, D., Laurent, D., González, V., & Minor, M. (1994). *Living a healthy life with chronic conditions*. Palo Alto, CA: Bull Publishing Company.

Lorig, K., Ritter, P., Stewart, A., Sobel, D., Brown, B, Jr., Bandura, A., et al. (2001). Chronic disease self-management program: 2-year health status and health care utilization outcomes. *Medical Care, 39*, 1217–1223.

Lorig, K., Sobel, D., Stewart, A., Brown, B, Jr., Bandura, A., Ritter, P., et al. (1999). Evidence suggesting that a chronic disease self-management program can improve health status while reducing hospitalization: A randomized trial. *Medical Care, 37*, 5–14.

Luthar, S., Cicinnati, D., & Becker, B. (2000). The construct of resilience: A critical evaluation and guidelines for future work. *Child Development, 71*, 534–562.

Manderscheid, R. (2014, April). From recovery to resilience via health activation. *Behavioral Healthcare*.

Masten, A. (2014). *Ordinary magic: Resilience in development*. New York: Guilford Press.

Masten, A., Best, K., & Garmezy, N. (1990). Resilience and development: Contributions from the study of children who overcome adversity. *Development and Psychopathology, 2*, 425–444.

Mazzucchelli, T. G., Kane, R. T., & Rees, C. S. (2010). Behavioral activation for well-being: A meta-analysis. *The Journal of Positive Psychology, 5*, 105–121.

Miller, W., & Rollnick, S. (2012). *Motivational interviewing* (3rd ed.). New York: Guilford Press.

Moemi, S., Kiyoto, E., Yoshiko, Y., Shin-Ichi, N., & Lieberman, R. (2013). Illness self-management for individuals in acute psychiatric care settings in Japan: Cross-cultural adaptation of an American program. *Psychiatric Rehabilitation Journal, 36*, 272–277.

Mosen, D., Schmittdiel, J., Hibbard, J., Sobel, D., Remmers, C., & Bellows, J. (2007). Is patient activation associated with outcomes of care for adults with chronic conditions? *Journal of Ambulatory Care Management, 30*, 21–29.

Mosolov, S., Potapov, A., & Ushakov, U. (2012). Remission in schizophrenia: Results of cross-sectional with 6-month follow-up period and 1-year observational therapeutic studies in an outpatient population. *Annals of General Psychiatry, 11*(1).

National Association of State Mental Health Program Directors Medical Directors Council. (2006). *Morbidity and mortality in people with serious mental people with serious mental illness*. Washington, DC: Author.

New Freedom Commission on Mental Health. (2003). *Achieving the promise: Transforming mental health care in America*. Rockville, MD: Department of Health and Human Services.

Nielsen-Bohlman, L., Panzer, A., & Kindig, D. (2004). *Health literacy: A prescription to end confusion*. Washington, DC: National Academy of Sciences.

Nutbeam, D. (2008). The evolving concept of health literacy. *Social Science Medicine, 67*, 2072–2078.

O'Connel, M. J., Tondora, J., Evans, A. C., Croog, G., & Davidson, L. (2005). From rhetoric to routine: Assessing recovery-oriented practices in a state mental health and addiction system. *Psychiaric Rehabilitation Journal, 28*(4): 378–386.

Osborne, H. (2004). *Health literacy from a to z: Practical ways to communicate your health message*. Sudbury, MA: Jones and Bartlett Publishers.

Palmer-Erbs, V., & Anthony, W. (1995). Incorporating psychiatric rehabilitation principles into mental health nursing: an opportunity to develop full partnership among nurses, consumers & families. *Journal of Psychosocial Nursing in Mental Health Services, 33* (3), 36–44.

Parekh, A. (2011). Winning their trust. *New England Journal of Medicine, 364*, e51.

Parks, J., Svendsen, D., Singer, P., & Foti, M. E. (2006). *Morbidity and mortality in people with serious mental*

*illness*. Washington, DC: National Association of State Mental Health Program Directors.
Peerson, A., & Saunders, M. (2009). Health literacy revisited: What do we mean and why does it matter? *Health Promotion International, 24*, 285–296.
Pignone, M., DeWalt, D., Sheridan, S., Berkman, N., & Lohr, K. (2005). Interventions to improve health outcomes for patients with low literacy. *Journal General Internal Medicine, 20*(2), 185–192.
Pollard, L., Gebhard, Y., Levy, G., & Gelkoph, M. (2008). Examining attitudes, beliefs and knowledge of effective practices in psychiatric rehabilitation in a hospital setting. *Psychiatric Rehabilitation Journal, 32*, 124–127.
Prochaska, J., & DiClemente, C. (1986). Toward a comprehensive model of change. In W. Miller & N. Heather (Eds.), *Treating addictive behaviors: Processes of change* (pp. 3–28). New York: Plenum Press.
Reich, J. (2015). *Mastering your self, mastering the world: Living by the serenity prayer*. Hants, UK: Psyche Books.
Reich, J., & Zautra, A. (1981). Life events and personal causation: Some relationships with satisfaction and distress. *Journal of Personality and Social Psychology, 41*, 1082–1112.
Reich, J., & Zautra, A. J. (1990). Dispositional control beliefs and the consequences of a control-enhancing intervention. *Journal of Gerontology: Psychological Sciences, 45*, 46–51.
Reich, J., & Zautra, A. (1995a). Spouse encouragement of self-reliance and other-reliance in rheumatoid arthritis patients. *Journal of Behavioral Medicine, 18*, 249–260.
Reich, J., & Zautra, A. (1995b). Other-reliance encouragement effects in female rheumatoid arthritis patients. *Journal of Social and Clinical Psychology, 14*, 119–133.
Reich, J., Zautra, A., & Hall, J. (2010). *Handbook of adult resilience*. New York: Guilford Press.
Rodin, J. (1986). Health, control, and aging. In M. Baltes & P. B. Baltes (Eds.), *The psychology of control and aging*. Hillsdale, NJ: Erlbaum.
Rodin, J., & Langer, E. (1977). Long-term effects of a control-relevant intervention with the institutionalized aged. *Journal of Personality and Social Psychology, 35*, 897–902.
Rollnick, S., Heather, N., & Bell, A. (1992). Negotiating behavior change in medical settings: The development of brief motivational interviewing. *Journal of Mental Health, 1*, 25–37.
Rollnick, S., Miller, W., & Butler, C. (2007). *Motivational interviewing in health care: Helping patients change behavior*. New York: Guilford Press.
Rothbaum, F., Weisz, J., & Snyder, S. (1984). Changing the world and changing the self: A two-process model of perceived control. *Journal of Personality and Social Psychology, 39*, 5–37.
Rotter, J. B. (1966). Generalized expectances for internal versus external locus of control. *Psychological Monographs, 80*(1), Whole No. 609.
Salyers, M., Matthias, M., Spann, C., Lydick, J., Rollins, A., & Frankel, R. (2009). The role of patient activation in psychiatric visits. *Psychiatric Services, 60*, 1535–1539.
Salyers, M., Teai, J., & Stutz, T. (2007). Measuring recovery orientation in a hospital setting. *Psychiatric Rehabilitation Journal, 31*(2), 131–137.
Saunders, T. (1906). *The maxims and reflections of Goethe*. New York: Macmillan.
Schillinger, D., Bindman, A., Wang, F., Stewart, A., & Piette, J. (2004). Functional health literacy and the quality of physician-patient communication among diabetes patients. *Patient Education and Counseling, 52*, 315–323.
Schneiderman, N., Ironson, G., & Siegel, S. (2005). Stress and health: Psychological, behavioral, and biological determinants. *Annual Review of Clinical Psychology, 1*, 607–628.
Schulz, R., & Hanusa, B. (1978). Long-term effects of control and predictability-enhancing interventions: Findings and ethical issues. *Journal of Personality and Social Psychology, 36*, 1194–1201.
Seubert, D. (2009). *Questions are the answer to improving health literacy and patient activation*. Madison, WI: Marshfield Clinic and Family Health Center of Marshfield Inc.
Shapiro, S., & Carlson, L. (2009). *The art and science of mindfulness: Integrating mindfulness into psychology and the helping professions*. Washington, DC: American Psychological Association.
Singh, N. N., Lancioni, G. E., Singh, A. N., Winton, A. S. W., Singh, J., McAleavey, K., et al. (2008). A mindfulness-based health wellness program for an adolescent with Prader-Willi syndrome. *Behavior Modification, 32*, 167–181.
Skodol, A. (2010) The resilient personality. In J. Reich, A., Zautra, & J. Hall (Eds.), *Handbook of adult resilience*. New York: Guilford Press.
Smith, S., Curtis, L., Wardle, J., von Wagner, C., & Wolf, M. (2013). Skill set or mind set? Associations between health literacy, patient activation and health. *PLoS ONE, 8*(9), e74373.
Spitzer, C., Barnow, S., Volzke, H., John, U., Freyberger, H., & Grabe, H. (2009). Trauma, posttraumatic stress disorder, and physical illness: Findings from the general population. *Psychosomatic Medicine, 71*, 1012–1017.
Sterling, P. (2004). Principles of allostasis. In J. Schulkin (Ed.), *Allostasis, homeostasis, and the costs of physiological adaptation*. New York, NY: Cambridge University Press.
Sterling, P., & Eyer, J. (1988). Allostasis: A new paradigm to explain arousal pathology. In S. Fisher & J. T. Reason (Eds.), *Handbook of life stress, cognition, and health*. New York: Wiley.
Substance Abuse and Mental Health Services Administration. (2002). *WHAM*. Rockville, MD: Author.
Substance Abuse and Mental Health Services Administration. (2010). *SAMHSA's working definition of recovery*. Rockville, MD: Author.

Substance Abuse and Mental Health Services Administration. (2014a). *Trauma informed care in behavioral health services*. Tip 57. Rockville, MD: Author.

Substance Abuse and Mental Health Services Administration. (2014b). *Eight dimensions of Wellness*. Rockville, MD: Author.

Swarbrick, M. (2006). A wellness approach. *Psychiatric Rehabilitation Journal, 29*(4), 311–314.

Vijayalakshmy, P., Smith, R., & Schefler, R. (2006). Facilitating discharge in the state psychiatric institutions: A group intervention strategy. *Psychiatric Rehabilitation Journal, 29*(3), 183–188.

Von Korff, M., Gruman, J., Schaefer, J., Curry, S. J., & Wagner, E. H. (1997). Collaborative management of chronic illness. *Annals of Internal Medicine, 127*, 1097–1102.

Wagner, E. (1998). Chronic disease management: What will it take to improve care for chronic illness? *Effective Clinical Practice, 1*, 2–4.

Webster, S., Harmon, S., & Paesler, B. (2005). Building a treatment mall: A first step in moving a state hospital to a culture of rehabilitation and recovery. *The Behavior Therapist, 28*(4), 71–77.

Williams, S., & Heller, A. (2007). Patient activation among Medicare beneficiaries: Segmentation to promote informed decision-making. *International Journal of Pharmacy and Healthcare Marketing, 1*(3), 199–213.

Wingfield, J. C. (2003). Control of behavioral strategies in capricious environments. *Animal Behavior, 66*(5), 807–816.

World Health Organization (WHO). (2005). *Preventing chronic diseases: A vital investment. WHO global report*. Geneva, Switzerland: WHO Press.

World Health Organizations (WHO). (1948, April). Preamble to the Constitution of the World Health Organization as adopted by the International Health Conference, New York.

Wright-Berryman, J., Salyers, M., O'Halloran, J., Kemp, A., Mueser, K., & Diazoni, A. (2013). Consumer and provider response to computerized version of the illness management and recovery program. *Psychiatric Rehabilitation Journal, 36*(4), 231–235.

Zautra, A. (2009). Resilience: One part recovery, two parts sustainability. *Journal of Personality, 77*(6), 935–1943.

Zautra, A., Arewasikporn, A., & Davis, M. (2010a). Resilience: Promoting well-being through recovery, sustainability, and growth. *Research in Human Development, 7*(3), 221–238.

Zautra, A., & Franczak, M. (2014). *Recovery is one milestone but not the only goal: A resilience paradigm for physical and behavioral health.* Paper presented at the Exploring Resiliency Conference. ASU Center for Applied Behavioral Health Policy, Phoenix, AZ.

Zautra, A., Hall, J., & Murray, K. (2010b) A new definition of health for people and communities. In J. Reich, A., Zautra, & J. Hall (Eds.), *Handbook of adult resilience*. New York: Guilford Press.

Zautra, A., Infurna, F., Zautra, E., Gallardo, C., & Velasco, L. (2015a). The humanization of social relations: Nourishment for resilience in did-life. In A. Ong, E. Corinna, & C. E. Löckenhoff (Eds.), *New developments in emotional aging*. Washington, DC: American Psychological Association.

Zautra, E. K., Zautra, A. J., Gallardo, E. C., & Velasco, L. (2015b). Can we learn to treat one another better? A test of a social intelligence curriculum. *PLoS ONE, 10* (6), e0128638.

# 18 Change and Systems Transformation

Scott Van Sant, Jack W. Barber and Nirbhay N. Singh

## Introduction

Great inroads into implementation of recovery-oriented practice have been made in many behavioral health systems. There are also many barriers to implementation as well as gaps in our knowledge about outcomes. Whether the impetus for this has been concern over evidence-based practice, civil rights, regulatory initiatives, and/or funding, this approach to provision of behavioral health services is becoming the standard. After all, it is difficult to argue with the goals of connectedness, hope, identity, meaning, self-determination, and empowerment. The premise is that all persons should have the opportunity to have productive, meaningful, and responsible lives in the community.

The focus has been on inpatient care, which by definition involves treatment for persons who are the most ill and most vulnerable. Often this care is involuntary and therefore presumably not compatible with "recovery". Hopefully, it is clear that regardless of the nature of the setting, the philosophy of recovery has to be the foundation for the involved person's interaction with the behavioral health system (Davidson et al. 2016). If the caregivers do not believe that people in their care can improve their lives and functioning, then there is no hope.

In this context, it is important to distinguish recovery from "recovery-oriented care" in that recovery is an unassailable and personal process that an individual goes through, and recovery-oriented care relates to the roles and responsibilities of behavioral health systems in providing care for persons with psychiatric disabilities (Davidson et al. 2006). Sowers (2005) compared system transformation to a process that is parallel to an individual's recovery, and correctly stated that it was a challenging process that requires, "… vigilance, dedication, skill, patience, humility, and a great deal of hard work." Sowers also stipulated that the organization has to be open to receiving help, specifically from persons in recovery as partners. The shift to this type of care requires that treatment goals identify and build upon an individual's assets, strengths, and areas of health and competence. In addition, the purpose is to support the person in managing his or her condition while regaining a meaningful and constructive life, and sense of membership in the broader community (Davidson et al. 2006).

S. Van Sant (✉) · N.N. Singh
Department of Psychiatry and Health Behavior, Medical College of Georgia, Augusta University, 997 St. Sebastian Way, Augusta, GA, USA
e-mail: svansant@gru.edu

J.W. Barber
Virginia Department of Behavioral Health and Developmental Services, Richmond, VA, USA



N.N. Singh et al. (eds.), *Handbook of Recovery in Inpatient Psychiatry*,
Evidence-Based Practices in Behavioral Health, DOI 10.1007/978-3-319-40537-7_18

## Impetus Behind Recovery Transformation

The President's New Freedom Commission on Mental Health (2003) stated that, "Recovery is possible for everyone with serious emotional disturbances to … live, work, learn, and participate fully in their communities," but that unfortunately for many supports and services to make this possible "remain fragmented, disconnected, and often inadequate." Unfortunately, the report concluded that the mental health system in the United States was not oriented to the most important outcome for the people it serves, which is the hope of recovery. It was determined that available evidenced-based care was not penetrating into the community and many people did not have access to quality individualized care, therefore reducing the opportunity they had for obtaining recovery.

It also stated that successful transformation within the mental health system required two principles. First, that care provision must be centered on real and meaningful choices for service-users, and not requirements of bureaucracies. Second, that care must increase coping abilities, facilitate recovery, and foster resilience, not just manage symptoms. In addition, service-users will contribute to the development of a recovery-oriented system by participating in planning, evaluation, research, training, and service delivery.

To aid in transforming the mental health system, the President's New Freedom Commission on Mental Health (2003) made the following recommendations: (a) Develop an individualized plan of care for every adult with a serious mental illness and child with a serious emotional disturbance; (b) Involve service-users and families fully in orienting the mental health system toward recovery; (c) Align relevant Federal programs to improve access and accountability for mental health services; (d) Create a Comprehensive State Mental Health Plan, and (d) Protect and enhance the rights of people with mental illnesses.

The *Institute of Medicine Committee on Crossing the Quality Chasm, Adaption to Mental Health and Addictive Disorders* (Institute of Medicine [IOM] 2006) also included statements that people with mental illness can recover as defined above even though the illness itself may not be cured. Unfortunately, they outlined the discrepancy between what research supports as evidenced-based care and what actually occurs, which has serious consequences for treated individuals, their families, and our society. They referenced studies that indicated only 27 % adherence with established practice guidelines for the most common disorders. They listed some of the primary barriers to the provision of quality care as follows: departures from known standards of care, variations in care in the absence of standards, failure to treat severe mental and addictive diseases, and lack of coordination among systems of care.

The IOM (2006) stipulated that service-users must be involved in decision-making, not just in individual care decisions, but in the development of systems of care. They outlined several concrete steps to reduce stigma by placing supported decision-making in policy and practices, involving service-users in service design, administration, and delivery, and supporting illness self-management programs. They stated that this should be embedded into the culture of an organization. Organizational leaders should demonstrate support of service-user decision-making in their interactions with employees; that the individual's right to make treatment decisions should be the default policy of the organization unless there is apparent danger; and this should permeate policy and procedure documents, mission statements of the organization itself.

Finally, though not necessarily in regulation, recovery-oriented care has permeated the philosophies of government regulatory bodies in the United States, such as the Centers for Medicare and Medicaid Services in the United States (Smith 2007) and governmental mental health strategic plans in many other western countries, including but not limited to Canada (Kirby and Keon 2006; Mental Health Commission of Canada 2009, 2012), England (HM Government 2009, 2011), New Zealand (Mental Health Commission 1998, 2012), and Australia

(Australian Health Ministers 2009) in relation to oversight of behavioral health systems of care. On review of these different strategic initiatives, there are multiple permutations of definition, focus, and level of incorporation of recovery concepts (Slade et al. 2012). There are cultural differences that can affect the development of these concepts such as the staunch American insistence on individualism versus other cultures' more collectivist view, structures of existing publicly funded healthcare entities, extent of nongovernmental advocacy organizations, and historical paths regarding civil rights (Amering et al. 2012; Bradstreet and McBrierty 2012; O'Hagan et al. 2012; Oades and Anderson 2012; Ostrow and Adams 2012; Piat and Sabetti 2012).

In some countries, such as Australia and New Zealand, the focus is shifting where recovery is being subsumed under positive psychology or general well-being (O'Hagan et al. 2012; Oades and Anderson 2012). This is carried even further with the melding in New Zealand with the Maori worldview of health and well-being, including an emphasis on extended family, as well as spiritual, physical, and psychological health (O'Hagan et al. 2012; Turia 2010). In the years since the governmental adoption of recovery-oriented mental health care, there have many political and economic upheavals that have changed direction of government sponsored health-care initiatives. One common theme that can be seen in these efforts is that, actual uptake of recovery-oriented concepts at the level where professionals are interacting with service-users can often miss the mark (O'Hagan et al. 2012; Oades and Anderson 2012; Piat and Sabetti 2012), or as stated by Oades and Anderson (2012) in discussing the relatively successful transformation in Australia: "There are significant limitations of the capacity of strategic initiatives to shape ground-level uptake of desired workplace practice. When values are espoused at the organizational level, or more broadly at the policy level, the risk is that these become distant, generic statements that are imposed on services and their staff. Value statements are unlikely to be experienced as meaningful in terms of translating the recovery vision into practice, or in answering the question how do we, as staff members, approach our work with individuals if we are to promote their recovery journey?"

## Change Management

There are many ways of transforming organizations. For example, Kotter (2007) presented several common major errors associated with organizational change in business organizations, but these errors are salient to behavioral healthcare systems as well (see Table 18.1). We discuss these errors in the context of implementing recovery-oriented care in behavioral healthcare systems.

### Urgency

Although there is clear service-user, advocacy, and governmental support behind the recovery movement, the issue is how to motivate leaders, managers, and frontline staff in behavioral healthcare organizations, including state and private inpatient psychiatric entities. All players within the organization must be on board with the

**Table 18.1** Eight errors in organizational transformation

| |
|---|
| 1. Not establishing a great enough sense of urgency |
| 2. Not creating a powerful enough guiding coalition |
| 3. Lacking a vision |
| 4. Under-communicating the vision by a factor of ten |
| 5. Not removing obstacles to the new vision |
| 6. Not systematically planning for, and creating, short-term wins |
| 7. Declaring victory too soon |
| 8. Not anchoring changes in the organization's culture |

Adapted from Kotter (2007)

change, and will have to give up the often-comfortable status quo. So, how is this going to make things better for them and the people who receive services from the organization? Kotter (2007) stipulated that change requires leadership, and that the leaders must make the "status quo seem more dangerous than launching into the unknown." Commensurate with our own experience in system change projects, new leadership is often required to accomplish this.

## Guiding Coalition

In addition to the leadership, managers, and clinical staff of a healthcare organization, service-users must be involved throughout the development of recovery-oriented systems from planning, evaluation, research, and training to service delivery (IOM 2006; US Department of Health and Human Services 2012). This core coalition has to provide the organization with the momentum and energy to see the transformation process through to completion. If not, either those who oppose change, or the entropy inherent to organizations, will overcome this effort (Kotter 2007). Opposition to change may be active or passive-aggressive, with those opposed to the change indulging in the blame game and fault finding with the change agents.

Consumer choice should be incorporated in all types of planning processes including, but not limited to treatment, service, transition, and development of recovery plans. The documents and processes should emphasize the identification and use of a person's strengths to design a plan to overcome their difficulties. Finally, systems of care should promote holistic approaches to health maintenance and recovery development that recognize the impact and interaction of cooccurring illnesses and the need to address them concurrently. Principles of recovery can be applied to diverse processes that disrupt mental health and can provide a common thread by which the return to mental health may be orchestrated. Respect for service-user participation, and efforts to obtain meaningful input from them, are hallmarks of recovery-oriented environments. This input should be solicited even when service-users are most debilitated and opportunities to make choices should be provided whenever possible (Sowers 2005).

## Mission/Vision

The guiding coalition must create a vision of the final product that is understandable and easy to convey. It must appeal to service-users, other stakeholders, and organizational staff. Without this vision, the transformation process can devolve into competing and incompatible initiatives (Kotter 2007).

Farkas et al. (2005) outlined the critical dimensions in establishing recovery-oriented, evidenced-based programs, with the hope of bridging the gap between traditional evidence-based practice and the vision of recovery. In addition to the overall picture of administration, they gave detailed requirements for structures such as mission statements, policies, procedures, record keeping, quality assurance, and employee selection, training and supervision. They stated that a values-based approach is applicable to all behavioral healthcare settings, and that this can significantly alter a person's individual experience within the program during his or her personal process of recovery.

The values Farkas et al. (2005) felt were key to supporting the recovery process included person-orientation, person-involvement, self-determination, and growth potential. To be person-oriented, a program must focus upon the individual rather than "the case", encouraging the person's strengths, talents, interests, and recognizing limitations. For persons to be involved, the program must acknowledge the right to full partnership in designing, planning, implementing, and evaluating the service. The program must recognize the person's right to make decisions about all aspects of their goals, outcomes, services utilized to achieve these outcomes, and when they will be engaged in services. Finally, the program must accept the capacity of individuals to recover no matter the state of disability they are in, i.e., in crisis in a hospital.

Promoting citizenship requires supporting individuals with mental illness to fully reintegrate into society as equal citizens. Contained within this domain are concepts such as viewing people as individuals who are not defined by their diagnosis or associated treatments. Also, this involves respecting and actually advocating for individuals' human rights, inclusion in community life, and support of meaningful and purposeful lives and occupations (Le Boutillier et al. 2011).

## Teaching by Example

Simply adding the phrase "Recovery is possible for everyone" to the letterhead of the organization will not accomplish this significant and difficult transformation. The leadership must actually believe in this transformation and let this conviction permeate their every action within the organization. If their actions, including policies, procedures, and practice within the organization are not consistent with the message they are conveying, the result will fuel organizational nihilism at every level (Kotter 2007). Person-centered, recovery-oriented care is focused on helping individuals build meaningful lives, not on the bureaucratic goals of a clinical organization. This requires a paradigm shift where care recipients are equal partners with care providers (Slade et al. 2014).

These values must permeate the structural components within the organization to provide a framework for recovery efforts. A system of care adapts to the needs of people instead of what services are available, including mission/vision, quality improvement programs, open access to services, and workforce planning (Farkas et al. 2005; Le Boutillier et al. 2011). The mission identifies intended recovery-based outcomes in behavioral terms, such as regaining employment, community membership, success, satisfaction, empowerment, well-being, self-esteem, and finally mitigating symptoms that interfere with these goals. Policies reflect respect for individuals using the service that espouses person-orientation, self-determination, and the potential for individual growth. Procedures ensure that these policies are implemented in a meaningful way and give detailed instructions to staff who provide services within the organization (Farkas et al. 2005). Organizational commitment requires creating a work environment and service structure that are conducive to promoting recovery-oriented practice. Practitioners must support individuals to personally define their recovery. This is the core of the organization and not an "add-on" to existing services. Individuals define their own goals, dreams, and plans to shape the care provided to them, not the other way around. This incorporates inclusion and respect for individuality, informed choice, peer support, strength-driven planning, and holistic care (Franczak and Dye 2016; Le Boutillier et al. 2011; Singh et al. 2016).

An aspect that is often ignored in healthcare organizations during the process of developing recovery-oriented programs is record keeping. Are the records designed and maintained in a matter that makes them easily accessible to the person receiving the services? Do they reflect the person's strengths, talents, and interests, as well as his difficulties? To take this even further, is the person able to comment in writing on the contents of a record? Furthermore, the physical environment where services are provided gives significant cues to those engaging in services. Of course, in hospital settings, there are many regulatory and safety concerns that have to be met, but service-users can give input into decoration, design, and physical plant resources in order to provide a welcoming and supportive environment (Farkas et al. 2005).

Within the organization, the employee training programs should ensure there is sufficient understanding of recovery concepts and of service-users perspectives and aspirations (Mabe et al. 2016). Professionals within the organization must have adequate exposure to service-users in nonclinical settings and exposure to recovery models, and the organization's training standards and competency requirements should reflect these values (Sowers 2005).

## Elimination of Obstacles

Assuming there is adequate leadership, vision, and communication, the process can still fail if obstacles to change are not removed, whether they are imagined or real (Kotter 2007). Are there policies and procedures that remain in place that contradict the effort? Has the organization retained old processes that interfere with the recovery philosophy? Does the organization have the resources to implement this potentially labor-intensive effort? Are there still managers, or influential frontline employees, in place who do not support the effort?

The people working within the organization must deliver service in a manner consistent with these values. Healthcare employees can be significant facilitators or, unfortunately, barriers to an individual's recovery. It is critical that employees have the basic knowledge, skills, and attitudes to promote recovery. Ideally, employee candidates who have personal experiences with their own recovery and/or mental health issues should be sought and included in organizational development (Franczak and Dye 2016). Furthermore, in keeping with person participation, service-users should be involved with selection criteria, interviewing, and the hiring process. Finally, ongoing staff development and supervision must encourage recovery-oriented knowledge, attitudes, and skills, including meaningful opportunities to meet individuals in recovery (Farkas et al. 2005). Finally, a working relationship entails a sincere belief on the part of service providers that individuals, and their families, can reach their potential and shape their own future. A working relationship supports recovery with genuine partnership and instills hope (Le Boutillier et al. 2011).

With specific regard to inpatient care, it is a mistake to assume that recovery concepts cannot be applied for the population receiving services (Davidson et al. 2016). Though much of the literature focuses on persons with schizophrenia and other psychoses, many pro-recovery interventions have been examined for a wide variety of other populations in acute crisis. Also, although treatment leading to amelioration of symptoms is important, this approach addresses only one aspect of a person's individual journey. The treatment we provide can unfortunately become a barrier to self-determination and community integration. In order for mental health systems to support individuals in their personal journeys, we will have to move away from care dominated by institutions, drug therapies, and coercion. Another paradigm shift is discarding the idea that the goal of treatment is to make people "normal", rather than helping include them as equal members of our society. This means creating inclusive communities where everyone is accommodated, and not imposing artificial societal restrictions on how people live (e.g., discharge to the community is predicated on day program attendance as the available "group home" requires this) (Slade et al. 2014).

One shift that may have to occur for members on the treatment team in the hospital is evaluating success for individuals on valued social roles such as residential stability, employment, and relationships, rather than the traditional view of symptom reduction and relapse rates. The traditional treatments we provide are just one component of how we can help individuals on their life's journey. In this conceptualization, our clinical focus on diagnosis, symptoms, and deficits actually can further stigmatize people instead of supporting them in their strengths, and aspirations that most people desire: stable housing, employment, and meaningful relationships (Bashor et al. 2016). This underlies the belief that people with mental illness are fundamentally similar to everyone, not patients who need treatment before they can get on with their lives. Examples of this dichotomy include, "housing first, no preconditions versus supported-housing" or "individual community job placement with appropriate supports versus sheltered workshops". This means supporting people's access to potential relationships where they can learn relationship building skills, both the positive aspects and the associated pitfalls, rather than focusing on social-skills training classes. In this view, "people with mental illness don't need treatment—they need a life. Treatment may contribute to the process of striving for a life worth living, but it is a means, not an end" (Slade 2012).

## Short-Term Successes

This transformation will take time, months to years, not days or weeks. It is human nature to seek feedback on efforts and few are able to delay this gratification in the interest of long-term outcomes. If the energy behind the effort is not maintained, many in the organization will lose interest and may even join the naysayers in sabotaging the initiative. In designing the transformation effort, the change leaders must establish periodic, obtainable, short-term goals. These accomplishments must be communicated to everyone involved in the effort, and rewards given that are realistic within the organization (Kotter 2007).

Similar findings were found in a study on successful implementation of translational research and evidence-based care in healthcare settings (Stetler 2003). For example, in this study, it was noted that this effort must be "institutionalized" so that it becomes part of both the organizations and employees' "way of doing business." The core components of a health system, including leadership, feedback systems, resources, capacities, competencies, and culture must be assessed for congruency of the goal, i.e., evidenced-based care or, in this case, recovery-oriented care. That is, the leadership of the organization must reinforce the culture of recovery or efforts will fail if their actions are incongruent with the messages being conveyed. In addition, employees must be provided with the tools and supports to deliver this type of care (Stetler 2003).

## Consolidation and Reinvigoration

It can be a mistake to declare victory too early in the battle. Successes should be celebrated, but the reality is that an actual cultural change usually takes years. The new organizational structure can be fragile during this time, and can slide back into the "old ways" of doing things. Sowers (2005) outlined elements with associated measurable indicators that would help ensure the quality of recovery-oriented transformation efforts. In these measures, Sowers stipulated that the organizational budget must allow for adequate resources to support service-user participation in administrative processes governing the organization and to create employment opportunities within the organization. Service-users and family members should be enlisted to participate in the decisions regarding resource allocation and service development. There also should be significant representation of persons in recovery on organization's treatment and support staff. In addition, persons in recovery should be involved in quality improvement efforts as equal partners and they should receive adequate compensation for the services they provide, just as the professional participants do. This recognizes the value of collaboration in establishing stable recovery environments. Stakeholders, including service-users, must be involved during the planning, development, and implementation of quality assurance programs. For example, outcomes that could be selected by service-users would be their personal goal attainment or satisfaction with services and processes (Farkas et al. 2005).

## Solidifying the New Culture

Once the recovery transformation is successfully completed, these processes must continue as the new "norm" instead of succumbing to degradation once the initial pressures for the change stop. Those involved must be shown how this change has improved the functioning within the organization and how their contributions made this possible. Moreover, new managers and leaders who join the organization must believe in recovery-oriented processes.

With the advent of recovery-oriented services across a broad spectrum of behavioral healthcare systems in North America, Europe, Australasia, and some parts of Asia, it has been noted that often agencies incorporate appropriate catch phrases in their organizational documents, such as mission statements and policies, but often fall short of actually changing practices. The Recovery Self-Assessment (RSA) was developed to evaluate the degree to which organizations have implemented recovery-oriented care and it has components tailored for various stake holders, including administrative directors, providers, persons in recovery, and significant others (O'Connell et al. 2005). They identified principles common to recovery and practices associated with these principles. From this, five factors were identified including: Life Goals, Involvement, Diversity of Treatment Options, Choice, and Individually Tailored Services. *Life Goals* looks at the extent to which the organization helps persons develop and pursue individually defined goals, such as employment and education. *Involvement* examines the extent to which persons in recovery participated in the development and provision of programs/services, staff training, and advisory board/management meetings. *Diversity of Treatment Options* indicates the extent to which an agency provides linkages to peer mentors and support, a variety of treatment options, and assistance with becoming involved in nonmental health activities. *Choice* looks at the extent to which service recipients have access to their treatment records, staff refrain from using coercive measures to influence choice, and decisions of service recipients are respected by staff. And finally, *Individually Tailored Services reflect* the extent to which services are tailored to individual needs, cultures, interest, and the building of community connections. There are other assessment tools, and it is important to determine whether the one chosen is valid regarding the service structure, population demographics, and cultural context (Williams et al. 2012). In the final analysis, the organization is responsible for formally evaluating its implementation efforts to ensure adequate penetrance of the desired concepts and outcomes.

## Examples Systems Transformation Efforts

There are a large number of system transformation efforts documented in the literature on recovery and recovery-oriented services. Familiarity with this literature will provide organizations that intend to implement recovery-oriented services with the strengths and limitations of various approaches to systems change. While a comprehensive review is beyond the scope of this chapter, we present a few selected examples.

### Connecticut

Davidson et al. (2007) reviewed a successful recovery-oriented transformation within the behavioral health system for the state of Connecticut that began in 2000. They saw this change as a shift from the medical model to a disability/civil rights model. Instead of focusing on "compliance", people with serious mental illness were encouraged to pursue their hopes and dreams. This entailed a shift from providers providing treatment and rehabilitation, to the system supporting people in their own efforts in overcoming their illness and in rebuilding their lives.

As part of this process, people with psychiatric disabilities described what recovery would look like for them, then they derived what practices and supports would be needed to promote this conceptualization of recovery, and finally how programs and systems needed to be structured and managed to provide this care. They determined that recovery-oriented systems must be included at all levels of care and there is no "wrong door" for accessing the system. In this initiative, they solicited input from people who were in recovery for developing the core values and then incorporated these values into the policy framework. There were several key themes in the core values they developed with service-users. People receiving services must have a say in the types of services that are provided and their choices respected, which includes involvement in boards, committees, and other decision-making bodies. In this system, service-users defined their goals and their choices were respected. They then focused on building workforce competencies and skills that were recovery-oriented, culturally diverse, and relevant. They also realigned their fiscal and administrative policies to recovery-oriented principles to support these programs. And finally, as with any successful change effort they established a formative evaluation system to monitor the status of the transformation and made adjustments, as needed. From these new systems, they were able to develop instruments for measuring recovery-oriented care, environments, and provider competencies. These instruments were then used in the next phase of monitoring, adjustment, and fine-tuning.

Of course, there were challenges associated with this effort and they shared several lessons. One mistake that could be extrapolated from their experience is to view inpatient hospitalizations as discrete episodes of illness rather than from the longitudinal perspective where people will require different levels of care at different times in their illness. Sometimes they will require more intense interventions such as hospitalization, and at times not. There has to be communication and fluidity among different services rather than the fragmented care that sometimes occurs. For persons that require periodic hospitalization, appropriate respectful relationships can mitigate some of the barriers to recovery-oriented care in times of crisis. This also encourages reliance on community-based resources, even outside the mental health system, hopefully encouraging normalization and reducing the impact of peoples' illness on their lives (Davidson et al. 2007).

People with mental illness fluctuate between the different stages of recovery during periods of their illness. Also, due to the heterogeneity of serious mental illness, people will progress at differing rates and accomplish varying degrees of recovery. Though the severity of a person's illness during hospitalization may preclude some basic tenets of shared decision-making temporarily, many will move past this and return to healthier functioning in the community (Duncan et al. 2016). The care provided during the inpatient episode should be seen as a part of a continuum, not an insulated microcosm, and recovery principles must infuse interventions at this time and be carried forward (Davidson et al. 2006; Liberman 2008). As Davidson et al. (2006) stated, "In terms of acute episodes, recovery doesn't start after the episode resolves, nor can it be put on hold while the person is receiving treatment. From the person's perspective, it is rather that the acute episode has temporarily disrupted his or her ongoing process of recovery (or it may be an anticipated part of the process), and care received during this period can more or less promote or undermine that process."

## Implementing Recovery Through Organizational Change (ImROC)

This transformation effort began in 2008, and was designed to manualize recovery-oriented systems change efforts in England, which can be reviewed in a series of detailed position papers published by the Sainsbury Centre for Mental Health and Mental Health Network of the National Health Service Confederation (Sainsbury Centre 2009). In these documents, the concept of recovery is developed further with an emphasis on "personalization" and shifting the power differential from clinician-driven services and treatments, to service-user choice in building/rebuilding their own lives. This effort began with a large body of stakeholders who were invested in recovery initiatives, but did not have an overall consistent model for development of a comprehensive recovery-oriented system of care. They developed a list of what they saw as the top ten organizational challenges associated with recovery-oriented system transformations (see Table 18.2). This was visualized as an immediate framework for systems change that could be used by all stakeholders, including the National Health Service, local private and government bureaucracies and administrations, services users, and carers.

One goal of this methodology was for stakeholders in individual localities to develop what

**Table 18.2** 11 key organizational challenges

| |
|---|
| 1. Changing the nature of day-to-day interactions and the quality of experience |
| 2. Delivering comprehensive, user-led education and training programs |
| 3. Establishing a Recovery Education Unit to drive the programs forward |
| 4. Ensuring organizational commitment, creating the culture |
| 5. The importance of leadership |
| 6. Increasing personalization and choice |
| 7. Changing the way we approach risk assessment and management |
| 8. Redefining user involvement |
| 9. Transforming the workforce |
| 10. Supporting staff in their recovery journey |
| 11. Increasing opportunities for building a life beyond illness |

Adapted from Sainsbury Centre (2009)

recovery-oriented services meant for that specific area, or the vision, before moving on to strategies for change, targets, and measurement. In establishing priorities for change efforts, they felt it was important for the organization to first assess what stage of change it was in, specifically termed "engagement", "development", or "transformation", ranging from the initial presence of philosophical support for efforts, to actual transformation of policies, processes, and practices imbedded at every level. Following this assessment, the organization would need to prioritize challenges salient to the organization, with the idea that conquering all 10 at one time would be unrealistic (Sheperd et al. 2009). There were several subsequent briefings included in this effort that cover details of various aspects of recovery implementation at the organizational level, which are briefly described below.

*Recovery Colleges* described innovative recovery education centers that have been piloted, which shift from the deficit-driven treatment model of day programs to a strengths-driven educational model. This is an attempt to "move beyond the narrow focus on symptom reduction to helping people to rebuild lives that they find satisfying, meaningful and valued" (Perkins et al. 2012).

*Recovery, Personalization and Personal Budgets* described the initiative to personalize public funding for persons receiving care, relying on the lived experience of individuals rather than the traditional clinician-driven assignment of treatment options (Alakeson and Perkins 2012). The goal of this effort was to give persons more control over the resources so they had more choice and freedom to pursue their own ambitions and aspirations as full citizens (see Table 18.3 for steps involved in developing a personal budget).

*Recovery, Public Mental-Health, and Well-being* introduced the concept of Health and Well-being Boards, which organize funding projects for community well-being, elements of which often fall outside the traditional clinical focus on healthcare resources (Boardman and Friedli 2012). This would include social resources, such as education, transportation, housing, employment, and leisure activities. Recovery is seen as an element of this, but the goal is to work beyond the traditional boundaries of behavioral health systems, providing opportunity for full citizenship and a "life beyond services." The hope is to address social inequalities, violence, racism, stigma, and exclusion, all of which affect both physical and mental health adversely. The eventual change that is hoped for is where professional services are available, but are in the background, and conditions are created where public attitude is improved, barriers are reduced, and healthy connections are supported.

*Recovery: A Carer's Perspective* is in reference to persons who provide unpaid supports to family members or friends who would have difficulty managing without this help (Machin and

**Table 18.3** Seven step personal budget process

| |
|---|
| 1. The first step is for individuals to complete an assessment or self-assessment questionnaire that identifies areas where they need support |
| 2. The assessment generates a score that is linked to a resource allocation system (RAS) to produce a personal budget amount. The RAS ensures that resources are allocated in a fair and transparent way to individuals according to need |
| 3. The personal budget amount provides the starting point for developing a recovery support plan, which identifies the goals a person has for his or her recovery and how those goals could be met. People can plan by themselves, with the support of friends and family, with peer support or with a professional broker. There is no set menu for support, allowing people and their supporters to develop highly personal, creative solutions |
| 4. The support plan is approved on the basis of being financially and clinically appropriate. Since there is no fixed menu, approval should focus on the likelihood that the support plan will contribute to a person's recovery |
| 5. Individuals can exercise as much or as little direct control over the money in their personal budget as they choose. They can receive it as a direct payment which they manage, they can use a third party to manage the money on their behalf or it can be held by a provider or commissioner |
| 6. With decisions about the money made, the services and supports in the plan can be put in place, either by the person themselves or by the organization that holds the budget in collaboration with them |
| 7. A person's support plan is reviewed on a regular basis and its effectiveness is judged on the basis of whether the goals identified in the plan are being met and the person is progressing in their recovery. If a person's needs change significantly, they will complete a new self-assessment and will be allocated a new personal budget amount |

Adapted from Alakeson and Perkins (2012)

Repper 2013). The guide provides direction on accessing supports available in England, including tackling stigma and discrimination, understanding the personal impact of this role, family interventions when needed, carer peer support, and education around carer issues

*Peer Support Workers: Theory and Practice* and *Peer Support Workers: A Practical Guide to Implementation* outline both the philosophical basis and practical steps required for peer support in mental healthcare organizations (Repper 2013a, b). In the first document, Repper (2013b) discussed the replacement of marginalization and exclusion through the companionship, empathy, and empowerment that peers can provide. This includes the different forms and roles of peer support, from informal relationships to government-supported staff positions in healthcare organizations. The core principles of peer support relationships include: mutual sharing of experiences; reciprocity (not expert/patient); being nondirective; recovery focused on inspiring hope, taking back control of individual challenges, and having access to opportunities the person values; strengths-based care planning; inclusion; progressive (in the shared journey of discovery); and negotiation of mutual emotional safety (Repper 2013b). In the second document, Repper (2013a) discussed the practical steps involved in incorporating peer support workers in the organization, including preparation (e.g., peer workers, existing employees, definition of roles, job descriptions), recruitment (e.g., advertisement, benefits, applications, interviews, human-resource issues), employment (e.g., selection, orientation, supervision, maintenance of well-being), and ongoing staff development (e.g., career coaching, training, and wider systems change).

The *Team Recovery Implementation Plan*: *A Framework for Creating Recovery-Focused Services* outlined a process where recovery ideas are embedded into the functioning and practice of care teams (care providers and recipients) utilizing the skills and resources of everyone involved (Repper 2013c). This process has four key elements, including an overview of the resources available, benchmarking of progress in implementing recovery-focused practice, prioritization of action items, and a method for systematic review and resetting of goals. This is seen as a ground-level effort, rather than a set of organizational top-down prescriptions. This allows staff and care recipients to identify progress, understand each other's perspectives and limitations, problem solve, develop solutions, and share responsibility for implementation of action plans.

*Risk Safety and Recovery* argued for a more collaborative approach while conducting risk assessments in the individual's context and the development of person-centered safety plans (Boardman and Roberts 2014). It also helps clarify the differences and tensions between positive risk-taking (as a basis for developing confidence, skills, and competence), dramatic risk (e.g., self-harm, suicide, violence, homicide), and safety promotion in general. This contrasts with the traditional risk assessment process that is driven by professionals utilizing population-based risk assessments, which then subsequently defaults to restrictive interventions.

*Making Recovery a Reality in Forensic Settings* addressed the inherent barriers to recovery-oriented care for individuals who have offended and are involved in the forensic system (Drennan and Wooldridge 2014). They provided guidance on implementing these concepts in a meaningful fashion while addressing prevalent challenges. They also described current best practices and hopeful progression of the criminal justice system, in general.

Finally, *Supporting Recovery in Mental Health Services*: *Quality and Outcomes* summarized their efforts to develop and/or implement existing quality measures to help organizations determine if they have fully realized recovery-oriented concepts (Sheperd et al. 2014). This was in the context of funding initiatives of the National Heath Service in England, in addition to other financial and political pressures, but of course many of the pressures are generalizable at least in the Western world. Difficulties mentioned included the cultural specificity of many of the measures that were available, i.e., tools may have been developed in the United States and were not validated for use in England. In addition, there is the over riding concern of taking recovery away from the people who really own it as it is "embedded in their unique and individual lives." They reviewed the differences between *individual* versus *organizational* quality measures and the validity of existing measures. At the individual level they distinguished recovery-promoting relationships (staff/care-recipient) and pro-recovery practices (e.g., WRAP, strengths rather than deficits focused care). Regarding organizational performance, they outlined four domains, which included quality of recovery-supporting care, achievement of individual recovery goals, subjective measures of personal recovery, and achievement of socially valued goals.

In summary, these examples illustrate the commonalities across system transformation efforts as well as the steps that can be taken to individualize the process that meets local conditions. The essence of these approaches seems to be that above all, input of the individuals with mental illness is paramount and the changes should flow from their perceptions of their needs so that they can reclaim meaning in their lives rather than be satisfied with clinician-driven treatment for the illness.

## Conclusion

This chapter provided a glimpse of the intensity of effort required to transform systems where they truly assist persons with mental illness on their paths to recovery. The focus has been on inpatient care, but this is only a small part of the continuum of interventions behavioral healthcare systems provide. Many of the traditional methodologies for treatment are still necessary elements that need to be used judiciously, such as validated psychosocial interventions (Jackman 2016; Myers 2016; Phillips 2016), psychotropic medications (Van Sant 2016), involuntary treatment (Elm and Devine 2016), and intensive inpatient care (Barber 2016; Myers 2016). Unfortunately, these same modalities have also historically created environments where persons are isolated, stigmatized, disempowered, and actually harmed (Bashor et al. 2016; Elm and Devine 2016; Spaulding et al. 2016).

The philosophy and science behind recovery and recovery-oriented care are still being debated and developed, but as with many disenfranchised populations there is a moral imperative for our societies to embrace full membership for all (Davidson et al. 2016; Spaulding et al. 2016). Although services can be recovery-oriented, recovery itself refers to what people with psychiatric disabilities can do for themselves to manage their illness and therefore return to a meaningful life. Recovery belongs to people with different abilities, and they have to define what it means to them and to lead the way in changing our behavioral healthcare systems (Franczak et al. 2016; Spaulding et al. 2016). This involves developing a positive vision of recovery-oriented care and working collaboratively with other stakeholders to develop a shared sense of where people in recovery and providers collectively are headed in this transformation. Finally, this effort cannot be an add-on to existing services, supports or behavioral healthcare systems; rather, it has to be the overarching goal.

## References


Alakeson, V., & Perkins, R. (2012). *Recovery, personalisation, personal budgets*. London, UK: Centre for Mental Health and NHS Confederation. Retrieved from http://www.imroc.org/latest-news/publications/imroc/

Amering, M., Mikus, M., & Steffen, S. (2012). Recovery in Austria: Mental health trialogue. *International Review of Psychiatry, 24*(1), 11–18.

Australian Health Ministers. (2009). *Fourth national mental health plan: An agenda for collaborative government action in mental helaht 2009–2014*. Canberra, Australia: Australian Government. Retrieved from https://www.health.gov.au/internet/main/publishing.nsf/Content/9A5A0E8BDFC55D3BCA257BF0001C1B1C/$File/plan09v2.pdf

Barber, J. W. (2016). Psychiatric services. In N. N. Singh, J. W. Barber, & S. Van Sant (Eds.), *Handbook of recovery in inpatient psychiatry*. New York: Springer.

Bashor, K., Junck, S., McGregor, C., & Anderson, C. (2016). Stigma and recovery. In N. N. Singh, J. W. Barber, & S. Van Sant (Eds.), *Handbook of recovery in inpatient psychiatry*. New York: Springer.

Boardman, J., & Friedli, L. (2012). *Recovery, public mental health and wellbeing*. London, UK: Centre for Mental Health and NHS Confederation. Retrieved from http://www.imroc.org/latest-news/publications/imroc/

Boardman, J., & Roberts, G. (2014). *Risk, safety and recovery*. London, UK: Centre for Mental Health and NHS Confederation. Retrieved from http://www.imroc.org/latest-news/publications/imroc/

Bradstreet, S., & McBrierty, R. (2012). Recovery in Scotland: Beyond service development. *International Review of Psychiatry, 24*(1), 64–69.

Davidson, L., Carr, E., Bellamy, C., Tondora, J., Fossey, E., Styron, T., et al. (2016). Principles for recovery-oriented inpatient care. In N. N. Singh, J. W. Barber, & S. Van Sant (Eds.), *Handbook of recovery in inpatient psychiatry*. New York: Springer.

Davidson, L., O'Connell, M., Tondora, J., Styron, T., & Kangas, K. (2006). The top ten concerns about recovery encountered in mental health system transformation. *Psychiatric Services, 57*(5), 640–645.

Davidson, L., Tondora, J., 'Connell, M. J., Kirk, T, Jr., Rockholz, P., & Evans, A. C. (2007). Creating a recovery-oriented system of behavioral health care: Moving from concept to reality. *Psychiatric Rehabilitation Journal, 31*(1), 23–31.

Drennan, G., & Wooldridge, J. (2014). *Making recovery a reality in forensic settings*. London, UK: Centre for Mental Health and NHS Confederation. Retrieved from http://www.imroc.org/latest-news/publications/imroc/

Duncan, G. N., Ahmed, A., Mabe, A., Anderson, B., Fenley, G., & Rollock, M. (2016). Shared decision-making. In N. N. Singh, J. W. Barber, & S. Van Sant (Eds.), *Handbook of recovery in inpatient psychiatry*. New York: Springer.

Elm, D. L., & Devine, J. L. (2016). Legal advocacy. In N. N. Singh, J. W. Barber, & S. Van Sant (Eds.), *Handbook of recovery in inpatient psychiatry*. New York: Springer.

Farkas, M., Gagne, C., Anthony, W., & Chamberlin, J. (2005). Implementing recovery oriented evidence based programs: Identifying the critical dimensions. *Community Mental Health Journal, 41*(2), 141–158.

Franczak, M., Barshter, D., Reich, J. W., Kent, M., & Zautra, A. (2016). In N. N. Singh, J. W. Barber, & S. Van Sant (Eds.), *Handbook of recovery in inpatient psychiatry*. New York: Springer.

Franczak, M., & Dye, C. (2016). Peer support services. In N. N. Singh, J. W. Barber, & S. Van Sant (Eds.), *Handbook of recovery in inpatient psychiatry*. New York: Springer.

HM Government. (2009). New horizons: A shared vision for mental health. London, UK: Department of Health. Retrieved from http://www.recoverydevon.co.uk/download/2010-02-04-299060_NewHorizons_acc2.pdf

HM Government. (2011). *No health without mental health: Delivering better mental health outcomes for people of all ages*. London, UK: Department of Health. Retrieved from https://www.gov.uk/government/uploads/system/uploads/attachment_data/file/213761/dh_124058.pdf

Institute of Medicine. (2006). *Improving the quality of health care for mental and substance-use conditions*. Washington, DC: National Academies Press.

Jackman, M. M. (2016). Occupational therapy services. In N. N. Singh, J. W. Barber, & S. Van Sant (Eds.), *Handbook of recovery in inpatient psychiatry*. New York: Springer.

Kirby, M. J., & Keon, W. J. (2006). *Out of the shadows at last: Transforming mental health, mental illness and addiction services in Canada.* Retrieved from http://ywcacanada.ca/data/research_docs/00000016.pdf

Kotter, J. P. (2007). Leading change: Why transformation efforts fail. *Harvard Business Review*, 92–107.

Le Boutillier, C., Leamy, M., Bird, V. J., Davidson, L., Williams, J., & Slade, M. (2011). What does recovery mean in practice? A qualitative analysis of international recovery-oriented practice guidance. *Psychiatric Services, 62*(12), 1470–1476.

Liberman, R. P. (2008). *Recovery from disability.* Washington, DC: American Psychiatric Publishing Inc.

Mabe, P. A., Rollock, M., & Duncan, G. (2016). Teaching clinicians the practice of recovery-oriented care. In N. N. Singh, J. W. Barber, & S. Van Sant (Eds.), *Handbook of recovery in inpatient psychiatry.* New York: Springer.

Machin, K., & Repper, J. (2013). *Recovery: A carer's perspective.* London, UK: Centre for Mental Health and NHS Confederation. Retrieved from http://www.imroc.org/wp-content/uploads/4ImROC_briefing_Carers_ImROC.pdf

Mental Health Commission. (1998). *Blueprint for mental health services in New Zealand.* Wellington, NZ: Mental Health Commission. Retrieved from http://www.moh.govt.nz/notebook/nbbooks.nsf/0/0E6493ACAC236A394C25678D000BEC3C/$file/Blueprint.pdf

Mental Health Commission. (2012). *Blueprint II: Improving mental health and wellbeing for all New Zealanders.* Wellington, NZ: Mental Health Commission. Retrieved from http://www.hdc.org.nz/media/207642/blueprintiihowthingsneedtobe.pdf

Mental Health Commission of Canada. (2009). *Toward recovery and well-being: A framework for a mental health strategy for Canada.* Retrieved from http://www.mentalhealthcommission.ca/English/system/files/private/document/FNIM_Toward_Recovery_and_Well_Being_Text_ENG.pdf

Mental Health Commission of Canada. (2012). *Changing directions, changing lives: the mental health strategy for Canada.* Retreived from http://strategy.mentalhealthcommission.ca/pdf/strategy-images-en.pdf

Myers, R. E. (2016). Mental health nursing services. In N. N. Singh, J. W. Barber, & S. Van Sant (Eds.), *Handbook of recovery in inpatient psychiatry.* New York: Springer.

New Freedom Commission on Mental Health. (2003). *Achieving the promise: Transforming mental health care in America.* Rockville, MD: Department of Health and Human Services.

O'Connell, M., Tondora, J., Croog, G., Evans, A., & Davidson, L. (2005). From rhetoric to routine: Assessing perceptions of recovery-oriented practices in a state mental health and addiction system. *Psychiatric Rehabilitation Journal, 28*(4), 378–386.

O'Hagan, M., Reynolds, P., & Smith, C. (2012). Recovery in New Zealand: An evolving concept? *International Review of Psychiatry, 24*(1), 56–63.

Oades, L. G., & Anderson, J. (2012). Recovery in Australia: Marshalling strengths and living values. *International Review of Psychiatry, 24*(1), 5–10.

Ostrow, L., & Adams, N. (2012). Recovery in the USA: From politics to peer support. *International Review of Psychiatry, 24*(1), 70–78.

Perkins, R., Repper, J., Rinaldi, M., & Brown, H. (2012). *Recovery colleges.* London, UK: Centre for Mental Health and NHS Confederation. Retrieved from http://www.imroc.org/latest-news/publications/imroc/

Phillips, J. (2016). Psychological services. In N. N. Singh, J. W. Barber, & S. Van Sant (Eds.), *Handbook of recovery in inpatient psychiatry.* New York: Springer.

Piat, M., & Sabetti, J. (2012). Recovery in Canada: Toward social equality. *International Review of Psychiatry, 24*(1), 19–28.

Repper, J. (2013a). *Peer support workers: a practical guide to implementation.* London, UK: Centre for Mental Health and NHS Confederation. Retrieved from http://www.imroc.org/latest-news/publications/imroc/

Repper, J. (2013b). *Peer support workers: Theory and practice.* London, UK: Centre for Mental Health and NHS Confederation. Retrieved from http://www.imroc.org/latest-news/publications/imroc/

Repper, J. (2013c). *The team recovery implementation plan: A framework for creating recovery-focused services.* London, UK: Centre for Mental Health and NHS Confederation. Retrieved from http://www.imroc.org/latest-news/publications/imroc/

Sainsbury Centre. (2009). *Implementing recovery: A new framework for organisational change.* London, UK: Sainsbury Centre for Mental Health. Retrieved from http://www.imroc.org/latest-news/publications/imroc/

Sheperd, G., Boardman, J., & Burns, M. (2009). *Implementing recovery: A methodology for organisational change.* Retrieved from http://www.imroc.org/latest-news/publications/imroc/

Sheperd, G., Boardman, J., Rinaldi, M., & Roberts, G. (2014). *Supporting recovery in mental health services: Quality and outcomes.* London, UK: Centre for Mental Health and NHS Confederation. Retrieved from http://www.imroc.org/latest-news/publications/imroc/

Singh, N. N., Lancioni, G. E., Harris, E., & Winton, A. S. W. (2016). Inpatient treatment planning. In N. N. Singh, J. W. Barber, & S. Van Sant (Eds.), *Handbook of recovery in inpatient psychiatry.* New York: Springer.

Slade, M. (2012). Everyday solutions for everyday problems: How mental health systems can support recovery. *Psychiatric Services, 63*(7), 702–704.

Slade, M., Amering, M., Farkas, M., Hamilton, B., O'Hagan, M., Panther, G., et al. (2014). Uses and abuses of recovery: Implementing recovery-oriented practices in mental health systems. *World Psychiatry, 13*(1), 12–20.

Slade, M., Leamy, M., Bacon, F., Janosik, M., Le Boutillier, C., Williams, J., et al. (2012). International differences in understanding recovery: Systematic review. *Epidemiology and Psychiatric Sciences, 21*(4), 353–364.

Smith, D. (2007). *State medicaid directors letter #07-11 (SMDL #07-011)*. Centers for Medicaid and State Operations. Retrieved from http://downloads.cms.gov/cmsgov/archiveddownloads/SMDL/downloads/SMD081507A.pdf

Sowers, W. (2005). Transforming systems of care: The American association of community psychiatrists guidelines for recovery-oriented services. *Community Mental Health Journal, 41*(6), 757–774.

Spaulding, W. D., Montague, E., Avila, A., & Sullivan, M. E. (2016). The idea of recovery. In N. N. Singh, J. W. Barber, & S. Van Sant (Eds.), *Handbook of recovery in inpatient psychiatry*. New York: Springer.

Stetler, C. B. (2003). Role of the organization in translating research into evidence-based practice. *Outcomes Management, 7*(3), 97–103.

Turia, T. (2010). *Whanau ora: Report of the taskforce on whanau-centred initiatives*. Report produced for Hon Tariana Turia, Minister for the Community and Voluntary Sector. Retreived from https://www.msd.govt.nz/documents/about-msd-and-our-work/publications-resources/planning-strategy/whanau-ora/whanau-ora-taskforce-report.pdf

US Department of Health and Human Services. (2012). *SAMHSA's working definition of recovery: 10 guiding principles recovery*. Rockville, MD: Author.

Van Sant, S. (2016). Psychopharmacological treatment. In N. N. Singh, J. W. Barber, & S. Van Sant (Eds.), *Handbook of recovery in inpatient psychiatry*. New York: Springer.

Williams, J., Leamy, M., Bird, V., Harding, C., Larsen, J., Le Boutillier, C., et al. (2012). Measures of the recovery orientation of mental health services: Systematic review. *Social Psychiatry and Psychiatric Epidemiology, 47*(11), 1827–1835.

# Index

*Note*: Page numbers followed by *f* and *t* indicate figures and tables respectively




N.N. Singh et al. (eds.), *Handbook of Recovery in Inpatient Psychiatry*,
Evidence-Based Practices in Behavioral Health, DOI 10.1007/978-3-319-40537-7